Prescription Drugs

Prescription

FAMILY ✚ MEDICAL

Drugs

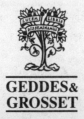

**GEDDES&
GROSSET**

ISBN 1 85534 877 2

Printed and bound in France
by Maury Eurolivres, Manchecourt

2 4 6 8 10 9 7 5 3 1

Introduction

This listing of prescription medicines provides an insight into the complexity of pharmaceutical preparations and medical diagnosis. It is not, however, intended as a tool for self-diagnosis or self-prescription and can in no way replace the medical practitioner or pharmacist. The book enables the patient to appreciate the vast array of medicines available and understand the likely action and effects of a particular medication. Each entry provides the name, manufacturer and salient details for each drug. Medical terms used are defined in the dictionary section or, failing that, in the body of the individual entry. The remaining categories in each entry, itemize conditions or goups where care should be exercised (*Special care*), cases where the drug should not be taken (*Avoid use*) and any interactions that may occur with other medications (*Possible interaction*). In *Side effects* are listed the primary possible effects of taking the drug.

No work of this nature can be totally comprehensive, and no one involved with the preparation of publication of this book can be held liable for any omissions, errors or for any consequences resulting from using the book.

Listed below are a number of abbreviations which you may meet and which, in conjunction with the accompanying medical dictionary, will help clarify the information presented.

ACE   angiotensin converting enzyme (ACE inhibitors are used in cardiac failure)

ß-blocker beta-blocker

BPH   benign prostatic hypertrophy (enlarged prostate gland)

BUN blood urea nitrogen

CNS central nervous system

GABA gamma-aminobutyric acid (an amino acid found in the brain, heart, lungs and kidney that acts as a neurotransmitter)

MAOI monamine oxidase inhibitor (antidepressant)

NSAID non-steroidal anti-inflammatory drug

SLE systemic lupus erythematosus (a chronic inflammatory disease that may be viral or an immune system dysfunction and tends to be commoner in women)

TCAD tricyclic antidepressant

UTI urinary tract infection

µg microgram (10^{-6}g)

CD signifies a controlled drug, that is, one that is subject to the specific restrictions and requirements of the Misuse of Drugs Regulations,1985.

The pharmaceuticals industry is constantly changing, with new drugs being developed all the time. In addition, drugs which previously were manufactured by, and carried the name of, a particular company may now appear under the banner of a different company. Because of this constant turnaround, a book of this nature can only represent the picture at a point in time. Nevertheless, every effort has been made in this edition to state the present manufacturer although the name appearing on a specific tablet or capsule may not reflect the current, but the previous company. However, the medication itself remains unchanged and the associated medical information remains valid.

A

ACCUPRO

Description: a proprietary preparation of the antihypertensive drug, quinapril; used in conjunction with a diuretic or cardiac glycoside. Available as brown tablets (oval, round or triangular according to strength). *Used for*: hypertension and congestive heart failure, especially after other treatments have been tried. *Dosage*: in adults only starts at 2.5mg per day usually increasing to 10–20mg per day. The maximum daily dose is 40mg. *Special care*: all elderly patients, impairment of kidney function, haemodialysis, severe congestive heart failure, some types of vascular disease and in patients having anaesthesia. *Avoid use*: children, pregnant and nursing mothers, some kidney and heart valve diseases. *Possible interaction*: potassium-containing supplements, diuretic drugs, NSAIDs, tetracyclines. *Side effects*: numerous including hypotension, abdominal, chest and muscle pains, headache, nausea, dizziness, rhinitis, upper respiratory tract infection and allergic reactions. *Manufacturer*: Parke-Davis.

ACEPRIL

Description: an ACE inhibitor and preparation of the antihypertensive drug captopril available as white tablets and marked A (12.5mg strength), or ACE and strength (for 25 and 50mg strengths). *Used for*: an addition to diuretic drugs and where appropriate digitalis in congestive heart failure. After heart attacks when there is a disorder of the left ventricle. *Dosage*: 6.25 or 12.5mg for heart failure, maintenance 25mg two or three times per day. Maximum 150mg per day. treatment to be commenced under close supervision. Diuretics to be reduced or stopped before treatment. Post heart attack-6.25mg, increasing slowly to 150mg per day in divided doses. Start 3 days after attack. For children, contact manufacturer. *Special care*: severe congestive heart failure, haemodialysis, kidney disease, anaesthesia, monitor kidney function, white cell count and urinary protein. *Avoid use*: pregnancy, lactation, narrowing of the aorta. *Possible interaction*: potassium supple-ments or potassium-sparing diuretics, vasodilators, NSAIDs, lithium, allopurinol, clonidine, probenecid, immunosuppressants. *Side effects*: anaemia, loss of taste, hypotension, proteinuria, pancreatitis, rash, angioneurotic oedema, neutropenia, thrombocytopenia. *Manufacturer*: Ashbourne.

ACEZIDE

Description: a combined diuretic/ACE inhibitor anti-hypertensive preparation. Contains captopril (50mg) and hydrochlorothiazide (25mg) in a white, scored tablet, code AZE 50/25. *Used for*: mild to moderate hypertension. *Dosage*: 1 tablet daily (maximum 2) (in patients who have first become accustomed to the two components given in the same amounts separately). *Special care*: patients with renal disorders or undergoing haemodialysis. *Avoid use*: in children, pregnant and breast feeding mothers, outflow obstruction of the heart, aortic stenosis and renovascular disease. *Possible interaction*: NSAIDs, potassium-containing supplements, antihypertensives, vasodilatory and immunosuppressant drugs. *Side effects*: protein in urine (proteinuria), rash, loss of sense of taste, fatigue, changes in constitution of the blood and, very unusually, a cough. *Manufacturer*: Ashbourne.

ACHROMYCIN

Description: a preparation of the antibiotic tetracycline hydrochloride used to treat a variety of conditions. Available as orange tablets. Also, as intramuscular injection and via intravenous drip. Effective against the bacterium *Haemophilus influenzae*. *Used for*: complications of chronic bronchitis. *Dosage*: 1 or 2 tablets at 6 hourly intervals. *Special care*: patients with any liver or kidney disease. May require avoidance of use in cases of renal impairment. *Avoid use*: in cases of impaired kidney function. It is absorbed into growing bone and stains teeth, hence must not be given to children less than 12 years or to pregnant women or nursing mothers. *Possible interaction*: consumption of milk which reduces absorption of tetracycline, contraceptive pill, antacids, iron, magnesium and calcium mineral supplements. *Side effects*: digestive upset—diarrhoea and vomiting, nausea, headache, disturb-ance of vision, possible allergic response. *Also used for*: acne vulgaris. *Description*: achromycin topical ointment containing 3% tetracycline hydrochloride. *Used for*: moderate to severe acne and effective against the bacterium *Propionbacterium acnes*. *Dosage*: apply to affected skin once a day or as directed by physician. *Special care*: in patients with kidney and liver disorders or perforated ear drum. *Avoid use*: as above. *Possible interaction*: as above. *Side effects*: possible additional infection, especially thrush. Occasionally diarrhoea. *Also used for*: mild bacterial skin infections. *Dosage*: apply once daily to affected area or as directed. *Side effects*: possible super infection (infection caused by different micro-organism, or a strain of the bacterium causing the original infection which has become resistant to Achromycin). Also available as sterile ointment containing 1% tetracycline hydrochloride. *Used for*: bacterial infections of the outer ear (otitis extrema) which are sensitive to tetracycline. *Dosage*: once or twice daily or as directed. *Special care*: patients with perforated ear drum and for short-term use. *Side effects*: localized allergic reactions and possible superinfection (see above). *Also used for*: infections of eyelids, e.g. styes, surface infections, e.g. conjunctivitis and chlamydial opthalmia (along with antibiotic preparations taken orally). Also following minor abrasions to the surface of the eye to prevent infections. *Dosage*: every 4 hours or as directed by physician. *Special care*: generally as above. *Side effects*: possible superinfection. *Manufacturer*: Wyeth.

ACTILYSE

Description: a fibrinolytic (disperses blood clots) drug available as a powder for reconstitution and injection. It can only be used under close medical supervision. *Used for*: thrombosis, embolisms and particularly myocardial infarction. *Dosage*: a total of 100mg, given intravenously over a 2 hour period in adults only. *Special care*: in patients with liver or kidney disease, diabetes or hypertension. *Avoid use*: in children, pregnant and nursing mothers, those with any form of bleeding (e.g. menstruation), recent surgery including dental treatment, or haemorrhage, any condition likely to bleed, e.g. active peptic ulcer or case of pancreatitis. Should not be administered to those having allergic reactions to streptokinase and anistreplase or who have recently been treated with these. *Possible interaction*: with other plasma protein-bound drugs, i.e. anticoagulants. *Side effects*: mainly nausea, vomiting and bleeding usually confined to puncture site but can occur elsewhere including intracerebral haemorrhage. Severe bleeding necessitates halting of treatment and possible administration of drugs to counter the fibrinolytic. Hence close monitoring is essential during treatment. *Manufacturer*: Boehringer Ingelheim.

ACTINAC

Description: an antibacterial steroid (corticosteroid) preparation with skin softening properties, available as a powder with solvent to be made up as a lotion. Contains the broad spectrum antibiotic chloramphenicol (4%), hydrocortisone acetate (4%) and also sulphur precipitate, allantoin and butoxyethyl nicotinate. *Used for*: acne. *Dosage*: apply to affected skin morning and night for 4 days then at night only for up to 3 weeks, continuing for 3 days after spots have disappeared. *Special care*: pregnant women, avoid contact with jewellery. *Side effects*: possible erythema, which may be severe. *Manufacturer*: Hoechst.

ACUPAN

Description: an analgesic non-narcotic drug available in the form of white tablets or as a solution for injection. Contains 30mg nefopam hydrochloride, tablets being marked APN. (Injection contains 20mg nefopam hydrochloride per ml in each ampoule). *Used for*: relief of moderate and severe pain, e.g. following surgery, muscle and joint pain, dental cancer. *Dosage*: tablets 3 times per day, adults only, total dose in the order of 30–90mg. Injection—one 20mg dose intramuscularly 3 times a day. *Special care*: elderly patients (1 tablet, 3 times a day initially), pregnant women, patients with kidney or liver disorders or suffering from urine retention. *Avoid use*: children, history of convulsions or heart attack (myocardial infarction) and also glaucoma. *Possible interaction*: drugs including sympathomimetics, tricyclics, anticholinergics and MAOIs (antidepressants). *Side effects*: nervousness, irritability, dry mouth, dizziness and nausea, headaches. Occasionally insomnia, irregular heartbeat and sweating. Urine may be tinged pink. *Manufacturer*: 3M Health Care.

ADALAT

Description: a calcium antagonist and vasodilator, available as liquid-filled orange capsules, containing the active ingredient nifedipine (5mg and 10mg). Also as sustained release tablets and as a preparation for injection. *Used for*: angina and Raynaud's phenomenon. *Dosage*: 10mg 3 times a day (5mg in elderly patients) in first instance, depending upon response, up to 60mg a day thereafter. Capsules taken with or immediately after food. *Special care*: patients with significant left ventricle disorders or congestive heart failure, low blood pressure, kidney and liver disease. *Avoid use*: if pain worsens during treatment, pregnant and nursing mothers, children, patients with very low blood pressure. *Possible interaction*: antihypertensive drugs; quinidine and cimetidine. *Side effects*: dizziness, flushing, nausea, palpitations, sweating, headaches, fluid retention, digestive upset, increased frequency of urination, drowsiness and insomnia. Rarely jaundice and swelling of gums. *Manufacturer*: Bayer. Nifedipine capsules also produced by Norton, Evans, APS, Ashbourne (Angiopine), CP, Eastern (Calcilat ®), Kerfoot, Cox.

ADCORTYL

Description: a potent topical steroid preparation (a corticosteroid), containing the active ingredient triamcinolone acetonide 0.1%, as cream or ointment. *Used for*: eczema and psoriasis, which has proved unresponsive to less potent preparations of corticosteroids. Can also be used to treat external ear infections and neurodermatitis. *Dosage*: apply sparingly to affected area 2–4 times each day and less frequently as condition improves. *Special care*: for children and babies, especially face and neck. *Avoid use*: acne (including acne rosacea), any skin conditions caused by ringworm, fungi, viruses, tuberculosis, leg ulcers, pregnant women and long term use. Also fungal or bacterial infections which have not been treated. *Side effects*: suppression of adrenal gland function, skin thinning and retention of fluid. *Also available*: adcortyl with graneodin (an antimicrobial agent) which includes the antibiotic neomycin. This contains 0.1% triamcinolone acetonide, 0.25% neomycin (as sulphate) and 0.025% gramicidin as cream. It is used as above but where a bacterial infection may additionally be present. **ADCORTYL IN OROBASE** is available as an oral paste used to treat mouth ulcers and other oral inflammations. It is applied 2 to 4 times daily and should not be used long term or by pregnant women. Adcortyl containing 10mg/ml triamcinolone acetonide is available for injection intradermally or into a joint. Used intradermally to treat scaly skin diseases, alopecia areata (patchy hair loss). Used intra-articularly to treat joint pain, stiffness and swelling caused especially by rheumatoid arthritis, bursitis, tenosynovitis and osteoarthrosis (osteoarthritis). *Manufacturer*: Squibb.

ADIFAX

Description: a preparation containing dexfenfluramine hydrochloride (fenfluramine is chemically related to amphetamine but is not a central nervous system stimulant and is less likely to cause dependence). It is an appetite suppressant which appears to affect the levels of serotonin (a naturally occurring compound in the body) in the brain. It is available in the form of 15mg white capsules marked S5614. *Used for*: severe obesity alongside other treatments, mainly control of diet. *Dosage*: 1 tablet in the morning and evening, at mealtimes. *Special care*: treatment should be limited to three months with gradual withdrawal over 1 or 2 weeks. Elderly patients. *Avoid use*: in children, pregnant and nursing mothers, patients with history of psychiatric illness, drug/alcohol abuse, anorexia, glaucoma, epilepsy, liver and kidney disorders. *Possible interaction*: anorectic drugs; MAOIs, antidepressants, sedatives, antihypertensive drugs, antidiabetics. *Side effects*: dependence effects possible on withdrawal including depression, breathlessness, headache, nervousness and irritability, sleep disturbance, dry mouth, dizziness, nausea, diarrhoela, constipation, more frequent urination. *Manufacturer*: Servier.

ADIZEM

Description: a calcium antagonist and vasodilator containing the active ingredient diltiazem hydrochloride. Available as tablets in 3 forms: **ADIZEM 60**—coded 60/DL, 60mg white capsules. **ADIZEM-SR**—white 90mg; brown 120mg; white/brown 180mg. Also as 120mg white tablets (DL/120). All continuous-release capsules. **ADIZEM XL**—pink/blue 120mg; pink/blue 180mg; red/blue 240mg; maroon/blue 300mg. All continuous-release capsules marked with strength. *Used for*: angina and hypertension. *Dosage*: 60mg 3 times a day increasing if required to a maximum of 480mg. Elderly, twice a day in first instance. *Special care*: patients with heart block, reduced function in left ventricle of heart, bradycardia, diabetes. *Avoid use*: in children, pregnant and nursing mothers, severe heart block or bradycardia, impairment of kidney and liver function. *Possible interaction*: digoxin, ß-blockers, antihypertensive drugs, cardiac depressants, diazepam, cyclosporin, cimetidine, theophylline and cartamazepine. *Side effects*: swelling of ankles, nausea, headache, bradycardia, rash, first degree heart block. *Manufacturer*: Napp.

AEROLIN AUTOHALER

Description: a preparation of a selective Beta$_2$-agonist (beta receptor stimulant) salbutamol which causes dilation or expansion of air passages in the lungs. Salbutamol (as sulphate) is present as 100µg per dose. *Used for*: prevention (prophylaxis) and treatment of bronchial asthma and breathing difficulties associated with bronchitis. *Dosage*: Aerolin is administered by means of a breath-activated aerosol inhalant which delivers a metered dose. Dose is 1–2 puffs 3–4 times daily for prevention. Half dose for children. *Special care*: thyroid gland disorders (hyperthyroidism) hypertension, heart disorders, e.g. myocardial insufficiency, during pregnancy and breast-feeding. May cause thyrotoxicosis with associated symptoms. *Possible interaction*: corticosteroids—increased risk of hypokalaemia with high doses. *Side effects*: headache, nervousness and irritability, fine tremor (in hands), vasodilation in peripheral areas of body. *Manufacturer*: 3M Health Care.

AKINETON

Description: an anticholinergic preparation containing the active ingredient biperiden hydrochloride, used to counter the effects of Parkinsonism. It is available as white, scored tablets with Knoll logo, containing 2mg biperiden hydrochloride and as a preparation containing biperiden lactate 5mg/ml, for slow intravenous or intramuscular injection. *Used for*: Parkinsonism and treatment of symptoms of drug-induced Parkinsonism. *Dosage*: *Tablets*: in adults, 1mg twice daily in first instance gradually increasing to 2mg 3 times a day. After initial period, the usual daily dose is in the order of 3–12mg 3 times a day. *Injection*: 2.5–4mg per ml up to 4 times per day. *Special care*: in patients with liver, kidney or heart disease. Treatment must be discontinued gradually. *Avoid use*: children, pregnant and nursing mothers, some types of glaucoma, patients with untreated urine retention or gastro-intestinal obstruction. *Possible interaction*: CNS depressant drugs and other anti-Parkinsonism drugs. *Side effects*: dry mouth, drowsiness, blurred vision and gastro-intestinal disorders. More rarely, urine retention and tachycardia and possible allergic reactions. *Manufacturer*: Knoll.

AKNEMIN

Description: an antibiotic drug, containing minocycline hydrochloride, available as 50mg red/fawn coloured capsules and 100mg red capsules. *Used for*: acne. *Dosage*: adults, twice daily dose of 50mg or 100mg. Tablets required for a minimum period of 6 weeks to 3 months with improvement not expected until after first month. *Special care*: liver or kidney disorders. *Avoid use*: pregnant and nursing mothers, children, kidney failure, SLE. *Possible interaction*: alcohol, antacid stomach preparations, mineral supplements, anticoagulant drugs, penicillin. *Side effects*: skin rashes, dizziness, blood abnormalities. Possible intracranial hypertension—drug should be discontinued. *Manufacturer*: Merck.

ALDACTIDE

Description: a proprietary preparation containing a potassium-sparing diuretic (encourages potassium to be retained and not eliminated in kidney) combined with a thiazide (a drug which inhibits the reabsorption of chloride and sodium in the kidney). The preparation is available in two strengths. **ALDACTIDE 25** contains 25mg spironalactone and 25mg hydroflumethiazide in buff-coloured tablets marked Searle 101. **ALDACTIDE 50** (Gold Cross) contains 50mg of each drug. *Used for*: congestive heart failure. *Dosage*: *Aldactide 25*: adults, 4 tablets daily with food in first instance with a maximum of eight. *Aldatide 50*: two tablets daily with a maximum of four. In children: 1.5–3mg per kg of body weight given at intervals through the day. *Special care*: elderly, liver and kidney disorders, pregnant mothers, diabetic patients, gout, long-term use in young people. Blood tests and monitoring of electrolyte levels may be required. *Avoid use*: nursing mothers, patients with liver or kidney failure, hypercalcaemia, hyperkalaemia, Addison's disease, sensititivity to sulphonamide drugs. *Possible interaction*: potassium supplements, other potassium-sparing diuretic drugs, NSAIDs, anti-diabetic drugs, antihypertensive drugs, ACE inhibitors and cardiac glycosides. *Side effects*: metabolic disorders, disturbance of electrolyte balance in blood, rash, drowsiness, sensitivity to light, gastro-intestinal upset, menstrual irregularities, deepening of voice. *Manufacturer*: Searle.

ALDACTONE

Description: a diuretic, potassium-sparing preparation containing spironolactone. Tablets available: 25mg buff marked Searle 39, 50mg off-white (Searle 916), 100mg buff (Searle 314). *Used for*: congestive heart failure, oedema caused by cirrhosis of the liver, malignancy or nephrotic syndrome, primary aldosteronism (over-production of the adrenal hormone, aldosterone). *Dosage*: in adults with congestive heart failure, 100mg daily in first instance increasing to 400mg taken with food. Thereafter, 75–200mg per day. Children, 3mg per kg of body weight in first instance in several doses. *Special care*: pregnant mothers, long-term use in young people patients with liver or kidney disorders. Blood electrolyte levels may need to be monitored. *Avoid use*: nursing mothers, patients with kidney failure, Addison's disease, and hyperkalaemia. *Side effects*: gastro-intestinal upset, rash, headache, disturbance of electrolyte levels, metabolic disturbance, breast enlargement, deepening of voice, menstrual irregularities, confusion, ataxia (unsteadiness). *Manufacturer*: Searle.

ALDOMET

Description: a centrally acting (on central nervous system), antihypertensive preparation containing the drug methyldopa. It is available as tablets or in ampoules for injection. May be used in combination with a diuretic drug. Aldomet tablets are available in three strengths all marked Aldomet and coloured yellow: Aldomet 125mg code 135; Aldomet 250mg code 401, Aldomet 500mg code 516. *Used for*: hypertension, especially useful for hypertension of pregnancy. *Dosage*: in adults, 250mg 2 to 3 times a day in first instance with an eventual maximum of 3 grams at 2-day intervals. In children, 10mg per kg of body weight each day in 2 to 4 separate doses. *Special care*: history of liver disease, kidney disorders, haemolytic anaemia, undergoing anaesthesia. *Avoid use*: liver disease, a disease of the adrenal glands called phaeochromocytoma, patients with depression. *Possible interaction*: sympathomimetics, other hypertensives, MAOIs, tricyclic antidepressants, lithium and phenothiazines. *Side effects*: depression, sleepiness, headache, dry mouth, nasal congestion, gastro-intestinal upsets, bradycardia, jaundice, haemolytic anaemia, positive Coombs test. *Manufacturer*: MSD.

ALFA D

Description: a manufactured form of vitamin D containing alfacalcidol (1α-hydroxycholcalciferol), a hydroxylated derivative. Since the conversion of vitamin D to its active form (which can be used by the body) requires hydroxylation by the kidneys, alfacalcidol is especially useful for patients suffering from any form of renal disorder. Alfa D is available in two strengths and contains 0.25μg of alfacalcidol in a pink capsule or 1μg in an orange capsule, each marked appropriately. *Used for*: rickets and osteomalacia (adult rickets, possibly caused by liver disease or malabsorption of vitamin D), overactivity of the parathyroid glands (and bone disease) (hyperparathyroidism), underactivity of the parathyroid glands (hypoparathyroidism), renal osteodystrophy (bone disease associated with chronic kidney failure). *Dosage*: adults: 1μg each day in first instance, adjusted according to response. Elderly patients: 0.5μg at first followed by adjustment of dose. Children over 20kg weight, 1μg daily, then adjusted dose. *Special care*: pregnant and breast-feeding mothers; vitamin D is passed into breast milk and can cause hypercalcaemia in infants. Patients with kidney failure. Monitoring of blood plasma levels of calcium is essential during treatment. *Avoid use*: children under 20kg body weight. *Possible interaction*: barbiturate and anticonvulsant drugs, digitalis, danazol, thiazides, mineral supplements, cholestyramine, sucralfate, colestipol. *Side effects*: (associated with overdose) diarrhoea, vomiting, nausea, weight loss, vertigo, headache, sweating, lethargy, thirst, elevated levels of calcium and phosphate in urine. *Manufacturer*: Berk.

ALGITEC

Description: a preparation, containing the H_2-receptor antagonist, cimetidine, which acts to reduce the production of gastric acid in the stomach. It is also a reflux suppressant which is available in chewable tablets called Chewtab and as a liquid suspension. Algitec tablets are off-white in colour and contain 200mg cimetidine and 500mg alginic acid and are marked ALGITEC 120. Also, **ALGITEC SUSPENSION** containing 100mg cimetidine and 250mg sodium alginate in each 5ml. *Used for*: gastric and duodenal ulcers, Zollingen-Ellison syndrome, reflux oesophagitis. *Dosage*: adults, one to two tablets chewed four times a day following meals, or 10–20mls of suspension, and at night time, for four to eight weeks. *Special care*: the presence of gastric cancer should first be eliminated. Patients suffering from kidney disorders and pregnant and nursing mothers. *Avoid use*: not for children. *Possible interaction*: oral anticoagulants, warfarin, phenytoin, theophylline or aminophylline. *Side effects*: generally few but dizziness, fatigue, rash, diarrhoea may occur, and rarely, headache, confusion, joint and muscle pains, reversible liver damage and gynaecomastia (breast enlargement). *Manufacturer*: SmithKline Beecham.

ALIMIX

Description: a preparation containing the active ingredient, asapride, which acts to promote stomach and intestine motility and emptying. It is thought to work by promoting the release of acetylcholine in the wall of gastro-intestinal tract. It is available as white scored tablets, marked J/Y and C and containing 10mg of cisapride (as monohydrate). *Used for*: gastro-oesophageal reflux, delayed gastric emptying accompanying such conditions as diabetes, systemic sclerosis and autonomic neuropathy (nerve supply to gastro-intestinal tract is disrupted), non-ulcer dyspepsia (short-term treatment). *Dosage*: depending upon condition being treated but usually 1 tablet 3 or 4 times daily, a quarter or half an hour before meals, for 6–12 weeks. *Special care*: nursing mothers, elderly patients, kidney and liver disorders. *Avoid use*: children and pregnant women, gastro-intestinal bleeding, obstruction or perforation. Any condition where stimulation of gastro-intestinal tract might prove to be harmful. *Possible interaction*: anticholinergic drugs, anticoagulants, sedatives, opiod analgesics, antimuscarines. *Side effects*: diarrhoea and abdominal pains, borborygmi (stomach and abdominal rumbling caused by fluid and gas), rarely headaches and convulsions. *Manufacturer*: Janssen.

ALKERAN

Description: a preparation of the alkylating, cytotoxic drug melphalan, for use by a physician skilled in cancer chemotherapy. It is available in tablets of two strengths, a white tablet coded A2A (2mg), and a white tablet coded B2A (5mg). Also available as a powder for reconstitution, containing 50mg melphalan (as hydrochloride), for injection. *Used for*: myeloma (or multiple myeloma, myelomatosis) a malignant bone marrow disease, ovarian and breast cancer. *Dosage*: 150–300g per kg of body weight each day for four to six days. This may be repeated after four to eight weeks. *Special care*: bone marrow suppression occurs but not immediately. Hence blood counts must be checked before each stage of treatment. Dose must be reduced in patients with impaired kidney function. *Possible interaction*: antibacterial drugs, nalidixic acid cyclosporin. *Side effects*: nausea, vomiting, hair loss, bone marrow suppression. *Manufacturer*: Glaxo Wellcome.

ALLEGRON

Description: a TCAD, nortriptyline, available in tablets of two strengths. It has less of a sedative efect than some other TCAD drugs. It is available as white scored tablets marked DISTA, containing 10mg nortriptyline hydrochloride, and orange scored tablets marked DISTA (25mg). *Used for*: depressive illnesses and bedwetting in children. *Dosage*: adults, 20 to 40mg each day in divided doses, increasing to 100mg if required. Maintenance, 30 to 75mg a day. Elderly persons; 10mg three times daily in first instance. Children (for bedwetting), seven to ten years, 10 to 20mg, 11 to 16 years, 25 to 50mg, given half an hour before bedtime. *Special care*: patients with heart disease, elderly people (reduced doses), nursing mothers, those with diabetes, thyroid disease, liver disorders, tumours of the medulla of adrenal glands, epilepsy, glaucoma, urine retention, psychosis, suicidal tendencies. Withdrawal should be gradual. May reduce ability to perform skilled tasks such as driving. *Avoid use*: pregnant mothers, heart block, heart attack, serious liver disorders. *Possible interaction*: alcohol, MAOIs, barbiturate drugs, anticholinergic drugs, other antidepressant and antihypertensive drugs, adrenaline, noradrenaline, oestrogens, cimetidine. *Side effects*: drowsiness, blurred vision, dry mouth, insomnia, urine retention, palpitations and shakiness, low blood pressure, weight changes, skin reactions, jaundice, blood changes, loss of libido. *Manufacturer*: King.

ALMEVAX

Description: a preparation of vaccine against German measles (Rubella) containing the live, but attenuated, strain Wistar RA 27/3 virus. It is available in one and ten dose vials for injection. *Used for*: immunization against Rubella in non-pregnant women and girls aged 10–14 who have not received MMR vaccine. *Dosage*: one dose given intramuscularly or subcutaneously. *Special care*: contraceptives should be used during the first three months although there is thought to be little risk of harm to the foetus. *Avoid use*: pregnancy, cancer, acute fevers, hypogamma globulinaemia (gamma globulin blood deficiency). *Possible interaction*: other live vaccines, transfusions, irradiation, cytotoxic drugs, corticosteroids, immunoglobulins. *Side effects*: sore throat, rash, malaise, aching joints, possible anaphylaxis. *Manufacturer*: Evans.

ALOMIDE

Description: a preparation containing Iodoxamide tromethamine with additives benzalkonium chloride and disodium edetate, available as 1% solution. *Used for*: allergic conjunctivitis. *Dosage*: one to two drops in each eye four times daily. *Special care*: pregnant and nursing mothers. *Avoid use*: those who wear soft contact lenses, children under four years of age. *Side effects*: irritation, stinging, watering of eyes. *Manufacturer*: Alcon.

ALPHADERM

Description: a moderately strong steroid with a hydrating agent (to moisten the skin). Alphaderm combines 1% hydrocortisone, 10% urea in a slightly oily cream. *Used for*: dermatitis and eczema. *Dosage*: wash and dry affected skin and apply thinly twice a day. *Special care*: short-term use only (especially in children or on face). *Avoid use*: acne, scabies, tuberculosis, ringworm, untreated bacterial and fungal infections, viral skin diseases, leg ulcers, pregnant mothers. *Side effects*: usually few but skin thinning, adrenal gland suppression, fluid retention possible. *Manufacturer*: Procter and Gamble.

ALPHOSYL HC

Description: a preparation of coal tar and hydrocortisone used in the treatment of psoriasis. It contains 5% coal tar extract, 0.5% hydrocortisone and 2%

allantoin in a water-based cream. *Used for*: psoriasis. *Dosage*: adults and children over 5 years, apply to affected skin twice each day. *Special care*: use should be limited to 5 days with children or on face. If treatment in adults is prolonged, withdrawal should be gradual. *Avoid use*: extensive or prolonged use in pregnant women, acne or untreated fungal and bacterial infections, tuberculosis, viral skin disease, leg ulcers, ringworm. Children under 5 years. *Side effects*: thinning of skin, suppression of adrenal glands, fluid retention. *Manufacturer*: Stafford-Miller.

ALRHEUMAT

Description: a NSAID preparation available as capsules and suppositories. Alrheumat contains 50mg ketoprofen and propionic acid in off-white cream-coloured capsules or as anal suppositories. *Used for*: pain and inflammation caused by musculo-skeletal diseases and rheumatoid and osteoarthritis, acute gout, pain following orthopaedic surgery, ankylosing spondylitis. *Dosage:* capsules—adults one 2–4 times each day with food. Suppositories—100mg at bedtime. Combined capsules and suppositories no more than 200mg daily. *Special care*: pregnancy and lactation, patients with heart, kidney or liver diseases, elderly people. *Avoid use*: children, patients with asthma, allergy to aspirin or NSAIDs, active peptic ulcer or history of peptic ulcer, gastrointestinal haemorrhage. *Possible interaction*: high doses of methotrexate, sulphonamide antibiotic drugs, quinolones, hydantoins and anticoagulant drugs. *Side effects*: gastrointestinal upsets, rash, rectal irritation (suppositories). *Manufacturer*: Bayer.

ALUPENT

Description: a bronchodilator, containing the partially selective drug orciprenaline sulphate. It is available as off-white scored tablets marked A7 containing 20mg orciprenaline sulphate. Also as alupent sugar-free syrup (10mg/5ml of solution) and alupent aerosol containing 0.75mg per metered dose. *Used for*: bronchial spasm due to asthma, chronic bronchitis and emphysema. *Dosage*: tablets and syrup: adults, one tablet or 10mls four times a day. Children under 1 year 2.5 to 5mls three times daily; 1–3 years, 2.5 to 5mls four times daily; 3–12 years, 5mls four times daily up to 10mls three times daily depending on age and symptoms. Aerosol: adults, 1–2 puffs which can be repeated after 30 minutes if required. Maximum dose 12 puffs in 24 hours. Children, 6 years and under, one puff, 6–12 years, one or two puffs. Must not be repeated within 30 minutes and maximum dose is four puffs in 24 hours. *Special care*: patients with diabetes or hypertension. Patients should follow instructions carefully. *Avoid use*: acute heart disease, hyperthyroidism or cardiac asthma. *Possible interaction*: sympathomimetic drugs, tricyclic antidepressants, MAOIs. *Side effects*: tachycardia, arrythmia, fine tremor, headache and nervous tension, dilation of blood vessels. *Manufacturer*: Boehringer Ingelheim.

AMBAXIN

Description: a broad-spectrum antibiotic preparation, containing a form of penicillin, available as scored, oblong-shaped tablets marked Upjohn and 130. *Used for*: respiratory, ear, nose, throat, soft tissue and skin infections. Also urinary tract infections and venereal diseases such as gonorrhoea. Para-typhoid fever. *Dosage*: adults, 1–2 tablets, 2 or 3 times a day. Venereal disease, 4 tablets plus 1g of probenecid as a single dose. Children over 5 years, half a tablet 3 times daily. *Special care*: patients suffering from liver and kidney diseases or infectious mononucleosis (glandular fever). *Avoid use*: children under five years. Allergy to penicillin. *Side effects*: gastro-intestinal upsets, possible allergic responses, e.g. rash (discontinue treatment). *Manufacturer*: Upjohn.

AMIKIN

Description: a preparation of the aminoglycoside antibiotic drug, amikacin, produced in the form of solutions for intramuscular or slow intravenous injection or infusion. Amikin contains 500mg per 2mls. **AMIKIN PAEDIATRIC** contains 100mg amikacin (as sulphate) per 2ml. *Used for*: serious bacterial infections particularly those caused by Gram-negative bacteria which are resistant to the more usual aminoglycosides, gentamicin and tobramycin. *Dosage*: adults, 15mg per kg of body weight intramuscularly or intravenously in two divided doses for up to 10 days. Maximum total dose 15g. For urinary tract infections, 7.5mg per kg of body weight each day in two divided doses. Children, 10mg–15mg per kg of body weight daily in two divided doses. *Special care*: patient should receive adequate fluid intake, caution with kidney disease. Monitor for toxicity. *Avoid use*: pregnant women. *Possible interaction*: anaesthetics, neuromuscular blocking drugs, ethacrynic acid, frusemide. *Side effects*: temporary kidney impairment and irreversible deafness can occur with prolonged or too high dosage. *Manufacturer*: Bristol-Myers.

AMIL-CO

Description: a potassium-sparing diuretic available in the form of peach-coloured, diamond-shaped tablets with the name and logo. They contain 5mg amiloride hydrochloride and 50mg hydrochlorothiazide (co-amilozide 5/50). *Used for*: cirrhosis of the liver (with fluid retention), congestive heart failure, hypertension. *Dosage*: adults, 1–2 tablets each day increasing up to 4, if required, in single or divided dose. *Special care*: patients with gout, kidney or liver disease, diabetes, acidosis. *Avoid use*: children, pregnant and nursing mothers, hyperkalaemia, severe or progressive kidney failure. *Possible interaction*: other potassium-sparing diuretics, potassium supplements, antihypertensive drugs, ACE inhibitors, lithium, digitalis (digoxin). *Side effects*: gout, rash, sensitivity to light, blood dyscrasias. *Manufacturer*: Baker-Norton.

AMOXIL

Description: preparations of the broad-spectrum antibiotic, amoxycillin, which is a derivative of ampicillin and available as maroon/gold capsules (250mg or 500mg amoxycillin trihydrate), marked with name and strength; dispersible, sugar-free tablets containing 500mg; **AMOXIL FIZTAB** chewable tablets, sugar-free (125mg). Not suitable for children under 3 years of age; **AMOXIL SYRUP SF** sugar-free, containing either 125mg or 250mg per 5ml for reconstitution with water; **AMOXIL PAEDIATRIC SUSPENSION**, 125mg amoxycillin (as trihydrate) per 1.25ml; **AMOXIL 3g SACHETS SF**—3g in sucrose-free sorbitol base as a powder in a sachet. **AMOXIL 750mg SACHET SF** containing 750mg in sugar-free, sorbitol base as a powder in a sachet; **AMOXIL INJECTION**—Either 250mg, 500mg or 1g amoxycillin (as sodium salts), in a vial as a powder for reconstitution. *Used for*: one or more of the different forms are used for soft tissue infections, urinary tract infections, respiratory, ear, nose, throat, infections, gonorrhoea, dental abscess and to prevent endocarditis during dental treatment. Glandular fever. *Dosage*: infants under 6 months, Amoxil Paediatric suspension is appropriate. Adults, 250–500mg three times each day, children half adult dose. Injection, (used for glandular fever), adults, 500mg intramuscularly at 8-hour intervals or 1g intravenously at 6-hourly intervals if infection is severe. Children, 50–100mg per kg of body weight in divided doses. *Special care*: patients with allergy to penicillin. *Side effects*: gastro-intestinal upsets, allergic responses, e.g. rash, especially in patients with glandular fever, HIV virus, lymphatic leukaemia. *Manufacturer*: Bencard.

AMPICLOX

Description: a broad-spectrum antibiotic ampicillin with cloxacillin available as capsules, black/purple (250mg ampicillin trihydrate) and 250mg cloxacillin (as sodium salt); Also **AMPICLOX SYRUP** containing 125mg/125mg per 5ml, available as powder for reconstitution; **AMPICLOX NEONATAL**, a sugar-free suspension containing 60mg/30mg per 0.6ml when reconstituted; **AMPICLOX NEONATAL INJECTION** containing 50mg/25mg as powder for reconstitution; **AMPICLOX INJECTION** containing 250mg/250mg as powder for reconstitution. *Used for*: emergency treatment of serious bacterial infections of urinary tract, ear, nose, throat, upper respiratory tract while bacteriology is being investigated. Also as a preventative against infection when the patient is to undergo major surgery. *Dosage*: adults, capsules, 1–2 every four to six hours; syrup, 10–20ml every four to six hours. Children, babies under one month, neonatal suspension, 0.6ml every four to six hours or neonatal injection intravenously or intramuscularly, 1 vial three times a day. Children 1 month to 2 years 2.5ml–5ml Ampiclox syrup both every 4 to 6 hours. Adults, Ampiclox injection, intravenously or intramuscularly, 1 to 2 vials every 4 to 6 hours. Children 1 month to 2 years, one-quarter adult dose, children 2 to 10 years, half adult dose. *Special care*: allergic patients, kidney disease, rashes especially in glandular fever, HIV, chronic lymphatic leukaemia. *Avoid use*: patients with known penicillin allergy. *Side effects*: gastro-intestinal upsets, allergic responses. *Manufacturer*: Beecham.

AMSIDINE

Description: a cytotoxic, antibiotic, anti-cancer preparation containing amsacrine. This is available as a preparation for intravenous infusion for use by a physician skilled in cancer therapy. Amsidine concentrate contains 5mg amsacrine (as lactate) per ml when reconstituted. *Used for*: acute myeloid leukaemia. *Dosage*: as directed by physician. Usually no more than 450mg/m² of body surface area as a total cumulative dose. *Special care*: patients with cardiac disorders, liver or kidney disease (reduced doses), elderly people, pregnant women. Caution in handling as irritant to tissues and skin; glass apparatus should be used for mixing. Cardiac monitoring and monitoring of electrolyte levels is essential during treatment. *Side effects*: suppression of bone marrow function (myelosuppression), hair loss, mucositis. Rarely, tachycardia associated with ventricles of heart. Heart disease and potentially fotal heart failure. *Manufacturer*: Goldshield.

AMYTAL^{CD}

Description: a barbiturate preparation containing amylobarbitone, available as white tablets containing 50mg amylobarbitone. *Used for*: severe intractable insomnia of a persistent nature for use by those patients already taking barbiturates. *Dosage*: adults, 100–200mg at bedtime. *Special care*: extremely dangerous, addictive drug with narrow margin of safety. Liable to abuse by overdose leading to coma and death or if combined with alcohol. Easily produces dependence and severe withdrawal symptoms. Drowsiness may persist next day affecting driving and performance of skilled tasks. *Avoid use*: should be avoided if possible in all patients. Not to be used for children, young adults, pregnant and nursing mothers, elderly pesons, those with drug or alcohol related problems, patients with liver, kidney or heart disease, porphyria, insomnia where the cause is pain. *Possible interaction*: alcohol, central nervous system depressant drugs, Griseofulvin, metronidazone, rifampicin, phenytoin, chloramphenicol. Anticoagulant drugs of the coumarin type, steroid drugs including contraceptive pill. *Side effects*: hangover with drowsiness, shakiness, dizziness, headache, anxiety, confusion, excitement, rash and allergic responses, gastrointestinal upsets, urine retention, loss of sexual desire. *Manufacturer*: Flynn.

ANAFRANIL

Description: a TCAD containing clomi-pramine hydrochloride, available as capsules, syrup and in ampoules for injection. There are three strengths: yellow/caramel (10mg), orange/caramel (25mg), grey/caramel (50mg) all marked Geigy. Also **ANAFRANIL SR** sustained release pink capsules containing 75mg, marked Geigy on one side and GD on the other. In addition, **ANAFRANIL SYRUP** containing 25mg per 5ml. Also, **ANAFRANIL INJECTION**, containing 25mg per 2ml in ampoules. *Used for*: depression, phobic and obsessional states. *Dosage*: adults, capsules for depression, 10mg each day gradually increasing to 30–150mg (maximum 250mg) in divided doses or as a single dose at bedtime. Obsession and phobia, 25mg at first increasing to 100–150mg daily. Elderly, 10mg each day at first increasing to a maximum of 75mg. Intramuscular injection, 25mg–50mg each day increasing by 25mg to 100–150mg. Intravenous infusion, 25–50mg then about 100mg for 7–10 days. *Special care*: nursing mothers, elderly, psychoses or suicidal tendencies. Persons with heart disease, liver disorders, thyroid disease (hyperthyroidism), epilepsy, diabetes, urine retention, glaucoma, tumour of the adrenal glands. Blood tests are advisable during therapy. *Avoid use*: children, pregnant women, patients with heart block, heart attack, serious liver disease. *Possible interaction*: MAOIs or within 14 days of their use, other antidepressant drugs, anticholinergic drugs, alcohol, adrenaline, noradrenaline (or anaesthetics containing these), antihypertensive drugs, barbiturates, cimetidine, oestrogens. *Side effects*: gastro-intestinal disturbances such as constipation, blurred vision, dry mouth, anxiety, drowsiness, insomnia, urine retention, sweating, tremor, disturbance of heartbeat rate, weight gain or loss. Also low blood pressure, allergic skin reactions, jaundice, loss of libido and impotence may occur. Occasionally, symptoms of schizophrenia and mania may be activated particularly in elderly persons. *Manufacturer*: Geigy.

ANAPOLON 50

Description: a preparation containing the anabolic steroid drug, oxymethalone. Available as white scored tablets containing 50mg and marked Syntex 50. *Used for*: certain types of anaemia (especially aplastic anaemias and hypoplastic anaemias which have not improved after other therapy). *Dosage*: children over 2 years, 2–4mg per kg of body weight daily. Adults, 2–5mg per kg of body weight in first instance reducing to half or less as condition improves. All in divided doses. *Special care*: patients with diabetes, cardiac failure, enlarged prostate gland in men. Liver tests should be carried out during therapy. *Avoid use*: children under 2 years, pregnant and nursing mothers, liver or kidney disease, men with breast or prostate cancer, women with breast cancer and hypercalcaemia. *Possible interaction*: anticoagulant and corticosteroid drugs. *Side effects*: vomiting, nausea, diarrhoea, sleeplessness, muscle cramps. Toxic effect on liver including jaundice, pruritis (itching), tumours, hepatic coma. Also oedema, congestive heart failure, mascu-linization in women and pre-pubertal children, loss of menstruation (amenorrhoea) in women, changes in blood, hypercalcaemia (therapy should be halted). *Manufacturer*: Syntex.

ANDROCUR

Description: an anti-androgen hormonal preparation containing cyproterone acetate, for use under hospital supervision. Available as white, scored tablets (50mg), marked BV in a hexagon. *Used for*: male sexual deviation and severe hypersexuality. (Also, acne and abnormal hair growth in women, prostate cancer in men). *Dose*: adult men only, 1 tablet in morning and evening after food. *Special care*: patient consent is vital. Drug inhibits sperm production resulting in reversible infertility. Abnormal sperm are produced and liver tumours have been produced in animals. Ability to drive and perform skilled tasks impaired. Ineffective where hypersexuality is caused by chronic alcoholism. Special care in patients with diabetes mellitus and disorders of adrenal glands. Blood (haemoglobin) and sperm tests and monitoring of liver and adrenal gland function is advisable. *Avoid use*: males under 18 years of age or those in whom bones and testes are not fully matured. Patients with thrombosis, embolism, severe liver disease, malignant or wasting diseases. Severe chronic depression. *Side effects*: depression, tiredness, weight gain, breast enlargement, changes in hair growth, rarely, osteoporosis. *Manufacturer*: Schering H.C.

ANECTINE

Description: a depolarizing muscle relaxant, the effect of which lasts for only 5 minutes and is used during anaesthesia. It is available as ampoules for injection, and contains 50mg suxamethonium chloride per ml. *Used for*: muscle relaxation during anaesthesia to facilitate the insertion, e.g. of a ventilator, into the windpipe. *Dosage*: according to body weight, usually 0.3–1.1mg/kg depending on degree of muscle relaxation needed. *Special care*: premedication with atropine is desirable. More prolonged muscle paralysis may occur in patients with dual block (after several doses of suxamethonium) and in those with low pseudocholinesterase enzymes in blood plasma, requiring continued artificial ventilation until normal muscle function is resumed. *Avoid use:* patients with burns and those with serious liver disease. *Manufacturer*: Glaxo Wellcome.

ANEXATE

Description: an antagonist to the effects of benzodiazepines used in anaestheseia, diagnostic procedures and intensive care. It contains 100μg of flumazenil per ml of solution and is administered by means of intravenous injection or infusion. *Used for*: reversal of sedative effects of benzodiazepines in anaesthesia, intensive care and diagnostic investigations. *Dosage*: by injection, 200μg given over 15 seconds. Repeated doses of 100μg at one minutes intervals if needed. Usual dose in the order of 300–600μg with a maximum of 1mg (possibly 2mg in intensive care procedures). By infusion (if drowsiness persists after initial injection), 100–400μg per hour according to patient response. *Special care*: rapid injection should be avoided especially in patients who have had major surgery, head injury or liver disorders. *Avoid use*: epileptic patients who have received sustained doses of benzodiazepines. *Side effects*: vomiting, nausea, flushing. If wakening is too rapid patient may be anxious, agitated and fearful. Intensive care patients may have short-lived increase in heart rate and blood pressure. Rarely, convulsions may occur especially in epileptic patients. *Manufacturer*: Roche.

ANHYDROL FORTE

Description: an anti-perspirant solution containing 20% aluminium chloride hexahydrate in an alcohol base. It is available as a solution in a bottle with a roll-on applicator. *Used for*: excessive sweating (hyperhidrosis) of armpits, hands and feet. *Dosage*: apply at night to dry skin and wash off the following morning. Use less as condition improves. *Special care*: avoid bathing immediately before use or use of depilatory creams and shaving of armpits within 12 hours of applying. Should only be used on feet in children. *Avoid use*: contact with eyes, broken or inflamed skin. Contact with clothing and jewellery. *Manufacturer*: Dermal.

ANQUIL

Description: an antipsychotic drug available as white tablets containing 0.25mg (butyrophenone) benperidol marked Janssen, A and 0.25. *Used for*: antisocial, deviant sexual behaviour. *Dosage*: adults, 0.25mg to 1.5mg per day in divided doses. Elderly or debilitated patients, half adult dose. *Special care*: patients with epilepsy, Parkinsonism, heart disease, kidney or liver disorders, glaucoma, acute infections, elderly persons, pregnant or nursing mothers. Also, those with history of jaundice, underactive thyroid gland, myasthenia gravis, enlarged prostate gland. Regular blood counts and tests of liver function should be carried out during extensive therapy. *Avoid use*: children, symptoms of central nervous system disturbance (pyramidal or extrapyramidal effects). *Possible interaction*: alcohol, antihypertensive, antidepressant and anticonvulsive drugs, analgesic drugs, central nervous system depressants, levodopa and antidiabetic drugs. *Side effects*: muscle spasms of eyes, neck, back, face, Parkinson-like symptoms (tremor and rigidity), dry mouth, nasal stiffness, irregular heartbeat, palpitations, blurring of vision, blood changes, jaundice, drowsiness, fatigue, low blood pressure, weight gain, impotence, breast enlargement, hypothermia (in elderly), constipation, rarely, fits. *Manufacturer*: Janssen-Cilag.

ANTABUSE

Description: a preparation containing the drug disulfiram, an enzyme (aldehyde dehydrogenase) inhibitor used in the treatment of alcoholism. It is available as white, scored tablets (200mg) marked ANY 200 and CP. *Used for*: adjunct in therapy for alcohol dependence. *Dosage*: adults, 800mg as single dose on first day. Afterwards reducing to 200–100mg over period of five days. Should not be used for longer than six months. *Special care*: liver or kidney disease, respiratory disease, diabetes mellitus, epilepsy. Careful counselling of patient essential before use as reaction of disulfiram with even a minute quantity of alcohol causes extremely unpleasant and possibly fatal consequences due to accumulation of acetaldehyde in body. With small amounts of alcohol reactions include severe throbbing headache, palpitations, nausea, vomiting, raised heartbeat, flushing of face. The quantity of alcohol in many medicines may be sufficient to precipitate this. Larger quantities of alcohol can cause hypotension, heart arrhythmias and collapse. No alcohol should be consumed until one week after stopping the drug or for 24 hours prior to start of treatment. *Avoid use*: patients with heart failure, coronary artery disease or high blood pressure. Children and pregnant women. Patients with severe mental disorders or suicidal tendencies. *Possible interaction*: alcohol, some TCADs, paraldehyde, warfarin, barbiturate drugs, antiepileptic drugs, metronidazole (antibacterial drug). *Side effects*: fatigue and drowsiness, vomiting and nausea, bad breath (halitosis), reduced libido, allergic skin reactions, liver damage. Rarely, mental disturbances (mania, paranoia, schizophrenia, depression). *Manufacturer*: Dumex.

ANTEPSIN

Description: a cytoprotectant (cell-surface protectant) preparation available in the form of tablets and suspension. The tablets are scored, white, oblong in shape and contain 1g sucralfate, marked Antepsin on one side and WY39 on reverse. **ANTEPSIN SUSPENSION** contains 1g/5ml of solution. *Used for*: gastric and duodenal ulcers, chronic gastritis, prevention of haemorrhage from stress, ulceration in patients who are seriously ill. *Dosage*: tablets, adults 2g twice a day in the morning and at bedtime or 1g four times a day one hour before meals. Maximum dose 8g per day. Treatment period usually 4–6 weeks, sometimes up to 12 weeks. Prevention (prophylaxis) of stress ulceration, 1g suspension 6 times a day with a maximum of 8g daily. *Special care*: patients with kidney failure, pregnancy and lactation. *Avoid use*: children and patients with severe kidney failure. *Possible interaction*: antibacterial drugs (ciproflxacin, ofloxacin, norfloxacin and tetracycline), warfarin, antiepileptics (phenytoin). *Side effects*: gastro-intestinal upsets—constipation, diarrhoea, indigestion, nausea, dry mouth, rash, back pain, dizziness, sleeplessness, drowsiness, vertigo are possible. *Manufacturer*: Wyeth.

ANTURAN

Description: a preparation containing the active ingredient, sulphinpyrazone, which promotes the excretion of uric acid by preventing its reabsorption in the kidney tubules. Anturan is available in the form of yellow, sugar-coated tablets marked Geigy in 2 strengths, (100mg and 200mg). *Used for*: hyperuricaemia (high blood levels of uric acid), chronic gout, recurrent gouty arthritis. *Dosage*: adults, 100mg to 200mg with food per day at first increasing over a 2–3 week period to 600mg. After this the amount is reduced (once uric acid level has dropped) to a maintenance dose which may be as low as 200mg daily. *Special care*: pregnant and breast-feeding mothers, kidney disease or heart failure. Plenty of fluids should be taken during treatment and blood and kidney function tests may be necessary. *Avoid use*: children. Patients with known allergies to anti-inflammatory drugs, severe liver or kidney disease, acute gout, history of peptic ulcers or acute peptic ulcer, blood disorders, porphyria. *Possible interaction*: salicylates, aspirin, hypoglycaemic drugs, anticoagulants, sulphonamides, penicillins, phenytoin, theophylline. *Side effects*: gastro-intestinal upset and bleeding, ulcers, acute gout, kidney stones, renal colic, liver and kidney disorders, rash, blood changes (treatment should stop). *Manufacturer*: Geigy.

ANUGESIC H-C

Description: a preparation containing corticosteroid combined with antiseptic and soothing properties, available in the form of a cream and as suppositories. The cream contains 1.25% benzyl benzoate, 0.875% bismuth oxide, 0.5% hydrocortisone acetate, 1.85% Peru balsam, 1% pramoxine hydrochloride and 12.35% zinc oxide. **ANUGESIC H-C SUPPOSITORIES** contain 33mg benzyl benzoate, 24mg bismuth oxide, 59mg bismuth subgallate, 5mg hydrocortisone acetate, 49mg Peru balsam, 27mg pramoxine hydrochloride and 296mg zinc oxide. *Used for*: haemorrhoids, anal itching and other ano-rectal disorders. *Dosage*: adults, 1 suppository or application of cream morning and night and after bowel movement. *Special care*: pregnant women. Avoid prolonged use—no more than 7 days. *Avoid use*: children. Fungal and viral infections. Tuberculosis. *Side effects*: systemic (affecting body as a whole) corticosteroid effects. *Manufacturer*: Parke-Davis.

ANUSOL HC

Description: an astringent antiseptic with soothing properties in the form of an ointment and suppositories. The ointment contains 1.25% benzyl benzoate, 0.875 bismuth oxide, 2.25% bismuth subgallate, 0.25% hydrocortisone acetate, 1.875% Peru balsam, 10.75% zinc oxide. The suppositories contain 33mg benzyl benzoate, 24mg bismuth oxide, 59mg bismuth subgallate, 10mg hydrocortisone acetate, 49mg Peru balsam and 296mg zinc oxide. *Used for*: haemorrhoids, anorectal inflammation. *Dosage*: adults, one application of ointment or one suppository night and morning and after bowel movement. *Special care*: pregnant women. Not to be used for longer than 7 days. *Avoid use*: children, patients with fungal or viral infections or suffering from tuberculosis. *Side effects*: systemic (affecting whole body) corticosteroid effects. *Manufacturer*: Parke-Davis.

APISATE[CD]

Description: a preparation which combines an appetite suppressant with vitamin B. It contains the central nervous system stimulant, and sympathomimetic agent, diethylproprion, which should only be taken for a few days as it can cause dependence and psychiatric effects. Apisate is available in the form of two-layer yellow, sustained-release tablets marked Wyeth containing 75mg diethylproprion hydrochloride, 5mg thiamine hydrochloride, 4mg riboflavine, 2mg pyridoxine hydrochloride, 30mg nicotinamide. *Used for*: patients suffering from obesity. *Dosage*: adults, 1 daily in early morning or mid-afternoon. *Special care*: patients with severe liver or kidney disorders, peptic ulcer, angina, heart arrhythmias, high blood pressure, enlargement of prostate gland, depression, first three months of pregnancy. May affect the performance of skilled tasks such as driving. Prolonged use should be avoided. *Avoid use*: children and elderly persons, patients with a history of psychiatric illness, drug or alcohol abuse, arteriosclerosis, glaucoma, severe high blood pressure, hyperthyroidism. *Possble interaction*: sympathomimetic drugs, MAOIs, psychotropic drugs, guanethidine, methyldopa, other anoretics. *Side effects*: dependence and tolerance, psychiatric disorders, anxiety, insomnia, agitation and nervousness. *Manufacturer*: Wyeth.

APRESOLINE

Description: a vasodilator available in the form of tablets of two strengths and as a powder for reconstitution for injection. It contains hydralazine hydrochloride. Yellow tablets (25mg) are sugar-coated and marked CIBA and GF, while the deep pink tablets are marked in the same way and contain 50mg. **APRESOLINE INJECTION** contains 20mg hydralazine hydrochloride as a powder in an ampoule for reconstitution. *Used for*: moderate and severe chronic heart failure. Also used for moderate to severe hypertension. *Dosage*: for hypertension in adults (along with ß-blocker and thiazide diuretic), 25mg twice a day at first increasing to a maximum of 200mg daily. For cardiac failure in adults (with diuretics and cardiac glycosides), 25mg 3–4 times each day increasing to 50–75mg 4 times a day every second day. *Special care*: patients with coronary or cerebrovascular disease, liver disorders, severe kidney failure, nursing mothers. Withdrawal should be gradual. *Avoid use*: children, first half of pregnancy, patients with certain heart disorders (aortic, mitral stenosis, tachycardia, idiopathic SLE, constructive pericarditis, dissecting aortic aneurysm, cor pulmonale). *Possible interaction*: anaesthetics, TCADs, MAOIs, antihypertensive drugs, diazoxide, CNS depressants. *Side effects*: hypotension, tachycardia, angina, headache, flushes, especially with daily dose exceeding 100mg. Protein in urine, blood in urine, kidney failure, urine retention. Possible though rare, liver damage, nerve disorders and blood changes. *Manufacturer*: CIBA.

APRINOX

Description: a thiazide preparation which has diuretic properties and is available as white tablets of two strengths containing 2.5mg or 5mg of bendrofluazide. *Used for*: hypertension, oedema such as occurs in mild to moderate heart failure. *Dosage*: adults, for oedema, 5–10mg in morning or on alternate days at first and then 5–10mg once or twice per week for maintenance. For hypertension, 2.5–5mg once each day. *Special care*: pregnancy and breastfeeding, elderly persons. Patients with liver or kidney disease, liver cirrhosis, gout, diabetes, SLE. Advisable to monitor fluid, electrolytes and glucose levels. *Avoid use*: children. Patients with severe liver or kidney failure, hypercalcaemia, Addisons disease, allergy to sulphonamide drugs. *Possible interaction*: alcohol, opioids, barbiturates, antidiabetic drugs, NSAIDs, corticosteroids, tubocurarine, carbenoxolone, cardiac glucosides, lithium. *Side effects*: metabolic disturbance and upset of electrolyte balance, gastro-intestinal disturbance, blood changes, rash, dizziness, impotence, pancreatitis, anorexia. *Manufacturer*: Knoll.

ARAMINE

Description: a sympathomimetiuc amine that acts as a vasoconstrictor available as ampoules for injection containing 10mg metraminol tartrate per ml. *Used for:* acute hypotension such as may occur in patients in severe shock or during general anaesthesia. *Dosage:* 15–100mg according to response. *Special care:* possible localized tissue death at injection site. *Avoid use:* pregnancy, heart attack. *Side effects:* reduced blood flow to kidneys, heart arrhythmias and tachycardia. *Manufacturer:* MSD.

AREDIA

Description: a preparation of the disophonate drug disodium pamidronate available as a powder for reconstitution and intravenous infusion. Vials contain 15mg or 30mg. *Used for:* hypercalcaemia caused by malignancy. *Dosage:* adults, depending upon levels of calcium in blood plasma, maximum dose of 90mg each treatment given by slow infusion at a rate not exceeding 30mg in two hours. Dose may be divided over 2–4 days. *Special care:* severe kidney disorders, may cause convulsions due to disturbance of electrolyte balance. *Avoid use:* pregnancy and breast-feeding. *Possible interaction:* other infusions containing calcium disophonates, drugs for hypocalcaemia, plicamycin. *Side effects:* diarrhoea, nausea, short-lived rise in body temperature, hypocalcaemia, lowering of magnesium levels, decrease in number of white blood cells (lymphocytes) in blood. *Manufacturer:* Ciba.

ARELIX

Description: a powerful diuretic (a *loop diuretic)* which acts on the parts of the kidney tubules known as the loops of Henle. It is available as orange/green sustained release capsules containing 6mg of piretanide. *Used for:* mild to moderate hypertension. *Dosage:* 1 or 2 capsules taken in the morning with food. *Special care:* hypokalaemia may develop and monitoring of electrolyte levels may be necessary especially in patients with impaired kidney or liver function. Also, in patients with enlarged prostate gland or impaired urination. Pregnancy and nursing mothers, persons with diabetes or gout. *Avoid use:* patients with severe imbalance of electrolytes, liver cirrhosis, children. *Possible interaction:* antihypertensive drugs, NSAIDs, digoxin, lithium, cephalosporin antibiotic drugs, aminoglycosides. *Side effects:* electrolyte imbalance, rarely gastrointestinal upset, muscle pain after high doses. *Manufacturer:* Hoechst.

ARFONAD

Description: trimetaphan camsylate, a ganglion blocker, available in ampoules for injection or infusion (50mg per ml). *Used for:* controlled lowering of blood pressure (hypotension) during surgery. *Dosage:* by intravenous infusion at a rate of 3–4mg per minute in first instance and thereafter adjusted according to the patient's response. *Special care:* patients with impaired liver or kidney function, coronary disease, cerebral vascular disease, degenerative conditions of the central nervous system, Addison's disease, reduced adrenal gland function. Also in elderly persons and patients with diabetes mellitus. *Avoid use*: pregnant women, serious heart disease, severe arteriosclerosis, pyloric stenosis. *Side effects*: depression of breathing (especially in combination with muscle relaxant drugs), tachycardia, dilation of pupils, increased intra-ocular pressure in eyes, constipation. *Manufacturer*: Cambridge.

ARPICOLIN

Description: an anticholinergic preparation of the drug procyclidine hydrochloride available in the form of a syrup in two strengths, containing 2.5mg or 5mg per 5ml. *Used for*: Parkinsonism, including that which is drug-induced. *Dosage*: 2.5mg–5mg 3 times each day at first. This is increased at 2 to 3 day intervals to a usual maximum of 30mg daily (exceptionally, 60mg). *Special care*: patients with obstruction of gastro-intestinal tract, enlarged prostate gland, heart disease, narrow-angle glaucoma. Drug should be withdrawn gradually. *Avoid use*: children, patients with a movement disorder called tardive dyskinesia. *Possible interaction*: antidepressant and antihistamine drugs. Phenothiazines. *Side effects*: anticholinergic effects, with high doses there may be mental confusion. *Manufacturer*: Rosemont.

ARTANE

Description: an anticholinergic containing benhexol hydrochloride, an antimuscarine drug used in the treatment of Parkinsonism. White-scored tablets are available in two strengths (2mg and 5mg) coded 4434 and 4436 respectively. Both are marked Lederle. *Used for*: Parkinsonism including drug-induced Parkinson's disease. *Dosage*: first day, 1mg, second day, 2mg, then increased by 2mg daily every 3 to 5 days. The maintenance dose is usually 5–15mg per day. *Special care*: patients with obstruction of gastro-intestinal tract, kidney or liver disease, heart disorders, enlargement of prostate gland, narrow angle glaucoma. *Avoid use*: children. *Possible interaction*: antihistamine and antidepressant drugs. Phenothiazine drugs. *Side effects*: anticholinergic effects. After high doses, agitation and confusion. *Manufacturer*: Lederle.

ARTHROTEC

Description: an NSAID containing diclofenac sodium, a phenylacetic acid prostaglandin analogue. Arthrotec tablets contain 50mg diclofenac sodium, 200 g misoprostol and are marked with a symbol and Searle 1411. *Used for*: osteoarthritis, rheumatoid arthritis. *Dosage*: adults, one tablet twice a day with food increasing to one three times a day if required. *Special care*: women of childbearing age should use effective contraception. Patients with gastric or duodenal ulcer, heart disease, coronary, cerebrovascular, peripheral vascular disease, kidney or liver disorders. Patients taking the drug for a long period should be monitored. *Avoid use*: children, pregnant women or those planning pregnancy, breast-feeding. Patients with gastro-intestinal bleeding, those with allergy to aspirin or other anti-inflammatory drugs. *Possible interaction*: NSAIDs, anticoagulants, quinolone, methotrexate, digoxin, lithium, steroids, diuretic drugs, oral hypoglycaemics. *Side effects*: gastro-intestinal upset, erosion of gastro-intestinal tract, heavy menstrual bleeding and intermenstrual bleeding, dizziness, headache, oedema, nausea, skin reactions. *Manufacturer*: Searle.

ARYTHMOL

Description: a class I antiarrhythmic drug used to treat disturbances of heart rhythm. Arythmol contains propafenone hydrochloride and is available in tablets of two strengths (150 and 300mg) which are white, scored and film-coated. *Used for*: treatment and prevention of ventricular arrhythmias. *Dosage*: adults, 150mg 3 times daily in first instance, gradually increasing at 3-day intervals to 300mg twice a day. Maximum dose is 300mg 3 times a day. *Special care*: patients with heart failure or who are fitted with pacemakers, those with liver or kidney disorders, elderly persons. *Avoid use*: children, pregnant women, some particular forms of heart rhythm disturbance, patients with uncontrolled congestive heart failure, electrolyte balance disturbances, obstructive lung disease, severe hypotension, myasthenia gravis. *Possible interaction*: other class I antiarrhythmic drugs, myocardial (heart muscle) depressant drugs, warfarin, digoxin, cimetidine rifampicin, propranolol, metoprolol. *Side effects*: gastro-intestinal upset including constipation, diarrhoea, vomiting, nausea, unpleasant bitter taste, fatigue, headache, allergic skin rashes, disturbances of heart rhythm. *Manufacturer*: Knoll.

ASACOL

Description: a preparation of the salicylate drug, mesalazine, available as tablets and suppositories. Tablets (400mg strength) are oblong, red and resin-coated. Suppositories are available in two strengths containing 250mg and 500mg. Also, **ASACOL FOAM ENEMA** is available. *Used for*: to induce and maintain remission in ulcerative colitis and to treat acute attacks of this condition. *Dosage*: adults, tablets, acute attack, 6 daily in divided doses. For maintenance, 3–6 tablets daily in divided doses. Asacol suppositories, adults 750–1500mg daily in divided doses with last dose at night. *Special care*: elderly persons, pregnant and nursing mothers, patients with kidney disease, elevated blood urea levels, proteinuria. *Avoid use*: children, patients with severe kidney disease. *Possible interaction*: lactulose, substance which increases acidity of motions. *Side effects*: gastro-intestinal upset, blood changes, headache, kidney failure. *Manufacturer*: SmithKline Beecham.

ASENDIS

Description: a TCAD preparation containing amoxapine, available in tablets of various strength, all seven-sided, scored tablets: 25mg, white, marked LL25; 50mg, orange, marked LL50; 100mg, blue, marked LL100 and 150mg, white, marked LL150. *Used for*: depression. *Dosage*: 100–150mg per day at first increasing to a maintenance dose in the region of 150–250mg. Maximum daily dose is 300mg. Elderly persons, 25mg twice a day at first increasing, after 5–7 days, to 50mg 3 times daily if required. *Special care*: patients with psychoses or suicidal tendencies, elderly persons, pregnant and nursing mothers, people with cardiac disorders, epilepsy, hyperthyroidism, urine retention, closed angle glaucoma, liver disease, tumours of adrenal gland, diabetes. *Avoid use*: children, patients with recent heart attack, heart arrhythmias, heart block, porphyria (rare blood disorder). *Possible interaction*: alcohol, barbiturate drugs, local anaesthetics (containing adrenaline or noradrenaline), antihypertensive and sympathomimetic drugs, anticholineric drugs, cimetidine, oestrogens. *Side effects*: anticholinergic effects including urine retention, dry mouth, constipation, blurred vision, rapid heartbeat, palpitations, nervousness, insomnia, sweating, dizziness, fatigue, weight changes, jaundice, blood changes, allergic skin rashes, changes in libido, breast enlargement and impotence. *Manufacturer*: Wyeth.

ASPAV

Description: a combined salicylate and opiate analgesic containing aspirin and papaveretum available as dissolvable tablets. Aspav white tablets contain 500mg aspirin, 10mg papaveretum. *Used for*: relief of post-operative pain and chronic pain caused by inoperable cancers. *Dosage*: adults, 1–2 tablets in water every four to six hours. Maximum daily dose, 8 tablets in 24 hours. *Special care*: women in labour, pregnant women and nursing mothers, elderly persons. Patients with head injury, liver or kidney disease, gastro-intestinal ulcers, heart failure, hypothyroidism, history of bronchospasm or allergy to anti-inflammatory drugs. *Avoid use*: children, patients in comatose states with depressed breathing, or obstructed airways. *Possible interaction*: central nervous system depressants, NSAIDs, anticoagulants, MAOIs, sulphonamide antibiotics, hypoglycaemic drugs, uric acid-lowering drugs, methotrexate. *Side effects*: allergic responses, asthma, bleeding of gastro-intestinal tract, confusion, nausea, constipation. *Manufacturer*: Hoechst.

ATARAX

Description: an antihistamine preparation containing hydroxyzine hydrochloride available as sugar-coated tablets of two strengths (10 and 25mg) coloured orange and green respectively and in the form of a syrup. **ATARAX SYRUP** contains 10mg hydroxyzine hydrochloride per 5ml. *Used for*: anxiety (short-term treatment) and itching caused by allergy (chronic urticaria and dermatitis). *Dosage*: anxiety, adults only, 50–100mg 4 times each day. Itching, adults, 25mg taken at night increasing to 25mg 3–4 times a day if required. Children, 6 months to 6 years, 5–15mg daily increasing to 50mg in divided doses if required; 6 years and over, 15–25mg daily increasing to 50–100mg in divided doses if required. *Special care*: patients with kidney disease. Patients must be warned that judgement and dexterity is impaired. Children should be given reduced doses for itching only. *Avoid use*: pregnant women. *Possible interaction*: central nervous system depressants, alcohol. *Side effects*: drowsiness, anticholinergic effects, if high doses are taken there may be involuntary muscle movements. *Manufacturer*: Pfizer.

ATIVAN

Description: an anxiolytic benzodiazepine, lorazepam, which is for short-term use only as it carries a risk of dependency. It is available as tablets of two strengths and also in the form of ampoules for injection. Blue, oblong, scored tablets, marked A1 contain 1mg and yellow, oblong, scored tablets, marked A2.5 contain 2.5mg. **ATIVAN INJECTION** contains 4mg lorazepam per ml. *Used for*: anxiety, status epilepticus (a condition where a person with epilepsy suffers a series of fits in close succession and is deprived of oxygen), a sedative premedication prior to full anaesthesia. *Dosage*: tablets, adults, for anxiety, 1–4mg each day in divided doses. Elderly persons, 0.5mg–2mg each day. For status epilepticus, adults, 4mg by intravenous injection, children half the adult dose. For premedication, adults, tablets, 2–4mg 1 or 2 hours prior to operation or 0.05mg per kg of body weight intravenously about 30–45 minutes before operation. *Special care*: women in labour, pregnancy, breast-feeding, elderly, liver or kidney disorders, lung disease. Short-term use only, withdraw gradually. *Avoid use*: children, acute lung diseases, depression of breathing, those with chronic psychoses, obsessional states and phobias. *Possible interaction*: CNS depressant drugs, alcohol, anticonvulsants. *Side effects*: lightheadedness, drowsiness, vertigo, confusion, unsteadiness in walking, gastrointestinal upset, disturbance of vision, rash, retention of urine, changes in libido, low blood pressure. Rarely, blood changes and jaundice. Risk of dependence especially with high doses. *Manufacturer*: Wyeth.

ATROMID-S

Description: an isobutyric acid derivative which lowers the concentration of cholesterol and other fats (lipids) found in blood plasma. Available as red, gelatin-coated capsules, marked ICI, containing 500mg of clofibrate. *Used for*: elevated plasma lipid levels (hyperlipidaemias) of types IIb, III, IV and V which have not been lowered by dietary changes or other appropriate treatments. *Dosage*: adults, 20–30mg per kg of body weight two to three times daily after meals in divided doses. *Special care*: patients with low levels of albumin (protein) in blood serum. Regu-lar blood checks may be carried out. *Avoid use*: children, pregnant women, patients with diseases of the gall bladder, liver or kidney disorders. *Possible interaction*: hypoglycaemics, phenytoin, anticoagulants. *Side effects*: gastro-intestinal upset, muscle pains, gallstones. *Manufacturer*: Zeneca.

ATROVENT

Description: an anticholinergic containing ipratropium bromide available available in various forms: aerosol inhalation, 20 g per dose delivered by metered dose inhaler; **ATROVENT AUTOTHALER**, 20μ g per dose delivered by breath-actuated metered dose aerosol; **ATROVENT FORTE**, 40μg per dose delivered by metered dose inhaler; **ATROVENT SOLUTION**, 250μg per ml, in preservative-free isotonic solution in unit dose vials for use with nebulizer. *Used for*: severe obstruction of airways, especially that caused by chronic bronchitis. *Dosage*: adults, inhaler, 1–2 puffs three or four times a day. Children under 6 years, one puff, 6–12 years, 1–2 puffs, both three times a day. Adults, Atrovent Forte, 1 or 2 puffs three to four times daily; children 6–12 years, 1 puff three times daily. Adults, Atrovent solution, 0.4–2ml nebulized up to four times each day. Children over 3 years, 0.4–2ml nebulized up to three times each day. *Special care*: patients with enlarged prostate gland (prostate hypertrophy), glaucoma. *Side effects*: urine retention, constipation, dry mouth. *Manufacturer*: Boehringer Ingelheim.

AUDICORT

Description: a combined antibacterial, antifungal and anti-inflammatory (corticosteroid) preparation available in the form of ear drops. Audicort contains 1mg triamcinolone acetate and neomycin undecylenate (antibiotic) (equivalent to 3.5mg neomycin base). *Used for*: chronic and acute inflammation and/or bacterial infection of the outer ear. *Dosage*: adults, 2–5 drops three of fopur times each day. *Special care*: pregnant and nursing mothers avoid prolonged use. *Avoid use*: children, patients with perforated ear drum. *Side effects*: localized irritation, additional infection. *Manufacturer*: Wyeth.

AUGMENTIN

Description: a broad-spectrum, penicillin-like antibiotic, amoxycillin as the trihydrate, with clavulanic acid as the potassium salt. The latter makes the antibiotic effective against a wider range of infections by combating certain enzymes produced by some bacteria. Available as white film coated tablets, Augmentin 375mg (250mg/125mg) and 625mg (500mg/125mg). Also, **AUGMENTIN DISPERSABLE** (250mg/125mg), white tablets marked Augmentin. Also **AUGMENTIN SUSPENSION 125/31 SF** (sugar-free) contains 125mg amoxycillin as trihydrate, 31mg clavulanic acid as potassium salt, per 5 ml when reconstituted with water. Similarly, **AUGMENTIN SUSPENSION 250/62 SF** (250/62mg). **AUGMENTIN INTRAVENOUS** is a powder for intravenous injection available in 2 strengths containing amoxycillin as sodium salt and clavulanic acid as potassium salt (500/100mg, and 1g/200mg). *Used for*: respiratory tract and ear, nose and throat infections, skin and soft tissue infections, urinary tract infections. *Dosage*: adults, tablets, 375mg three times a day (severe infections 625mg) for 14 days. Children, use suspension, under 6 years use lower strength 125/31. Under one year 25mg per kg body weight each day; 1–6 years, 5ml three times a day for 14 days. 6–12 years use 250/62 suspension, 5ml 3 times each day for 14 days. Intravenous injection: adults, 1.2g or by intermittent infusion 6 to 8-hourly for 14 days. Children, under 3 months, 30mg per kg of body weight every 12 hours in newborns increasing to every 8 hours in older infants. 3 months–12 years, 30mg per kg of body weight every 8 or 6 hours. By intravenous or intermittent infusion for up to 14 days. *Special care*: pregnant and breast-feeding mothers, patients with liver and kidney disease, glandular fever. Review after 14 days. *Avoid use*: allergy to penicillin. *Side effects*: gastro-intestinal upset, allergic responses, rarely cholestatic jaundice, hepatitis, phlebitis at site of injection. *Manufacturer*: Beecham.

AUREOCORT

Description: a combined antibacterial and steroid preparation available in the form of cream or ointment, containing 0.1% of the corticosteroid triamcinolone acetonide and 3% of the tetracycline antibiotic, chlortetracycline hydrochloride. *Used for*: inflammation and irritation of the skin where infection is present also. *Dosage*: apply sparingly to affected skin two or three times daily. *Special care*: limit use to a short time period. In children and on face, treatment should not exceed 5 days. *Avoid use*: on extensive areas of skin or for long time periods or for prevention. Acne (including rosacea), urticaria, scabies, leg ulcers, viral skin infections, tuberculosis, ringworm. *Side effects*: thinning of skin and skin changes, adrenal gland suppression, fluid retention. *Manufacturer*: Wyeth.

AUREOMYCIN

Description: a broad-spectrum antibiotic preparation, containing chlortetracycline hydrochloride, available as cream and ointment both of which contain 3% chlortetracycline hydrochloride. Aureomycin is also available as an eye ointment containing 1% tetracycline hydrochloride. *Used for*: superficial skin infections with bacterial origin. Eye infections sensitive to tetracycline. *Dosage*: skin infections, apply on gauze once or twice daily. Eye infections, apply into eye every two hours then reduce frequency as condition improves. Continue to use for 48 hours after symptoms have disappeared. *Avoid use*: Possible interaction: *Side effects*: additional infections. *Manufacturer*: Wyeth.

AVLOCLOR

Description: an antimalarial drug containing chloroquine phosphate, available as white, scored tablets containing 250mg chloroquine phosphate. *Used for*: prevention and treatment of malaria, rheumatoid arthritis, lupus erythematosus (inflammatory disease of skin and some internal organs), amoebic hepatitis. *Dosage*: prevention of malaria; adults, 2 tablets as one dose on the same day each week commmencing 2 weeks before entering affected area and continuing for 4 weeks after leaving. Children should take in the same way at a dose rate of 5mg per kg of body weight. Treatment of hepatitis, adults only, four tablets each day for two days then one tablet twice daily for two to three weeks. *Special care*: pregnancy, liver or kidney disease, breast-feeding, patients with epilepsy and some other neurological conditions, psoriasis, porphyria, severe gastro-intestinal disorders. Regular eye tests may be needed during treatment. *Side effects*: gastro-intestinal upset, headache, hair loss, loss of pigment, skin rashes, blurred vision, opacity of cornea, retinal damage. *Manufacturer*: Zeneca.

AXID

Description: a preparation containing nizatidine (an H_2 blocker) available in the form of capsules: pale, yellow/dark yellow, coded 3144 (150mg) and yellow/brown coded 3145 (300mg). **AXID INJECTION** contains 25mg nizatidine per ml. *Used for*: duodenal and benign gastric ulcers and their prevention. Gastro-oesophageal reflux disease. *Dosage*: adults, for duodenal and gastric ulcers, 300mg taken in the evening or 150mg morning and evening for 4–8 weeks. Prevention, 150mg in evening for up to one year. Adults, for gastro-oesophageal reflux disease, 150mg–300mg twice a day for up to 12 weeks. Axid injection, adults, dilute before use, 100mg by slow intravenous injection three times each day or 10mg per hour by intravenous infusion. Maximum 480mg per day. *Special care*: patients with liver or kidney disease, pregnant or breast-feeding mothers. *Avoid use*: children. *Possible interaction*: salicylates. *Side effects*: sweating, sleepiness, itchiness, headache, muscle and joint pain, jaundice, raised levels of liver enzymes, hepatitis, anaemia. *Manufacturer*: Lilly.

AXSAIN

Description: a topical counter-irritant analgesic preparation available as a cream containing 0.075% capsaicin. *Used for*: post-herpetic neuralgia. *Dosage*: adults only, massage in 3 to 4 times daily once lesions have healed. *Avoid use*: children, on broken, irritated skin. *Side effects*: local skin irritation. *Manufacturer*: Euroderma.

AZACTAM

Description: a powder for injection and infusion, containing 500mg aztreonam available as 1g or 2g powder in vials. *Used for*: serious infections caused by Gram-negative bacteria, including those of the lower respiratory tract and lung infections in cystic fibrosis sufferers. Also, soft tissue, skin, joint, bone, gynaecological and abdominal infections. Urinary tract infections and gonorrhoea, meningitis (where *II. influenzae* or *N. Menigitidis* is the causal organism), septicaemia and bacteraemia (bacteria in blood indicating infection). *Dosage*: adults, 1g by intramuscular or intravenous injection every eight hours or 2g intravenously every 12 hours. If infection is severe, 2g six to eight hourly intravenously. Maximum daily dose is 8g. For urinary tract infections, 0.5–1g intramuscularly or intravenously every eight to twelve hours. For cystitis, 1g intramuscularly as a single dose. Children, one week to two years, 30mg per kg of body weight every six to eight hours. Severe infections in children over two years, 50mg per kg of body weight every six to eight hours. Maximum dose is 8g each day. *Special care*: patients with allergy to penicillin or cephalospoin. Persons with kidney or liver disease. *Avoid use*: children under one year, pregnant or breast-feeding mothers. *Side effects*: gastro-intestinal upset, vomiting and diarrhoea, local skin inflammation at injection site. *Manufacturer*: Squibb.

AZAMUNE

Description: an immunosuppressant, cytotoxic preparation containing azathioprine available as yellow, scored tablets marked AZA 50 (50mg). *Used for*: to lessen the likelihood of rejection following organ transplants and donor skin grafts. Also, some auto-immune diseases. *Dosage*: adults and children, following transplant, 5mg per kg of body weight at first then 1–4mg per kg of body weight each day for 3 months in divided doses. For chronic hepatitis, 1–1.5mg per kg of body weight daily. Auto-immune diseases, 2–2.5mg per kg of body weight daily. *Special care*: Azathioprine causes suppression of bone marrow function, hence careful monitoring of blood count for toxic effects is necessary and dosage must be adjusted accordingly. Pregnant women, patients with overexposure to sun, any infection, kidney disorders. *Avoid use*: toxic hepatitis, stoppage of bile flow. *Possible interaction*: muscle relaxant drugs, cytostatics, allopurinol. *Side effects*: bone marrow suppression, liver toxicity, gastro-intestinal upset, rashes. *Manufacturer*: Penn Pharmaceuticals.

B

BACTRIM

Description: a preparation combining an antibacterial sulphonamide with a folic acid inhibitor. Elongated, orange, film-coated capsules marked Roche contain 80mg trimethoprim and 400mg sulphamethoxazole. Also, **BACTRIM DISPERSIBLE**: yellow tablets, scored, containing 480mg co-trimoxazole. **BACTRIM DOUBLE STRENGTH**: white scored tablets containing 160mg trimethoprim and 800mg sulphmethoxazole and marked Roche 800 and 160. **BACTRIM ADULT SUSPENSION** is a yellow syrup containing 480mg co-trimoxazole per 5ml and **BACTRIM PAEDIATRIC SYRUP** contains 40mg trimethoprim and 200mg sulphmethoxazole per 5ml (sugar-free and fruit-flavoured). *Used for*: urinary tract infections, infections of joints, bones and skin, gastro-intestinal and respiratory tract. *Dosage*: adults, ordinary strength tablets, 1–3 tablets twice each day; children 6 to 12 years, 1 twice a day. Children under 6 years use paediatric syrup. Six weeks to 5 months, 2.5ml; 6 months to 5 years, 5ml. Six to 12 years, 10ml, all doses twice each day. Adults, double strength tablets, 1/2 to 11/2 tablets twice each day. *Special care*: breast-feeding, elderly, kidney disease (reduce dose, increase interval between doses). Regular blood tests should be carried out. *Avoid use*: children under 6 weeks, pregnant women, patients with severe kidney or liver disease or blood changes. *Possible interaction*: antidiabetics, anticoagulants, antiepileptic drugs, antimalarial drugs, cyclosporin, cytotoxics, folate inhibitors. *Side effects*: vomiting, nausea, blood changes, skin rashes, inflammation of the tongue (glossitis), folate (folic acid) deficiency. Rarely, Lyell syndrome, erythema multiformae (circular red patches on skin). *Manufacturer*: Roche.

BACTROBAN

Description: a broad-spectrum antibiotic preparation containing 2% mupirocin in the form of an ointment. **BACTROBAN NASAL** is an ointment containing 2% mupirocin in a soft white paraffin base. *Used for*: bacterial skin infections. Nasal ointment, infections of the nose and nostrils caused by staphlocci bacteria. *Dosage*: ointment, apply to skin 3 times a day for up to 10 days. Nasal ointment, apply to the inner surface of nostrils 2 or 3 times daily. *Special care*: patients with kidney disorders, avoid eyes. *Side effects*: may sting on application. *Manufacturer*: SmithKline Beecham.

BAMBEC

Description: a preparation containing bambuterol hydrochloride which is a selective β_2-agonist used in the treatment of asthma. Bambec is available as tablets of 2 strengths containing 10mg (marked A/BA) and 20mg (marked A/BM). Tablets are oval, white and scored. *Used for*: asthma (bronchospasm) and reversible airways obstruction. *Dosage*: 10mg as one dose taken at night increasing to 20mg once a day if necessary. If the patient has been used to treatment with a β_2-agonist, then 20mg may be taken from the start. *Special care*: pregnant women and breast-feeding mothers, diabetics, moderate or severe kidney disorders, heart disorders, thyrotoxicosis. In cases of severe asthma, potassium levels in blood should be monitored. *Avoid use*: children. *Possible interaction*: Other ß-blockers, suxamethonium. *Side effects*: headache, palpitations, cramps, tremor, hypokalaemia. *Manufacturer*:Novex.

BARATOL

Description: an antihypertensive, alpha-adrenoreceptor blocking drug, indoramin hydrochloride, available in 2 strengths, blue tablets (25mg, marked MPL020 and 25) and green tablets (50mg, marked MPL 021 and 50). Both are film-coated and scored. *Used for*: hypertension (high blood pressure). *Dosage*: adults, 25mg twice each day at start increasing by 25mg or 50mg each fortnight. Maximum dose is 200mg per day in 2 or 3 divided doses. *Special care*: patients with liver or kidney disorders, Parkinson's disease, epilepsy, history of depression. Patients with incipient heart failure should be treated with digoxin and diuretics. Performance of skilled tasks such as driving may be impaired. *Avoid use*: children, cardiac failure. *Possible interaction*: alcohol, antihypertensive drugs, MAOIs. *Side effects*: drowsiness, dizziness, depression, dry mouth, blocked nose, weight gain, failure to ejaculate. *Manufacturer*: Monmouth.

BAXAN

Description: a cephalosporin antibiotic preparatiton available as tablets and as powder for reconstitution with water, in 3 strengths. Baxan white capsules contain 500mg cefadroxil (as monohydrate) and are marked 7244. **BAXAN SUS-**

PENSION contains either 125mg, 250mg or 500mg per 5ml when reconstituted with water, available as powder to make 60ml. *Used for*: various infections of skin, urinary and respiratory tracts, ear and soft tissues. *Dosage*: adults, 500mg–1g twice each day (1 to 2 tablets); children under 1 year, 25mg per kg of body weight in divided doses; 1 to 6 years, 250mg twice each day; 6 years and over, 500mg twice each day. *Special care*: patients with penicillin allergy or kidney disease. *Avoid use*: cephalosporin allergy, porphyria. *Possible interaction*: some diuretics. *Side effects*: gastro-intestinal upset, allergic responses. *Manufacturer*: Bristol-Myers.

BAYCARON

Description: a thiazide-like diuretic preparation, mefruside, available as white scored tablets marked Bayer and L/1 (strength 25mg). *Used for*: oedema and hypertension. *Dosage*: 1–2 tablets as a single dose taken in the morning for 10–14 days, then 1 daily or on alternate days for maintenance. Maximum dose for oedema is 4 tablets daily. *Special care*: elderly, pregnancy and breast-feeding, liver or kidney disease, gout, diabetes, liver cirrhosis. Fluid, electrolytes and glucose levels should be monitored. *Avoid use*: children, patients with liver or kidney failure, Addison's disease, hypercalcaemia, sensitivity to sulphonamide drugs. *Possible interaction*: alcohol, opioids, barbiturates, NSAIDs, antidiabetic drugs, tubocurarine, lithium, corticosteroids, cardiac glycosides, carbenoxolone. *Side effects*: gastro-intestinal upset, rash, blood changes, disturbance of electrolyte levels and metabolism, dizziness, sensitivity to light, pancreatitis, anorexia, impotence. *Manufacturer*: Bayer.

BECLAZONE

Description: a corticosteroid preparation containing either 50 or 100µg beclomethasone dipropionate per dose, delivered by metered dose aerosol. Also **BECLAZONE 250**, containing 250µg per metered dose. *Used for*: chronic reversible obstructive airways disease (asthma). *Dosage*: adults, 100 g 3 to 4 times each day. If very severe, 600–800µg (maximum 1g) in divided doses each day. Children, 50–100µg 2 to 4 times each day. Beclazone 250, adults only, 250µg twice each day or 250µg 4 times each day. This may be increased to 1500–2000µg each day in divided doses if required. *Special care*: pulmonary tuberculosis, pregnant women, patients who have been taking systemic steroid drugs. *Side effects*: hoarseness, fungal infections of throat and mouth. *Manufacturer*: Baker Norton.

BECLOFORTE

Description: a corticosteroid preparation in a variety of forms for inhalation containing 250µg beclomethasone dipropionate per dose delivered by metered dose aerosol. **BECLOFORTE VM** is available as a pack consisting of 2 Becloforte inhalers and Volumatic. Also, **BECLOFORTE DISKHALER** consisting of blisters containing 400µg beclomethasone dipropionate per dose delivered by breath-actuated inhaler. *Used for*: patients with chronic and severe asthma, emphysema or chronic bronchitis who require high doses of Beclomethasone. *Dosage*: adults only, 500µg twice each day or 250µg 4 times a day. May be increased to 500µg 3 or 4 times each day if necessary. Diskhaler, adults, 2 blisters each day. *Special care*: pregnancy, patients with active or quiescent pulmonary tuberculosis, those transferring from systemic steroids. *Avoid use*: children. *Side effects*: hoarseness, fungal infections of throat and mouth. *Manufacturer*: A & H.

BECODISKS

Description: a corticosteroid preparation available as a dry powder for inhalation with Diskhaler. Beige disks contain 100µg beclomethasone dipropionate; brown disks contain 200µg; light brown disks contain 400µg. *Used for*: bronchial asthma. *Dosage*: adults, 400 g twice each day or 200µg 3 to 4 times each day. Children, 100µg 2 to 4 times each day or 200µg twice each day. *Special care*: pregnant women, patients with active or quiescent pulmonary tuberculosis, those transferring from systemic steroids. *Side effects*: hoarseness, fungal infections of throat and mouth. *Manufacturer*: A & H.

BECOTIDE

Description: a corticosteroid preparation, beclomethasone diproprionate, available in the form of an aerosol of different strengths for inhalation. Becotide-50 (50µg per metered inhalation), Becotide-100 (100µg) and Becotide-200 (200µg). *Used for*: bronchial asthma. *Dosage*: adults, 400µg each day in 2, 3 or 4 divided doses. If asthma is severe, 600–800µg may be required in first instance in daily divided doses. This should be reduced as condition improves. Children, 200µg twice each day using Becotide-50 or 100 only. *Special care*: pregnant women, patients with active or quiescent pulmonary tuberculosis, those transferring from systemic steroids. *Side effects*: hoarseness, fungal infections of throat and mouth. *Manufacturer*: A & H.

BECOTIDE ROTACAPS

Description: a corticosteroid preparation, beclomethasone diproprionate, available as a dry powder in capsules for inhalation: buff/clear (100µg), brown (200µg), dark brown/clear (400µg), all marked with name and strength and each is a single dose for use with a Rotahaler. *Used for*: bronchial asthma. *Dosage*: adults, 400µg twice each day or 200µg 3 or 4 times each day. Children, 100µg 2 or 4 times each day or 200µg twice each day. *Special care*: pregnant women, patients with active or quiescent pulmonary tuberculosis, those transferring from systemic steroids. *Side effects*: hoarseness, fungal infections of throat and mouth. *Manufacturer*: A & H.

BENEMID

Description: a uricosuric preparation (one which enhances the excretion of uric acid from the kidneys), available as white, scored tablets containing 500mg probenecid, and marked MSD 501. *Used for*: gout, hyperuricaemia (elevated

uric acid levels in blood). Also, with certain antibiotics (e.g. penicillin) to pro-
long their effects and maintain high blood levels. This occurs because excretion
of the antibiotic is inhibited. *Dosage*: for gout and hyperuricaemia, half a tablet twice a day for 1 week then 1 twice daily. Adults, with certain antibiotics, 4
tablets daily in divided doses. Children over 2 years, with antibiotics, 25mg per
kg of body weight, then 40mg per kg each day in divided doses. *Special care*:
pregnancy, elderly, history of peptic ulcer or kidney disorders. Plenty of fluids
should be taken. *Avoid use*: children under 2 years, patients during acute attack
of gout (the start of treatment should be delayed), uric acid stones in kidneys,
blood changes. *Possible interaction*: ß lactam antibiotics, methotextrate, indomethacin, sulphonamides, salicylates, pyrazinamide, sulphonylureas. *Side
effects*: gastro-intestinal upset, headache, sore gums, flushes, frequency of urination, hypersensitivity, kidney colic, kidney stones, acute gout. *Manufacturer*:
M.S.D.

BEROTEC 100

Description: a proprietary bronchodilator and short-acting $ß_2$-agonist that acts
rapidly to relax smooth muscle in the walls of the airways and relieves symptoms for about 3 to 6 hours. Berotec is produced in the form of an aerosol of 2
strengths or as a solution for use with a nebulizer, for inhalation. Berotec 100
contains 0.1mg fenoterol hydrobromide per metered dose inhalation. **BEROTEC
200** contains 0.2mg per metered dose inhalation. **BEROTEC NEBULIZER**
solution contains 0.5% fenoterol hydrobromide. *Used for*: reversible obstruction of airways as in bronchial asthma, emphysema and bronchitis. *Dosage*:
adults, aerosol starting with lower strength (100), 1 to 2 puffs up to 3 times
each day with a maximum of 2 puffs every 6 hours. Berotec 200, 1 to 2 puffs up
to 3 times each day with a maximum of 2 puffs every 6 hours. Nebulized solution, 0.5–1.25mg us to 4 times a day with strength adjusted as necessary by
dilution with sterile sodium chloride solution. Children, lower strength 100
aerosol, over 6 years of age, 1 puff up to 3 times each day with a maximum of
2 puffs every 6 hours. Berotec 200 and nebulizer solution should not be given to
children under 16 years of age. *Special care*: pregnant women, patients with
hypertension, heart arrhythmias, heart disorders, angina, hyperthyroidism. *Avoid
use*: children under 6 years. *Possible interaction*: sympathomimetic drugs. *Side
effects*: headache, dilation of blood vessels in skin, nervousness. *Manufacturer*:
Boehringer Ingelheim.

BETA-ADALAT

Description: a cardio-selective ß-blocker/Class II calcium antagonist containing atenolol and nifedipine available as red-brown capsules marked with the
Bayer cross and name and containing 50mg atenolol and 20mg nifedipine. *Used
for*: hypertension, angina (where therapy with a calcium-channel blocker or
beta-blocker alone proves to be ineffective). *Dosage*: for hypertension, 1 capsule each day increasing to 2 if required. Elderly persons, 1 capsule. Angina, 1

capsule twice each day. *Special care*: weak heart, liver or kidney disease, diabetes, anaesthesia. *Avoid use*: children, pregnancy, breast-feeding, heart block, heart shock or heart failure. *Possible interaction*: cardiac depressant drugs, cimetidine, quinidine. *Side effects*: headache, dizziness, flushing, dryness of eyes, skin rashes, oedema, swelling of gums, allergic jaundice. *Manufacturer*: Bayer.

BETA-CARDONE

Description: a non-cardioselective ß-blocker, sotalol hydrochloride, available as tablets in 3 strengths: green-scored tablets marked Evans/BC4 (40mg) ; pink-scored tablets marked Evans/BC8 (80mg) and white-scored tablets marked Evans/BC20 (200mg). *Used for*: heart arrhythmias, angina, hypertension and as an additional therapy for thyrotoxicosis. *Dosage*: heart arrhythmias, 40mg 3 times daily for 7 days increasing to 120–240mg each day either all at once or in divided doses. Angina, 80mg twice each day in first instance for 1 week to 10 days, increasing to 200–600mg daily either all at once or in divided doses. Hypertension, 80mg twice each day in first instance for 1 week to 10 days, increasing to 200–600 mg daily, either all at once or in divided doses. Thyrotoxicosis, 120–240 mg each day as a single amount or in divided doses. *Special care*: patients with diabetes, liver or kidney disorders, those undergoing general anaesthesia (drug may need to be stopped). Pregnant women and nursing mothers. Patients with weak hearts may need to be treated with digitalis and diuretic drugs. *Avoid use*: children, patients with asthma or history of bronchospasm, those with heart block, heart attack, heart shock and some other cardiac disorders. Drug should be stopped gradually. *Possible interaction*: verapamil, clonidine withdrawal, hyperglycaemics, class I anti-arrhythmic drugs, some anaesthetics, reserpine, sympathomimetics, antidepressants, ergotamine, indomethacin, cimetidine. *Side effects*: slow heartbeat, disruption of sleep, cold hands and feet, fatigue in exercise, gastro-intestinal upset, wheezing, heart failure, skin rash, dry eyes (withdraw drug gradually). *Manufacturer*: Evans.

BETAGAN

Description: a ß-blocker in the form of eye drops containing 0.5% levobunolol hydrochloride and 1.4% polyvinyl alcohol, and as single dose units. *Used for*: chronic simple open-angle glaucoma, reduction of intra-ocular pressure. *Dose*: adults, 1 drop once or twice each day. *Special care*: patients with breathing disorders, breast-feeding mothers, diabetics. *Avoid use*: children, patients with asthma, pregnant women, those with various heart disorders including heart block, heart failure, heart shock, slow heartbeat, history of obstructive lung disease. *Possible interaction*: ß-blockers, reserpine. *Side effects*: local allergic irritation or dry eyes, respiratory difficulties, dizziness, headache, ß-blocker effects. *Manufacturer*: Allergan.

BETA-PROGRANE

Description: a non-cardioselective ß-blocker produced in the form of sustained-release capsules which are white and contain 160mg propranolol hydrochloride. Also available, **HALF BETA-PROGRANE** white sustained-release capsules containing 80mg propranolol hydrochloride. *Used for*: angina, high blood pressure, as additional therapy for overactive thyroid gland (thyrotoxicosis), prevention of migraine. *Dosage*: angina, 80–160mg each day increasing to a maximum of 240mg if needed. Hypertension, 160mg each day increasing to 320mg by 80mg each day if necessary. Thyrotoxicosis, 80mg to 160mg each day increasing to 240mg if necessary. Prevention of migraine, 80mg–160mg each day increasing to 240mg if necessary. *Special care*: pregnancy and lactation, diabetes, liver or kidney disease, metabolic acidosis, those undergoing general anaesthesia, patients with weak hearts should be treated with digitalis and diuretics. The drug should be stopped gradually. *Avoid use*: children, patients with various heart disorders including heart shock, heart block, heart failure, asthma. *Possible interaction*: some anaesthetics, antidiabetic drugs, antihypertensives, sympathomimetics, sedatives, indo-methacin, reserpine, class I antiarrhythmics, verapamil, clonidine withdrawal. *Side effects*: disturbance of sleep, cold feet and hands, slow heartbeat rate, fatigue with exercise, wheezing, heart failure, gastro-intestinal disorders; dry eyes or skin rash (gradually withdraw drug). *Manufacturer*: Tillomed.

BETALOC

Description: a cardioselective ß-blocker, metaprolol tartrate, available as tablets of 2 strengths, as modified-release tablets and in ampoules for injection. Betaloc tablets are white, scored and contain 50mg (marked A/BB) or 100mg (marked A/ME). Also, **BETALOC-SA** modified-release tablets (Durules®), containing 200mg and marked AMD. Also, **BETALOC INJECTION** containing 1mg per ml in 5ml ampoules. *Used for*: heart arrhythmias, angina, maintenance therapy in heart attack, hypertension, additional therapy in thyrotoxicosis, prevention of migraine. *Dosage*: heart attack, 200mg each day; heart arrhythmias, 50mg 2 or 3 times each day increasing to maximum daily dose of 300mg. Angina, 50–100mg twice or three times each day. Hypertension, 50mg twice each day at first increasing to 400mg if required. Thyrotoxicosis, 50mg 4 times each day; migraine prevention, 100mg–200mg each day in divided doses. *Special care*: pregnancy, breast-feeding, liver or kidney disease, diabetes, metabolic acidosis, those undergoing anaesthesia; patients with weak hearts should be treated with digitalis and diuretics. Drug should be stopped gradually. *Avoid use*: children, patients with asthma, heart diseases including heart block, heart shock, slow heartbeat rate, heart failure. *Possible interaction*: cardiac depressant, anaesthetics, reserpine, sedatives, antihypertensives, sympathomimetics, cimetidine, indomethacin, ergotamine, class I antiarrhythmic drugs, verapamil, clonidine withdrawal, hypoglycaemics. *Side effects*: sleep disturbance, cold feet and hands, slow heartbeat, fatigue on exercise, wheeziness, heart failure, gastro-intestinal disorders; dry eyes or skin rash (stop use gradually). *Manufacturer*: Astra.

BETHANIDINE

Description: an antihypertensive drug, bethanidine sulphate, which acts by blocking the release of noradrenaline (a neurotransmitter) from nerve endings. It is available in the form of tablets containing 10mg bethanidine sulphate. *Used for*: hypertension, especially that which has failed to respond to other antihypertensive drugs. It is usually used in conjunction with a diuretic (e.g. a thiazide) or beta-blocker. *Dosage*: adults, 10mg, 3 times each day after food at first increasing by 5mg once a week to a maximum daily dose of 200mg. *Special care*: kidney disease, pregnant women, asthma, peptic ulcer or history of peptic ulcer, cerebral or coronary arteriosclerosis. Low blood pressure when rising from a prone position may cause falls in elderly people. *Avoid use*: children, patients with kidney or heart failure, phaeochromocytoma. *Possible interaction*: tricyclic antidepressants, sympathomimetics, MAOIs. *Side effects*: low blood pressure associated with lying down (postural hypotension), blocked nose, headache, drowsiness, oedema, failure of ejaculation.

BETIM

Description: a non-cardioselective beta-blocker available as white, scored tablets containing 10mg timolol maleate and marked with 102 and symbol. *Used for*: prevention of second heart attack following initial episode, angina, hypertension, prevention of migraine. *Dosage*: adults, prevention of secondary heart attack, 5mg twice each day for first 2 days, thereafter 10mg twice each day. Angina, 10mg twice each day at first, adjusted according to response to a maximum of 60mg. Hypertension, 10mg a day at first in single or divided dose increasing by 10mg every 3 to 4 days to a maximum of 60mg. Usual maintenance dose is in the order of 10–30mg. Prevention of migraine, 10–20mg each day in 1 or 2 divded doses. *Special care*: pregnancy, breast-feeding, liver or kidney disease, diabetes, those undergoing general anaesthesia, patients with weak hearts should receive digitalis and diuretics. Drug should be stopped gradually. *Avoid use*: children, patients with asthma or history of breathing difficulties, those with various forms of heart disease including heart block, heart shock, slow heartbeat, heart failure. *Possible interaction*: class I antiarrhythmics, cardiac depressant anaesthetics, ergotamine, sedatives, sympathomimetics, cimetidine, indomethacin, reserpine, hypoglycaemic drugs, clonidine withdrawal, verapamil. *Side effects*: sleep disturbance, cold feet and hands, slow heartbeat, fatigue in exercise, wheeziness, heart failure, gastro-intestinal upset, dry eyes or skin rash (stop drug gradually). *Manufacturer*: Leo.

BETNELAN

Description: a corticosteroid preparation containing the glucocorticoid betmethasone, in the form of white, scored tablets (0.5mg strength) and marked with the name and Evans. *Used for*: allergic conditions, severe asthma, rheumatoid arthritis, collagen diseases. *Dosage*: adults, 0.5mg–5mg daily then reduce to effective maintenance dose according to response. Children, 1 to 7 years, quarter to half adult dose, 7 to 12 years, half to three-quarters adult dose. *Special care*: pregnant women, patients who have recently undergone intestinal surgery, some cancers, inflamed veins, peptic ulcer, active infections and those with viral or fungal origin, tuberculosis. High blood pressure, kidney diseases, osteoporosis, diabetes, glaucoma, epilepsy, underactive thyroid, liver cirrhosis, stress, psychoses. Patients should avoid contact with chicken pox or *Herpes zoster* virus while on steroid treatment and for 3 months afterwards. In the event of exposure to chicken pox, patients should be immunized within 3 days (if chicken pox is contracted specialist care is required). Drug should be stopped gradually. *Avoid use*: children under 12 months. *Possible interaction*: NSAIDs, anticoagulants taken by mouth, diuretics, hypoglycaemics, cardiac glycosides, anticholinesterases, phenobarbitone, phenytoin, rifampicin, ephedrine. *Side effects*: mood swings (euphoria and depression), hyperglycaemia, osteoporosis, peptic ulcers, Cushing's syndrome caused especially by high doses. *Manufacturer*: Evans.

BETNESOL

Description: a corticosteroid containing the glucocorticoid betmethasone (as sodium phosphate), available as soluble tablets— pink, scored and marked with the name and Evans and containing 0.5mg. Also, **BETNESOL INJECTION** containing 4mg per ml in 1ml ampoules. *Used for*: allergic conditions, severe asthma, rheumatoid arthritis, collagen diseases. Injection: adrenal crisis and shock. *Dosage*: adults, 0.5mg–5mg in water as daily dose reducing to minimum effective dose for maintenance. Children, 1 to 7 years, one quarter to half adult dose; 7 to 12 years, half to three-quarters adult dose. Injection: adults, 4–20mg intravenously 3 or 4 times a day if needed. Children, 1 year and under, 1mg; 1 to 5 years, 2mg; 6 to 12 years, 4mg by intravenous injection. *Special care*: pregnancy, recent intestinal surgery, some cancers, inflamed veins, peptic ulcer, active infections and those with fungal or viral origin, tuberculosis, high blood pressure, kidney diseases, osteoporosis, diabetes, glaucoma, epilepsy, underactive thyroid, liver cirrhosis, stress, psychoses. Patients should avoid contact with chicken pox or *Herpes zoster* while on steroids and for 3 months after treatment has ceased. In the event of exposure to chicken pox, patients should be immunized within 3 days. (If chicken pox is contracted, specialist care is required). Drug should be stopped gradually. *Avoid use*: children under 12 months. *Possible interaction*: NSAIDs, oral anticoagulants, diuretics, hypoglycaemics, cardiac glycosides, anticholinesterases, phenobarbitone, phenytoin, rifampicin, ephedrine. *Side effects*: mood swings (euphoria and depression), hyperglycaemia (elevated blood sugar levels), osteoporosis, peptic ulcers, Cushings syndrome, especially caused by high doses. *Manufacturer*: Evans.

BETNOVATE

Description: a group of moderate to potent corticosteroid preparations containing betmethasone and available as ointment, cream or lotion. Betnovate cream and ointment both contain 0.1% betmethasone (as valerate); **BETNO-VATE SCALP APPLICATION**, (0.1%) **BETNOVATE C** cream and ointment contains an antimicrobial drug (antifungal and antibacterial), 3% clinoquinol and 0.1% betmethasone (as valerate); **BETNOVATE N** cream and ointment also contain an antimicrobial (antibacterial) drug, 0.5% neomycin sulphate and 0.1% betmethasone (as valerate). **BETNOVATE RD** cream and ointment are less potent containing 0.025% betmethasone (as valerate). *Used for*: eczema, seborrhoeic and contact dermatitis, psoriasis, other skin disorders (lichen simplex and planus). For infected conditions, Betnovate C or N are used depending upon causal organism. *Dosage*: adults, apply sparingly 2 or 3 times each day. More potent preparations may be used first with Betnovate RD then used for maintenance treatment. Children over 1 year same as adult dose. *Special care*: should not be used extensively or for a prolonged period. Should be used for only 5 days on children or on face. Stop use gradually. *Avoid use*: children under 1 year, continuous use especially by pregnant women, any conditions caused by ringworm, fungi, viruses, tuberculosis, acne, leg ulcers, scabies. *Side effects*: thinning of skin, suppression of adrenal glands, hair growth, symptoms associated with Cushings syndrome, e.g. reddening of skin on face and neck. *Manufacturer*: Glaxo Wellcome.

BETNOVATE RECTAL

Description: a steroid, vasoconstrictor and local anaesthetic preparation produced in the form of an ointment with applicator. The ointment contains 2.5% lignocaine hydrochloride, 0.1% phenylephrine hydrochloride and 0.05% betmethasone valerate. *Used for*: haemorrhoids and mild proctitis (inflammation of the rectum). *Dosage*: adults, apply 2 or 3 times daily at first and then once each day. *Special care*: avoid use for a long period, especially pregnant women. *Avoid use*: children, patients with tuberculosis, bacterial, viral or fungal infections. *Side effects*: systemic corticosteroid effects. *Manufacturer*: Glaxo.

BETOPTIC

Description: a cardio-selective beta-blocker that reduces pressure within the eye. Betoptic contains 0.5% betaxolol hydrochloride in the form of eye drops. *Used for*: chronic open angle glaucoma and hypertension of eyes. *Dosage*: 1 drop twice each day into eye. *Special care*: patients with diabetes, thyrotoxicosis, blocked airways disease, those undergoing general anaesthetic. *Avoid use*: children, patients with certain heart diseases including heart shock, cardiac failure, slow heart beat, those using soft contact lenses. *Side effects*: passing slight discomfort, rarely staining or reddening of cornea and decreased sensitivity of cornea. *Manufacturer*: Alcon.

BEZALIP

Description: a preparation used to reduce high levels of fats (lipids) in the bloodstream, and available in the form of white, film-coated tablets marked BM/G6, containing 200mg bezafibrate. Bezalip-MONO are white, film-coated, modified-release tablets marked BM/D9 containing 400mg bezafibrate. *Used for*: hyperlipidaemias (high blood levels of lipids, classified as type IIa, IIb, III, IV and V) which are resistant to changes in diet. *Dosage*: adults, Bezalip-MONO, 1 tablet after food at night or in morning. Bezalip, 1 tablet 3 times each day with food. *Special care*: patients with kidney disease. *Avoid use*: children, patients with serious kidney or liver disease, nephrotic disease, pregnant and breastfeeding women. *Possible interaction*: MAOIs, antidiabetic and anticoagulant drugs. *Side effects*: gastro-intestinal upset, rash, muscle pain. *Manufacturer*: B.M.UK.

BICILLIN

Description: a preparation of 2 types of penicillin used in the treatment of a variety of infections. Bicillin is available as a powder for reconstitution and injection containing 1.8g procaine penicillin and 360mg benzylpenicillin (300mg procaine penicillin, 60mg benzylpenicillin per ml). *Used for*: gonococcal, streptococcal, pneumococcal, meningococcal infections, gas-gangrene, anthrax, syphilis, tetanus, diphtheria, yaws, Lyme disease in children. Other penicillin-sensitive infections where prolonged effect of antibiotic in tissues is desirable. *Dosage*: adults, 1ml given by intramuscular injection once or twice each day. Early syphilis, 3ml by intramuscular injection (or 4ml for patients over 80kg), each day for 10 days. Gonorrhoea, up to 12ml as a single intramuscular injection. Children, under 25kg body weight dose adjusted in proportion to that given to a light adult. Over 25kg, same as adult dose. *Special care*: patients with history of allergy or kidney disease. *Avoid use*: patients with penicillin allergy. *Side effects*: allergic responses including rash, fever, joint pains (anaphylactic shock in patients with penicillin allergy), gastro-intestinal upset. *Manufacturer*: Yamanouchi.

BICNU

Description: an alkylating cytotoxic drug used in the treatment of certain cancers and produced in the form of a powder for reconstitution and injection. Bicnu contains 100mg carmustine as a powder in a vial, with 3ml sterile ethanol for reconstitution. *Used for*: leukaemia, lymphomas, myelomas, brain tumours. *Dosage*: as directed by skilled cancer specialist. *Special care*: patients should receive regular checks for blood count. *Side effects*: vomiting and nausea, hair loss, bone marrow suppression (onset of which is delayed) necessitating regular blood checks, adverse effects on fertility. Possible kidney and liver damage may occur. *Manufacturer*: Bristol-Myers.

BINOVUM

Description: a combined oestrogen/progesterone oral contraceptive preparation produced as a course of 21 tablets: 7 white tablets marked C over 535 contain 0.5mg (500 g) norethisterone and 35 g ethenyloestradiol; 14 peach tablets, marked

C over 135, contain 1mg nore-thisterone and 35 g ethinyloestradiol. *Used for*: oral contraception. *Dosage*: 1 tablet each day starting with white tablets on first day of period. There are 7 tablet-free days before the process is repeated. *Special care*: hypertension, asthma, diabetes, varicose veins, multiple sclerosis, Raynaud's disease, kidney dialysis, chronic kidney disease, obesity, severe depression. Family history of heart disease, inflammatory bowel disease, Crohn's disease. Risk of arterial thrombosis especially in older women, those who smoke and those who are obese. Regular checks on blood pressure, breasts and pelvic organs should be carried out at intervals. *Avoid use*: pregnancy, history of heart disease or thrombosis, hypertension, sickle cell anaemia, liver disease, cholestatic jaundice of pregnancy, abnormalities of liver function, porphyria, undiagnosed vaginal bleeding, some cancers, (hormone-dependent ones), infectious hepatitis, recent trophoblastic disease. *Possible interaction*: barbiturates, tetracycline antibiotics, rifampicin, griseofulvin, carbamezapine, chloral hydrate, primidone, phenytoin, ethosuximide, glutethimide, dichloralphenazone. *Side effects*: oedema and bloatedness, leg cramps, reduction in sexual desire, headaches, depression, weight gain, vaginal discharge, breakthrough bleeding, cervical erosion, nausea, chloasma (brownish patches on skin). *Manufacturer*: Janssen-Cilag.

BIOPLEX

Description: a cytoprotectant produced in the form of granules for reconstitution with water to form a mouthwash. Bioplex contains 1% carbenoxolone sodium (20mg per 2g sachet). *Used for*: mouth ulcers. *Dosage*: use as mouthwash 3 times each day and at night. *Special care*: do not swallow. *Manufacturer*: Thames.

BIORPHEN

Description: an antimuscarine or anticholinergic preparation used in the treatment of Parkinsonism. It is thought that antimuscarine drugs act to correct the excess of acetylcholine believed to be the result of dopamine deficiency in Parkinsonism. Biorphen is produced as a sugar-free liquid containing 25mg orphenadrine hydrochloride per 5ml. *Used for*: Parkinsonism including drug-induced symptoms. *Dosage*: adults and children, 150mg each day at first in divided doses, increasing by 25–50mg every 2 or 3 days. Usual maintenance dose is in the order of 150–300mg. *Special care*: heart disorders, gastro-intestinal blockage, liver or kidney disease, avoid abrupt withdrawal of treatment. *Avoid use*: narrow or closed angle glaucoma, enlarged prostate gland, some disorders of movement (tardive dyskinesia). *Possible interaction*: antidepressants, antihistamines, phenothiazines. *Side effects*: euphoria, agitation, confusion, anticholinergic effects and rash (high doses). *Manufacturer*: Bioglan.

BLOCADREN

Description: a non-cardioselective beta-blocker produced in the form of blue scored tablets, marked MSD 135, containing 10mg timolol maleate. *Used for*: prevention of secondary heart attack, angina, prevention of migraine, hypertension. *Dosage*: adults, prevention of secondary heart attack, starting 1 to 4 weeks after first heart attack, 5mg twice each day for 2 days, then 10mg. Adults, angina, 5mg 2 or 3 times each day at first, increasing if required to 10–15mg daily every 3 days. Usual maintenance dose is in the order of 35–45mg. Adults, hypertension, 10mg each day at first as single or divided doses, increasing to a maximum of 60mg daily if required. Adults, prevention of migraine, 10–20mg each day, either as a single or as divided doses. *Special care*: patients with kidney or liver disease, diabetes, metabolic acidosis, those undergoing general anaesthesia, pregnant women and nursing mothers. Persons with weak hearts should receive diuretics and digitalis. May need to halt drug before planned surgery. Withdraw gradually. *Avoid use*: children, patients with asthma, heart block, heart failure, slow heartbeat, heart shock, severe peripheral arterial disease. *Possible interaction*: cardiac depressant anaesthetic drugs, antihypertensives, sedatives, class I antiarrhythmic drugs, verapamil, clonidine withdrawal, ergotamine, cimetidine, indomethacine, sympathomimetics. *Side effects*: disturbance of sleep, cold hands and feet, fatigue on exercise, slow heartbeat, bronchospasm, heart failure, rash, dry eyes (withdraw gradually). *Manufacturer*: MSD.

BONEFOS

Description: a preparation of the drug, sodium clodronate (a diphosphonate) which affects bone metabolism, preventing the increased rate of bone turnover associated with certain malignant conditions. Bonefos is available in the form of capsules and as a solution for intravenous infusion. Yellow capsules contain 400mg and intravenous solution contains 60mg per ml in 5ml ampoules. *Used for*: hypercalcaemia of malignancy. Bone pain and lesions associated with secondary bone growths as a result of multiple myeloma (malignant bone marrow disease) or breast cancer. *Dosage*: adults, 4 tablets each day as single or divided dose avoiding food for 1 or 2 hours before and after treatment, especially anything containing calcium, mineral supplements or iron. Infusion, adults, 1500mg as single infusion over 4 hours or 300mg given by slow intravenous infusion for up to 7 days. Afterwards, capsules should be taken. *Special care*: moderate kidney disorders. Ensure adequate fluid intake, monitor blood calcium levels and kidney function. *Avoid use*: children, pregnancy, breast-feeding, severe kidney failure. *Possible interaction*: other diphosphonates, NSAIDs, mineral supplements, antacid preparations. *Side effects*: skin rashes, gastro-intestinal upset, disturbance of kidney function, parathyroid hormone, lactic acid dehydrogenase, creatinine, transaminase, alkaline phosphatase (enzymes) levels may be elevated for a time. Rarely, there may be hypocalcaemia which does not cause symptoms. There may be transient proteinurea. *Manufacturer*: Boehringer Ingelheim.

BRETYLATE

Description: a proprietary class III antiarrhythmic drug used to treat irregularities of heartbeat and available in the form of a solution for injection containing

50mg bretylium tosylate per ml in 10ml ampoules. *Used for*: heartbeat irregu-larities (ventricular arrhythmias) especially those resistant to other forms of treatment. *Dosage*: 5–10mg per kg of body weight at first given intramuscularly or intravenously and repeated after 1–2 hours if necessary. The treatment is continued every 6 to 8 hours for up to 5 days. *Special care*: patients with kidney disorders. *Avoid use*: children, patients with phaeochromocytoma. *Possible in-teraction*: noradrenaline, other sympathomimetics. *Side effects*: passing wors-ening of arrhythmia, hypotension, vomiting and nausea. *Manufacturer*: Glaxo Wellcome.

BREVIBLOC

Description: a cardio-selective beta-blocker available in the form of a solution for injection. Brevibloc contains either 10mg esmolol hydrochloride per ml in a 10ml vial or 250mg per ml (for dilution before use) in 10ml ampoules. *Used for*: cardiac arrhythmias of various types, (sinus tachycardia; atrial flutter, atrial fibrillation), raised heartbeat rate and hypertension. *Dosage*: 50–200μg per kg body weight per minute by intravenous infusion. *Special care*: women in late pregnancy, breast-feeding, liver disease, kidney disease, angina, diabetes. *Avoid use*: asthma, history of obstructive airways disease, heart failure, heart block, heart shock. *Possible interaction*: other antiarrhythmic drugs. *Manufacturer*: Sanofi Winthrop.

BREVINOR

Description: a combined oestrogen/progestogen contraceptive preparation avail-able as white tablets, marked B and Syntex contain 35μg ethinyloestradiol and 0.5mg norethisterone. *Used for*: contraception. *Dosage*: 1 each day for 21 days starting on 5th day of period, then 7 tablet-free days. *Special care*: women with asthma, hypertension, Raynaud's disease, diabetes, multiple sclerosis, chronic kidney disease, kidney dialysis, varicose veins, depression, smoking, age and obesity increase the risk of thrombosis. *Avoid use*: pregnant women, patients with history of thrombosis or who may be at risk of this, heart disease, sickle cell anaemia, liver diseases, infectious hepatitis, history of cholestatic jaundice (caused by a failure of bile to reach the small intestine), porphyria, chorea, ostosclerosis, haemolytic uraemic syndrome, hormone-dependent cancers, re-cent trophoblastic disease, undiagnosed vaginal bleeding. *Possible interaction*: tetracycline antibiotics, barbiturates, chloral hydrate, griseofulvin, rifampicin, carbamazepine, phenytoin, primidone, dichloralphenazone, ethosuximide glu-tethimide. *Side effects*: oedema and bloatedness, leg cramps, enlargement of breasts, loss of libido, headaches, nausea, depression, weight gain, breakthrough bleeding, cervical erosion, vaginal discharge, brownish patches on skin (ch-loasma). *Manufacturer*: Searle.

BRICANYL

Description: a bronchodilator and a selective β₂-agonist (a selective beta receptor stimulant) and muscle relaxant containing terbutaline sulphate. Bricanyl is available as tablets, a syrup and as a variety of preparations suitable for use with different kinds of inhaler. *Dosage*: Bricanyl white scored tablets, marked 5 contain 5mg. Adult dose: 1 tablet twice each day or at 8-hour intervals. Children: 7 to 15 years, half adult dose. Young children under 7 should use syrup. Also, **BRICANYL SA** (sustained release) tablets, white, marked A/BD, contain 7.5mg. Adult dose: 1 twice each day. Aerosol inhalation, capsules contain 0.25mg per metered dose aerosol. Adults and children: 1 to 2 puffs as required, maximum dose 8 puffs in 24 hours. **BRICANYL TURBOHALER** is a breath-actuated dry powder inhaler containing 0.5mg per metered dose. Adults and children, 1 inhalation as needed with a maximum of 4 in 24 hours. **BRICANYL SPACER INHALER** (with extended mouthpiece which is collapsible) contains 0.25mg per dose. Adults and children, 1 to 2 puffs as required with a maximum of 8 in 24 hours. **BRICANYL RESPULES** (for use with nebulizer) contain 5mg per 2ml solution as single dose units. Adults: 5–10mg 2, 3 or 4 times each day. Children over 25kg body weight: 5mg 2, 3 or 4 times daily. Both with nebulizer. **BRICANYL RESPIRATOR SOLUTION** (for use with power-operated nebulizer) contains 10mg per ml (diluted before use with sterile physiological saline). Adults and children 2–10mg diluted and used with nebulizer. **BRICANYL SYRUP** (sugar-free) contains 1.5mg per 5ml. Adults: 10–15ml; children under 3 years: 2.5ml; 3 to 7 years, 2.5–5ml, 7 to 15 years, 5–10ml. All at 8-hour intervals. **BRICANYL INJECTION** contains 0.5mg per ml in ampoules. Adults; 0.25–0.5mg by subcutaneous, intramuscular or slow intravenous injection. Children; 2 to 15 years, 10 g per kg of body weight, subcutaneously, intramuscularly or by slow intravenous injection. *Special care*: pregnancy, angina, heart disorders and arrhythmias, hypertension, hyperthyroidism. Caution in diabetic persons if given intravenously. *Possible interaction*: sympathomimetics. *Side effects*: headache, nervous tension, trembling, dilation of blood vessels. *Manufacturer*: Astra.

BRITAJECT

Description: a dopamine agonist used in the treatment of Parkinson's disease. Britaject contains 10mg apomorphine hydrochloride per ml in ampoules for injection. *Used for*: treatment of involuntary muscle movements in Parkinson's disease which have not responded to other methods of treatment. *Dosage*: as directed by hospital physician. *Special care*: patients require 3 or more days of treatment prior to start of therapy. *Manufacturer*: Britannia

BRITIAZEM

Description: a vasodilator which is a class III calcium antagonist, available as white tablets, scored on one side contain 60mg diltiazem hydrochloride. *Used for*: angina. *Dosage*: 1 tablet 3 times daily increasing if required to a maximum of 6 each day in divided doses. Elderly, 1 tablet twice each day. *Special care*: monitoring of heartbeat rate may be required during therapy especially in elderly patients, those with a slow heartbeat and those with kidney or liver disorders. *Avoid use*: children, pregnant women, those with marked bradycardia, heart block (2nd- and 3rd-degree atrio-ventricular block) sick sinus syndrome. *Possible interaction*: beta-blockers, carbamazepine, digoxin, cardiac depressants, other antihypertensive drugs, cyclosporin, diazepam, lithium, cimetidine, dantrolene infusion. *Side effects*: bradycardia, 1st degree heart block (atrio-ventricular block), headache, rash, nausea, swelling of ankles caused by oedema. *Manufacturer*: Thames.

BRITLOFEX

Description: a preparation acting on the central (sympathetic) nervous system available as peach, film-coated tablets with 0.2mg lofexidine hydrochloride. *Used for*: control of withdrawal symptoms in patients undergoing detoxification from opioid drug dependency. *Dosage*: adults, 1 tablet twice each day in first instance increasing by 1 or 2 daily if necessary. Maximum daily dose is 12 tablets. Therapy usually should be carried out over a period of 7 to 10 days and then is gradually withdrawn over 2 to 4 days. *Special care*: pregnancy, breast-feeding, heart and circulatory diseases, recent heart attack or chronic kidney failure, severe bradycardia, depression. *Avoid use*: children. *Possible interaction*: alcohol, sedatives. *Side effects*: dry mouth throat and nose, drowsiness, hypotension, rebound hypertension on withdrawal. *Manufacturer*: Britannia.

BROFLEX

Description: an antimuscarine or anticholinergic preparation, produced in the form of a pink syrup containing 5mg benzhexol hydrochloride per 5ml. *Used for*: Parkinsonism including drug-induced. *Dosage*: adults, 1mg each day at first increasing over a period of days by 1 or 2mg to a usual maintenance dose of 5–15mg. Maximum daily dose is 20mg. *Special care*: narrow angle glaucoma, enlarged prostate gland, obstruction of gastro-intestinal tract, heart, liver or kidney disease. Withdraw drug slowly. *Avoid use*: children, tardive dyskinesia (movement disorder), closed angle glaucoma, severe gastro-intestinal obstruction, untreated urinary retention. *Possible interaction*: antidepressants, antihistamines, phenothiazines. *Side effects*: gastro-intestinal disturbances, dry mouth, dizziness, blurred vision, sometimes nervousness, hypersensitivity, tachycardia (raised heart beat rate), urinary retention. In susceptible patients and/or with higher doses, psychiatric disturbances, mental confusion, excitability which may require treatment to be discontinued. *Manufacturer*: Bioglan.

BRONCHODIL

Description: a bronchodilator and selective beta$_2$-agonist available in the form of an aerosol containing 0.5mg reproterol hydrochloride per metered dose inhalation. *Used for*: reversible airways obstruction in bronchitis, bronchial asthma and emphysema. *Dosage*: adults, 1 or 2 puffs every 3 to 6 hours. Prevention of symptoms, 1 puff 3 times each day. Children, 6 to 12 years, 1 puff 3– to 6–hourly; prevention of symptoms, 1 puff 3 times each day. *Special care*: pregnant women, patients with weak hearts, heart arrhythmias, hypertension, angina, hyperthyroidism. *Avoid use*: children under 6 years. *Possible interaction*: sympathomimetics. *Side effects*: headache, dilation of blood vessels, fine tremor of hands, nervous tension. *Manufacturer*: ASTA Medica.

BRUFEN

Description: an NSAID used as an analgesic to treat a variety of disorders and available as tablets, granules and syrup containing ibuprofen: magenta-coloured, oval, sugar-coated tablets are available in 3 strengths; coded BRUFEN (200mg);coded BRUFEN 400 (400mg) and coded BRUFEN 600 (600mg). **BRUFEN GRANULES** are effervescent, orange-flavoured granules in sachet containing 600mg. **BRUFEN SYRUP** contains 100mg per 5ml and **BRUFEN RETARD**, contain 800mg as white, oval film-coated sustained release tablets. *Used for*: pain and inflammation in such conditions as rheumatic disorders, joint pain, juvenile arthritis, periarticular disorders, rheumatoid arthritis, seronegative arthritis, ankylosing spondylitis, osteoarthrosis, post-operative pain, period pain, soft tissue injuries. *Dosage*: adults, 1200–1800mg each day in divided doses (after food) with a maximum daily dose of 2400mg. A maintenance dose in the region of 600–1200mg may be sufficient. Children, over 7kg body weight, use syrup. Age 1 to 2 years, 2.5ml; 3 to 7 years, 5ml; 8 to 12 years, 10ml. All 3 to 4 times each day. *Special care*: pregnancy, nursing mothers, elderly, asthma, gastro-intestinal disorders, heart, liver or kidney disease. Patients on long-term therapy should receive monitoring. *Avoid use*: patients with known allergy to aspirin or anti-inflammatory drugs, those with peptic ulcer. Children under 7kg body weight. *Possible interaction*: quinolones, anticoagulants, thiazide diuretics. *Side effects*: gastro-intestinal upset and bleeding, rash, low levels of blood platelets. *Manufacturer*: Knoll.

BUCCASTEM

Description: an anti-emetic and dopa-mine antagonist belonging to a group called the phenothiazines, available as pale yellow (buccal) tablets containing 3mg prochlorperazine maleate. *Used for*: severe nausea, vomiting, vertigo due to labyrinthine disorders or Ménière's disease. *Dosage*: 1 to 2 tablets twice each day, the tablet being placed high up between upper lip and gum and left to dissolve. *Special care*: pregnancy, nursing mothers. *Avoid use*: children under 14 years of age (may cause dystonia, a movement disorder, and other extra-pyramidal symptoms in children and young people). Patients with Parkinson's disease, blood changes, narrow angle glaucoma, enlarged prostate gland, liver or kidney disease, epilepsy. *Possible interaction*: alcohol, alpha-blockers, CNS depressants (sedatives). *Side effects*: hypotension (low blood pressure), especially in elderly persons or dehydrated patients, anticholinergic effects, drowsiness, skin reactions, insomnia. Rarely extra-pyramidal symptoms may occur and parkinsonism, especially in elderly patients. *Manufacturer*: Reckitt & Colman.

BURINEX

Description: a loop diuretic preparation, (acting on the part of the kidney tubules called loops of Henle), available in the form of tablets, liquid and in ampoules for injection containing bumetanide. White, scored tablets marked 133 and with logo contain 1mg, those marked with strength contain 5mg. **BURINEX LIQUID** contains 1mg per 5ml. **BURINEX INJECTION** contains 0.5mg per ml in ampoules. *Used for*: oedema caused by congestive heart failure, liver and kidney disease including nephrotic syndrome. *Dosage*: adults, tablets or liquid, 1mg daily according to response. Injection, 1–2mg given intravenously (for pulmonary oedema), repeated after 20 minutes if necessary. *Special care*: pregnancy, breast-feeding, diabetes, gout, liver or kidney disease, enlarged prostate gland, impaired micturition (urination). Potassium supplements may be needed. *Avoid use*: children, patients in precomatose states as a result of liver cirrhosis. *Possible interaction*: digoxin, lithium, antihypertensives, aminoglycosides. *Side effects*: gastro-intestinal upset, cramps, skin rash, blood changes, enlarged breasts, thrombocytopenia. *Manufacturer*: Leo.

BURINEX A

Description: a combined loop and potassium-sparing diuretic preparation available as scored, cream, oval-shaped tablets, marked with lion and 149, containing 1mg bumetanide and 5mg amiloride hydrochloride. *Used for*: patients requiring immediate diuresis, especially those in whom hypokalaemia may be a problem. *Dosage*: adults, 1 to 2 tablets each day. *Special care*: pregnancy, breast-feeding, diabetes, impaired micturition (urination). Blood electrolyte levels should be monitored. *Avoid use*: children, patients with severe imbalance of electrolyte levels (salts), kidney or liver disease, disorders of adrenal glands, hepatic pre-coma. *Possible interaction*: antihypertensive drugs, digitalis, potassium supplements, potassium-sparing diuretics, lithium, ACE inhibitors, cephalosporins, aminoglycosides. *Side effects*: gastro-intestinal upset, skin rash, cramps, thrombocytopenia. *Manufacturer*: Leo.

BURINEX K

Description: a combined loop diuretic, potassium supplement preparation available in the form of white, oval tablets, containing 0.5mg bumetanide, and 573mg potassium in a slow release wax core. *Used for*: oedema accompanying congestive heart failure, kidney and liver disease in which a potassium supplement is needed. *Dosage*: adults, 1 to 4 tablets each day. *Special care*: pregnancy, breast-feeding, gout, diabetes, kidney or liver disorders, enlarged prostate gland, impaired micturition (urination). *Avoid use*: children, patients with Addison's disease, hyperkalaemia, precomatose states in liver cirrhosis. *Possible interaction*: aminoglycosides, digitalis, lithium, antihypertensives, potassium-sparing diuretics. *Side effects*: gastro-intestinal upset, cramps, skin rash, enlarged breasts, thrombocytopenia. Drug should be discontinued if obstruction of ulceration of small bowel occurs. *Manufacturer*: Leo.

BUSPAR

Description: an anxiolytic (anxiety-relieving) preparation, and an azapirone. It is thought to be less open to abuse than the benzodiazepine drugs which are also used to relieve severe anxiety, and also to be less sedating in its effect. Buspar is produced in tablets of 2 strengths, containing 5mg or 10mg buspirone hydrochloride. The tablets are white, oval-shaped and marked with strength. *Used for*: short-term relief of severe anxiety, i.e. that which is causing extreme distress and inability to function normally. This may be accompanied by depression. *Dosage*: adults, 5mg 2 or 3 times each day at first, increasing every 2 or 3 days to a usual dose in the order of 10mg twice daily. Maximum dose is 45mg daily. *Special care*: if patient has been taking a benzodiazepine this should be slowly withdrawn before starting Buspirone therapy. Special care in patients with liver or kidney disorders. *Avoid use*: children, patients with severe kidney or liver disease, epilepsy, pregnant women, breast-feeding mothers. *Possible interaction*: *Side effects*: headache, nervous tension, dizziness. Rarely, confusion, fatigue, dry mouth, chest pain, tachycardia. *Manufacturer*: Bristol-Myers.

C

CAFERGOT

Description: an analgesic preparation containing ergotamine which is available as white, sugar-coated tablets containing 1mg ergotamine tartrate and 100mg caffeine. **CAFERGOT SUPPOSITORIES** contain 2mg ergotamine tartrate and 200mg caffeine. *Used for*: migraine. *Dosage*: 1 or 2 tablets at start of attack with no more than 4 in 24 hours; should not be repeated within 4 days. Suppositories, 1 at start of attack with maximum of 2 in 24 hours. Must not repeat within 4 days. *Avoid use*: children, pregnancy, breast-feeding, liver or kidney disease, coronary, occlusive or peripheral vascular disease, sepsis, severe hyptertension. *Possible interaction*: ß-blocker, erythromycin. *Side effects*: vomiting, nausea, abdominal pains, impairment of circulation, weakness in legs. If pleural or retroperitoneal fibrosis occurs drug should be immediately stopped. *Manufacturer*: Sandoz.

CALCIPARINE

Description: an anticoagulant available in the form of pre-filled syringes containing 25,000 units heparin calcium per ml for use as subcutaneous injection only. *Used for*: deep vein thrombosis, pulmonary embolism and prevention of these before surgery. *Dosage*: 5000 units 2 hours before surgery then every 8 to 12 hours for 7 days. *Special care*: pregnancy, kidney or liver disease. Blood platelet counts are required and therapy should be halted in patients who develop thrombocytopenia. *Avoid use*: patients with allergy to heparin, those with haemophilia, haemorrhagic disorders, severe hypertension, peptic ulcer, cerebral aneurysm, recent eye surgery or concerning central nervous system, serious liver disease. *Side effects*: haemorrhage, thrombocytopenia, allergic reactions. After prolonged use, osteoporosis and rarely, baldness may occur. *Manufacturer*: Sanofi Winthrop.

CALCITARE

Description: a preparation of thyroid hormone (derived from pig), available as a powder for reconstitution and injection, consisting of 160 units porcine calcitonin in a vial with gelatin diluent. *Used for*: Paget's disease of bone, hypercalcaemia. *Dosage*: Paget's disease, 80 units 3 times a week to 160 units daily in single or divided doses, but subcutaneous intramuscular injection. Hypercalcaemia, 4 units per kg of body weight daily by subcutaneous or intramuscular injection, adjusted according to response. Children per kg of body weight in similar way but should not receive treatment for periods exceeding a few weeks. *Special care*: if history of allergy, scratch skin test should be carried out. Pregnant women, breast-feeding mothers. *Possible interaction*: cardiac glycosides. *Side effects*: vomiting and nausea, tingling in hands, flushing, unpleasant taste in mouth. *Manufacturer*: R.P.R.

CALMURID HC

Description: a topical, moderately potent steroid with keratolytic and hydrating agents which have a softening and moistening effect on the skin. Available as a cream containing 1% hydrocortisone, 10% urea and 5% lactic acid. *Used for*: dry eczemas and dermatoses. *Dosage*: wash and dry affected skin, apply thinly twice a day at first and reduce frequency as condition improves. *Special care*: limit use in children to 5 to 7 days, use extreme care with infants (napkin rash and infantile eczema). Also, use on face should be limited to 5 to 7 days. If stinging occurs, dilute to half-strength with water-based cream for 1 week before reverting to full strength preparation. *Avoid use*: long-term use especially in pregnant women, patients with acne or skin conditions caused by tuberculosis, viral, fungal, bacterial infections which are untreated or ringworm, leg ulcers. *Side effects*: not usually severe but thinning of skin, lines in skin (striae), blotchy red patches caused by distended blood vessels (capillaries) (telangiectasia), suppression of adrenal glands may occur. *Manufacturer*: Galderma.

CALSYNAR

Description: a manufactured form of a hormone, calcitonin, which is concerned with the regulation of calcium levels in the body. It is produced in ampoules for injection and contains 100 units salcatonin per ml in saline, (salcatonin is synthetic salmon calcitonin). Calcitonin lowers levels of calcium in blood plasma by inhibiting resorption of bone. *Used for*: osteoporosis in post-menopausal women, Paget's disease, hypercalcaemia, in bone cancer, bone pain resulting from cancer. *Dosage*: hypercalcaemia, 5–10 units per kg of body weight each day to 400 units 6- to 8-hourly according to response, by subcutaneous or intramuscular injection. Paget's disease of bone, 50 units 3 times each week to 100 units daily in single or divided doses, by subcutaneous or intramuscular injection. Post-menopausal osteoporosis, 100 units each day by subcutaneous or intramuscular injection along with 600mg calcium and 400 units vitamin D taken by mouth. Bone pain in cancer, 200 units every 6 hours or 400 units every 12 hours, for 48 hours by subcutaneous or intramuscular injection. Children should not receive therapy for more than a few weeks, as directed by physician. *Special care*: history of allergy, perform scratch skin test. Pregnant women, breast-feeding mothers. *Possible interaction*: cardiac glycosides. *Side effects*: vomiting and nausea, tingling sensation in hands, flushing, allergic responses, unpleasant taste in mouth. *Manufacturer*: R.P.R.

CAMCOLIT

Description: an antidepressant preparation of lithium salts available as tablets of 2 strengths. Camcolit 250® tablets are white, scored, film-coated and contain 250mg lithium carbonate (equivalent to 6.8mmol Li^+). CAMCOLIT 400® tablets are white, scored, modified release, film-coated and contain 400mg lithium carbonate (10.8mmol Li^+), marked S and CAMCOLIT. *Used for*: treatment and prevention of mania, recurrent bouts of depression, manic depression, aggressive and self-mutilating behaviour. *Dosage*: adults, prevention 0.5–1.2g each day at first (elderly patients 0.5–1g). Maintain serum levels of lithium in range of 0.5 to 1mmol per litre. Treatment: 1.5 to 2g each day at first, (elderly patients, 0.5 to 1g). Maintain serum levels of lithium in range of 0.6 to 1.2 mmol per litre. Camcolit 250 should be given in divided doses; Camcolit 400 in single or divided doses. *Special care*: treatment should be started in hospital with monitoring of plasma lithium concentrations at regular intervals. (Overdosage usually with plasma concentrations in excess of 1.5mmol Li^+ per litre can be fatal). Adequate fluid and salt intake should be maintained. Monitor thyroid function. *Avoid use*: children, pregnancy, breast-feeding, heart or kidney disease, hypothyroidism, Addison's disease, imbalance in sodium levels. *Possible interaction*: NSAIDs, diuretics, haloperidol, phenytoin, metodopramide, carbamazepine, flupenthixol. *Side effects*: oedema, hypo and hyperthyroidism, weight gain, gastro-intestinal upset, diarrhoea and nausea, trembling in hands, muscular weakness, heart and central nervous system disturbance, skin reactions, intense thirst, large volumes of dilute urine. *Manufacturer*: Norgine.

CANESTEN-HC

Description: a mildly potent steroid with an antifungal and antibacterial drug in the form of a cream containing 1% hydrocortisone and 1% clotrimazole. *Used for*: fungal infections accompanied by inflammation. *Dosage*: apply to affected skin twice each day. *Special care*: limit use on face or in children to 5 to 7 days, especially on infants. Withdraw gradually, short term use only. *Avoid use*: prolonged or extensive use on pregnant women, patients with untreated bacterial or fungal infections, acne, leg ulcers, scabies, viral skin infections, tuberculosis, ringworm, peri-oral dermatitis. *Side effects*: slight burning or irritation, allergic reactions. *Manufacturer*: Bayer.

CAPASTAT

Description: a peptide antituberculous preparation available as a powder for reconstitution and injection. Capastat consists of 1 mega unit (million units) of capreomycin sulphate (equivalent to approximately 1g capreomycin). *Used for*: treatment of tuberculosis which has failed to respond to other drugs. *Dosage*: usually 1g each day given by deep intramuscular injection for a period of 60–120 days. Thereafter, 1g 2 or 3 times a week by intramuscular injection. *Special care*: pregnancy, breast-feeding, kidney and hearing disorders, history of liver disease or allergy. Liver, kidney and vestibular (concerned with balance and controlled by organs in the inner ear) functions should be monitored and hearing tests carried out. *Avoid use*: children. *Possible interaction*: other antibacterial drugs, streptomycin, viomycin, vancomycin, colistin, aminoglycosides. *Side effects*: allergic reactions, e.g. skin rash and urticaria, changes in blood (thrombocytopenia, leucocytosis—an increased number of white blood cells, leucopenia), nephrotoxicity (toxic effects on the kidney), ototoxicity (damage to the organs of hearing and balance), liver damage, electrolyte level disturbances, loss of hearing accompanied by tinnitus and vertigo. *Manufacturer*: King.

CAPOTEN

Description: an antihypertensive preparation, captopril, which is an ACE inhibitor, produced in tablets of 3 strengths: white (12.5mg); mottled white square (25mg); mottled white oval (50mg). *Used for*: mild to moderate hypertension (with diuretics and digitalis), severe hypertension, where other methods have not been successful, congestive heart failure, heart attack, diabetic nephropathy in insulin-dependent diabetes. *Dosage*: adults, mild to moderate hypertension, 12.5mg twice each day at first with usual maintenance dose in the order of 25mg twice daily. Maximum dose is 50mg twice each day. Addition of a thiazide may be needed. Severe hypertension, 12.5mg twice each day at first, increasing to a maximum of 50mg 3 times each day if needed. Diabetic nephropathy, 75–100mg each day in divided doses. Heart failure, 6.25–12.5mg daily at first increasing to usual maintenance in the order of 25mg 2 or 3 times each day. Maximum dose is 150mg each day. N.B. therapy should be initiated in hospital under strict medical supervision with any diuretics being stopped or reduced before treatment begins. Post heart attack, 6.25mg daily at first beginning 3 days after attack increasing to 150mg daily in divided doses. *Special care*: severe congestive heart failure, kidney disease, reno-vascular hypertension, undergoing dialysis or anaesthesia. Those with collagen vascular disease. White blood cell counts and checks on protein in urine and kidney function should be carried out before and during therapy. Contact manufacturer before use in children. *Avoid use*: pregnancy, breast-feeding, various heart disorders (aortic stenosis, outflow obstruction). *Possible interaction*: NSAIDs, potassium supplements, potassium-sparing diuretics, immunosuppressants, vasodilators, allopurinol, probenecid, clonidine, procainamide. *Manufacturer*: Squibb.

CAPOZIDE

Description: a combined thiazide diuretic with an ACE inhibitor, produced in the form of white, scored tablets marked SQUIBB containing 25mg hydrochlorothiazide and 50mg captopril. **CAPOZIDE LS** tablets are white, scored and contain 12.5mg hydrochlorothiazide and 25mg captopril and are marked SQUIBB 536. *Used for*: mild to moderate hypertension in patients who are stable when taking the same proportions of captopril and hydrochlorothiazide individually. *Dosage*: adults, 1 tablet daily with a possible maximum of 2. Capozide LS, 1 tablet each day. *Special care*: patients with kidney disease or receiving dialysis, liver disease, gout, collagen vascular disease, diabetes, undergoing asnaesthesia. Kidney function, urinary protein and white blood cell count shoudl be checked before and during treatment. *Avoid use*: pregnant women, breast-feeding mothers, patients with certain heart diseases (aortic stenosis, outflow obstruction), anuria. *Possible interaction*: NSAIDs, potassium supplements, potassium-sparing diuretics, immunosuppressants, vasodilators, allopurinol, probenecid, clonidine, procainamide. *Side effects*: blood dyscrasias (blood changes), hypotension, rash, proteinuria, loss of sensation of taste, sensitivity to light, pancreatitis, tiredness, rarely, a cough. *Manufacturer*: Squibb.

CARACE

Description: an ACE inhibitor produced in the form of blue, oval tablets marked NSD15 containing 2.5mg lisinopril; white, oval, scored tablets contain 5mg lisinopril; yellow, oval, scored tablets contain 10mg lisinopril; orange, oval, scored tablets contain 20mg lisinopril. All except 2.5mg tablets are marked with name and strength. *Used for*: congestive heart failure (in conjunction with diuretics and possibly digitalis), hypertension. *Dosage*: adults, congestive heart failure, (reduce dose of any diuretic being taken before start of treatment) 2.5mg once each day at first increasing gradually to maintenance dose in the order of 5–20mg once daily, after 2 to 4 weeks. Hypertension, (discontinue any diuretic being taken 2 to 3 days before treatment starts); 2.5mg once a day increasing to a maintenance dose in the order of 10–20mg once daily. Maximum daily dose, 40mg. *Special care*: breast-feeding, patients with kidney disease, receiving dialysis, renovascular hypertension, severe congestive heart failure, undergoing anaesthesia. Kidney function should be monitored before and during treatment. Treatment should begin under hospital supervision for heart failure patients. *Avoid use*: pregnancy, children, patients with various heart disorders (aortic stenosis, outflow obstruction), cor pulmone (a lung disorder), angioneurotic odema as a result of previous ACE inhibitor treatment. *Possible interaction*:

potassium supplements, potassium-sparing diuretics, antihypertensives, indomethacin, lithium. *Side effects*: headache, dizziness, diarrhoea, nausea, tiredness, palpitations, hypotension, rash, angioedema, asthenia (weakness), cough. *Manufacturer*: DuPont.

CARACE PLUS

Description: an ACE inhibitor with a thiazide diuretic produced in the form of blue, hexagonal tablets marked 145 containing 10mg lisinopril and 12.5mg hydrochlorothiazide. **CARACE 20 PLUS** are yellow, hexagonal scored tablets containing 20mg lisinopril and 12.5mg hydrochlorothiazide. *Used for*: mild to moderate hypertension in patients who are stable when taking the same proportions of lisinopril and hydrochlorothiazide individually. *Dosage*: adults, 1 Carace Plus or Carace 20 Plus each day with a possible maximum of 2 tablets. *Special care*: patients with liver or kidney disease receiving dialysis, heart and circulatory diseases, gout, hyperuricaemia (excess uric acid levels in blood), undergoing anaesthesia or surgery, with imbalances in salts (electrolytes) or fluid levels, children. *Avoid use*: pregnancy, breast-feeding, anuria, angioneurotic oedema as a result of previous ACE inhibitor treatment. *Possible interaction*: potassium supplements, hypoglycaemics, NSAIDs, lithium, tubocurarine. *Side effects*: cough, headache, nausea, weariness, hypotension, diarrhoea, angioneurotic oedema, impotence, dizziness. *Manufacturer*: Du Pont.

CARBO-CORT

Description: a mildly potent topical steroid combined with a cleansing agent, produced in the form of an antipsoriatic cream. Carbo-Cort contains 0.25% hydrocortisone and 3% coal tar solution. *Used for*: eczema, lichen planus (a type of skin disease). *Dosage*: apply to affected skin 2 or 3 times each day. *Special care*: use in children or on face should be limited to 5 to 7 days. Special care in infants. Extensive or prolonged use should be avoided and the preparation withdrawn gradually. *Avoid use*: patients with acne, untreated fungal or bacterial infections, tuberculosis, ringworm, viral skin infections, leg ulcers, scabies, peri-oral dermatitis. *Side effects*: adrenal gland suppression, skin thinning, striae (lines on skin), telangiectasia (red blotches on skin). *Manufacturer*: Lagap.

CARDENE

Description: a Class II calcium antagonist produced in the form of capsules: blue/white capsules contain 20mg nicardipine hydrochloride and pale blue/blue capsules containing 30mg . *Used for*: chronic angina which is stable. *Dosage*: adults, angina, 20mg 3 times each day in first instance increasing with 3-day intervals to a maintenance dose in the order of 30mg 3 times daily. Maximum daily dose, 120mg. *Special care*: congestive heart failure, liver or kidney disease, weak heart. *Avoid use*: children, pregnancy, breast-feeding, advanced aortic stenosis (a heart valve disease). *Possible interaction*: cimetidine, digoxin. *Side effects*: headache, dizziness, nausea, palpitations, flushing and feeling of warmth;

chest pain within half an hour of taking dose or on increasing dose, drug should be withdrawn. *Manufacturer*: Roche.

CARDENE SR

Description: a Class II calcium antagonist produced in the form of sustained-release capsules: white capsules marked SYNTEX 30 contain 30mg nicardipine hydrochloride; blue capsules marked SYNTEX 45 contain 45mg. *Used for*: mild to moderate hypertension. *Dosage*: adults, 30mg twice each day at first increasing to 60mg twice daily if required. *Special care*: congestive heart failure, liver or kidney disease, weak heart. *Avoid use*: children, pregnant women, breast-feeding mothers, patients with advanced aortic stenosis (a heart valve disease). *Possible interaction*: cimetidine, digoxin. *Side effects*: headache, dizziness, nausea, palpitations, flushing and feeling of warmth; chest pain within half an hour of taking dose or on increasing dose, drug should be withdrawn. *Manufacturer*: Roche.

CARDURA

Description: an antihypertensive alpha-blocker, doxazosin mesylate, available as white, pentagonal tablets, marked DXP1 (1mg); white, oval tablets, marked DXP2 (2mg); white, square tablets, marked DXP4 (4mg). All tablets are marked Pfizer. *Used for*: hypertension. *Dosage*: adults, 1mg once a day at first increasing to 2mg after 1 or 2 weeks and then to 4mg once each day if needed. Maximum daily dose is 16mg. *Special care*: pregnant women. *Avoid use*: children, breast-feeding. *Side effects*: headache, weariness, dizziness, vertigo, postural hypotension, asthenia (weakness), oedema. *Manufacturer*: Invicta.

CARISOMA

Description: a carbamate preparation which acts as a muscle relaxant and available as white tablets containing 125mg carisoprodol and white tablets marked with P in a hexagon contain 350mg carisoprodol. *Used for*: muscle spasm resulting from bone and muscle disorders. *Dosage*: 350mg, elderly, 125mg, both 3 times each day. *Special care*: history of drug abuse or alcoholism, liver or kidney disease. Long-term treatment should be avoided and the drug withdrawn gradually. *Avoid use*: children, pregnancy, breast-feeding, acute intermittent porphyria. *Possible interaction*: oral contraceptives, steroids, CNS depressants, tricyclics, griseofulvin, phenothiazines, rifampicin, phenytoin, anticoagulants. *Side effects*: nausea, constipation, flushes, rash, weariness, drowsiness, headache. *Manufacturer*: Pharmax.

CATAPRES

Description: an antihypertensive preparation, clonidine hydrochloride, produced in the form of tablets of 2 strengths, modified release capsules and in ampoules for injection. White scored tablets, marked with symbol and C over C, contain 0.1mg; white scored tablets marked with symbol and C over 03C, contain 0.3mg. Also, **CATAPRES PERLONGETS** are yellow/red sustained-release capsules marked with name, 11P and symbol and contain 0.25mg. Additionally, **CATAPRES INJECTION** contains 0.15mg per ml in ampoules. *Used for*: hypertension. *Dosage*: tablets, 0.05–1mg 3 times each day, gradually increasing every second or third day. Perlongets, 1 at night increasing, if required, to 1 tablet night and morning. *Special care*: breast-feeding, depression, peripheral vascular disease. Tablets should be stopped gradually especially if beta-blockers are being withdrawn. *Avoid use*: children. *Possible interaction*: other antihypertensives, tricyclics, CNS depressants, alpha-blockers. *Side effects*: dry mouth, oedema, drowsiness, dizziness. *Manufacturer*: Boehringer Ingelheim.

CELANCE

Description: a dopamine agonist, pergolide mesylate, produced in the form of tablets: ivory, marked 4131 contain 0.05mg , green marked 4133, contain 0.25mg, and pink tablets, marked 4135 contain 1mg. All are rectangular, scored and marked LILLY. *Used for*: additional therapy (to levodopa) in treatment of Parkinson's disease. *Dosage*: 0.05mg each day at first increasing every third day by 0.1–0.15mg for a period of 12 days. Then the dose is increased by 0.25mg every third day until the best response is achieved. Maximum daily dose is 5mg. Levodopa dose should be carefully reduced. *Special care*: pregnancy, breast-feeding, heart disease, heart arrhythmias, history of hallucinations. Drug should be gradually withdrawn. *Avoid use*: children. *Possible interaction*: anticoagulants, antihypertensives, other dopamine antagonists. *Side effects*: disturbances of heartbeat, movement disorder (dyskinesia), drowsiness, hypotension, inflammation of the nose, dyspepsia, nausea, dyspnoea (laboured breathing), diplopia. *Manufacturer*: Lilly.

CELECTOL

Description: an antihypertensive preparation which is a cardioselective beta$_1$-blocker and partial beta$_2$-agonist. It is produced in heart-shaped tablets of 2 strengths, yellow scored tablets contain 200mg celiprolol hydrochloride and white tablets contain 400mg. The tablets are film-coated and marked with logo and strength. *Used for*: mild to moderate hypertension. *Dosage*: adults, 200mg once each day half an hour before food, maximum dose 400mg. *Special care*: pregnancy, nursing mothers, anaestheseia or planned surgery, diabetes, liver or kidney disease, metabolic acidosis. Patients with weak hearts should receive diuretic and digitalis. Patients with history of bronchospasm. Drug should be gradually withdrawn. *Avoid use*: children, patients with various forms of heart disease including heart block, heart failure, slow heart beat rate; sick sinus syndrome, peripheral arterial disease. Patients with obstructive airways disease (unless absolutely no alternative). *Possible interaction*: sympathomimetics, central nervous system depressants, indomethacin, antihypertensives, ergotamine, reserpine, cimetidine, cardiac depressant anaesthetics, hypoglycaemics, verapamil, Class I antiarrhythmics, clonidine withdrawal. *Side effects*: gastro-intestinal disorders, fatigue with exercise, cold feet and hands, disruption of sleep, slow heartbeat rate. If dry eyes or skin rash occur, drug should be gradually withdrawn. *Manufacturer*: R.P.R.

CEPOREX

Description: a cephalosporin antibiotic produced in the form of tablets, capsules and syrup. Pink, film-coated tablets, containing 250mg, 500mg and 1g cephalexin are marked GLAXO and with name and strength. **CEPOREX CAPSULES** coloured grey/caramel contain 250mg and 500mg and are marked GLAXO and with capsule name and strength. **CEPOREX ORANGE SYRUP** (produced as granules for reconstitution), contains 125mg, 250mg and 500mg per 5ml when made up with water. **CEPOREX SUSPENSION** coloured yellow, contains 125mg or 250mg per 5ml. **CEPOREX PAEDIATRIC DROPS** coloured orange contain 125mg per 1.25ml solution (produced as granules for reconstitution with 10ml water). *Used for*: urinary tract infections, gonorrhoea, middle ear infections, respiratory tract, skin and soft tissue infections. *Dosage*: adults, 1–2g daily in 2, 3 or 4 divided doses. Children, under 3 months, 62.5mg–125mg twice each day; 4 months to 2 years, 250–500mg each day; 3 years to 6 years, 1–2g each day, all in 2, 3 or 4 divided doses. *Special care*: patients with allergy to penicillins or kidney disease. *Side effects*: allergic reactions, gastrointestinal upset. *Manufacturer*: Glaxo Wellcome.

CESAMET

Description: an anti-emetic preparation, which is a cannabinoid drug thought to have an effect in the central nervous system involving opiate receptors. It is produced as blue/white capsules, for hospital use only, containing 1mg babilone. *Used for*: nausea and vomiting caused by cytotoxic drugs. *Dosage*: 1mg twice each day increasing to 2mg twice daily if required. First dose is taken the night before and the second, 1 to 3 hours before cytotoxic therapy begins. Maximum dose is 6mg in 3 divided doses. If necessary, it may be continued for 48 hours after cytotoxic therapy has ceased. *Special care*: elderly persons, patients with heart disease, severe liver disorders, hypertension, history of psychiatric disorders. Performance of skilled tasks, e.g. driving may be affected. *Possible interaction*: alcohol, hypnotics and sedatives (enhances the effect of drowsiness). *Side effects*: dry mouth, disturbance of vision, headache, drowsiness, vertigo, inability to concentrate, sleep disturbances, unsteady gait, hypotension, nausea. Mental disturbances including confusion, euphoria, disorientation, hallucinations, psychosis, depression, lack of co-ordination, loss of appetite, increased heartbeat rate, tremor, abdominal pain. *Manufacturer*: Lilly.

CHEMOTRIM PAEDIATRIC

Description: an antibiotic preparation produced in the form of a suspension specifically intended for children. It combines a sulphonamide with a folic acid inhibitor, containing 200mg sulphamethoxazole and 40mg trimethoprim per 5ml of suspension. *Used for*: urinary tract, skin, respiratory and gastro-intestinal infections. *Dosage*: children 6 weeks to 5 months, 2.5ml; 6 months to 5 years, 5ml; 6 years to 12 years, 10ml. All twice each day. *Special care*: elderly, breast-feeding, kidney disease (reduce and/or increase time between doses). During long-term therapy, regular blood counts should be carried out. *Avoid use*: neonates (babies from birth to 1 month of age), pregnancy, patients with serious liver or kidney disease or blood changes. *Possible interaction*: hypoglycaemics, anticoagulants, anticonvulsants, folate inhibitors. *Side effects*: skin rashes, glossitis (inflammation of tongue), nausea, vomiting, blood changes, folate deficiency. Rarely erythema multiforme, Lyell syndrome. *Manufacturer*: Rosemont.

CHENDOL

Description: a bile acid preparation produced in the form of orange/ivory capsules, marked CHENDOL contain 125mg chenodeoxycholic acid. *Used for*: to dissolve cholesterol gallstones which are not calcified. *Dosage*: adults 10–15mg per kg of body weight as a single nightly dose or divided doses. Continue for 3 months after gallstones have been dissolved. *Special care*: liver function should be carefully monitored. *Avoid use*: children, women planning a pregnancy, patients with chronic liver disease or inflammatory intestinal disease. *Possible interaction*: oral contraceptives. *Side effects*: pruritis (itching), diarrhoea. *Manufacturer*: CP Pharmaceuticals.

CHENOFALK

Description: a bile acid preparation produced in the form of tablets and available as white capsules containing 250mg chenodeoxycholic acid. *Used for*: to dissolve cholesterol gallstones which are not calcified. *Dosage*: adults, 15mg per kg of body weight each day in divided doses. Should be continued for 3 to 6 months after stones have been dissolved. *Special care*: liver function should be carefully monitored. *Avoid use*: women planning pregnancy or who are not using contraception. Patients with non-functioning gall bladder, inflammatory intestinal disease, chronic liver disease. *Possible interaction*: oral contraceptives. *Side effects*: pruritis (itching), diarrhoea. *Manufacturer*: Thames.

CHLORDIAZEPOXIDE

Description: an anxiolytic and long-acting benzodiazepine produced in the form of tablets of strengths 5mg, 10mg and 25mg chlordiazepoxide. Also, **CHLORDIAZEPOXIDE HYDROCHLORIDE** tablets are available in strengths of 5mg, 10mg and 25mg and **CHLORDIAZEPOXIDE CAPSULES**, available in strengths of 5mg and 10mg. *Used for*: relief of anxiety. *Dosage*: adults, 30mg each day in divided doses increasing to 40–100mg if symptoms are severe. Elderly persons, 10mg each day at first, carefully increased if needed. *Special care*: use for short-term relief of severe and disabling anxiety (for a period of 2–4 weeks). Lowest possible dose and withdraw drug gradually. Special care needed for elderly persons, pregnant women, breast-feeding mothers, women in labour.

Patients with lung, liver or kidney disease. *Avoid use*: patients with severe lung disease or depressed respiration. Those with psychiatric disorders including obsessional and phobic states and psychosis. *Possible interaction*: alcohol, CNS depressants, anticonvulsant drugs. *Side effects*: gastro-intestinal upset, drowsiness, light headedness, unsteadiness, vertigo, confusion, impaired judgment and dexterity. Disturbance of vision, hypotension, skin rashes. Urine retention, changes in libido. Rarely, jaundice and blood changes. Risk of dependency with higher doses or longer period of use. *Manufacturer*: non-proprietary.

CHLOROMYCETIN

Description: a broad-spectrum antibiotic, chloramphenicol, produced in the form of capsules, as a suspension and as a powder for reconstitution and injection. White/grey capsules marked PARKE-DAVIS contain 250mg, **CHLOROMYCETIN PALMITATE SUSPENSION** contains 125mg per 5ml. **CHLOROMYCETIN INJECTION** produced as a powder in vials for reconstitution contains cholamphenicol (as sodium succinate). *Used for*: severe infections where there are no effective alternatives, typhoid fever, influenzae meningitis. *Dosage*: adults, 50mg per kg of body weight each day in divided doses at 6 hourly intervals. Children under 2 weeks of age, half adult dose; over 2 weeks, same as adult. *Special care*: regular blood tests are advisable during course of treatment. *Avoid use*: for minor infections or for prevention. *Possible interaction*: paracetamol, anticonvulsants, anticoagulants. *Side effects*: gastro-intestinal upset, allergic reactions, blood changes, neuritis, and optic (eye) neuritis with prolonged use. Newborn babies may develop Grey syndrome. *Manufacturer*: Forley.

CICATRIN

Description: an aminoglycoside, antibacterial preparation available in the form of a cream, dusting powder and aerosol. The cream and powder contain 3300 units neomycin sulphate, 250 units bacitracin zinc, 2mg l-cysteine, 10mg glycine and 1mg threonine per g. The aerosol contains 16,500 units neomycin sulphate, 1250 units bacitracin zinc, 12mg l-cysteine, 60mg glycine/g in the form of a spray powder. *Used for*: minor bacterial skin infections. *Dosage*: adults and children, cream, aerosol and dusting powder, apply 3 times each day to affected skin for 3 weeks. *Special care*: on large areas of affected skin. Do not repeat for 3 months. *Side effects*: allergic responses, ototoxicity (damage to organs of hearing and balance). *Manufacturer*: Glaxo Wellcome.

CIDOMYCIN

Description: an aminoglycoside antibiotic preparation containing gentamicin as sulphate and produced in a variety of different forms for injection. Cidomycin injection contains 40mg gentamicin (as sulphate) per ml produced in ampoules and vials. **CIDOMYCIN PAEDIATRIC INJECTION** contains 10mg/ ml in 2ml vials. **CIDOMYCIN INTRATHECAL INJECTION** contains 5mg/ml in ampoules. *Used for*: serious infections sensitive to gentamicin; urinary tract infections. *Dosage*: adults, 5mg per kg of body weight by intramuscular or intravenous injection each day in 3 or 4 divided doses. Children, up to 2 weeks of age, 3mg per kg of body weight at 12 hour intervals; over 2 weeks, 2mg per kg of body weight at 8-hour intervals. Both intramuscularly or intravenously for a period of 7–10 days. *Special care*: patients with kidney disease, myasthenia gravis; regular blood tests are necessary as blood concentrations over 10 g per ml can cause damage to the organs of hearing and balance. *Avoid use*: pregnant women. *Possible interaction*: anaesthetics, neuromuscular blocking drugs, frusemide, ethacrynic acid. *Manufacturer*: Hoechst.

CIDOMYCIN CREAM AND OINTMENT

Description: an aminoglycoside antibiotic preparation containing 0.3% gentamicin (as sulphate) in the form of a cream or ointment. *Used for*: skin infections (including impetigo), of a primary and secondary nature. *Dosage*: apply to affected skin 3 or 4 times each day. *Special care*: large areas of affected skin. *Side effects*: allergic reactions, ototoxicity. *Manufacturer*: Hoechst.

CIDOMYCIN EYE AND EAR DROPS

Description: an antibiotic preparation containing 0.3% gentamicin (as sulphate) in the form of ear and eye drops. Also, **CIDOMYCIN EYE OINTMENT** containing 0.3% gentamicin as sulphate. *Used for*: bacterial infections of the external ear and eye. *Dosage*: ear drops, adults and children, 2 to 4 drops 3 or 4 times each day and at night. Eye drops and ointment, adults and children, 1 to 3 drops or applications of ointment 3 to 4 times each day. *Avoid use*: ear infections where drum is perforated. *Side effects*: risk of superinfection (another infection occurring during treatment). *Manufacturer*: Hoechst.

CILEST

Description: a combined oestrogen/progestogen contraceptive preparation containing 35µg ethinyloestradiol and 0.25mg norgestimate in the form of blue tablets marked C250. *Used for*: oral contraception. *Dosage*: 1 tablet each day for 21 days starting on first day of period, followed by 7 tablet-free days. *Special care*: patients with asthma, diabetes, Raynaud's disease, varicose veins, hypertension, serious kidney disease, kidney dialysis, multiple sclerosis, hyperprolactinaemia (an excess of prolactin, a hormone, in the blood), serious depression. The risk of thrombosis increases with age and if woman smokes or is obese. Pelvic organs, breasts and blood pressure should be checked regularly during the time oral contraceptives are being taken. *Avoid use*: pregnancy, history of thrombosis, those with heart disease, heart valve disease and angina. Patient with sickle cell anaemia, infectious hepatitis, certain liver and kidney disorders, hormone-dependent cancers, undiagnosed vaginal bleeding. *Possible interaction*: tetracyclines, barbiturates, carbamazepine, primidone, griseofulvin, phenytoin, chloral hydrate, glutethimide, ethosuximide, dichloralphenazone. *Side effects*: nausea, headaches, bloatedness due to fluid retention, enlargement of breasts, cramps and leg pains, reduction in libido, depression, weight gain, bleeding, vaginal discharge, erosion of cervix. *Manufacturer*: Janssen-Cilag.

CINOBAC

Description: a quinolone antibiotic drug produced as green/orange capsules containing 500mg cinoxacin and marked LILLY 3056. *Used for*: infections of the urinary tract. *Dosage*: 1 tablet twice each day for 7 to 14 days. For prevention of infection, 1 tablet at night. *Special care*: patients with kidney disorders or history of liver disease. *Avoid use*: children, pregnancy, breast-feeding, severe kidney disorders. *Possible interaction*: NSAIDs, anticoagulant drugs taken by mouth, theophylline. *Side effects*: gastro-intestinal upset, disturbance of CNS, allergic reactions. *Manufacturer*: Lilly.

CIPROXIN

Description: A 4-quinolone antibiotic preparation, ciprofloxacin hydrochloride monohydrate, produced in the form of tablets of 3 different strenths and as a solution for infusion. White, film-coated tablets, marked with BAYER logo and CIP 250 contain 250mg; BAYER logo and CIP 500 (500mg); marked with BAYER logo and CIP 750 (750mg). **CIPROXIN INFUSION** contains 2mg ciprofloxacin (as lactate) per ml. *Used for*: ear, nose, throat, respiratory tract infections. Skin, bone, joint, soft tissue and eye infections. Also, pelvic and gastro-intestinal infections, gonorrhoea and pneumonia caused by Gram-negative bacteria. Prevention of infection in endoscopy and surgery on upper gastrointestinal tract. *Dosage*: adults, tablets, 250mg to 750 mg twice each day for 5 to 10 days. For gonorrhoea, one 250mg dose. For prevention of infection, 750mg 1 hour to 1½ hours before operation. Infusion, 100–200mg twice each day by intravenous infusion for 5 to 7 days. For gonorrhoea, 100mg by intravenous infusion. *Special care*: severe kidney and liver disorders, epilepsy or disorders of central nervous system, history of convulsions. Plenty of fluids should be drunk. *Avoid use*: children and adolescents (except in exceptional circumstances), pregnancy, breast-feeding. *Possible interaction*: alcohol, NSAIDs, opiates, theophylline, cyclosporin, glibenclamide, iron, magnesium or aluminium salts. *Side effects*: headache, tremor, dizziness, confusion, impaired judgment and dexterity (ability to drive and operate machinery may be affected), disturbance of sleep, convulsions. Sensitivity to light, skin rash, pains in joints, disturbance of vision, tachycardia. There may be changes in liver, kidneys and in blood. *Manufacturer*: Bayer.

CITANEST

Description: a local anaesthetic preparation produced as solutions of various strengths, for injection and containing prilocaine hydrochloride. Citanest is available in strengths of 0.5% (5mg prilocaine hydrochloride per ml), 1% (10mg per ml), 2% (20mg per ml) and 4% (40mg per ml). Also, **CITANEST WITH OCTAPRESSIN** containing 3% and 0.03 units per ml of felypressin. *Used for*:

local anaesthesia. *Dosage*: adults, (adjusted according to patient response and nature of operation), maximum 400mg if used alone or 600mg with felypressin or adrenaline. Children according to body weight and nature of operation. *Special care*: patients with liver, kidney or respiratory disorders, epilepsy or conduction disturbances. *Avoid use*: patients with anaemia, methaemoglobinaemia (presence in the blood of methaemoglobin derived from the blood pigment, haemoglobin, which results in a lack of oxygen being carried in the blood and various symptoms arising from this). *Side effects*: allergic reactions, rarely, whole body (systemic) effects. *Manufacturer*: Astra.

CLAFORAN

Description: a cephalosporin antibiotic preparation produced in the form of a powder for reconstitution and injection. Claforan contains 500mg, 1g or 2g of cefotaxime (as sodium salt), as powder in vials. *Used for*: urinary tract and soft tissue infections, septicaemia, meningitis and respiratory tract infections. *Dosage*: adults, 1g by intravenous or intramuscular injection at 8-hourly intervals. For serious infections dose may need to be increased to 6g (maximum 12g) daily in 3 or 4 divided doses. The 2g dose should be given intravenously. Children, newborn babies, 50mg per kg of body weight daily in 2, 3 or 4 divided doses; older infants and children, 200mg per kg of body weight daily in 2, 3 or 4 divided doses. *Special care*: pregnancy, breast-feeding, penicillin allergy and serious kidney failure. *Possible interaction*: aminoglycosides, loop diuretics. *Side effects*: gastro-intestinal upset, pain at injection site, allergic reactions, candidosis, blood changes, haemolytic anaemia, rise in liver enzymes and blood urea. *Manufacturer*: Hoechst.

CLARITYN

Description: an antihistamine preparation produced in the form of oval, white, scored tablets containing 10mg loratadine, and marked with strength and logo. Also, **CLARITYN SYRUP** containing 5mg per 5ml. *Used for*: relief of symptoms of allergic rhinitis, e.g. hay fever, urticaria. *Dosage*: adults, 1 tablet each day, or 10ml syrup. Children, syrup only, 2 to 7 years, 5ml; 7 to 12 years, 10ml, both once each day. *Avoid use*: children under 2 years of age, pregnancy, breast-feeding. *Side effects*: headache, nausea, fatigue. *Manufacturer*: Schering-Plough.

CLEXANE

Description: an anticoagulant preparation produced in pre-filled syringes for injection containing either 20mg (low molecular weight heparin) enoxaparin per 0.2ml or 40mg enoxaparin per 0.4ml. *Used for*: prevention of deep vein thrombosis especially associated with orthopaedic and general surgery. Prevention of blood clot formation during haemodialysis. *Dosage*: adults, low to medium risk of thrombosis (in general surgery), 20mg 2 hours before operation by deep subcutaenous injection and then 20mg once each day for 7 to 10 days. High risk of thrombosis (orthopaedic surgery), 40mg 12 hours before operation by deep subcutaenous injection, and 40mg once a day for 7 to 10 days. Haemodialysis, 1mg per kg of body weight with a further dose of 0.5 to 1mg/kg if process lasts for longer than 4 hours. *Special care*: pregnancy, breast-feeding, hypertension, history of liver disorders or ulcers. *Avoid use*: children, patients with peptic ulcer, serious bleeding disorders (e.g. haemophilia), those at risk of haemorrhage, thrombocytopenia, cerebral aneurysm, severe liver disease. Patients who have had recent CNS or eye surgery. *Possible interaction*: aspirin, NSAIDs, dextran, anticoagulants taken by mouth, antiplatelet drugs. *Side effects*: effects on liver, thrombocytopenia, less commonly, bruising and haemorrhage. *Manufacturer*: R.P.R.

CLIMAGEST

Description: a combined oestrogen, progestogen hormonal preparation, produced in the form of tablets. Climagest 1mg consists of 16 blue-grey tablets containing 1mg oestradiol valerate, coded E1, and 12 white tablets, containing 1mg oestradiol valerate and 1mg norethisterone, coded N1. Also, **CLIMAGEST 2MG** consists of 16 blue tablets containing 2mg oestradiol valerate, coded E2, and 12 yellow tablets containing 2mg oestradiol valerate and 1mg norethisterone, coded N2. *Used for*: relief of menopausal symptoms. *Dosage*: 1 tablet daily starting with oestradiol valerate (coded E) on first day of period (if present), and finishing with the 12 tablets (coded N), containing norethisterone. *Special care*: patients considered to be at risk of thrombosis, those with diabetes, epilepsy, hypertension, multiple sclerosis, migraine, fibroids in uterus, ostosclerosis, tetany, liver disease, porphyria, gallstones. Regular examination of breasts and pelvic organs should be carried out and blood pressure checked. Drug should be stopped if there are any signs of jaundice, headaches which are severe, migraine, rise in blood pressure before planned surgery. *Avoid use*: pregnancy, breast-feeding, hormone-dependent cancers, breast or uterus cancer, endometriosis, undiagnosed vaginal bleeding, sickle cell anaemia. Serious heart, kidney or liver disease, thrombosis. Patients suffering from Dublin-Johnson syndrome or Rotor syndrome. *Possible interaction*: drugs which induce liver enzymes. *Side effects*: weight gain, enlargement and tenderness of breasts, fluid retention, cramps, gastro-intestinal upset, nausea and vomiting, headaches, breakthrough bleeding, dizziness. *Manufacturer*: Sandoz.

CLIMAVAL

Description: a hormonal oestrogen preparation produced in tablets of 2 strengths. Climaval 1mg are grey/blue tablets containing 1mg oestradiol valerate marked E1; Climaval 2mg are blue tablets containing 2mg oestradiol valerate and marked E2. *Used for*: treatment of menopausal symptoms in women who have had a hysterectomy. *Dosage*: 1 tablet each day either 1mg or 2mg according to response. May be taken continuously for up to 2 years. *Special care*: only in elderly women for post-menopausal symptoms, otherwise avoid use; patients considered to be at risk of thrombosis, those with diabetes, epilepsy, hypertension, multiple sclerosis, migraine, fibroids in uterus, ostosclerosis, tetany, liver disease, porphyria, gallstones. Regular examination of breasts and pelvic organs should be carried out and blood pressure checked. Drug should be stopped if there are any signs of jaundice, severe headaches and migraine, a rise in blood pressure and before planned surgery. *Avoid use*: pregnancy, breast-feeding, hormone-dependent cancers, breast and uterine cancer, endometriosis, undiagnosed vaginal bleeding, sickle cell anaemia, serious heart, kidney or liver disease, thrombosis. Patients suffering from Dublin-Johnson syndrome or Rotor syndrome. *Possible interaction*: drugs which induce liver enzymes. *Side effects*: weight gain, enlargement and tenderness of breasts, fluid retention, cramps, gastrointestinal upset, nausea and vomiting, headaches, dizziness. *Manufacturer*: Sandoz.

CLINORIL

Description: a proprietary analgesic NSAID produced in the form of hexagonal yellow scored tablets containing 100mg or 200mg sulindac and marked MSD 943 and MSD 942 respectively. *Used for*: inflammation and pain in rheumatic diseases including gout, rheumatoid arthritis and osteoarthritis. *Dosage*: adults, 200mg twice each day with food or drink. *Special care*: elderly persons with history of lithiasis (gallstones, kidney stones, stones in lower urinary tract), patients with heart failure, liver or kidney disease, history of gastro-intestinal haemorrhage or ulcers. Plenty of fluids should be taken and liver function monitored. *Avoid use*: children, pregnancy, breast-feeding, allergy to aspirin or anti-inflammatory drugs, those with gastro-intestinal bleeding or peptic ulcer. *Possible interaction*: aspirin, anticoagulants, diflunisal, hypoglycaemic drugs, methotrexate, dimethyl sulphoxide, cyclosporin. *Side effects*: allergic responses including liver failure and fever (stop drug immediately). Disturbance of vision, central nervous system effects, heart arrythmias, changes in blood, kidney stones and disturbance of kidney function, pancreatitis, hyperglycaemia, gastrointestinal bleeding and upset. Also rash, dizziness, glossitis (inflammation of tongue), tinnitus, muscle weakness, effects on urine including discolouration, proteinuria (protein in urine), crystals in urine (crystalluria), oedema. *Manufacturer*: MSD.

CLOBAZAM

Description: an anxiolytic long-acting benzodiazepine drug also used as an additional treatment for epilepsy. It is produced in the form of capsules containing 10mg clobazam. *Used for*: short-term relief of symptoms of anxiety; additional therapy for epilepsy. *Dosage*: anxiety, 20–30mg each day in divided doses or as 1 dose taken at night. In severe cases (under hospital supervision) dose may be increased to 60mg each day in divided doses. Elderly or debilitated persons, reduced daily dose of 10–20mg. Adults, epilepsy, 20–30mg each day (maximum 60mg) in divided doses. Children, for epilepsy only, age 3 to 12 years, half adult dose. *Special care*: children under 3 years (epilepsy) and not for children in cases of anxiety, pregnancy, women in labour, breast-feeding, elderly (reduced dose), patients with liver or kidney disease or respiratory disorders. Prolonged use and abrupt withdrawal of drug should be avoided. *Avoid use*: severe respiratory or lung disorders. *Possible interaction*: CNS depressants, alcohol, anticonvulsant drugs. *Side effects*: impaired judgment and dexterity interfering with performance of skilled tasks, lightheadedness, confusion, drowsiness, unsteadiness, vertigo. Also disturbance of vision, gastro-intestinal upset, retention of urine, skin rashes, change in libido, hypotension. Rarely, jaundice and blood changes. *Manufacturer*: non-proprietary but available from Hoechst as Frisium.

CLOMID

Description: an anti-oestrogen hormonal preparation produced in the form of pale yellow scored tablets, containing 50mg clomiphene citrate, and marked with a circle containing the letter M. *Used for*: treatment of sterility in women due to failure of ovulation. *Dosage*: 1 tablet each day for 5 days starting on the fifth day of menstruation. *Special care*: ensure patient is not pregnant before and during the course of treatment. *Avoid use*: women with large ovarian cyst, cancer of the womb, undiagnosed uterine bleeding, liver disease. *Side effects*: hot flushes, enlargement of ovaries, abdominal discomfort, blurring of vision (withdraw drug). *Manufacturer*: Hoechst.

CLOPIXOL

Description: an antipsychotic drug and thioxanthene produced in the form of tablets and as solutions for injection. Tablets are produced in various strengths and all are film-coated; pink tablets contain 2mg zuclopenthixol hydrochloride; light brown tablets contain 10mg; brown tablets contain 25mg. **CLOPIXOL INJECTION** contains 200mg per ml (as oily injection) contained in ampoules and vials. **CLOPIXOL CONCENTRATED INJECTION** contains 500mg per ml (as oily injection) contained in ampoules. **CLOPIXOL ACUPHASE** contains 50mg per ml (as oily injection) contained in ampoules. *Used for*: psychoses, particularly schizophrenia and especially when accompanied by aggression and agitated behaviour. *Dosage*: tablets, 20–30mg each day in divided doses in first instance. Usual maintenance dose is in the order of 25–50mg each day with a maximum daily dose of 500mg. Clopixol injection, 200–400mg every 2 to 4 weeks by deep intramuscular injection with a maximum weekly dose of 600mg. Clopixol concentrated injection, 250–500mg every 1 to 4 weeks by deep intramuscular injection with a maximum weekly dose of 600mg. Clopixol acuphase (for immediate treatment of acute psychoses), 50–150mg by deep intramuscular injection repeated after 1, 2 or 3 days if required. Maximum total dose is 400mg and maintenance should be by means of tablets or other Clopixol injections. *Special care*: pregnancy, breast-feeding, heart and circulatory disorders, liver or kidney disease, Parkinsonism, an intolerance to neuroleptic drugs taken by mouth. *Avoid use*: children, coma, states of withdrawal and apathy.

Possible interaction: alcohol, antidiabetic drugs, levodopa, anticonvulsant drugs, analgesics, CNS sedatives, antihypertensive drugs. *Side effects*: Parkinsonism-like effects, spasms in muscles and involuntary, repetitive movements, rapid heartbeat rate, vision disturbance, tremor. Also hypotension, changes in weight, difficulty in passing urine, dry mouth and stuffiness in nose, impotence, enlargement of breasts, hypothermia (especially in elderly persons). There may be blood changes, dermatitis, weariness and lethargy, fits and jaundice. *Manufacturer*: Lundbeck.

CLOSTET

Description: a preparation of tetanus toxoid vaccine (40iu per 0.5ml) adsorbed onto aluminium hydroxide and contained in pre-filled (0.5ml) syringes. *Used for*: immunization against tetanus and for "booster" injections to reinforce immunity. *Dosage*: adults, a course of 0.5ml by subcutaneous or intramuscular injection given a total of 3 times at 4 week intervals. After 10 years, a "booster" reinforcing dose of 0.5ml may be given by subcutaneous or intramuscular injection. If an injury is received which might give rise to tetanus, a booster reinforcing dose should be given to patients previously immunized. Those who have not, should be given a first dose of the primary course and an injection of antitetanus immunoglobin at a different site. Children normally receive a combined triple vaccine consisting of adsorbed tetanus, diphtheria and pertussis (whooping cough) vaccine, and can later receive booster reinforcing doses against tetanus. *Special care*: allergic reactions especially in persons receiving vaccine within 1 year of receiving a previous booster dose. Normally, 10 years should have elapsed before a reinforcing dose is given. *Avoid use*: patients with serious infections unless there is a wound likely to be prone to tetanus. *Side effects*: malaise, fever, slight soreness and local reactions. *Manufacturer*: Evans.

CLOZARIL

Description: an antipsychotic drug and dibenzodiazepine, clozapine, produced as yellow scored tablets (25mg strength) and marked CLOZ 25, and 100mg strength, marked CLOZARIL 100. *Used for*: schizophrenia which has failed to respond to, or patient is intolerant of other conventional antipsychotic drugs. *Dosage*: first day, 12.5mg once or twice. Second day, 25mg once or twice; dose is gradually increased over a period of 2 to 3 weeks by 25–50mg each day until patient is receiving 300mg daily in divided doses. Depending upon response, a further increase may be required by giving an additional 50–100mg every 4 to 7 days to a maximum of 900mg each day in divided doses. Usual maintenance dose is in the order of 150–300mg in divided doses. Elderly persons, 12.5mg each day in first instance slowly increasing by 25mg daily. *Special care*: patient, prescribing doctor and pharmacist must be registered with Sandoz Clorazil Patient Monitoring Service (CPMS). Patients should report signs of infection and must take contraceptive precautions. Special care in pregnant women, patients with enlarged prostate gland, liver disease, glaucoma, paralytic ileus. Persons with epilepsy should be monitored. Regular blood counts of leucocytes should be carried out before and during treatment. Drug should be immediately withdrawn if whole blood count falls below 3000/mm³ or neutrophil (a type of white blood cell) count below 1500/mm³. *Avoid use*: children; patients with history of drug induced blood disorders—neutropenia, agranulocytosis (a serious fall in the number of white blood cells called eosinophils, basophils and neutrophils), bone marrow disorders. Also, patients with history of drug intoxication, toxic and alcoholic psychoses, CNS depression or those in comatose states. Avoid use in breast-feeding mothers, persons with serious kidney or liver disease or circulatory collapse and cardiac failure. *Possible interaction*: benzodiazepines, alcohol, MAOIs, CNS depressants, other drugs which cause agranulocytosis, anticholinergics, antihistamines, hypotensive drugs, lithium, phenytoin, warfarin, cimetidine. *Side effects*: neutropenia leading to agranulocytosis (characterized by fever, collapse, bleeding ulcers of vagina, rectum and mouth) which may be fatal, effects on heart muscle and brain activity, tachycardia, fits, fatigue, dizziness, headache, over-production of saliva in mouth, retention of urine, gastro-intestinal upset, disturbance of body temperature regulation. *Manufacturer*: Sandoz.

CO-BETALOC

Description: an antihypertensive preparation combined with a cardioselective ß-blocker with a thiazide diuretic as white scored tablets, marked A/MH, contain 100mg metoprolol tartrate and 12.5mg hydrochlorothiazide. Also **CO-BETALOC SA** are yellow, film-coated tablets, marked A/MC, containing 200mg metoprolol tartrate and 25mg hydrochlorothiazide and having a sustained-release core. *Used for*: mild to moderate hypertension. *Dosage*: adults, 1 to 3 tablets each day in single or divided doses, or 1 Co-Betaloc SA tablet daily. *Special care*: pregnancy, breast-feeding, diabetes, kidney or liver disorders, metabolic acidosis, undergoing general anaesthesia, (may need to be withdrawn before planned surgery). Monitor electrolyte levels. Patients with weak hearts may need treatment with digitalis and diuretics. Withdraw drug gradually. Potassium supplements may be required. *Avoid use*: children, patients with history of obstructive airways disease, bronchospasm, asthma, heart block, heart shock, heart failure, severe peripheral arterial disease, sick sinus syndrome, severe kidney failure, anuria. *Possible interaction*: sympathomimetics, cardiac depressant anaesthetics, clonidine withdrawal, hypoglycaemics, class I antiarrhythmic drugs, other antihypertensives, verapamil, ergotamine, reserpine, indomethacin, cimetidine, CNS depressants, lithium, digitalis. *Manufacturer*: Astra.

CO-DANTHRAMER

Description: a preparation which combines a stimulant laxative and faecal softener produced in the form of a liquid. It contains 200mg of Poloxamer '188' and 25mg of danthron per 5ml of liquid. Also, **STRONG CO DANTHRAMER** which contains 1g Poloxamer '188' and 75mg danthron per 5ml of liquid. *Used* *for*: treatment and prevention of constipation in terminally ill persons (which has been caused by analgesic drugs). Also, constipation in elderly persons and patients with coronary thrombosis or cardiac failure. *Dosage*: adults, 5–10ml Co-Danthramer or 5ml Strong Co-Danthramer taken at night. Children, 2.5–5ml Co-Danthramer only, taken at night. *Special care*: pregnant women, patients suffering from incontinence (avoid prolonged contact with skin as irritation and soreness may occur). *Avoid use*: babies in nappies, breast-feeding, severe painful abdominal disorders, any intestinal obstruction. *Side effects*: red discolouration of urine and skin with which urine comes into contact. *Manufacturer*: non-proprietary, available from Napp as variations of Codalax.

CO-DANTHRUSATE

Description: a preparation which combines a stimulant laxative and faecal softener produced in the form of capsules and as a suspension. The capsules contain 50mg danthron and 60mg docusate sodium and **CO-DANTHRUSATE SUSPENSION** contains 50mg danthron and 60mg docusate sodium per 5ml. *Used for*: treatment and prevention of constipation in terminally ill patients (which has been caused by analgesic drugs). Also, constipation in elderly persons and patients with coronary thrombosis and cardiac failure. *Dosage*: adults, 1 to 3 capsules or 5–15ml suspension taken at night. Children over 6 years of age, 1 capsule or 5ml suspension taken at night. *Special care*: pregnancy, breast-feeding. *Avoid use*: children under 6 years, patients with intestinal obstruction. *Side effects*: red discoloration of urine and skin with which urine may come into contact. *Manufacturer*: non-proprietary, available from Evans as Normax.

CO-DYDRAMOL

Description: a compound opiate analgesic preparation combining 10mg dihydrocodeine tartrate with 500mg paracetamol in the form of tablets. *Used for*: relief of mild to moderate pain. *Dosage*: adults, 1 to 2 tablets every 4 to 6 hours with a maximum of 8 daily. *Special care*: pregnant women, elderly persons, patients with allergies, under-active thyroid, liver or kidney disease. *Avoid use*: children, patients with obstructive airways disease or respiratory depression. *Possible interaction*: CNS sedatives, alcohol. *Side effects*: headaches, constipation, nausea. *Manufacturer*: Non-proprietary, available from several companies.

CO-PROXAMOL

Description: a compound opiate analgesic preparation combining 32.5mg dextropropoxyphene hydrochloride and 325mg paracetamol in tablet form. *Used for*: relief of mild to moderate pain. *Dosage*: adults, 2 tablets 3 or 4 times each day. *Special care*: pregnant women, elderly persons, patients with liver or kidney disease. *Avoid use*: children. *Possible interaction*: CNS sedatives, alcohol, anticonvulsant and anticoagulant drugs. *Side effects*: risk of dependence and tolerance, dizziness, rash, nausea, constipation, drowsiness. *Manufacturer*: non-proprietary, available from several companies.

COBADEX

Description: a mildly potent topical corticosteroid preparation produced in the form of a cream containing 1% hydrocortisone and 20% dimethicone. *Used for*: mild inflammatory skin conditions such as eczema which are responsive to steroids. Also, anal and vulval pruritis (itching). *Dosage*: apply thinly 2 or 3 times daily to affected area. *Special care*: use in children or on face should be limited to a maximum period of 5 days. Should be gradually withdrawn after prolonged use. *Avoid use*: various skin conditions including acne, leg ulcers, scabies, viral skin disease, ringworm, tuberculosis, untreated bacterial or fungal infections. Continuous use or long-term use in pregnancy. *Side effects*: thinning of skin, suppression of adrenal glands, hair growth. *Manufacturer*: Cox.

COBALIN-H

Description: a preparation of vitamin B_{12} produced in ampoules for injection containing 1000µg hydroxocobalamin per ml. *Used for*: B_{12} responsive macrocytic anaemia (a disorder of the blood characterized by reduced production of red blood cells and the presence of large, fragile red blood cells), megaloblastic anaemia, tobacco amblyopia (an eye disorder). *Dosage*: for anaemias, 250-1000µg by intramuscular injection on alternate days for 1 to 2 weeks. Afterwards, 250µg once a week until normal blood count is achieved. Maintenance dose is 1000µg every 2 to 3 months. *Special care*: should only be given when cause of anaemia (either lack of vitamin B_{12} or of folate) has been established. *Manufacturer*: Link.

CODAFEN CONTINUS

Description: a combined opiate analgesic and NSAID produced as pink/white tablets containing 20mg codeine phosphate and 300mg of sustained-release ibuprofen. *Used for*: relief of pain including post-operative, dental and period pain. *Dosage*: adults, 2 tablets every 12 hours at first increasing to 3 tablets every 12 hours if needed. Maintenance dose is 1 to 3 tablets each 12 hours. *Special care*: Pregnancy, elderly, allergy to anti-inflammatory drugs or aspirin. Those with liver or kidney disease, heart failure, hypotension, hypothyroidism, head injury, history of bronchospasm. *Avoid use*: children, patients with peptic ulcer or history of peptic ulcer, respiratory depression, breathing disorders. *Possible interaction*: CNS sedatives, anticoagulants taken by mouth, thiazides, MAOIs, quinolones. *Side effects*: dizziness, blurring of vision, headache, gastrointestinal upset and bleeding, peptic ulcer, drowsiness. Rarely, disturbance of liver and kidney function, thrombocytopenia, agranulocytosis (abnormal blood disorder in which there is a reduction in the number of certain white blood cells). *Manufacturer*: Napp.

CODALAX

Description: a preparation which combines a stimulant laxative and faecal softener produced in the form of a solution of 2 different strengths. It contains

200mg Poloxamer '188' and 25mg danthron per 5ml. **CODALAX FORTE** contains 1g Poloxamer '188' and 75mg danthron per 5ml. *Used for*: treatment and prevention of constipation in terminally ill persons (which has been caused by analgesic drugs). Also, constipation in elderly persons and patients with coronary thrombosis or cardiac failure. *Dosage*: adults, Codalax, 5–10ml taken at night; Codalax Forte, 5ml taken at night. Children, Codalax only, 2.5–5ml taken at night. *Special care*: pregnancy, incontinence. *Avoid use*: babies in nappies, patients suffering from severe painful conditions of the abdomen or intestinal blockage. *Side effects*: red discoloration of urine and skin with which urine comes into contact. *Manufacturer*: Napp.

CODEINE PHOSPHATE

Description: an opiate analgesic preparation which additionally acts as a cough suppressant, and is available in the form of tablets and as a solution. The tablets are available in 3 strengths of 15mg, 30mg and 60mg codeine phosphate. The solution contains 25mg codeine phosphate per 5ml. *Used for*: relief of mild to moderate pain. *Dosage*: adults, 10–60mg every 4 hours with a maximum dose of 200mg each day. Children, 1 to 12 years, 3mg per kg of body weight, in divided doses, each day. *Special care*: elderly persons, women in labour, patients with hyperthyroidism or serious liver disease. *Avoid use*: children under 1 year of age, patients with obstructive airways disease or respiratory depression. *Possible interaction*: central nervous system sedatives, MAOIs. *Side effects*: blurred vision, drowsiness, dry mouth, dependence and tolerance, constipation. *Manufacturer*: non-proprietary.

COGENTIN

Description: an anticholinergic preparation produced as tablets and in ampoules for injection. White, scored tablets, contain 2mg benztropine mesylate and are coded MSD 60. **COGENTIN INJECTION** contains 1mg per ml in 2ml ampoules. *Used for*: treatment of Parkinsonism including drug-induced symptoms of tremor and involuntary muscle movements (dyskinesia). *Dosage*: tablets 0.5mg each day at first, increasing gradually as required by 0.5mg every 5 or 6 days. Maximum dose is 6mg daily. Children over 3 years consult manufacturer. Adults, injection (for emergency treatment), 1–2mg given intramuscularly or intravenously. *Special care*: narrow angle glaucoma, tachycardia, enlarged prostate gland, gastro-intestinal blockage. Drug should be withdrawn slowly. *Avoid use*: patients with movement disorder (tardive dyskinesia) or children under 3 years. *Possible interaction*: antidepressants, phenothiazines, antidopaminergic drugs. *Side effects*: agitation and confusion, anticholinergic effects; with higher doses, rash. *Manufacturer*: MSD.

COLESTID

Description: a form of a resin which is a bile acid sequestrant acting as a lipid-lowering agent. Colestid is available as 5g yellow granules in sachets containing colestipol hydrochloride. Also, **COLESTID ORANGE** granules consisting of 5g orange-flavoured powder containing colestipol hydrochloride with aspartame. *Used for*: hyperlipidaemias (high fat levels in blood) particularly type IIa. *Dosage*: adults, 5–30g each day in 1 or 2 divided doses taken with liquid. Children, consult manufacturer. *Special care*: pregnancy, nursing mothers, additional vitamins A, D and K may be needed. *Avoid use*: complete biliary blockage (total obstruction of bile duct). *Possible interaction*: diuretics, digitalis, antibiotics. Any drug should be taken 1 hour before or 4 hours after Colestid as there may be intereference with absorption. *Side effects*: constipation. *Manufacturer*: Pharmacia & Upjohn.

COLIFOAM

Description: a corticosteroid produced in the form of an aerosol foam containing 10% hydrocortisone acetate in mucoadherent foam. *Used for*: ulcerative colitis and inflammation of the bowel. *Dosage*: adults, 1 applicatorful into rectum once or twice each day for 2 or 3 weeks. Afterwards the same dosage every second day. *Special care*: pregnant women, patients with severe ulcerative disease. Avoid use for prolonged periods. *Avoid use*: children, patients with intestinal obstruction, abscess, perforation, peritonitis. Also, patients with recent anastomoses within the intestine, or extensive fistulas. Patients suffering from fungal or viral infectioins or tuberculosis. *Side effects*: systemic corticosteroid effects including mood changes, thinning of bones, mood swings, elevated blood sugar levels. *Manufacturer*: Stafford-Miller.

COLOFAC

Description: an anticholinergic, antispasmodic preparation produced in the form of tablets and as a liquid. White, sugar-coated tablets contain 135mg mebeverine hydrochloride. Yellow banana-flavoured, sugar-free **COLOFAC SUSPENSION** contains mebeverine pamoate (equivalent to 50mg mebeverine hydrochloride per 5ml). *Used for*: bowel spasm and gastro-intestinal spasm in irritable bowel syndrome and gastro-intestinal disorders. *Dosage*: adults, 1 tablet or 15ml suspension 20 minutes before a meal 3 times each day. Children over 10 years, same as adult dose. *Avoid use*: children under 10 years. *Manufacturer*: Solvay.

COLOMYCIN

Description: a polymyxin antibiotic preparation produced in the form of powder in vials for reconstitution with water and injection, syrup, tablets and as a powder for topical application. Colomycin powder for injection consists of 500,000 units colistin sulphomethate sodium or 1 million units colistin sulphomethate sodium in vials. **COLOMYCIN SYRUP** contains 250,000 units colistin sulphate per 5ml. **COLOMYCIN TABLETS** are quarter-scored and white containing 1.5 million units colistin sulphate and are marked with P inside a hexagon. **COLOMYCIN POWDER** for topical application contains 1g colistin sulphate in vial. *Used for*: burns and wounds, surgery, skin infections,

ENT infections, gram negative infections, aerosol therapy. *Dosage*: adults (over 60kg body weight), injection, 2 mega units every 8 hours; children 50,000 units/kg body weight each day 8-hourly. Adults, tablets, 1 to 2 8-hourly; children, syrup, up to 15kg body weight, 5–10ml; 15–30kg, 15–30ml; over 30kg same as adult. All taken 8-hourly. *Special care*: patients with kidney disease, porphyria. *Avoid use*: pregnancy, breast-feeding, myasthenia gravis. *Possible interaction*: muscle relaxant drugs, other antibiotic drugs, anticoagulants, cytotoxics, cholinergics, diuretics, bisophonates, cyclosporin. *Side effects*: paruesthesia ("pins and needles"), vertigo, muscle weakness, apnoea (temporary halt in breathing), toxic effects on kidneys. Rarely, confusion, slurred speech, psychosis, bronchospasm (on inhalation). *Manufacturer*: Pharmax.

COMBIDOL

Description: a bile acid preparation available in the form of white, film-coated tablets containing 125mg chenodeoxycholic acid marked COMBIDOL 60. *Used for*: to dissolve small or medium sized radiolucent gallstones in patients who have slight symptoms and unimpaired gall bladder function. *Dosage*: adults, 2 or 3 tablets each day (5mg per kg of body weight) either as single night time dose, or in divided doses after meals with final dose taken before bedtime. If patient is 120% or more above ideal body weight, 6 tablets (7.5mg per kg of body weight) should be taken daily. *Avoid use*: children, pregnancy, breast-feeding, women who are not using contraception, patients with non-functioning or impaired gall bladder, those with inflammatory diseases of colon and small intestine, peptic ulcer, chronic liver disease. *Possible interaction*: bile acid sequestrants, antacids, oestrogens, oral contraceptives, other drugs which influence cholesterol levels. *Side effects*: minor effects on liver and a rise in serum levels of transaminases (enzymes), diarrhoea, pruritis (itching), gallstones may become opaque. *Manufacturer*: CP Pharmaceuticals.

CONCORDIN

Description: a TCAD preparation available as pink film-coated tablets containing 5mg protryptyline hydrochloride and marked MSD 26, and white, film-coated tablets contain 10mg and marked MSD 47. *Used for*: depression. *Dosage*: adults, 15–60mg each day in divided doses. Reduced dose of 5mg 3 times each day in elderly persons. *Special care*: breast-feeding, liver or kidney disease, epilepsy, heart and circulatory diseases, diabetes, hyperthyroidism, tumours of adrenal gland, retention of urine, glaucoma. Also, certain psychiatric conditions, suicidal tendencies and psychoses. *Avoid use*: pregnant women, children, patients with serious liver disease, heart attack or heart block. *Possible interaction*: alcohol, barbiturates, other antidepressant drugs, antihypertensives, cimetidine, oestrogens, local anaesthetics containing adrenaline or noradrenaline, anticholinergic drugs. *Side effects*: nervousness, drowsiness, dizziness, sweating, tremor, weariness, gastro-intestinal upset, insomnia, hypotension. Anticholinergic effects including constipation, urine retention, blurring of vision, dry mouth. Allergic skin rashes, blood changes, jaundice, heart arrhythmias, weight gain or loss, changes in libido, enlargement of breasts, production of milk, blood sugar changes. Mania and schizophrenic symptoms may be activated, especially in elderly persons. *Manufacturer*: MSD.

CONDYLINE

Description: a preparation available in the form of a solution with applicators containing 0.5% podophyllotoxin in alcoholic base. *Used for*: genital warts. *Dosage*: adults, apply solution twice each day for 3 days directly on to warts. Repeat at 4 day intervals if required for a maximum of 5 weeks. *Avoid use*: children, open wounds. *Side effects*: irritation at site of application. *Manufacturer*: Nycomed.

CONVULEX

Description: an anticonvulsant carboxylic acid preparation produced in the form of soft enteric-coated gelatin capsules of 3 different strengths containing 150mg, 300mg and 500mg of valproic acid. *Used for*: epilepsy. *Dosage*: adults and children, 15mg per kg of body weight at first in divided doses, gradually increasing by 5–10mg/kg body weight each day as required. *Special care*: pregnant women, coagulation tests and liver function tests should be carried out before starting therapy or increasing dose and also at 2-monthly intervals. Urine tests give false positives for ketones. *Avoid use*: patients with liver disease. *Possible interaction*: alcohol, barbiturates, antidepressants, other antiepileptic drugs, anticoagulants, neuroleptic drugs. *Side effects*: gastro-intestinal upset, central nervous system effects, toxic effects on liver coagulation. Rarely, there may be short-lived hair loss, pancreatitis. *Manufacturer*: Pharmacia & Upjohn.

CORACTEN

Description: an antianginal and antihypertensive preparation which is a class II calcium antagonist available as sustained-release capsules of 2 different strengths. Grey/pink capsules contain 10mg nifedipine and pink/brown capsules contain 20mg nifedipine. Both are marked with the strength and name. *Used for*: prevention of angina, hypertension. *Dosage*: adults, 20mg every 12 hours, adjusted according to response within the range of 10–40mg each 12 hours. *Special care*: patients with weak hearts, diabetes, liver disease, hypotension, hypovolaemia (abnormally low volume of circulating blood). *Avoid use*: children, pregnant women, patients with cardiogenic (heart) shock. *Possible interaction*: cimetidine, quinidine, antihypertensive drugs. *Side effects*: flushing, headache, dizziness, oedema, lethargy, nausea, rash, pain in eyes, frequency of urination, gum hyperplasia (increase in number of cells); rarely, allergic-type jaundice. *Manufacturer*: Evans.

CORDARONE X

Description: a proprietary class III antiarrhythmic preparation produced in the form of tablets of 2 different strengths. White, scored tablets, marked with strength and action potential symbol contain 100mg or 200mg of amiodarone hydrochloride. Also, **CORDARONE X** intravenous injection comprising 50mg per ml of solution in ampoules for injection. *Used for*: various heart rhythm disorders especially those which do not respond to other drugs. Tachycardia associated with Wolfe-Parkinson-White syndrome. *Dosage*: adults, 200mg 3 times each day for first week then 200mg twice each day for the following week. Maintenance dose is usually in the order of 200mg each day and the minimum necessary should be used. Children, manufacturer should be consulted. *Special care*: pregnancy, heart failure, elderly, liver or kidney disease, enlargement of prostate gland, glaucoma, sensitivity to iodine. Liver, kidney and thyroid function should be tested throughout the course of treatment. Eyes should also be monitored and therapy started under hospital supervision. *Avoid use*: breast-feeding, patients with heart block, shock, history of thyroid disease, serious bradycardia. *Possible interaction*: other antiarrhythmic drugs, ß-blockers, diuretics, digoxin, phenytoin, calcium antagonists, anticoagulants taken by mouth, anaesthetics. *Side effects*: micro-deposits on cornea of eyes, sensitivity to light, effects on eyes, heart, thyroid, liver and nervous system, pulmonary fibrosis or alveolitis (inflammation of alveoli of lungs). *Manufacturer*: Sanofi Winthrop.

CORDILOX

Description: an antihypertensive and antiarrhythmic preparation which is a class I calcium antagonist produced as tablets of 3 different strengths and as a solution for intravenous injection. Yellow, film-coated tablets, marked with the name and strength, contain 40mg, 80mg and 120mg of verapamil hydrochloride. **CORDILOX INTRAVENOUS** contains 2.5mg verapamil hydrochloride per ml in ampoules for injection. *Used for*: supraventricular heart arrhythmias, hypertension, angina. *Dosage*: adults, heart arrhythmias, 40–120mg 3 times each day; children under 2 years, 20mg 2 or 3 times daily; over 2 years, 40–120mg 2 or 3 times each day. Adults, hypertension, 240–480mg each day in 2 to 3 divided doses. Adults, angina, 8–120mg 3 times each day. *Special care*: patients with weak heart should take digitalis and diuretics; persons with first degree heart block, kidney or liver disease, heart attack, heart conduction disorders, bradycardia, hypotension. *Avoid use*: severe bradycardia, second or third degree heart block, heart failure, heart shock, sick sinus syndrome. *Possible interaction*: ß-blockers, digoxin, quinidine. *Side effects*: flushes and constipation. *Manufacturer*: Baker Norton.

CORGARD

Description: an antihypertensive, non-cardioselective ß-blocker produced in the form of pale blue tablets of 2 different strengths containing either 40 or 80mg of nadolol and marked 207 or 241 respectively. *Used for*: heart arrythmias, angina, hypertension, additional therapy in thyroid gland disease (thyrotoxicosis), prevention of migraine. *Dosage*: heart arrhythmias, 40mg each day at first increasing as required to maximum of 160mg; angina, 40mg each day at first increasing as required with usual daily dose in the order of 40–240mg; hypotension, 80mg each day at first increasing as needed with usual daily dose in the order of 80–240mg; thyrotoxicosis, 80–160mg once each day; prevention of migraine, 40mg each day at first increasing if necessary to a usual daily dose in the order of 80–160mg. *Special care*: pregnancy, breast-feeding, patients with weak hearts should receive diuretics and digitalis, liver or kidney disease, diabetes, metabolic acidosis. Persons undergoing general anaesthesia may need to be withdrawn before planned surgery. Withdraw drug gradually. *Avoid use*: children, patients with obstructive airways disease or history of bronchospasm (asthma), various heart disorders including heart block, heart shock, heart failure, sick sinus syndrome, serious peripheral arterial disease, sinus bradycardia. *Possible interaction*: cardiac depressant anaesthetics, antihypertensives, ergotamine, sympathomimetics, verapamil, clonidine withdrawal, CNS depressants, class I antiarrhythmic drugs, cimetidine, reserpine, indomethacin, hypoglycaemics. *Side effects*: bradycardia, fatigue on exercise, cold hands and feet, disturbance of sleep, gastro-intestinal upset, bronchospasm, heart failure. Withdraw drug gradually if dry eyes or skin rash occur. *Manufacturer*: Sanofi Winthrop.

CORGARETIC 40

Description: a combined antihypertensive, non-cardioselective ß-blocker and thiazide diuretic produced in the form of white, mottled, scored tablets, marked SQUIBB 283, and containing 40mg nadolol and 5mg bendrofluazide. Also, **CORGARETIC 80**, white, mottled, scored tablets marked 284, and containing 80mg nadolol and 5mg bendrofluazide. *Used for*: hypertension. *Dosage*: adults, 1 to 2 tablets a day (Corgaretic 40), increasing if required to a maximum dose of 2 Corgaretic 80 tablets. *Special care*: pregnancy, breast-feeding, weak hearts (should receive digitalis and diuretics), liver or kidney disease, diabetes, metabolic acidosis, gout. Persons undergoing general anaesthesia, may require to be withdrawn before planned surgery. Electrolyte levels should be monitored. *Avoid use*: children, patients with obstructive airways disease or history of bronchospasm (asthma), various heart disorders including heart block, heart shock, heart failure, sick sinus syndrome, serious peripheral arterial disease, sinus bradycardia. Severe or progressive kidney failure, anuria. *Possible interaction*: cardiac depressant anaesthetics, antihypertensives, ergotamine, sympathomimetics, verapamil, clonidine withdrawal, central nervous system depressants, class I antiarrhythmic drugs, cimetidine, reserpine, indomethacin, hypoglycaemics, lithium, digitalis. *Side effects*: bradycardia, fatigue on exercise, cold hands and feet, disturbance of sleep, gastro-intestinal upset, bronchospasm, heart failure, blood changes, sensitivity to light, gout. Withdraw drug gradually if skin rash or dry eyes occur. *Manufacturer*: Sanofi Winthrop.

CORTISYL

Description: a glucocorticoid-mineralocorticoid (corticosteroid) preparation produced in the form of white, scored tablets containing 25mg of cortisone acetate. *Used for*: replacement therapy following removal of adrenal glands and in Addison's disease (a failure of the cortex of the adrenal glands to produce their hormones). *Dosage*: adults, acute attacks, up to 300mg each day with usual maintenance in the order of 12.5mg to 37.5mg daily. *Special care*: pregnancy, liver cirrhosis, glaucoma, epilepsy, diabetes, hypertension, acute glomerulonephritis (inflammation of part of the kidney tubules), peptic ulcer, active infections, tuberculosis, fungal and viral infections. Patients with osteoporosis, recent intestinal anastomoses, thrombophlebitis, nephritis, secondary cancers, infectious diseases which cause skin spots or rash. Patients should avoid contact with chicken pox or *Herpes zoster* virus while receiving therapy and for 3 months after treatment. In the event of contact or contracting chicken pox, further specialist treatment should be given. Withdraw drug gradually. *Avoid use*: children. *Possible interaction*: hypoglycaemics, NSAIDs, anticoagulants taken by mouth, anticholinesterases, diuretics, cardiac glycosides, ephedrine, phenytoin, rifampicin, phenobarbitone. *Side effects*: hypertension, skin changes, fluid retention, hyperglycaemia, loss of potassium, osteoporosis, peptic ulcer, mood changes—euphoria and depression. *Manufacturer*: Hoechst.

CORWIN

Description: a sympathomimetic heart muscle stimulant which is a partial β_1-agonist, produced in the form of yellow, film-coated tablets containing 200mg of xamoterol (as fumerate) marked with symbol and CORWIN. *Used for*: chronic mild heart failure. *Dosage*: adults, start treatment in hsopital with 1 tablet daily in first instance, increasing to 1 tablet twice daily if there is a favourable response. *Special care*: withdraw drug if there is a deterioration in the progress of the disease. Patients with obstructive airways disease, disease of heart muscle and a heart valve (aortic stenosis), kidney disease. *Avoid use*: children, pregnancy, breast-feeding, more severe forms of heart failure, fatigue when resting and breathlessness, hypotension, tachycardia. Patients with fluid in lungs (pulmonary oedema) or other fluid retention. Those needing ACE inhibitor drugs or taking higher doses of loop diuretics (equivalent to 40mg frusemide). *Side effects*: muscle cramps, rash, gastro-intestinal upset, headache, dizziness, palpitations. *Manufacturer*: Zeneca.

COSMEGEN LYOVAC

Description: a cytoloxic antibiotic drug produced in the form of a powder in vials for reconstitution and injection, containing 0.5mg actinomycin D. *Used for*: cancers in children e.g. leukaemia. *Dosage*: fast running intravenous infusion at 3 week intervals or as directed by cancer specialist. *Side effects*: leakage at injection site causes severe tissue death and damage, vomiting, nausea, baldness, suppression of bone marrow, inflammation of mucous membranes, e.g. in nose and throat. *Manufacturer*: M.S.D.

COVERSYL

Description: an antihypertensive preparation which is an ACE inhibitor and is produced as tablets of 2 different strengths. White tablets contain 2mg perindopril tert-butylamine and white, scored oblong tablets contain 4mg. *Used for*: additional therapy with digitalis and/or diuretics in congestive heart failure, hypertension. *Dosage*: adults, heart failure, treatment should start in hospital under close supervision with 2mg once daily taken in the morning increasing to 4mg once each day. Any diuretic should be withdrawn 3 days before the start of treatment. Hypertension, 2mg once each day before food increasing to daily maintenance dose of 4mg (8mg a day is maximum dose). Elderly persons should take a reduced dose of 2mg each day under close medical supervision. Any diuretic should be withdrawn 3 days before start of treatment. *Special care*: patients with kidney disorders or receiving dialysis. Kidney function should be monitored before and during treatment; patients undergoing anaesthesia and surgery. *Avoid use*: children, pregnancy, breast-feeding. *Possible interaction*: antidepressants, other antihypertensives, lithium, potassium supplements, potassium-sparing diuretics. *Side effects*: hypotension, skin rashes and itching, flushing, loss of sense of taste, oedema, headache, malaise, fatigue, nausea, pain in abdomen, weakness, slight cough, blood changes, protein in urine. *Manufacturer*: Servier.

CROMOGEN

Description: an anti-inflammatory, non-steroidal, bronchodilator produced in the form of an aerosol for inhalation containing 5mg of sodium cromoglycate per metered dose aerosol. Also, **CROMOGEN STERI-NEB**, a preservative-free solution containing 10mg sodium cromoglycate per ml, available as a single dose for use with nebulizer. *Used for*: prevention of asthma. *Dosage*: adults and children, 2 puffs 4 times each day in first instance with a maintenance dose of 1 puff 4 times daily. Cromogen Steri-Neb, 20mg with power-operated nebulizer 4 times each day at 3 to 6 hourly intervals. If necessary frequency can be increased to 5 or 6 times each day and, to be effective, therapy must be continuous. *Side effects*: irritation of throat and short-lived cough (due to inhalation of powder). Rarely, short-lived bronchospasm. *Manufacturer*: Baker-Norton.

CRYSTAPEN

Description: a preparation of benzylpenicillin or penicillin G, an antibiotic which is inactivated by the penicillinase enzymes produced by certain bacteria. It is inactivated by stomach (gastric) juices and poorly absorbed from the gut and hence is produced as a solution for intravenous or intramuscular injection. Crystapen 600mg benzylpenicillin sodium (unbuffered) as powder in vials for reconstitution and injection. *Used for*: gonorrhoea, septicaemia, endocarditis, osteomyelitis, meningitis, respiratory tract, ear, nose and throat, skin and soft tissue infections. *Dosage*: adults, 600–1200mg by intravenous or intramuscular injection each day in 2, 3 or 4 divided doses. (For meningitis, up to 14.4g daily in divided doses may be needed). Children, newborns, 30mg per kg of body weight in 2, 3 or 4 divided doses; 1 month to 12 years, 10–20mg per kg each day in 2, 3 or 4 divided doses. For meningitis, age 1 week and under, 60–90mg per kg, in 2 divided doses; 1 week to 1 month, 90–120mg per kg each day in 3 divided doses; 1 month to 12 years, 150–300mg per kg each day in 4, 5 or 6 divided doses. All doses are delivered by intravenous or intramuscular injection. *Special care*: history of penicillin allergy or kidney disease. *Avoid use*: allergy to penicillin. *Side effects*: allergic responses including rash, joint pains, fever, blood changes and anaphylactic shock in hypersensitive persons. *Manufacturer*: Britannia.

CYCLIMORPH^{cd}

Description: a strong analgesic preparation which combines an opiate with an anti-emetic and is available as solutions of 2 different strengths in 1ml ampoules for injection. Cyclimorph 10 contains 10mg morphine tartrate and 50mg cyclizine tartrate per ml; **CYCLIMORPH 15** contains 15mg morphine tartrate and 50mg cyclizine tartrate per ml. *Used for*: acute and chronic intractable pain. *Dosage*: adults, Cyclimorph 10, 1ml by subcutaneous, intravenous or intramuscular injection which can be repeated after 4 hours but maximum dose is 3ml in 24 hours. Children, age 1 to 5 years, 0.25–0.5ml as 1 single dose; 6 to 12 years, 0.5–1ml as 1 single dose. Adults, Cyclimorph 15, 1ml by subcutaneous, intravenous or intramuscular injection which may be repeated after 4 hours but maximum dose is 3ml in 24 hours. *Special care*: women in labour, elderly, liver disease or hypothyroidism. *Avoid use*: children under 1 year, patients with blocked airways or respiratory depression. *Possible interaction*: central nervous system sedatives, MAOIs. *Side effects*: drug dependence and tolerance may develop and Chief Medical Officer should be notified in cases of addiction. Rash, constipation, dizziness, nausea. *Manufacturer*: Glaxo Wellcome.

CYCLO-PROGYNOVA

Description: a combined oestrogen/progestogen hormonal preparation available as tablets in 2 different strengths. Cyclo-Progynova 1mg consists of a course of sugar-coated tablets; 11 beige ones contain 1mg oestradiol valerate and 10 brown ones contain 1mg oestradiol valerate and 0.25mg levonorgestrel. **CYCLO-PROGYNOVA 2mg** consists of a course of sugar-coated tablets; 11 white ones contain 2mg oestradiol valerate and 10 brown ones contain 2mg oestradiol valerate and 0.5mg norgestrel (= 0.25mg levonorgestrel). *Used for*: menopausal symptoms including the prevention of osteoporosis. *Dosage*: 1 oestradiol tablet each day for 11 days (beginning on fifth day of period, if present), followed by 1 combined oestradiol/levonorgestrel tablet for 10 days. Then there are 7 tablet-free days before course is repeated. The lower strength preparation should be tried first. *Special care*: women at any risk of thrombosis and those with liver disease. Liver function should be monitored every 2 to 3 months during treatment. Patients with diabetes, porphyria, migraine, epilepsy, hypertension, fibroids in the uterus, multiple sclerosis, ostosclerosis, gallstones, tetany. These persons should be closely monitored. Also, women with a family history of breast cancer or fibrocystic disease of the breast should be carefully monitored. Breasts and pelvic organs should be examined and blood pressure checked regularly before and during the period of treatment. *Avoid use*: pregnancy, breast-feeding, endometriosis, undiagnosed vaginal bleeding, hormone-dependent cancers, breast cancer, serious heart, liver or kidney disease, thromboembolism. Also, women with kidney, liver or heart disease and Rotor or Dublin-Johnson syndromes. Drug should be stopped 6 weeks before planned surgery and during any condition which makes thrombosis more likely. *Possible interaction*: drugs which induce liver enzymes. *Side effects*: breakthrough bleeding, weight gain, tenderness in breasts, gastro-intestinal upset, dizziness, nausea, headache, vomiting. Drug should be stopped immediately in the event of frequent severe headaches, migraine, disturbance of vision, thromboembolism or thrombophlebitis, jaundice or sudden blood pressure rise, pregnancy. *Manufacturer*: Asta Medica.

CYCLOGEST

Description: a hormonal preparation in the form of suppositories containing either 200mg or 400mg of progesterone. *Used for*: premenstrual syndrome, depression following childbirth (but effectiveness is controversial and subject to debate). *Dosage*: adults, 200 or 400mg via rectum or vagina once or twice each day from the twelfth or fourteenth day of monthly cycle until period begins. *Special care*: use rectally if barrier contraceptives are being used or if patient has thrush infection. Breast-feeding mothers and women with liver, kidney, heart disease, diabetes, hypertension. *Avoid use*: women with abnormal and undiagnosed vaginal bleeding or who have a history of, or are at risk from, thromboembolic disorders. Also, those suffering from breast cancer, porphyria, serious arterial disease. *Possible interaction*: cyclosporins. *Side effects*: gastro-intestinal upset, weight changes, breast tenderness, change in libido, alteration in menstrual cycle, rash, acne. *Manufacturer*: Shine.

CYKLOKAPRON

Description: an antifibrinolytic preparation produced in the form of tablets, syrup and as a solution for injection. White, oblong, film-coated scored tablets, marked C-Y, contain 500mg tranexamic acid. **CYKLOKAPRON SYRUP** contains 500mg tranexamic acid per 5ml; also **CYKLOKAPRON INJECTION** contains 100mg tranexamic acid per ml in ampoules for injection. *Used for*: local or general fibrinolytic disorders, i.e. those characterized by haemorrhage; menorrhagia (abnormally heavy menstrual bleeding or prolonged periods). *Dosage*: local fibrinolysis, 15–25mg per kg of body weight 2 or 3 times each day. (For more general fibrinolytic states, as directed by physician). Children, 25mg per kg of body weight 2 or 3 times each day. Adults, menorrhagia, 1 to $1^1/_2$g 3 or 4 times each day for up to 4 days. *Special care*: patients with kidney disorders, haematuria (blood in urine), especially associated with haemophilia. Patients suffering from angioneurotic oedema require eye and liver function tests during the course of long-term treatment. *Avoid use*: history of thrombosis. *Side effects*: gastro-intestinal upset. If disturbance in colour vision occurs, drug should be withdrawn. *Manufacturer*: Pharmacia & Upjohn.

CYMEVENE

Description: an antiviral preparation available as a powder in vials for reconstitution and injection containing 500mg ganciclovir. *Used for*: life-threatening viral infections or those which threaten sight, caused by cytomegalovirus in patients with reduced immunity. *Dosage*: adults and children, 5mg per kg of body weight given by intravenous infusion over 1-hour period every 12 hours for a period of 14 to 21 days. 6mg per kg of body weight may be required for patients who have sight-threatening infection. *Special care*: polythene gloves and safety glasses must be worn while handing the preparation and accidental splashes on skin should be washed off immediately with soap and water. Regular blood counts required due to toxic effects on blood; potential carcinogen. Patients with kidney disease. Should be administered carefully into veins with good bloodflow and patient's fluid level should be maintained after infusion. *Avoid use*: pregnant women, lactating mothers should not breast-feed until 72 hours have elapsed since last dose, allergy to ganciclovir or acyclovir. Patients with abnormally low neutrophil (a type of white blood cell) counts. *Possible interaction*: other antiviral drugs, zidovudine. *Side effects*: effects on blood including anaemia and severe reduction in levels of white blood cells, elevated levels of serum creatinine and blood urea nitrogen. Effects on all body systems and functions, fever, rash, malaise. *Manufacturer*: Roche.

CYPROSTAT

Description: an anti-androgen preparation used to treat prostate cancer, a type which is hormone-dependent and develops under the influence of the male sex hormone, androgen. The drug blocks androgens produced by the adrenal glands and testes. Cyprostat is available in the form of tablets of 2 strengths; white scored tablets, marked BV within a hexagon, contain 50mg cyproterone acetate. White scored tablets, marked LA within a hexagon, contain 100mg cyproterone acetate. *Used for*: cancer of the prostate. *Dosage*: 300mg each day in 2 or 3 divided doses after food. *Special care*: diabetes, liver disease, history of thrombosis, severe depression. *Side effects*: weariness, infertility, liver disorders, breast enlargement, anaemia. *Manufacturer*: Schering HC.

CYSTRIN

Description: an anticholinergic and antispasmodic preparation available as white tablets containing 3mg oxybutynin hydrochloride and white scored tablets, marked L11, containing 5mg oxybutynin hydrochloride. *Used for*: incontinence, urgency and frequency of urination and night-time bedwetting in children. *Dosage*: 5mg 2 or 3 times each day (with a maximum daily dose of 20mg), in divided doses. Elderly persons, 3mg twice each day adjusted according to response. Children, 5 years and over, 3mg twice each day in first instance, adjusted according to response to usual dose in the order of 5mg 2 or 3 times daily. For night-time bedwetting, last dose should be taken at bedtime. *Special care*: pregnant women, disease of the autonomic nervous system, liver or kidney disease, heart arrhythmias, heart failure, enlarged prostate, tachycardia, hyperthyroidism, hiatus hernia. *Avoid use*: breast-feeding, blocked gastro-intestinal tract or bladder, other intestinal diseases, glaucoma, myasthenia gravis, severe ulcerative colitis. *Possible interaction*: other anticholinergics, TCADs, digoxin, levodopa, amantadine, phenothiazines, butyrophenones. *Side effects*: facial flushing, anticholinergic effects. *Manufacturer*: Pharmacia & Upjohn.

CYTAMEN

Description: a proprietary vitamin B_{12} preparation produced as a solution in 1ml ampoules for injection containing 1000 g cyanocobalamin per ml. *Used for*: vitamin B_{12} responsive macrocytic anaemias (characterized by the presence of fragile enlarged red blood cells), megaloblastic anaemia. *Dosage*: adults and children, 250–1000 g by intramuscular injection every other day for 1 or 2 weeks and then 250 g once a week until normal blood count is achieved. Usual maintenance dose is 1000 g each month. *Possible interaction*: oral contraceptives, chloramphenicol. *Side effects*: rarely, allergic reactions. *Manufacturer*: Evans.

CYTOSAR

Description: a powerful cytotoxic antimetabolite produced as a powder in vials for reconstitution and injection, containing 100mg or 500mg cytarabine. *Used for*: to induce remission in acute myeloblastic anaemia. *Dosage*: given subcutaneously or intravenously, as directed by physician skilled in cancer chemotherapy. *Special care*: requires careful monitoring of blood counts. *Side effects*: severe myelosuppression (bone marrow suppression), loss of hair, nausea and vomiting; early menopause in women and sterility in men if therapy is prolonged, local tissue death if there is leakage at the injection site. *Manufacturer*: Pharmacia & Upjohn.

CYTOTEC

Description: a synthetic form of prostaglandin (a naturally occurring hormone-like substance present in many body tissues) which inhibits the seretion of gastric juice and promotes the healing of ulcers. It is produced in the form of white, hexagonal tablets, containing 200 g misoprostol, and marked SEARLE 1461. *Used for*: stomach and duodenal ulcers, ulceration caused by NSAIDs, prevention of NSAID ulceration. *Dosage*: adults, 4 tablets each day with meals, in divided doses, with last taken at bedtime for 1 to 2 months. Prevention of ulcers, 1 tablet 2, 3 or 4 times each day during the period that NSAID is being taken. *Special care*: women should use effective contraception, patients with circulatory diseases including peripheral or coronary vascular disease and cerebrovascular disease. *Avoid use*: children, pregnancy, women planning pregnancy, breast-feeding. *Side effects*: gastro-intestinal upset, diarrhoea, pain in abdomen, vaginal bleeding and disturbance of menstrual cycle, dizziness, rash. *Manufacturer*: Searle.

D

DAKTACORT

Description: an antifungal/antibacterial agent with mild steroid, comprising miconazole nitrate (2%) and hydrocortisone (1%). Available as cream and ointment. *Used for*: fungal and bacterial (Gram-positive) infections where there is associated inflammation. *Dosage*: to be applied 2 or 3 times daily. *Special care*: use on face or for children should be limited to 5 days maximum. Withdraw gradually after prolonged use. *Avoid use*: on acne, leg ulcers, tuberculous, ringworm or viral skin disease, peri-oral dermatitis, untreated infections whether fungal or bacterial. Extensive or prolonged use during pregnancy. *Side effects*: skin atrophy, striae and telangiectasia (permanent widening of superficial blood vessels), suppression of adrenal glands, Cushingoid changes (see Cushing's syndrome). *Manufacturer*: Janssen-Cilag.

DALACIN CREAM

Description: an antibacterial cream (clindamycin phosphate) available as a 2% cream. *Used for*: bacterial vaginosis. *Dosage:* 1 applicatorful intravaginally each night for 7 days. *Special care*: less effectiveness from barrier contraceptives. *Avoid use*: in cases of lincomycin sensitivity. *Side effects*: vaginal irritation, gastrointestinal upset. Discontinue with colitis or diarrhoea. *Manufacturer*: Pharmacia & Upjohn.

DALACIN C

Description: a lincosamide, clindamycin hydrochloride as 75mg (lavender) and 150mg maroon/lavender capsules. Also **DALACIN PAEDIATRIC**, clindamycin palmitate, containing 75mg per 5ml available as 100mg powder. *Used for*: serious infections sensitive to clindamycin. *Dosage*: 150–450mg every 6 hours. Children under 12 months, 2.5ml every 6 or 8 hours; 1 to 3 years, 2.5–5ml; 4 to 7 years, 5–7.5ml; 8 to 12 years, 7.5–10ml, all every 6 hours. Also **DALACIN PHOSPHATE**, available as ampoules, 150mg/ml, of clindamycin phosphate. *Dosage*: 600mg–2.7g in divided doses each day, by intramuscular injection or intravenous infusion. Children over 1 month, 15–40mg/kg daily in divided doses.

Special care: kidney or liver disease, cease use should colitis or diarrhoea occur. *Avoid use*: in cases of lincomycin sensitivity. *Possible interaction*: neuromuscular blocking agents. *Side effects*: jaundice and blood disorders, gastro-intestinal upsets. *Manufacturer*: Pharmacia & Upjohn.

DALACIN T

Description: antibiotic clindomycin phosphate in a 10mg/ml solution. Also, **DALACIN T LOTION** available as an aqueous solution in a roll-on bottle. *Used for*: moderate to severe acne vulgaris. *Dosage*: apply twice daily. *Special care*: avoid eyes and mucous membranes. *Avoid use*: in cases of lincomycin sensitivity. *Possible interaction*: keratolytics (applies to the solution). *Side effects*: dermatitis, dry skin, folliculitis (solution). Discontinue should colitis or diarrhoea occur. *Manufacturer*: Pharmacia & Upjohn.

DALMANE

Description: a long-acting benzodiazepine (hypnotic) prepared as flurazepam hydrochloride in strengths of 15mg (grey/yellow capsules) and 30mg (black/grey capsules) marked with ROCHE and strength. *Used for*: short-term treatment of severe or disabling insomnia. *Dosage*: 15–30mg at bedtime (elderly, 15mg). *Special care*: chronic liver, kidney or lung disease, the elderly. Also during pregnancy, labour or lactation. To be withdrawn gradually. May impair judgement. *Avoid use*: acute lung disease, depression of the respiration, obsessional states, chronic psychosis. Not for children. *Possible interaction*: anticonvulsants, CNS depressants, alcohol. *Side effects*: confusion, vertigo, drowsiness, ataxia, light-headedness, gastro-intestinal upsets, skin rashes, hypotension, disturbance in vision. Urine retention, changes in libido. Dependence is possible. *Manufacturer*: Roche.

DANOL

Description: a gonadotrophin release inhibitor, danazol, available in capsules of 100mg (white/grey) and 200mg (white/pink), marked with name and strength. *Used for*: menorrhagia (long or heavy menstruation). *Dosage*: 200mg daily for 3 months starting on the first day of menstruation. *Also used for*: endometriosis and as a pre-operative preparation for endometrial ablation. *Dosage*: 400mg daily for 6 to 9 months. 400–800mg daily for 3 to 6 weeks before ablation. *Also used for*: severe mastalgia, benign breast cysts, gynaecomastia. *Dosage*: 200–400mg daily for up to 6 months depending upon the condition. *Special care*: migraine, epilepsy, hypertension, other cardiovascular diseases, diabetes, polycythaemia (increase in blood erythrocytes), conditions adversely affected by fluid retention. *Avoid use*: pregnancy, lactation, porphyria, severe kidney, heart or liver disease, vaginal bleeding, androgen-dependent tumour, thromboembolic disease. *Possible interaction*: steroids, anticonvulsants, anticoagulants, cyclosporin, antihypertensives, hypoglycaemics. *Side effects*: backache, flushes, muscle spasms, nausea, rashes, male hormone effects, fluid retention, menstrual disturbances, headache, emotional disturbance, cholestatic jaundice (due to blockage of bile flow through any part of the biliary system). *Manufacturer*: Sanofi Winthrop.

DANTRIUM

Description: a muscle relaxant, dantrolene sodium, available in capsules (orange with light brown cap) of strength 25mg and 100mg, marked 0030 and 0033 respectively. *Used for*: severe or chronic spasticity of skeletal muscle. *Dosage*: 25mg daily to start, increasing to a maximum of 100mg 4 times per day. *Special care*: lung or heart disease, pregnancy. Liver to be checked before and 6 weeks after the start of treatment. *Avoid use*: liver disease, where spasticity is useful for movement. *Possible interaction*: CNS depressants, alcohol. *Side effects*: diarrhoea, drowsiness, weakness, fatigue. *Manufacturer*: Procter & Gamble.

DAONIL

Description: a sulphonylurea, glibenclamide, available as white oblong tablets (5mg) marked LDI with symbol. Also **SEMI-DAONIL** (2.5mg white tablet). *Used for*: maturity-onset diabetes (non-insulin-dependent diabetes mellitus). *Dosage*: 5mg daily at breakfast increasing by 2.5–5mg weekly to a maximum of 15mg. *Special care*: kidney failure, the elderly. *Avoid use*: juvenile, growth-onset or unstable brittle diabetes (all now called insulin-dependent diabetes mellitus), severe liver or kidney disease, ketoacidosis, stress, infections, surgery, endocrine disorders. Pregnancy or lactation. *Possible interaction*: MAOIs, corticosteroids, corticotrophin, oral contraceptives, alcohol, ß-blockers. Also glucagon, chloramphenicol, rifampicin, sulphonamides, aspirin, phenylbutazone, cyclophosphamide, oral anticoagulants, clofibrate, benzafibrate. *Side effects*: sensitivity including skin rash. *Manufacturer*: Hoechst.

DARANIDE

Description: a preparation of dichlor-phenamide in yellow tablet form (50mg, marked MSD 49) which is a weak diuretic, reducing fluid in the aqueous humour of the eye. *Used for*: treatment of glaucoma. *Dosage*: 2 to 4 tablets initially then 2 every 12 hours. Thereafter ½ to 1 up to 3 times daily. *Avoid use*: with children or with patients suffering from kidney or liver disease, pulmonary obstruction, low sodium or potassium levels. During pregnancy. *Possible interaction*: with steroids, local anaesthetics, anticoagulants, anticonvulsants, antidiabetics, salicylates, digitalis, hypoglycaemics and ACTH (adrenocorticotrophic hormone). *Side effects*: gastro-intestinal upsets, weight loss, frequent urination, headache, lassitude, itching, abnormal blood condition (dyscrasia). *Manufacturer*: Merck, Sharp and Dohme.

DDAVP

Description: The acetate of desmopressin, an analogue of the hormone vasopressin and an antidiuretic compound. *Used for*: it is administered as nose drops for the treatment of diabetes insipidus and enuresis (bedwetting, the involuntary passing of urine). *Dosage*: adults, 0.1–0.2ml once or twice daily. Children, 0.05–0.2ml at the same rate. (Lower dosage for infants). Also available as white tablets: 0.2–0.4mg at bedtime for adults and children over 5 with enuresin; 0.1mg thrice daily for diabetes insipidus. Injection also available. *Avoid use*: in pregnancy and for patients with epilepsy, migraine, asthma or chronic kidney disease. *Side effects*: may cause fluid retention, headache, nausea and vomiting. *Manufacturer*: Ferring.

DECA-DURABOLIN

Description: a form of the anabolic steroid nandrolone, in ampoules or syringes. *Used for*: its protein-building properties (in conjunction with a nourishing diet), particularly after major surgery or debilitating disease. It was administered for osteoporosis but is no longer advocated as its value is dubious. It may be used to treat cancers linked to sex hormones. *Dosage*: 50mg every 3 weeks, by intramuscular injection. *Special care*: in case of heart, liver or kidney impairment, hypertension, migraine, epilepsy and diabetes. *Possible interaction*: with anticoagulants, hypoglycaemics. *Side effects*: oedema, hypercalcaemia, some virilization in women (i.e. appearance of male features such as deepening of the voice, growth of body hair and increase in musculature). *Manufacturer*: Organon.

DECA-DURABOLIN 100

Description: The same form of the anabolic steroid nandrolene as is found in Deca-Durabolin. *Used for*: the treatment of some forms of anaemia, e.g. aplastic anaemia, also post-cytotoxic therapy anaemia, and anaemia associated with chronic kidney failure. *Dosage*: all administered by intramuscular injection: 50–150mg weekly (aplastic); 200mg per week from 2 weeks before cytotoxic therapy until the blood returns to normal; 100mg (females) or 200mg (males) weekly for kidney failure. *Special care*: in cases of heart, liver or kidney impairment, hypertension, migraine, epilepsy and diabetes. *Avoid use*: in pregnancy, also where there is a known or suspected prostate or mammary cancer in males. *Possible interaction*: with anticoagulants, hypoglycaemics. *Side effects*: oedema, hypercalcaemia, some virilization in women (i.e. appearance of male features such as deepening of the voice, growth of body hair and increase in musculature). *Manufacturer*: Organon.

DECADRON

Description: a corticosteroid preparation available as white (0.5mg) tablets marked MSD 41, or injection. *Used for*: treatment of inflammation, particularly in allergic or rheumatic conditions. *Dosage*: often a daily dose; magnitude varies with the case. *Special care*: to be taken in numerous conditions including nephritis, osteoporosis, peptic ulcer and metastatic carcinoma. Also viral/fungal infections, tuberculosis, hypertension, glaucoma, epilepsy, diabetes, cirrhosis and hypothyroidism. Also pregnancy and stress. To be withdrawn gradually. *Possible interaction*: NSAIDs, diuretics, hypoglycaemics, oral anticoagulants, phenobarbitone, ephedrine, phenytoin, anticholinesterases and others. *Side effects*: osteoporosis, depression, hyperglycaemia, euphoria, peptic ulceration. *Manufacturer*: M.S.D.

DECASERPYL

Description: an alkaloid (methoserpidine) compound originally derived from the dried root of the shrub *Rauwolfia serpentina*. It is available in tablet form, 5mg (white) and 10mg (pink), marked D/5 and D/10 respectively, both with RL on reverse. *Used for*: treatment of high blood pressure. *Dosage:* 10mg 3 times per day initially. This can be increased by 5–10mg daily on a weekly basis up to a maximum of 50mg per dose. *Special care*: during pregnancy or lactation. *Avoid use*: in patients with a history of mental depression; peptic ulcer, ulcerative colitis or severe kidney disease; Parkinson's disease. It should not be given to children. *Possible interaction*: anticonvulsants. *Side effects*: vertigo, tremor, lethargy, nasal congestion, and gastro-intestinal upset. *Manufacturer*: Roussel.

DECLINAX

Description: The sulphate of debrisoquine available in (white) tablet form marked ROCHE 10 at 10mg strength, and used for moderate to severe hypertension. *Used for*: treatment of high blood pressure. *Dosage*: 10–20mg once or twice daily to begin with. This may be increased to a daily dose of 120mg. *Special care*: with cases of kidney disease. *Avoid use*: in cases of recent heart attack; phaeochromocytoma. Not to be used for children. *Possible interaction*: sympathomimetics (drugs that stimulate the sympathetic nervous system and whose action resembles noradrenaline), some antidepressants. *Side effects*: headache, general malaise, postural hypotension (i.e. low blood pressure on standing) and failure to ejaculate. *Manufacturer*: Roche.

DELTACORTRIL

Description: a corticosteroid preparation containing the glucocorticoid steroid, prednisolone. It is available as 2 enteric-coated tablets, brown (2.5mg) and red (5mg) marked Pfizer. *Used for*: allergic conditions, collagen disorders or inflammation. *Dosage*: 5–60mg daily, reducing to a minimum for maintenance. *Special care*: with numerous conditions including nephritis, osteoporosis, peptic ulcer and metastatic carcinoma. Also viral/fungal infections, tuberculosis, hypertension, glaucoma, epilepsy, diabetes, cirrhosis and hypothyroidism. Also pregnancy and stress. To be withdrawn gradually. Not to be given to children under 12 months. *Possible interaction*: NSAIDs, diuretics, hypoglycaemics, oral anticoagulants, phenobarbitone, ephedrine, phenytoin, anticholinesterases and others. *Side effects*: osteoporosis, depression, hyperglycaemia, euphoria, peptic ulceration. *Manufacturer*: Pfizer.

DELTASTAB

Description: a corticosteroid preparation containing prednisolone acetate, a glucocorticoid steroid. Available as white tablets (1mg and 5mg) and ampoules of an aqueous solution (25mg/ml). *Used for*: (tablets) treatment of inflammation associated with rheumatic and allergic conditions and collagen disorders. Solution injected into joints for rheumatic conditions and intramuscularly for systemic therapy. *Dosage*: tablets initially 10–20mg daily (up to 60mg for severe cases), reducing as soon as possible to a maintenance daily dose of 2.5–15mg. Injection of solution in range 5–25mg depending on joint size up to 3 times daily. Intramuscular injection 25–100mg once or twice weekly. Children should receive only minimal doses and for the shortest possible time and even then only when specifically indicated. *Special care*: with numerous conditions including nephritis, osteoporosis, peptic ulcer and metastatic carcinoma. Also viral/fungal infections, tuberculosis, hypertension, glaucoma, epilepsy, diabetes, cirrhosis and hypothyroidism. Also pregnancy and stress. To be withdrawn gradually. Not to be given to children under 12 months. *Possible interaction*: NSAIDs, diuretics, hypoglycaemics, oral anticoagulants, phenobarbitone, ephedrine, phenytoin, anticholinesterases and others. *Side effects*: osteoporosis, depression, hyperglycaemia, euphoria, peptic ulceration. *Manufacturer*: Knoll.

DENTOMYCIN

Description: an antibacterial available as a 2% gel of minocycline hydrochloride. *Used for*: periodontitis (disease causing formation of spaces 'pockets' between gums and teeth and loss of bone and connective fibres) where pockets are 5mm or more. *Dosage*: using the applicator, the gel is put into the pockets 2 or 3 times at 14-day intervals. After completion of treatment, not to be repeated within 6 months. *Special care*: in cases of liver or kidney impairment. Pregnancy, nursing mothers. No intake of food or drink and no rinsing of mouth (including cleaning of teeth) for 2 hours after treatment. *Avoid use*: not suitable for children. *Possible interaction*: anticoagulants. *Side effects*: local irritation. *Manufacturer*: Wyeth.

DEPIXOL

Description: a thioxanthene antipsychotic drug available in several forms. Yellow tablets (marked LUNDBECK) contain 3mg flupenthixol dihydrochloride. **DEPIXOL INJECTION** is available as the decanoate of flupenthixol in ampoules, vials and syringes (20mg/ml). **DEPIXOL CONC.** and **DEPIXOL LOW VOLUME** are concentrated forms of the decanoate (100mg/ml and 200mg/ml respectively), for injection. *Used for*: schizophrenia and other mental disorders, especially for apathetic and withdrawn patients. *Dosage*: Depixol—1 to 3 tablets twice daily (6 maximum); Depixol injection—deep intramuscular injection of 20–40mg every 2 to 4 weeks; Depixol Conc. and Depixol Low Volume—50mg 4-weekly up to 300mg every 2 weeks by deep intramuscular injection. *Special care*: with the elderly, sufferers of Parkinsonism or kidney, liver, respiratory or cardiovascular disease and anyone with an intolerance to neuroleptic drugs taken orally. *Avoid use*: in pregnancy and lactation. Patients who are comatose, excitable or overactive. Not for children. *Possible interaction*: alcohol, analgesics and central nervous system depressants. Also anticonvulsants, antidiabetics, levodopa and antihypertensives. *Side effects*: muscular spasms, rigidity and tremor, dry mouth and nasal stuffiness, urine retention, increased heart rate, constipation, weight gain, drowsiness, lethargy, fatigue, blood and skin changes, menstrual changes and galactorrhoea. *Manufacturer*: Lundbeck.

DEPO-MEDRONE

Description: a corticosteroid preparation containing the glucocorticoid steroid methylprednisolone acetate as vials of 40mg/ml. Also, **DEPO-MEDRONE WITH LIDOCAINE**, which in addition contains 10mg/ml lignocaine hydrochloride local anaesthetic. *Used for*: severe allergic rhinitis, asthma, osteo- and rheumatoid arthritis, collagen disorders and skin diseases (Depo-Medrone). Local use for rheumatic or inflammatory conditions (Depo-Medrone with Lidocaine). *Dosage*: by injection into joints or soft tissue, 4–80mg (according to joint size or amount of tissue) repeated 1–5 weekly depending upon response. *Special care*: with numerous conditions including nephritis, osteoporosis, peptic ulcer and metastatic carcinoma. Also viral/fungal infections, tuberculosis, hypertension, glaucoma, epilepsy, diabetes, cirrhosis and hypothyroidism. Also pregnancy and stress. To be withdrawn gradually. Not to be given to children under 12 months. *Possible interaction*: NSAIDs, diuretics, hypoglycaemics, oral anticoagulants, phenobarbitone, ephedrine, phenytoin, anticholinesterases and others. *Side effects*: osteoporosis, depression, hyperglycaemia, euphoria, peptic ulceration. *Manufacturer*: Pharmacia & Upjohn.

DEPO-PROVERA

Description: a depot-injectable preparation of the progestogen medroxyprogesterone acetate available in vials as a suspension of 150mg/ml and 50mg/ml. *Used for*: contraception for women who cannot use other methods and endometriosis. (Also used in treatment of certain types of carcinoma.) *Dosage*: for contraception: 50mg by deep intramuscular injection during the first 5 days of the cycle or within 5 weeks of giving birth, repeated 3-monthly; for endometriosis: 50mg weekly or 100mg 2-weekly by intramuscular injection over 6 months and longer if necessary. *Special care*: undiagnosed abnormal vaginal bleeding, diabetes or severe depression. Also, wait 6 weeks after birth if lactating; not for genital malignancy. *Avoid use*: pregnancy. Also hormone-dependent carcinoma. *Side effects*: temporary fertility with continuous treatment, irregular or heavy vaginal bleeding during early cycles, weight gain, back pain and fluid retention. *Manufacturer*: Pharmacia & Upjohn.

DEPOSTAT

Description: a depot progestogen available as 2ml ampoules of gestronol hexanoate (100mg/ml). *Used for*: benign hyperplasia of the prostate and endometrial cancer. *Dosage*: 200–400mg by intramuscular injection every 5 to 7 days for both conditions. *Special care*: migraine, epilepsy, asthma and diabetes, kidney disease. *Avoid use*: liver disease, severe arterial disease, carcinoma of the breast or genital tract. *Side effects*: nausea, fluid retention, weight gain. *Manufacturer*: Schering H.C.

DERMOVATE

Description: a potent steroid, clobetasol proprionate, available as 0.05% cream and ointment. Also available as DERMOVATE SCALP APPLICATION (solution), and DERMOVATE-NN which is also an antifungal/antibacterial agent containing, in addition, 0.5% neomycin sulphate and 100,000 units/g nystatin. *Used for*: psoriasis, eczemas that are hard to control, inflammatory skin diseases. Dermovate-NN is for such conditions when infection is present or suspected. *Dosage*: to be applied sparingly once or twice daily for a maximum of 4 weeks (maximum of 50g weekly for Dermovate-NN), then review. *Special care*: limit use of face to 5 days. Withdraw gradually. *Avoid use*: on acne, scabies, leg ulcers or prolonged use in pregnancy. Not for children. *Side effects*: Cushingoid (see Cushing's syndrome) changes, skin atrophy, telangiectasia (multiple telangiectases, collections of distended blood capillaries). *Manufacturer*: Glaxo Wellcome.

DESERIL

Description: The maleate of methysergide which acts as a serotonin antagonist. Serotonin is active in inflammation (similar to histamine) and also acts as a neurotransmitter and is released by the liver and certain tumours. Available as white tablets of 1mg strength marked DSL. *Used for*: diarrhoea associated with carcinoid disease, i.e. a tumour in certain glands in the intestine. For relief of recurring severe migraine, histamine (cluster) headaches and headaches where other treatments have failed. *Dosage*: for diarrhoea: 12 to twenty daily with meals, in divided doses. For migraine: 1 or 2 tablets 3 times per day with meals. *Special care*: anyone with a history of peptic ulcer. In treating migraine, 6 months of therapy should be followed by a month's interval and the dosage reduced 2 to 3 weeks before withdrawal. Patient should be monitored regularly. *Avoid use*: pregnancy or lactation; coronary, peripheral or occlusive vascular disorders; heart or lung disease; severe hypertension; liver or kidney impairment; disease of the urinary tract; poor health, weakness and malnutrition (cachexia); sepsis; phlebitis or cellulitis (skin infection leading to abscess and tissue destruction) of the lower extremities. Not recommended for children. *Possible interaction*: vasopressors and vasoconstrictors; ergot alkaloids (alkaloids derived from the fungus *Laviceps purpurea*). *Side effects*: dizziness, nausea, oedema, lassitude, leg cramps, drowsiness, weight gain, rashes, hair loss, CNS disturbances, abdominal discomfort, arterial spasm. Discontinue in the event of inflammatory fibrosis. *Manufacturer*: Sandoz.

DESFERAL

Description: desferrioxamine mesylate as 500mg powder in a vial for reconstitution and injection. Desferal acts as a chelating agent with the iron, i.e. it locks up the iron chemically, enabling it to be removed from the system. *Used for*: iron poisoning, haemochromatoses (excess deposits of iron in the body due to faulty iron metabolism), excess aluminium in dialysis patients. *Dosage*: depending upon condition and circumstances—by mouth, intramuscular injection or intravenous infusion. *Special care*: kidney dysfunction; pregnancy and lactation; patients with aluminium-related encephalopathy may have seizures (treat first with Clonazepam). *Possible interaction*: erythropoietin, prochlorperazine. *Side effects*: hypotension if given too rapidly intravenously; cardiovascular, gastro-intestinal and neurological disturbances; changes in lens and retina; urine has red colouration; leg cramps; liver and kidney dysfunction; blood conditions, e.g. anaemia. *Manufacturer*: Ciba.

DESTOLIT

Description: a bile acid, visodeoxycholic acid, available as white tablets (150mg) marked DESTOLIT. *Used for*: dissolution of small cholesterol gallstones. *Dosage*: 3 to 4 daily in 2 doses after meals, 1 after an evening meal. To be continued for 3 to 4 months after stones have been dissolved. *Avoid use*: active gastric or duodenal ulcer; liver and intestine conditions affecting recycling of bile between intestine and liver; if gall bladder not functioning; women if not using contraception (non-hormonal methods ideally). Not for children. *Possible interaction*: oestrogens; oral contraceptives; agents lowering cholesterol levels. *Manufacturer*: Hoechst.

DETECLO

Description: a compound tetracycline preparation containing chlortetracycline hydrochloride (115.4mg), tetracycline hydrochloride (115.4mg) and demeclocycline hydrochloride (69.2mg) in blue film-coated tablets, marked LL, and 5422 on the reverse. *Used for*: ear, nose and throat infections; infection of respiratory, gastro-intestinal and urinary tracts and soft tissues; severe cases of acne vulgaris. *Dosage*: 1 tablet 12-hourly. *Special care*: impaired liver. *Avoid use*: during pregnancy and lactation; kidney impairment; SLE. *Possible interaction*: penicillins; anticoagulants; oral contraceptives; milk, antacids or mineral supplements. *Side effects*: allergic reactions; gastro-intestinal upsets; superinfection (i.e. one infection arising during the course of another); withdraw in the case of intracranial hypertension. *Manufacturer*: Wyeth.

DEXA-RHINASPRAY

Description: a metered dose aersol for nasal inhalation consisting of a corticosteroid (dexamethasone-21 isonicotinate, 20mg per dose), antibiotic (neomycin sulphate, 100mg) and the sympathomimetic (i.e. something that mimics the effects of organ stimulation by the sympathetic nervous system) tramazoline hydrochloride (120mg). *Used for*: allergic rhinitis (e.g. hay fever). *Dosage*: 1 dose per nostril up to 6 times per 24 hours. One dose twice daily for children 5 to 12 years. Not recommended for children under 5 years. *Special care*: not to be used over a prolonged period. *Side effects*: nasal irritation. *Manufacturer*: Boehringer Ingelheim.

DEXEDRINE^{CD}

Description: a sympathomimetic, dexamphetamine sulphate, available as a white tablet (5mg strength), marked EVANS DB5. *Used for*: narcolepsy, untreatable hyperactivity in children. *Dosage*: 1 tablet twice daily increasing weekly by 10mg to a maximum of 60mg daily. For the elderly, 5mg daily increasing by 5mg every week. Not recommended for children under 3 years; 2.5mg daily increasing by 2.5mg every week for children aged 3 to 5 and 5–10mg daily for children aged 6 to 12 years, increasing at weekly intervals by 5mg. A maximum of 20mg daily is customary. *Special care*: pregnancy. *Avoid use*: glaucoma; hypertension; hyperexcitability; hyperthyroidism; in cases of cardiovascular disease; where there is a history of drug abuse. *Possible interaction*: guanethidine, MAOIs. *Side effects*: restlessness and insomnia; retarded growth; euphoria; dry mouth; sweating, palpitations; tachycardia; disturbances of the central nervous system and stomach; raised blood pressure. Also, possible dependence. *Manufacturer*: Evans.

DEXTROPROPOXYPHENE

Description: an opiate and weak analgesic, dextropropoxyphene napsylate, available as capsules (60mg strength). *Used for*: mild to moderate pain anywhere in the body. *Dosage*: 3 to 4 capsules per day. *Special care*: pregnancy, elderly; liver or kidney impairment. *Avoid use*: in children. *Possible interaction*: anticoagulants; anticonvulsants; alcohol or depressants of the central nervous system. *Side effects*: constipation; rash; nausea and dizziness; drowsiness. May develop tolerance and dependence. *Manufacturer*: Lilly.

DHC CONTINUS

Description: an opiate, dihydrocodeine tartrate, available as white capsules for sustained (prolonged) release and in strengths of 60, 90 and 120mg, marked with DHC and strength. *Used for*: chronic severe pain e.g. as associated with cancer. *Dosage*: 60-120mg 12-hourly. *Special care*: chronic liver disease; kidney impairment; in pregnancy or the elderly; allergies; hypothyroidism; raised intracranial pressure. *Avoid use*: depression of respiration; disease causing obstruction of the airways. *Possible interaction*: MAOIs, alcohol and central nervous system depressants. *Side effects*: headache; vertigo; nausea; constipation. *Manufacturer*: Napp.

DIABINESE

Description: a sulphonylurea, and hypoglycaemic agent containing chlorpropamide and available as white tablets of strength 100 and 250mg. Marked with DIA, strength and Pfizer. *Used for*: type II non-insulin dependent diabetes, adult-onset diabetes mellitus (when the pancreas is still active to some extent). *Dosage*: usually 100–250mg daily with breakfast, maximum 500mg. *Special care*: the elderly or patients with kidney failure. *Avoid use*: during pregnancy or lactation; juvenile, growth-onset or unstable brittle diabetes (insulin-dependent diabetes mellitus); ketoacidosis; severe kidney or liver disorders; stress, infections or surgery; endocrine disorders. *Possible interaction*: MAOIs, corticosteroids, ß-blockers, diuretics, corticotrophin (ACTH), oral contraceptives, alcohol. Also aspirin, oral anticoagulants, bezafibrate, clofibrate, phenylbutazone, cyclophosphamide, rifampicin, sulphonamides and chloramphenicol. Also glucagon. *Side effects*: skin rash and other sensitivity reactions. Other conditions tend to be rare, e.g. hyponatraemia (low blood sodium concentration) or aplastic anaemia. *Manufacturer*: Pfizer.

DIAMICRON

Description: a sulphonylurea, and hypoglycaemic agent, containing gliclazide and available as white tablets (80mg strength). *Used for*: type II non-insulin-dependent diabetes, adult-onset diabetes mellitus (when the pancreas is still active to some extent). *Dosage*: half to 1 daily up to a maximum of 4 (2 divided doses if above 2 tablets). *Special care*: the elderly or patients with kidney failure. *Avoid use*: during pregnancy or lactation; juvenile, growth-onset or unstable brittle diabetes (insulin-dependent diabetes mellitus); ketoacidosis; severe kidney or liver disorders; stress, infections or surgery; endocrine disorders. *Possible interaction*: MAOIs, corticosteroids, ß-blockers, diuretics, corticotrophin (ACTH), oral contraceptives, alcohol. Also aspirin, oral anticoagulants, and the generic drugs bezafibrate, clofibrate, phenylbutazone, cyclophosphamide, rifampicin, sulphonamides and chloramphenicol. Also glucagon. *Side effects*: skin rash and other sensitivity reactions. Other conditions tend to be rare, e.g. hyponatraemia (low blood sodium concentration) or aplastic anaemia. *Manufacturer*: Servier.

DIAMOX

Description: a carbonic anhydrase inhibitor, acetazolamide, available as white tablets (250mg strength) marked LEDERLE 4395. *Used for*: congestive heart failure and oedema; epilepsy; glaucoma. *Dosage*: for heart failure, oedema: 250–375mg to start, each morning or on alternate days. For premenstrual oedema, 125–375mg in 1 dose 5 to 10 days before menstruation. For epilepsy: 250–1000mg each day. Children under 24 months 125mg daily; 2 to 12 years 125–750mg daily. For glaucoma: 250–1000mg daily. Children, 125–750mg daily; infants, 125mg daily. All in divided doses. Also **DIAMOX SR** *Description:* as for Diamox, but available as 250mg strength sustained-release orange capsule. *Used for:* glaucoma. *Dosage:* 1 to 2 daily. Also **DIAMOX PARENTERAL** *Description:* as for Diamox, but available as powder in a vial, 500mg strength. *Used for:* congestive heart failure and oedema; epilepsy; glaucoma. *Dosage:* intravenous or intramuscular injection of equivalent oral dose. *Special care:* diabetes, lactation, gout, potassium supplements may be required. Monitor blood, electrolytes and fluid. Also for glaucoma treatment: emphysema and pulmonary obstruction, any unusual rashes to be reported. *Avoid use:* pregnancy, certain kidney conditions, chronic closed angle glaucoma, adrenal insufficiency, hypersensitivity to sulphonamides, depletion of sodium or potassium. Also for glaucoma—*liver impairment*. *Possible interaction*: oral anticoagulants, hypoglycaemics, folic acid antagonists. *Side effects*: headache, drowsiness, thirst, flushing, polyuria, blood dyscrasias, rash, excitability, paraesthesia (tingling, "pins and needles"). *Manufacturer*: Storz.

DIANETTE

Description: the oestrogen/anti-androgen ethinyloestradiol (35 g) with 2mg cyproterone acetate, available as beige tablets. *Used for*: severe acne in women; for prolonged oral antibiotic therapy; idiopathic hirsutism. *Dosage*: 1 daily for 3 weeks starting on first day of cycle (then 7 days without). *Special care*: diabetes, varicose veins, hypertension, Raynaud's disease (numbness in the fingers due to spasm of arteries), asthma, chronic kidney disease (or dialysis), severe depression, multiple sclerosis. *Avoid use*: not recommended for children. Also with cardiovascular conditions such as angina, ischaemia, heart valve disease, sickle cell anaemia, those at risk of and with a history of thrombosis. Patients with liver disorders; hormone-dependent carcinoma, undiagnosed vaginal bleeding, pregnancy, chorea, otosclerosis (bone overgrowth in the inner ear causing deafness), haemolytic uraemic syndrome (sudden destruction of red blood cells causing acute kidney failure). *Possible interaction*: tetracyclines, barbiturates, phenytoin, griseofulvin, primidone, carbamazepine, rifampicin, chloral hydrate, ethosuximide, glutethimide, dichloralphenazone. *Side effects*: leg pains and cramps, depression, enlargement of breasts, fluid retention, headaches, nausea, weight gain, loss of libido, vaginal discharge. *Manufacturer*: Schering H.C.

DIAPHINE^{CD}

Description: The analgesic opiate, diamorphine hydrochloride available as powder in ampoules in strengths of 5, 10, 30, 100 and 500mg. *Used for*: severe pain. *Dosage*: 5–10mg subcutaneously or intramuscularly, to be varied according to patient response. *Special care*: liver or kidney impairment, hypotension, hypothyroidism, myxoedema, reduced respiratory capacity, depression of the CNS, toxic psychoses, prostatic hypertrophy, stricture of the urethra, acute alcoholism, delirium tremens, severe diarrhoea, the elderly. *Avoid use*: in children. With head injuries, raised intracranial pressure, acute liver disease, acute respiratory depression, diseases causing obstruction of the airways. *Possible interaction*: depressants of the central nervous system, MAOIs. *Side effects*: shock, cardiac arrest, vomiting, nausea, constipation, depression of respiration. Possible tolerance and dependence. *Manufacturer*: Napp.

DIARREST

Description: a combined opiate, antispasmodic and electrolyte containing 5mg codeine phosphate, 2.5mg dicyclomine hydrochloride, 40mg potassium chloride, 50mg sodium chloride, 50mg sodium citrate per 5ml. Available in 200ml bottles. *Used for*: diarrhoea and to maintain levels of electrolytes during attacks. *Dosage*: 20ml 4 times per day with water. Children, at the same frequency: 10 to 13 years, 15ml; 6 to 9 years, 10ml; 4 to 5 years, 5ml; under 4 years, contact the manufacturer. *Special care*: cardiac failure, liver or kidney malfunction, glaucoma, thyrotoxicosis, ulcerative colitis. *Avoid use*: diverticular disease, pseudomembranous colitis (severe colitis occurring in debilitated patients taking broad-spectrum antibiotics). *Possible interaction*: MAOIs. *Side effects*: sedation. *Manufacturer*: Galen.

DIAZEMULS

Description: a long-acting anxiolytic, benzodiazepine, available as an emulsion of 10mg in 2ml. *Used for*: severe acute anxiety, delirium tremens; acute muscle spasms; anticonvulsant for status epilepticus (continual seizures resulting in brain damage if not stopped); and as a premedication. *Dosage*: 10mg (5mg for elderly) by infusion or intravenous injection at 4-hourly intervals; 0.2mg/kg for children by the same means. As an anticonvulsant, 0.15–0.25mg/kg by intravenous injection, repeated after half to one hour and then up to 3mg/kg over 24 hours by intravenous infusion. For premedication, 0.1–0.2mg/kg by intravenous injection. *Special care*: chronic lung insufficiency, chronic liver or kidney disease, the elderly, pregnant, during labour or lactation. Judgement and dexterity may be affected, long-term use is to be avoided. To be withdrawn gradually. *Avoid use*: acute lung insufficiency, depression of respiration (escept in cases of acute muscle spasms). Also when treating anxiety, obsessional states or chronic psychosis. *Possible interaction*: alcohol and other CNS depressants, anticonvulsants. *Side effects*: vertigo, gastro-intestinal upsets, confusion, ataxia, drowsiness, light-headedness, hypotension, disturbance of vision, skin rashes. Also urine retention, changes in libido. Dependence a potential problem. *Manufacturer*: Dumex.

DIAZEPAM

Description: an anxiolytic, long-acting benzodiazepine, available as 2, 5 and 10mg tablets and as **DIAZEPAM ELIXIR** (2mg/5ml). *Used for*: severe anxiety in the short term, acute alcohol withdrawal, night terrors and sleepwalking in children. *Dosage*: 6–30mg daily (elderly 3–15mg); children 1–5mg at bedtime. *Special care*: chronic lung insufficiency, chronic liver or kidney disease, the elderly, pregnant, during labour or lactation. Judgement and dexterity may be affected, long-term use is to be avoided. To be withdrawn gradually. *Avoid use*: acute lung insufficiency, depression of respiration, obsessional states or chronic psychosis. *Possible interaction*: alcohol, other CNS depressants, anticonvulsants. *Side effects*: vertigo, gastro-intestinal upsets, confusion, ataxia, drowsiness, light-headedness, hypotension, disturbance of vision, skin rashes. Also urine retention, changes in libido. Dependence a potential problem. *Manufacturer*: nonproprietary.

DIBENYLINE

Description: an anti-adrenaline antihypertensive, phenoxybenzamine hydrochloride, available as 10mg red and white capsules marked SKF. Also as **DIBENYLINE INJECTION** (50mg/ml) in 2ml doses. *Used for*: vasodilation to treat high blood pressure associated with phaeochromocytoma. *Dosage*: 1 capsule daily increasing by 1 each day to achieve control. Children, 1–2mg/kg daily in divided doses. *Special care*: the elderly, kidney disease, cardiovascular or cerebrovascular disease, congestive heart failure. *Avoid use*: after myocardial infarction, cerebrovascular accident (i.e. heart attack or stroke). *Side effects*: dizziness, tachycardia, low blood pressure on standing, failure to ejaculate, pinpoint pupils (miosis). *Manufacturer*: Forley.

DICLOMAX RETARD

Description: White, sustained-release capsules containing diclofenac sodium (100mg). *Used for*: osteoarthritis, rheumatoid arthritis, ankylosing spondylitis, musculoskeletal disorders such as sprains and strains, back pains. Acute gout. *Dosage*: 1 tablet daily with food. *Special care*: kidney, liver or heart disorders, pregnancy or lactation, the elderly, blood disorders, hepatic porphyria (production of excess porphyrins in the liver producing abdominal pain, neuropathy and photosensitivity), and those with a history of gastro-intestinal lesions. Patients on long-term treatment should be monitored. *Avoid use*: active peptic ulcer, asthma, aspirin or anti-inflammatory drug-induced allergy, during last 3 months of pregnancy. Not recommended for children. *Possible interaction*: steroids, NSAIDs, anticoagulants, antidiabetics, quinolones, diuretics, salicylates, lithium, digoxin, methotrexate, cyclosporin. *Side effects*: headache, oedema, gastro-intestinal upsets, peptic ulcer, liver and kidney malfunction, skin reactions. *Manufacturer*: Parke-Davis.

DICONAL[cd]

Description: an opiate and antiemetic containing cyclizine hydrochloride (30mg) and dipipanone hydrochloride (10mg) and available as a pink tablet, coded WELLCOME F3A. *Used for*: moderate to severe pain. *Dosage*: 1 initially, then as advised. *Special care*: in pregnancy or with severe liver or kidney diseases. *Avoid use*: respiratory depression, diseases causing obstruction of the airways. Not suitable for children. *Possible interaction*: alcohol, depressants of the central nervous system, MAOIs. *Side effects*: dry mouth, drowsiness, blurred vision. Tolerance and dependence may occur. *Manufacturer*: Glaxo Wellcome.

DICYNENE

Description: a haemostatic drug and preparation of ethamsylate, available as ampoules (250mg/2ml) and 500mg white capsules. *Used for*: prevention and treatment of periventricular bleeding in low birth weight infants. Also menorrhagia (abnormally heavy menstrual bleeding). *Dosage*: for the newly born, 12.5mg/kg body weight 6 hourly within 2 hours of birth given intravenously or intramuscularly, continuing for 4 days. For menorrhagia, one 500mg capsule 4 times per day from the start of bleeding to the end of menstruation. *Side effects*: headache, nausea, rash. *Manufacturer*: Delandale.

DIDRONEL PMO

Description: a diphosphonate/calcium supplement available as white capsule-shaped tablets containing 400mg etidronate disodium marked NE and 406; with 1250mg calcium carbonate (Cacit) as pink effervescent tablets with an orange taste. *Used for*: vertebral osteoporosis. *Dosage*: 1 tablet daily for 14 days taken with water in the middle of a 4-hour fast, followed by 1 Cacit tablet daily in water for 76 days. The 90-day cycle is repeated for 3 years. Also **DIDRONEL INJECTION** *Description*: ampoules of 50mg/ml etidronate disodium. *Used for*: hypercalcaemia associated with malignant tumours. *Dosage*: slow intravenous infusion of 7.5mg/kg daily for 3 days. Interval of 7 days thereafter. Also **DIDRONEL TABLETS** *Description*: 200mg of etidronate disodium in white rectangular tablets. *Used for*: Paget's disease after treatment for hypercalcaemia of malignancy. *Dosage*: 5mg/kg daily taken in the middle of a 4-hour fast over 6 months maximum (for Paget's disease). For hypercalcaemia, 20mg/kg for 30 days. *Special care*: pregnancy, lactation, enterocolitis (inflammation of the colon and small intestine). Monitor kidney function and ensure adequate intake of calcium and vitamin D. *Avoid use*: severe kidney disease. Not recommended for children. *Side effects*: diarrhoea, nausea. *Manufacturer*: Procter & Gamble Pharmaceuticals.

DIFLUCAN

Description: a triazole, fluconazole, available as blue and white (50mg), purple and white (200mg) capsules and **DIFLUCON SUSPENSION** (50mg and 200mg/5ml) and **DIFLUCAN INFUSION** (bottles with 2mg/ml). Both capsules marked with FLU, strength and PFIZER. *Used for*: candidiasis (thrush) whether oral or vaginal, systemic candidiasis, cryptococcosis (infection, with *Cryptococcus*, of the lungs and possibly the brains and CNS), oral/oropharyngeal candidosis, prevention of fungal infections following cytotoxic radio- or chemotherapy, for maintenance in AIDS sufferers to prevent relapse of cryptococcal meningitis. *Dosage*: oral/vaginal candidiasis, 50–100mg daily for 14 to 30 days. Systemic candidiasis, 400mg on first day, and 200–400mg daily thereafter. Oropharyngeal, 50–100mg daily for 7 to 14 days. Maintenance against meningitis, 100–100mg daily. Prevention of fungal infections, 50–100mg daily. Doses delivered orally or by intravenous infusion. For children over 1 year, only in the case of life-threatening infections, 3–6mg/kg daily. *Special care*: kidney damage with multiple doses. *Avoid use*: during pregnancy or lactation. *Possible interaction*: oral sulphonylureas, phenytoin, cyclosporin, rifampicin, theophylline, anticoagulants. *Side effects*: gastro-intestinal upsets. *Manufacturer*: Pfizer.

DIGIBIND

Description: an antidote for digoxin comprising 40mg of antibody fragments in a vial for reconstitution. *Used for*: digoxin overdose. *Dosage*: seek advice. *Special care*: kidney disease. *Avoid use*: allergy to ovine protein. *Side effects*: hypokalaemia. *Manufacturer*: Glaxo Wellcome.

DIHYDROCODEINE

Description: an analgesic opiate, dihydrocodeine tartrate, available as tablets (30mg strength). Also as **DIHYDROCODEINE ORAL SOLUTION**, a syrup containing 10mg per 5ml. *Used for*: moderate to severe pain. *Dosage*: 1 tablet or 5–15ml 4 to 6-hourly, after food and as required. Children, 4 to 12 years, 0.5–1mg/kg body weight, 4 to 6-hourly. Not suitable for children under 4 years. Also **DIHYDROCODEINE INJECTION** as 50mg/ml in ampoules. *Dosage*: up to 50mg by deep subcutaneous or intramuscular injection. Children, same details as for dihydrocodeine/oral solution. *Special care*: kidney disease or chronic liver disease, allergies, hypothyroidism. The elderly or pregnant. *Avoid use*: respiratory depression, or diseases that cause obstruction of the airways. *Possible interaction*: MAOIs, alcohol, depressants of the CNS. *Side effects*: nausea, headache, vertigo, constipation. *Manufacturer*: Knapp.

DILZEM SR

Description: an antihypertensive/antianginal calcium ion antagonist prepared as diltiazem hydrochloride. Available as beige sustained-release capsules of strengths 60, 90 or 120mg, marked with strength. *Used for*: angina, mild to moderate hypertension. *Dosage*: 90mg twice daily initially increasing to 180mg if required. For the elderly 60mg twice daily. Also **DILZEM XL**, white capsules of diltiazem hydrochloride available as 120, 180 or 240mg strengths. *Dosage*: 180mg daily increasing to 360mg. For the elderly, 120mg daily. *Special care*: diabetes, mild bradycardia, impaired left ventricular function, 1st degree AV block or porolonged P-R interval. *Avoid use*: pregnancy or lactation, 2nd or 3rd degree AV block, left ventricular failure, bradycardia, liver or kidney disease, sick sinus syndrome (syndromes associated with dysfunction of the sinus (sinoatrial) node, the heart tissue that generates the cardiac electrical impulse). *Possible interaction*: infusion of dantrolene, other cardiac depressants or hypertensives, also cyclosporin, digoxin, lithium, diazepam, cimetidine, theophylline, carbamazepine. *Side effects*: ankle oedema, nausea, rash, headache, flushes, gastro-intestinal upset, SA or AV block. *Manufacturer*: Elan.

DIMETRIOSE

Description: a gonadotrophin release inhibitor, gestrinone, in white capsules (2–5mg). *Used for*: endometriosis. *Dosage*: 1 twice weekly on the first and fourth day of the cycle, then on the same days of the week throughout the treatment. *Special care*: diabetes, hyperlipidaemia. *Avoid use*: in pregnancy, lactation. Severe heart, kidney or liver disease, metabolic or vascular disorders. *Possible interaction*: rifampicin, oral contraceptives, anticonvulsants. *Side effects*: gastro-intestinal upsets, cramp, hirsutism, depression, voice changes, acne, weight gain. *Manufacturer*: Hoechst.

DINDEVAN

Description: an anticoagulant, phenindione, of strengths 10 (white, marked D10), 25 (green, marked D25) and 50mg (white, marked D50). *Used for*: thromboembolic conditions. *Dosage*: 200mg to start, then 100mg the following day and subsequent daily maintenance dose of 50–150mg. *Special care*: the elderly, acute illness, vitamin K deficiency. Hypertension, weight changes, kidney disease. *Avoid use*: severe liver or kidney disease, haemorrhagic conditions, within 24 hours of surgery or labour. Pregnancy or lactation. *Possible interaction*: corticosteroids, NSAIDs, sulphonamides, oral hypoglycaemics, quinidine, antibiotics, phenformin, drugs affecting liver enzymes, cimetidine. *Side effects*: diarrhoea, hepatitis, kidney damage, urine discoloured, fever, rash, leucopenia, agranulocytosis (abnormal blood condition involving a reduction in the number of granulocytes). *Manufacturer*: Goldshield.

DIODERM

Description: a topical steroid, hydrocortisone, available as a 0.1% cream. *Used for*: allergic, pruritic or inflammatory skin conditions. *Dosage*: to be applied sparingly. Rub in well twice daily. *Special care*: maximum 5 days use on face or for children. Withdraw gradually after prolonged use. *Avoid use*: acne (and rosacea), scabies, leg ulcers, peri-oral dermatitis, untreated fungal or viral infections, tuberculous, ringworm or viral skin disease. Extensively or for prolonged period in pregnancy. *Side effects*: skin atrophy, striae, telangiectasia (multiple telangiectases, which are collections of distended blood capillaries), Cushingoid changes (see Cushing's syndrome). *Manufacturer*: Dermal.

DIPENTUM

Description: a salicylate, olsalazine sodium, available as a 250mg caramel capsule. *Used for*: acute mild ulcerative colitis. *Dosage*: 4 daily with food to begin, maximum 12 daily (all in divided doses). For maintenance, 2 twice daily with food. Not recommended for children. *Avoid use*: pregnancy, severe kidney disease, hypersensitivity to salicylates. *Side effects*: headache, rash, arthralgia (joint pain), gastro-intestinal upset. *Manufacturer*: Pharmacia & Upjohn.

DIPRIVAN

Description: a general anaesthetic, propofol, containing 10mg/ml as an emulsion in vials and ampoules. Associated with rapid recovery without a hangover effect. *Used for*: general anaesthesia at the start of surgery, and its maintenance. *Dosage*: by intravenous injection, 2–2.5mg/kg (less in the elderly) at 20–40mg per 10 seconds; adjusted for children. Maintenance, 4–12mg/kg/hour. *Side effects*: occasionally convulsions and brachycardia. *Manufacturer*: Zeneca.

DIPROSALIC

Description: a potent steroid and keratolytic (causing shedding of outer skin layer) ointment, containing betamethasone dipropionate (0.05%) and salicylic acid (3%). *Used for* hard skin and dry skin disorders. *Dosage*: apply thinly once or twice per day. Also **DIPROSALIC SCALP APPLICATION** comprising betamethasone dipropionate (0.05%), salicylic acid (2%) in solution. *Dosage*: apply a few drops to the scalp and rub in, twice daily. *Special care*: limit use on face to 5 days. Withdraw gradually after prolonged use. *Avoid use*: leg ulcers, scabies, peri-oral dermatitis, untreated fungal or viral infections, tuberculous, ringworm or viral skin diseases, acne. Lengthy or extensive use in pregnancy. Not for children. *Side effects*: skin striae and atrophy, telangiectasia (multiple telangiectases, which are collections of distended blood capillaries), Cushingoid changes (see Cushing's syndrome), adrenal gland suppression. *Manufacturer*: Schering-Plough.

DIPROSONE

Description: a potent steroid, betamethasone dipropionate, as 0.05% cream and ointment. *Used for*: skin diseases that respond to steroid treatment. *Dosage*: apply sparingly once or twice per day. Also **DIPROSONE LOTION**, 0.05% betamethasone dipropionate in alcoholic solution. *Used for*: scalp skin diseases *Dosage*: apply a few drops twice daily *Special care*: limit use on face to 5 days. Withdraw gradually after prolonged use. *Avoid use*: leg ulcers, scabies, peri-oral dermatitis, untreated fungal or viral infections, tuberculous, ringworm or viral skin diseases, acne. Lengthy or extensive use in pregnancy. Not for children. *Side effects*: skin striae and atrophy, telangiectasia (multiple telangiectases, which are collections of distended blood capillaries), Cushingoid changes (see Cushing's syndrome), adrenal gland suppression. *Manufacturer*: Schering-Plough.

DIRYTHMIN SA

Description: an antiarrhythmic, disopyramide phosphate, available as a white 150mg film-coated sustained-release tablet, marked A over DR. *Used for*: heart arrhythmias. *Dosage*: 2 every 12 hours, maximum 5 per day. *Special care*: kidney and liver failure, pregnancy, prostatic hypertrophy, glaucoma, urine retention, hypokalaemia, 1st degree AV block. *Avoid use*: cardiomyopathy, cardiogenic shock (low cardiac output), disease of the sinoatrial node when there is no pacemaker, 2nd or 3rd degree AV block. Not recommended for children. *Possible interaction*: ß-blockers, other antiarrhythmics in the same class, erythromycin, agents causing potassium reduction, anticholinergics (inhibiting the action of acetylcholine). *Side effects*: anticholinergic effects. *Manufacturer*: Astra.

DISIPAL

Description: an anticholinergic, orphenadrine hydrochloride, available in yellow, sugar-coated tablets, strength 50mg, marked DISIPAL. *Used for*: Parkinsonism. *Dosage*: 50mg 3 times per day initially, increased by 50mg every 2 to 3 days. Maintenance 100–300mg per day. Maximum 400mg daily. *Special care*: heart disorders, gastro-intestinal obstructions. Withdraw slowly. *Avoid use*: prostatic hypertrophy (enlarged prostate), glaucoma, tardive dyskinesia (repetitive muscular movements of the limbs, face or trunk). *Possible interaction*: antihistamines, antidepressants, phenothiazines. *Side effects*: confusion, agitation, rashes with high dosages, euphoria, anticholinergic effects. *Manufacturer*: Yamanouchi.

DISTACLOR MR

Description: a cephalosporin, cefaclor, available as a blue sustained-release tablet (375mg strength) marked with name and strength. *Used for*: infections of the skin, soft tissue and respiratory tract, otitis media, infections of the urinary tract. *Dosage*: 1 twice daily or 2 twice daily for the treatment of pneumonia. Not recommended for children. Also **DISTACLOR CAPSULES** available in white/violet (250mg), violet/grey (500mg) capsules; and Distaclor Suspension (125, 250mg/5ml.) *Dosage*: 250mg every 8 hours up to a maximum of 4g per day. Children from 1 month–1 year, 62.5mg; 1 to 5 years, 125mg; over 5 years, 250mg. All 3 times per day to a maximum of 1g. *Special care*: pregnancy or lactation. Kidney disease, hypersensitivity to penicillins. *Possible interaction*: anticoagulants. *Side effects*: gastro-intestinal upsets, hypersensitivity reactions, pseudomembranous colitis (a severe form of colitis). *Manufacturer*: Lilly.

DISTALGESIC

Description: an analgesic and compound opiate containing dextropropoxyphene hydrochloride (32.5mg) and paracetamol (325mg), available in white oblong film-coated tablets marked DG. *Used for*: mild to moderate pain. *Dosage*: 2, 3 or 4 times per day. Not recommended for children. *Special care*: kidney or liver disease, pregnancy or the elderly. *Possible interaction*: anticonvulsants, anticoagulants, alcohol, depressants of the central nervous system. *Side effects*: constipation, drowsiness, dizziness, nausea, rash, tolerance and dependence. *Manufacturer*: Dista.

DISTAMINE

Description: a penicillin derivative penicillamine, available as white tablets of strengths 50, 125 (marked DS and 125) and 250mg (marked DM and 250). *Used for*: severe active rheumatoid arthritis, heavy metal poisoning, chronic hepatitis, cystinuria (abnormal occurrence of cystine, an amino acid, in the urine), Wilson's disease (a defect in copper metabolism causing deposition of copper in the liver or brain, producing jaundice and cirrhosis, and mental retardation respectively). *Dosage*: 125–250mg daily for 4 weeks increasing by 125–2500 mg at intervals of 4 to 12 weeks. Maximum daily dose 1.5g. Maintenance dose 500–750mg. For the elderly, 50–125mg daily increasing to 500–750mg and a maximum of 1g per day. Children, 50mg per day for 1 month increasing 4-weekly. Maintenance 15–20mg/kg of body weight per day. *Special care*: kidney disease, sensitivity to penicillin, blood, urine and functioning of kidneys should be monitored during treatment. *Avoid use*: pregnancy, lactation, agranulocytosis (abnormal blood condition involving a reduction in the number of granulocytes), thrombocytopenia, lupus erythematosus (an inflammatory disease affecting the skin and some internal organs, regarded as an autoimmune disease). *Possible interaction*: antacids, gold, zinc or iron salts, cytotoxic or antimalarial drugs, phenylbutazone. *Side effects*: fever, rash, anorexia, nausea, blood disorders, loss of taste, proteinuria, myasthenia gravis, haematuria, SLE, nephrotic syndrome. *Manufacturer*: Dista.

DITROPAN

Description: an anticholinergic/antispasmodic, oxybutynin hydrochloride, available as blue tablets in strengths 2.5mg and 5mg. All marked with tablet name, strength and company initials. Also **DITROPAN ELIXIR** as 2.5mg/5ml. *Used for*: nocturnal enuresis (involuntary urination/bedwetting), urinary frequency and incontinence, neurogenic bladder instability (often relating to the detrusor muscle of the bladder). *Dosage*: 5mg 2 or 3 times per day to a daily maximum of 20g. 5mg twice daily for the elderly. Not recommended for children under 5; 5mg 2 or 3 times per day for children over 5. Last dose to be given at bedtime for nocturnal enuresis. *Special care*: liver or kidney disease, hyperthyroidism, congestive heart failure, coronary artery disease, cardiac arrhythmias, tachycardia, hiatus hernia, prostatic hypertrophy, autonomic neuropathy. The frail, elderly or in pregnancy. *Avoid use*: bladder or bowel obstruction, severe ulcerative colitis, glaucoma, lactation, myasthenia gravis, intestinal atony (weak), toxic megacolon (a serious complication of ulcerative colitis, involving massive dilatation of the colon). *Possible interaction*: levodopa, digoxin, butyrophenones, amantadine, phenothiazines, tricyclic antidepressants, anticholinergics. *Side effects*: facial flushes, anticholinergic effects (limit transmission of parasympathetic nerve impulses). *Manufacturer*: Lorex.

DIUMIDE-K CONTINUS

Description: a loop diuretic (a powerful, short-duration drug that acts on the loop of Henle in the kidney) and potassium ion supplement, available as frusemide (40mg) and sustained-release potassium chloride (600mg) in white and orange film-coated tablets marked DK. *Used for*: kidney and liver disease where a potassium supplement is required, oedema including that associated with congestive heart failure. *Dosage*: 1 tablet per day, taken in the morning. *Special care*: diabetes, pregnancy, lactation. Gout, prostatic hypertrophy, liver or kidney disease, impaired urination. *Avoid use*: hyperkalaemia, Addison's disease, precomatose states in cases of liver cirrhosis. *Possible interaction*: NSAIDs, cephalosporins, antihypertensives, lithium, digitalis, aminoglycosides, potassium-sparing diuretics. *Side effects*: gout. To be discontinued if small bowel appears to be ulcerated or obstructed. *Manufacturer*: ASTA Medica.

DIUREXAN

Description: a thiazide-like diuretic, xipamide, available as 20mg, white tablets, marked A. *Used for*: oedema, hypertension, congestive heart failure. *Dosage*: 1 each morning for hypertension; 2 each morning for oedema initially, then 1 to 4 daily as required. Not recommended for children. *Special care*: liver or kidney disease, liver cirrhosis, diabetes, SLE, gout. The elderly, during pregnancy or lactation. Monitor fluid glucose and electrolytes. *Avoid use*: severe liver or kidney failure, hypercalcaemia, sensitivity to sulphonamides, Addison's disease. *Possible interaction*: NSAIDs, corticosteroids, carbenoxolone, tubocurarine, antidiabetic agents, alcohol, barbiturates, opioids, lithium, cardiac glycosides. *Side effects*: gastro-intestinal upset, photosensitivity, rash, blood disorders, pancreatitis, dizziness, impotence, disturbance of electrolytes and metabolism. *Manufacturer*: ASTA Medica.

DOBUTREX

Description: a β_1-antagonist (acts on beta$_1$ receptors in cardiac muscle) dobutamine hydrochloride available in vials, as a solution of 12.5mg/ml. *Used for*: cardiac surgery, cardiomyopathies, septic and cardiogenic shock (low cardiac output with acute myocardial infarction and congestive heart failure), inotropic (i.e. affecting heart muscle contraction) support in infarction. *Dosage*: intravenous infusion of 2.5–10mg/kg/minute varying with response. *Special care*: severe hypotension complicating cardiogenic shock. *Side effects*: tachycardia, increase in systolic blood pressure indicating overdosage. *Manufacturer*: Lilly.

DOLMATIL

Description: a substitute benzamide, sulpiride, available as white tablets (200mg) marked D200. *Used for*: chronic schizophrenia. *Dosage*: over 14 years, 400–800mg initially per day in divided doses then 200–1200mg twice daily varying with required result. Not recommended for children under 14 years. *Special care*: epilepsy, pregnancy, kidney disease, hypomania (a mental state of hyperactivity and irritability). *Avoid use*: phaeochromocytoma. *Possible interaction*: alcohol, analgesics, depressants of the CNS, antidepressants, antidiabetics, levodopa, anticonvulsants, antihypertensives. *Side effects*: muscle spasms, restlessness, rigidity and tremor, urine retention, tachycardia, constipation, dry mouth, hypotension, blurred vision, impotence, weight gain, galactorrhea, hypothermia, amenorrhoea, blood and skin disorders, lethargy, jaundice. *Manufacturer*: Delandale.

DOLOBID

Description: a salicylate analgesic and anti-inflammatory drug containing diflurisal and available as peach (250mg) and orange (500mg) film-coated tablets, marked DOLOBID. *Used for*: acute and chronic pain; rheumatoid arthritis and osteoarthritis. *Dosage*: 500mg twice daily then 250–500mg twice daily for maintenance. For arthritis, 500–1000mg daily, in 1 or 2 doses and varying according to the response. Not recommended for children. *Special care*: kidney or liver disease, heart failure, the elderly, a history of gastro-intestinal ulcers or haemorrhage. Kidneys and liver to be monitored during long-term treatment. *Avoid use*: pregnancy, lactation, active peptic ulcer, aspirin or anti-inflammatory-induced allergy or asthma. *Possible interaction*: anticoagulants, indomethacin. *Side effects*: diarrhoea, dyspepsia, headache, rash, tinnitus, dizziness, gastro-intestinal pain. *Manufacturer*: Morson.

DOLOXENE

Description: an opiate, dextropropoxyphene napsylate, available as pink capsules (60mg) marked LILLY H64. *Used for*: mild to moderate pain. *Dosage*: 1, 3 or 4 times per day. *Special care*: pregnancy, the elderly, kidney or liver disease. *Possible interaction*: anticonvulsants, anticoagulants, alcohol, CNS depressants. *Side effects*: drowsiness, constipation, nausea, dizziness, rash. Also tolerance and dependence. *Manufacturer*: Lilly.

DOLOXENE CO

Description: an analgesic comprising an opiate, salicylate and xanthine containing dextropropoxyphene napsylate (100mg), aspirin (375mg) and caffeine (30mg) and available as red and grey capsules marked H91. *Used for*: mild to moderate pain. *Dosage*: 1, 3 to 4 times per day. *Special care*: kidney or liver disease (monitor during long-term treatment), heart failure, the elderly, anti-inflammatory induced allergies or a history of bronchospasm. *Avoid use*: haemophilia, active peptic ulcer, hypoprothrombinaemia (lack of prothrombin in the blood, upsetting clotting function). *Possible interaction*: alcohol, CNS depressants, anticonvulsants, anticoagulants, hypoglycaemics, uricosurics (drugs for elimination of uric acid or relief of pain due to gout). *Side effects*: nausea, rash, drowsiness, constipation, dizziness. Also tolerance and dependence. *Manufacturer*: Lilly.

DOPACARD

Description: a catecholamine, dopexamine hydrochloride, available in ampoules as a solution (50mg/5ml). *Used for*: inotropic (i.e. affecting heart muscle contraction) support and vasodilation in heart failure during cardiac surgery. *Dosage*: 0.5mg/kg/minute by intravenous infusion which may be increased to 6mg/kg/minute. *Special care*: myocardial infarction, recent angina, hyperglycaemia, hypokalaemia. Monitor pulse, blood pressure etc. *Avoid use*: thrombocytopenia, phaeochromocytoma, obstruction of the left ventricular outlet. *Side effects*: increased heart rate, nausea, vomiting, tremor, anginal pain. *Manufacturer*: Speywood.

DOPRAM

Description: a respiratory stimulant, doxapram hydrochloride, available in 5ml ampoules (20mg/ml). Also **DOPRAM INFUSION** (2mg/ml). *Used for*: ventilatory failure in cases of chronic obstructive airways disease. *Dosage*: 1.5–

4mg per minute by intravenous infusion, varying according to patient's condition and response. *Special care*: epilepsy, liver impairment; used only under precise, expert supervision in hospital. *Avoid use*: coronary artery disease, severe hypertension, thyrotoxicosis, status asthmaticus (asthma attack lasting over 24 hours). *Possible interaction*: sympathomimetics, theophylline. *Side effects*: dizziness, increase in heart rate and blood pressure. *Manufacturer*: Anpharm.

DORALESE

Description: a selective a_1 blocker, indoramin, available as pale yellow traingular film-coated tablets (20mg strength). *Used for*: obstruction of urine outflow due to benign prostatic hypertrophy. *Dosage*: 1 tablet twice daily. *Special care*: liver or kidney disease, patients with poor heart function, epilepsy, depression, Parkinsonism. *Avoid use*: in cases of heart failure. *Possible interaction*: antihypertensives, MAOIs. *Side effects*: drowsiness, dry mouth, blocked nose, ejaculation failure, weight gain. *Manufacturer*: Bencard.

DOVONEX

Description: an ointment and vitamin D analogue, containing 0.005% calcipotriol, also available as **DOVONEX CREAM**. *Used for*: mild to moderate psoriasis. *Dosage*: to be applied twice daily up to a maximum of 100g per week. *Special care*: during pregnancy and lactation. Avoid the face. *Avoid use*: calcium metabolism disorders. *Side effects*: temporary irritation, facial (including peri-oral) dermatitis. *Manufacturer*: Leo.

DOZIC

Description: an antipsychotic drug, butyrophenone available as a liquid preparation of haloperidol in 2 strengths, 1 and 2mg/ml. *Used for*: mania, schizophrenia, psychoses, delirium tremens, alcohol withdrawal syndrome, childhood behavioural disorders. *Dosage*: psychosis in the elderly: 0.5 0 2mg initially, others 0.5–5mg, both 2 to 3 times per day, increasing as required to a daily maximum of 200mg. This is reduced when control is gained, to a daily dose of 5–10mg. For anxiety, 0.5mg twice daily. For children, 0.05mg/kg daily in 2 divided doses. *Special care*: liver or kidney failure, epilepsy, Parkinsonism, pregnancy, thyrotoxicosis and severe cardiovascular disease. *Avoid use*: if patient is unconscious. *Possible interaction*: alcohol, analgesics, CNS depressants, anticonvulsants, antidiabetics, antidepressants, antihypertensives, levodopa. *Side effects*: spasms of eye, face, neck and back muscles, dry mouth, blocked nose, restlessness, tremor and rigidity, tardive dyskinesia (involuntary, repetitious muscle movements), urine retention, tachycardia, constipation, blurred vision, weight gain, impotence, hypothermia, menstrual changes, skin and blood changes, drowsiness, lethargy, sometimes fits. *Manufacturer*: Rosemont.

DRICLOR

Description: a 20% solution of aluminium chloride hexahydrate in roll-on bottle. *Used for*: very heavy sweating (hyperhidiosis) of hands, feet and armpits.

Dosage: apply at night and wash off in the morning. Reduce applications as sweating lessens. Use only on feet for children. *Special care*: area to be treated should be dry and not shaved. Contact with clothes and jewellery to be avoided. *Avoid use*: on broken or inflamed skin. *Side effects*: skin irritation. *Manufacturer*: Stiefel.

DROGENIL

Description: an anti-androgen and form of flutamide available as a 250mg yellow tablet. *Used for*: advanced prostatic cancer. *Dosage*: 1 tablet 3 times per day. *Special care*: fluid retention in patients with heart disease. Liver function tests should be performed periodically. *Possible interaction*: warfarin. *Side effects*: gynaecomastia, breast tenderness, gastro-intestinal upsets, galactorrhea. Increased appetite, tiredness and insomnia. *Manufacturer*: Schering-Plough.

DROLEPTAN

Description: a butyrophenone, droperidol, available as a 10mg yellow tablet marked JANSSEN and D10. Also **DROLEPTAN LIQUID** as 1mg/ml of droperidol. *Used for*: the rapid soothing of manic, agitated patients. *Dosage*: 5–20mg every 4 to 8 hours. Children 0.5–1mg daily. Adjusted to match response. Also **DROLEPTAN INJECTION** available as 2ml ampoules (5mg/ml). *Dosage*: 5–15mg intravenously or up to 10mg intramuscularly every 4 to 6 hours. Children 0.5–1mg daily, intramuscularly. Adjust to match response. Also available as 2ml ampoules containing 5mg/ml. *Used for*: post-operative or chemotherapy-induced nausea. *Dosage*: 5mg intravenously or intramuscularly postoperatively. 1–10mg by the same means 30 minutes before chemotherapy then 1–3mg/hr by continuous intravenous infusion or 1–5mg intramuscularly or intravenously every 1 to 6 hours. Children 0.02–0.075mg/kg by the same means. *Special care*: Parkinsonism, epilepsy, pregnancy, lactation, severe liver disease. *Avoid use*: severe depression or comatose states. *Possible interaction*: alcohol, analgesics, depressants of the CNS, anticonvulsants, antidiabetics, antidepressants, antihypertensives, levodopa. *Side effects*: spasms of eye, face, neck and back muscles, dry mouth, blocked nose, restlessness, tremor and rigidity, tardive dyskinesia (involuntary, repetitious muscle movements), urine retention, tachycardia, constipation, blurred vision, weight gain, impotence, hypothermia, menstrual changes, skin and blood changes, drowsiness, lethargy, sometimes fits. *Manufacturer*: Janssen-Cilag.

DTIC-DOME

Description: a cytotoxic drug and preparation of dacarbazine available as powder in vials for reconstitution (100 and 200mg). *Used for*: soft tissue sarcomas and in combination for Hodgkin's disease. *Dosage*: by intravenous injection. *Special care*: an anti-emetic should be given simultaneously to lessen the risk of nausea and vomiting. Kidney function and hearing should be monitored. *Avoid use*: again within 4 weeks. *Side effects*: severe nausea and vomiting, alopecia, bone marrow suppression (necessitating blood counts), skin irritation. *Manufacturer*: Bayer.

DUOVENT

Description: a ß$_2$ agonist and anticholinergic consisting of 100 g ipratropium bromide in a metered dose aerosol. Also **DUOVENT AUTOHALER**. *Used for*: obstruction to airways; for bronchodilation. *Dosage*: 1 or 2 puffs 3 to 4 times daily. Children over 6, 1 puff 3 times per day. Not recommended for children under 6. Also **DUOVENT UDVS**, 1.25mg fenoterol hydrobromide and 500 g ipratropium bromide per 4ml of solution, in vials. *Used for*: acute severe asthma. *Dosage*: over 14 years, 1 vial nebulized immediately. Repeat under supervision. Maximum of 4 vials in 24 hours. *Special care*: angina, arrhythmias, hyperthyroidism, heart muscle disease, hypertension, glaucoma, prostatic hypertrophy. *Possible interaction*: sympathomimetics. *Side effects*: headache, dry mouth, peripheral dilatation. *Manufacturer*: Boehringer Ingelheim.

DUPHASTON

Description: a progestogen, dydrogesterone, available as a white tablet (10mg strength) marked DUPHAR 155. *Used for*: dysmenorrhoea (painful menstruation), dysfunctional (abnormal) bleeding, endometriosis, premenstrual syndrome (PMS), as part of hormone replacement therapy (HRT), habitual and threatened abortion. *Dosage*: 1 twice daily from day 5 to 25 of the cycle (dysmenorrhoea); 1 tablet 2 or 3 times per day from days 5 to 25 or continuously (endometriosis); 1 twice daily from days 12 to 26 (PMS), 1 twice daily for the first 12 to 14 days of the month (HRT). *Special care*: high blood pressure, tendency to thrombosis, liver abnormalities, ovarian cysts, migraine, diabetes. *Avoid use*: pregnancy, severe heart or kidney disease, previous ectopic pregnancy, benign liver tumours, undiagnosed vaginal bleeding. *Possible interaction*: cyclosporin. *Side effects*: breast tenderness, irregular menstruation, acne, fluid retention and weight gain. *Manufacturer*: Solvay.

DUROMINE^{CD}

Desription: a CNS stimulant, phentermine, available as sustained-release capsules, 15mg (green/grey) and 30mg (maroon/grey), both marked with name and strength. *Used for*: obesity. *Dosage*: 15–30mg daily, at breakfast. *Special care*: angina, arrhythmias, hypertension. *Avoid use*: pregnancy, lactation, arteriosclerosis, hyperthyroidism, severe hypertension, drug/alcohol abuse, past psychiatric illness. *Possible interaction*: antihypertensives, sympathomimetics, MAOIs, psychotropics (mood-affecting drugs). *Side effects*: oedema, tachycardia, raised blood pressure, restlessness, hallucinations. Possible tolerance, dependence, psychoses—avoid prolonged use. *Manufacturer*: 3M Health Care.

DYAZIDE

Description: a potassium-sparing thiazide diuretic, consisting of 50mg triamterene and 25mg hydrochlorothiazide in peach tablets coded SKF E93.

Used for: oedema, mild to moderate hypertension. *Dosage*: 1 twice daily after meals, falling to 1 daily (oedema), daily maximum of 4. Initially 1 daily for hypertension. *Special care*: diabetes, acidosis, gout, pregnancy, lactation, pancreatitis, liver or kidney disease. *Avoid use*: Addison's disease, hypercalcaemia, hyperkalaemia, severe liver or kidney failure. *Possible interaction*: potassium supplements, potassium-sparing diuretics, lithium, digitalis, NSAIDs, ACE inhibitors, antihypertensives. *Side effects*: diarrhoea, nausea, vomiting, headache, dry mouth, weakness, cramps, rash, hypercalcaemia, hyperglycaemia, low blood pressure. *Manufacturer*: S.K.F.

DYSPAMET

Description: a form of cimetidine in white square chewable tablets (200mg). Also, DYSPAMET SUSPENSION (200mg/5ml). *Used for*: persistent acid-related dyspeptic conditions. *Dosage*: 2 chewed thoroughly (or 10ml) twice daily, at breakfast and bedtime. Minimum recommended course, 4 weeks. *Special care*: exclude malignancy first; pregnancy, lactation, impaired kidneys, monitor for long-term treatment. *Possible interaction*: phenytoin, theophylline, oral anticoagulants. *Side effects*: tiredness, dizziness, rash, diarrhoea, gynaecomastia, confusion. *Manufacturer*: SmithKline Beecham.

DYSPORT

Description: a bacterial, botulinum, toxin, type A-haemagglutinin complex (500 units as pellets in vial). *Used for*: eyelid and hemifacial spasm. *Dosage*: 120 units for affected eye, by subcutaneous injection, spread over 4 sites around the eye (see accompanying literature). Repeat as necessary or every 8 weeks. *Special care*: pregnancy, lactation, caution to inject accurately. *Side effects*: minor bruising and eyelid swelling, paralysis of mid-facial muscles, reduced blinking giving dry eyes and keratitis (inflammation of the cornea), double vision, eyelid droop (ptosis). *Manufacturer*: Speywood.

DYTAC

Description: a potassium-sparing diuretic, triamterene, available as 50mg capsules marked SKF. *Used for:* oedema in congestive heart failure, liver or kidney disease. *Dosage*: 3 to 5 per day in divided doses. Use on alternate days after first week. *Special care*: elderly, gout, pregnancy, lactation, liver or kidney disease, acidosis, diabetic nephropathy (kidney disease related to diabetes). *Avoid use*: Addison's disease, hyperkalaemia, progressive kidney or liver disease. *Possible interaction*: potassium supplements, potassium-sparing diuretics, ACE inhibitors, antihypertensives, indomethacin. *Side effects*: weakness, headache, cramps, nausea, diarrhoea, dry mouth, rash, blood dyscrasias (abnormal blood or bone marrow condition e.g. leukaemia), metabolic disturbances. *Manufacturer*: Pharmark.

DYTIDE

Description: a potassium-sparing thyazide diuretic comprising 50mg triamterene and 25mg benzthiazide in capsules (clear/maroon) marked SKF. *Used for*: oedema. *Dosage*: 2 after breakfast and 1 after lunch to begin with, then 1 or 2 on alternate days for maintenance. *Special care*: liver or kidney disease, gout, elderly, pregnancy, lactation, diabetes. *Avoid use*: severe kidney failure or progressive liver or kidney disease, Addison's disease, hypercalcaemia, diabetic keto-acidosis (acute side effects of uncontrolled diabetes mellitus with electrolyte imbalance, very high blood glucose and acidosis). *Possible interaction*: potassium supplements, potassium-sparing diuretics, indomethasin, ACE inhibitors, antihypertensives, digitalis, lithium. *Side effects*: weakness, headache, nausea, cramps, diarrhoea, rash, dry mouth, blood dyscrasias (abnormal blood or bone marrow conditions, e.g. leukaemia), metabolic disturbances. *Manufacturer*: Pharmark.

E

ECONACORT

Description: a combined topical steroid and antifungal antibacterial preparation produced in the form of a cream containing 1% hydrocortisone and 1% econazole nitrate. *Used for*: Gram-positive bacterial and fungal skin infections with inflammation. *Dosage*: massage into affected skin morning and night. *Special care*: use in children or on face should be limited to a period of 5 days; short-term use only and withdraw gradually. *Avoid use*: continuous or prolonged use especially in pregnant women, untreated bacterial or fungal infections, infections caused by tuberculosis, viruses or ringworm, acne, leg ulcers, scabies, peri-oral dermatitis. *Side effects*: adrenal gland suppression, thinning of skin, fluid retention. *Manufacturer*: Squibb.

EDECRIN

Description: a proprietary loop diuretic (one which acts on part of the loops of Henle of the kidney tubules), in the form of white scored tablets, marked MSD 90, containing 50mg ethacrynic acid. Also **EDECRIN INJECTION** containing sodium ethacrynate equivalent to 50mg ethacrynic acid as powder in vial for reconstitution. *Used for*: oedema including that which accompanies liver and kidney diseases and congestive heart failure. *Dosage*: adults, 1 tablet daily after breakfast in first instance increasing by half to 1 each day as required. Usual dose is in the order of 1 to 3 tablets daily with maximum of 8 in divided doses. Injection: 50mg given intravenously. Children, 2 to 12 years, half tablet each day after breakfast, increasing by half tablet to the minimum effective dose required. *Special care*: pregnancy, gout, enlarged prostate gland, liver disease, diabetes, impaired urination. Electrolyte levels should be monitored and potassium supplements may be needed. *Avoid use*: children under 2 years, breast-feeding mothers, patients suffering from anuria, liver cirrhosis, serious kidney failure. *Possible interaction*: antihypertensives, corticosteroids, digitalis, lithium, warfarin, aminoglycosides. *Side effects*: blood changes, gastro-intestinal upset, jaundice, gout. *Manufacturer*: M.S.D.

EFALITH

Description: a proprietary anti-inflammatory preparation produced as an ointment containing 8% lithium succinate and 0.05% zinc sulphate. *Used for*: seborrhoeic dermatitis. *Dosage*: apply thinly to affected skin and rub in, twice each day in the morning and at night. *Special care*: patients with psoriasis; avoid eyes and mucous membranes. *Avoid use*: children. *Side effects*: local irritation at site of application. *Manufacturer*: Searle.

EFAMAST

Description: a fatty acid preparation in soft gelatin, oblong-shaped capsules containing 40mg gamolenic acid. *Used for*: mastalgia (breast pain). *Dosage*: adults, 3 to 4 capsules twice each day. *Special care*: patients suffering from epilepsy. Possibility of breast cancer should be eliminated before treatment begins. *Side effects*: headache, nausea. *Manufacturer*: Searle.

EFCORTELAN

Description: a topical corticosteroid preparation produced as cream and ointment of different strengths containing 0.5%, 1% or 2.5% hydrocortisone. Mildly potent. *Used for*: dermatitis, inflammation and itching in anal and urinongenital areas, neurodermatitis (an itching skin disorder seen in nervous, anxious persons). *Dosage:* rub into affected areas 2 or 3 times each day. *Special care*: use in children or on face should be limited to 5 days. Short-term use and withdraw gradually. *Avoid use*: long-term or extensive use, especially in pregnant women. Untreated fungus or bacterial skin infections or those which are viral or tuberculous in origin, ringworm, acne, leg ulcers, scabies. *Side effects*: thinning of skin, adrenal gland suppression, hair growth. *Manufacturer*: Glaxo Wellcome.

EFCORTELAN SOLUBLE

Description: a glucocorticoid-mineralocorticoid preparation produced as a powder in vials for reconstitution and injection and containing 100mg hydrocortisone (as sodium succinate). *Used for*: severe shock, adrenal gland failure, status asthmaticus (very severe and prolonged asthma attack which may prove life-threatening). *Dosage*: adults, 100–500mg by slow intravenous injection repeated according to patient's response. Children up to 1 year, 25mg; 1 to 5 years, 50mg; 6 to 12 years, 100mg, all given by slow intravenous injection. *Special care*: pregnancy, hypertension, various inflammatory kidney disorders (nephritis, glomerulonephritis), diabetes, osteoporosis, epilepsy, secondary cancers, recent intestinal anastomoses, liver cirrhosis, thrombophlebitis, peptic ulcer, exanthematous diseases (characterized by rash). Also, stress or psychoses. Contact with chicken pox should be avoided (and specialist care is required for those contracting this disease). Drug should be withdrawn gradually. *Possible interaction*: NSAIDs, anticholinesterases, diuretics, anticoagulants taken by mouth, cardiac glycosides, phenobarbitone, phenytoin, rifampicin, ephedrine. *Side effects*: hypertension, weakness, depression and euphoria, hyperglycaemia, peptic ulcer, potassium loss, fluid retention, Cushingoid changes (as in Cushing's Syndrome). *Manufacturer*: Glaxo.

EFCORTESOL

Description: a glucocorticoid-mineralocorticoid preparation produced as a solution in ampoules for injection, containing 100mg hydrocortisone (as sodium phosphate) per ml. Efcortesol is available in 1ml and 5ml ampoules. *Used for*: severe shock, adrenal gland failure, status asthmaticus (very severe and prolonged asthma attack which may prove life-threatening). *Dosage*: adults, 100–500mg by slow intravenous injection repeated according to patient's response. Children, up to 1 year, 25mg; 1 to 5 years, 50mg; 6 to 12 years, 100mg, all given by slow intravenous injection. *Special care*: pregnancy, hypertension, various inflammatory kidney disorders (nephritis, glomerulonephritis), diabetes, osteoporosis, epilepsy, secondary cancers, recent intestinal anastomoses, liver cirrhosis, thrombophlebitis, peptic ulcer, exanthematous diseases (characterized by rash); patients suffering from stress or psychoses. Avoid contact with chicken pox (specialist care is required for those contracting this disease). Drug should be withdrawn gradually., *Possible interaction*: NSAIDs, anticholin-esterases, diuretics, anticoagulants taken by mouth, cardiac glycosides, phenobarbitone, phenytoin, rifampicin, ephedrine. *Side effects*: hypertension, weakness, depression and euphoria, hyperglycaemia, peptic ulcer, potassium loss, fluid retention, Cushingoid changes (as in Cushing's Syndrome). *Manufacturer*: Glaxo Wellcome.

ELDEPRYL

Description: a proprietary preparation of an anti-Parkinsonism drug which is a monoamine oxidase-B inhibitor (monoamine oxidase B is an enzyme which breaks down dopamine). A deficiency in dopamine accompanies Parkinson's disease and the drug prolongs dopaminergic function in the brain. Eldepryl is produced as white, scored tablets of 2 strengths containing 5mg and 10mg selegiline hydrochloride. *Used for*: Parkinsonism; (sometimes given along with levodopa). *Dosage*: adults, 10mg daily either as a single morning dose, or in divided doses in the morning and middle of the day; taken with meals. *Special care*: if taken with levodopa, side effects of this may be increased and the dosage of levodopa may need to be reduced. *Side effects*: nausea, confusion, agitation, vomiting, hypotension. *Manufacturer*: Orion.

ELDISINE

Description: a cytotoxic drug which is a vinca alkaloid produced in the form of a powder in vials for reconstitution and injection. Eldisine contains 5mg vindesine sulphate in vial and in addition, 5ml diluent. *Used for*: leukaemia, lymphomas and some other forms of solid tumour, e.g. those which may affect the lung or breast. *Dosage*: as directed by physician skilled in cancer chemotherapy. *Special care*: precautions must be observed in handling. Powder should be reconstituted by skilled staff wearing protective clothing and gloves under controlled conditions. Contact with skin and eyes should be avoided. *Side effects*: vomiting, hair loss, bone marrow suppression, possible early menopause in women, sterility in men. *Manufacturer*: Lilly.

ELOCON

Description: a topical and potent steroid produced as an ointment and cream containing 0.1% mometasone furoate. Also **ELOCON LOTION** (same strength). *Used for*: atopic dermatitis (extremely itchy, damaged skin (caused by scratching in allergic individuals), psoriasis including that of the scalp, seborrhoeic dermatitis. *Dosage*: apply thinly once each day. *Special care*: pregnancy, hypertension, various inflammatory kidney disorders (nephritis, glomerulonephritis), diabetes, osteoporosis, epilepsy, secondary cancers, recent intestinal anastomoses, liver cirrhosis, thrombophlebitis, peptic ulcer, exanthematous diseases (characterized by rash). Also, stress or psychoses. Contact with chicken pox should be avoided (and specialist care is required for those contracting this disease). Drug should be withdrawn gradually. *Possible interaction*: NSAIDs, diuretics, anticholinesterases, anticoagulants taken by mouth, cardiac glycosides, phenobarbitone, phenytoin, rifampicin, ephedrine. *Side effects*: hypertension, weakness, depression and euphoria, hyperglycaemia, peptic ulcer, potassium loss, fluid retention, Cushingoid changes (as in Cushing's Syndrome). Any adverse reactions should be reported to Committee on Safety of Medicines. *Manufacturer*: Schering-Plough.

ELTROXIN

Description: a preparation of thyroid hormone, thyroxine sodium, produced in the form of tablets of 2 strengths: 50 g (white, scored) and 100 g (white) both marked with name and strength. *Used for*: hypothyroidism in children and adults, including cretinism and myxoedema. *Dosage*: adults, 50–100 g each day in first instance increasing every 3 to 4 weeks by 50 g according to response until optimum dose is achieved. Maximum dose is 100–100 g each day. Children 25 g each day in first instance, increasing every 2 to 4 weeks by 25 g according to response. Dose should then be slightly reduced. *Special care*: pregnancy, breastfeeding, elderly, patients with weak hearts or with reduced adrenal gland function. *Possible interaction*: anticonvulsants, sympathomimetics, antidiabetics, tricyclics, cardiac glycosides, anticoagulants. *Side effects*: tachycardia, muscular cramps, chest pains, sweating, flushing, arrhythmias, severe weight loss. *Manufacturer*: Goldshield.

ELYZOL

Description: an antibacterial preparation produced in the form of a gel with applicator containing 25% metronidazole. *Used for*: additional therapy in severe periodontal disease. *Dosage*: apply gel to affected area and repeat after 1 week. *Special care*: pregnant women. *Avoid use*: do not repeat therapy until 6 months have elapsed. Not for children. *Possible interaction*: alcohol, disulfiram, anticoagulants taken orally. *Side effects*: local inflammation, headache. *Manufacturer*: Dumex.

EMCOR

Description: an antianginal and anti-hypertensive preparation, which is a cardioselective ß-blocker, produced in the form of heart-shaped, orange, film-coated tablets containing 10mg bisoprolol fumarate. Also, EMCOR LS (5mg) which are yellow, scored, film-coated tablets. *Used for*: angina, hypertension. *Dosage*: 10mg once each day with a maximum daily dose of 20mg. *Special care*: pregnancy, breast-feeding, liver or kidney disease, diabetes, metabolic acidosis, general anaesthesia. May require to be withdrawn before planned surgery and should be stopped gradually. Patients with weak heart should receive diuretics and digitalis. *Avoid use*: children, patients with obstructive airways disease or history of bronchospasm, heart and circulatory diseases including heart block, heart failure, heart shock, sick sinus syndrome, sinus bradycardia and peripheral arterial disease. *Possible interaction*: CNS depressants, cardiac-depressant anaesthetics, ergotamine, indomethacin, reserpine, sympathomimetics, some other anti-hypertensives, clonidine withdrawal, cimetidine, hypoglycaemic, verapamil, class I antiarrhythmics. *Side effects*: cold feet and hands, fatigue on exertion, disturbance of sleep, gastro-intestinal upset, bradycardia, bronchospasm, heart failure. Withdraw gradually if dry eyes or skin rash appear. *Manufacturer*: Merck.

EMESIDE

Description: an anticonvulsant preparation produced as capsules and as a flavoured syrup. Orange capsules contain 250mg ethosuximide and blackcurrant or orange-flavoured **EMESIDE SYRUP** contains 250mg per 5ml. *Used for*: epilepsy. *Dosage*: adults, 500mg each day in first instance increasing by 250mg at 5 to 7-day intervals until condition is controlled. Maximum daily dose is 2g. Children under 6 years, 250mg each day in first instance adjusted every few days by small amounts until condition is controlled. Maximum daily dose is 1g. Children over 6 years receive adult dose. *Special care*: pregnancy, breast-feeding; liver or kidney disease. Drug should be withdrawn gradually. *Side effects*: blood changes, central nervous system effects, gastro-intestinal upset, SLE, skin rashes. *Manufacturer*: L.A.B.

EMFLEX

Description: an NSAID which is a form of indomethacin and is produced as orange/yellow capsules containing 60mg acemetacin. *Used for*: osteoarthritis, rheumatoid arthritis, pain and inflammation following surgery and lower back pain. *Dosage*: adults, 2 tablets daily in divided doses taken with meals, a glass of milk, or with an antacid preparation. The maximum daily dose is 3 capsules. *Special care*: liver or kidney disease, congestive heart failure, elderly persons, septic infections, epilepsy, Parkinsonism, psychiatric illness, imbalance in fluid or electrolyte levels. Patients on long-term treatment should receive checks on liver and kidney function, blood count and eyes. *Avoid use*: children, pregnancy, breast-feeding, certain gastro-intestinal disorders, peptic ulcer, angioneurotic oedema. Also, allergy to NSAID or aspirin. *Possible interaction*: thiazides, salcylates, lithium, anticoagulants, frusemide, probenecid, ACE inhibitors, methotrexate, ß-blockers, triamterene haloperidol, quinolones. *Side effects*: blood changes, dizziness, blurring of vision, headache, tinnitus, gastro-intestinal upset, oedema. *Manufacturer*: Merck.

EMINASE

Description: a fibrinolytic preparation produced in the form of a powder in vials for reconstitution and injection, containing 30 units anistreplase. *Used for*: myocardial infarction. *Dosage*: adults, one 30-unit dose within 6 hours of myocardial infarction, given over a period of 4 to 5 minutes by slow intravenous injection. *Special care*: pregnancy, breast-feeding, heart arrhythmias, risk of bleeding, increased risk of thrombi or emboli. *Avoid use*: children, treatment should not be repeated after first 5 days for 12 months, patients who have had surgery within past 10 days, those with menorrhagia, aneurysm, serious hypertension, peptic ulcer, CVA. *Side effects*: vomiting, fever, nausea, allergic responses, flushing, hypotension, bleeding, bradycardia. *Manufacturer*: Monmouth.

EMLA

Description: a local anaesthetic preparation produced in the form of a cream containing 25mg lignocaine, 25mg prilocaine per g. *Used for*: local anaesthesia of skin and genital area (removal of genital warts). *Dosage*: adults and children, minor surgery, 2g applied to affected area for a minimum of 1 hour and a maximum of 5 hours. For larger areas, 1.5–3g per 10cm^2 of skin for minimum of 2 hours and maximum of 5 hours. (Cream is applied as a thick layer under a dressing). Genital warts, 10g applied for 5 to 10 minutes before surgical removal. *Avoid use*: infants, patients with atopic dermatitis, on wounds or mucous membranes. *Side effects*: local slight skin reactions. *Manufacturer*: Astra.

ENDOBULIN

Description: a preparation of human normal immunoglobin (HNIG) available as a concentrate which is freeze-dried plus diluent, for reconstitution and intravenous infusion. *Used for*: replacement therapy in patients with deficient immunoglobulins (gamma globulins) which are antibodies present in blood serum. *Dosage*: depending upon particular syndrome or disease being treated, in the order of 0.4g to 1g/kg body weight by intravenous infusion for 4 or 5 days, or within first 2 weeks. Some conditions require maintenance doses in the order of 0.1–0.6g/kg body weight each month in 1 or 2 doses. *Special care*: pregnant women, patients with diabetes. Monitor closely during infusion for signs of anaphylaxis. Special care in patients with selective immunoglobulin A deficiency who are sensitized and carry antibodies to IGA. *Avoid use*: patients known to have certain types of antibody to immunoglobulin. *Possible interaction*: live vaccines. *Side effects*: fever, chills, headache, fatigue; rarely, anaphylaxis. *Manufacturer*: Immuno.

ENDOXANA

Description: an alkylating cytotoxic drug produced as a powder in vials containing 100mg, 200mg, 500mg or 1g of cyclophosphamide, for reconstition and injection. It is also available as white sugar-coated tablets (50mg). *Used for*: malignant diseases e.g. lymphoma, leukaemia and some solid tumours. *Dosage*: adults, taken with Uromitexan as directed by physician skilled in cancer chemotherapy. *Special care*: patients with diabetes, elderly or debilitated persons. *Avoid use*: children. *Possible interaction*: sulphonylureas, radiotherapy, doxorubicin. *Side effects*: vomiting, hair loss, nausea, bone marrow suppression and suppression of the reticulo-endothelial system, toxic effects on heart and urinary tract, haematuria, male sterility (Azoospermia—a lack of spermaztozoa in the semen), amenorrhoea. *Manufacturer*: Asta Medica.

ENGERIX B

Description: a genetically derived suspension of hepatitis B surface antigen (from yeast cells) containing 20 micrograms per ml adsorbed onto aluminium hydroxide, in vials or pre-filled syringes. *Used for*: immunization against the Hepatitis B virus. *Dosage*: adults, first dose 1ml by intramuscular injection into the deltoid muscle (upper arm) repeated after an interval of 1 month and 6 months. Children, first dose of 0.5ml by intramuscular injection into the thigh repeated after an interval of 1 month and 6 months. *Special care*: pregnant women, patients receiving kidney dialysis or who have a deficient immune system may need to receive additional doses. *Avoid use*: severe infections accompanied by fever. *Side effects*: slight short-lived soreness at injection site, with inflammation and hardening, dizziness, feverishness, nausea, malaise. *Manufacturer*: SmithKline Beecham.

EPANUTIN

Description: an anticonvulsant available as capsules and suspension, which belongs to a group called hydantoins which are similar in composition to barbiturates. White/purple, white/pink and white/orange capsules contain 25mg, 50mg and 100mg of phenytoin sodium respectively. All marked with capsule name and strength. Also, **EPANUTIN SUSPENSION** containing 30mg phenytoin per 5ml and **EPANUTIN INFATABS** containing 50mg phenytoin in the form of triangular, scored, yellow, chewable tablets. *Used for*: prevention and treatment of grand mal (tonic clonic) epileptic seizures, partial (focal) epileptic seizures and seizures which may follow trauma to the brain due to neurosurgery or head injury. Also, trigeminal neuralgia. *Dosage*: adults, capsules, 3–4mg/kg body weight in first instance each day, gradually increasing until condition is controlled. Maintenance dose is in the order of 200–500mg in divided doses each day. Suspension: 15ml 3 times each day. Infatabs: 2 tablets 2, 3 or 4 times each day. Children, capsules, (all except newborn babies), 5mg/kg body weight in 2 divided doses, with a maintenance dose in the order of 4–8mg/kg body weight each day. Suspension, under 6 years of age, 5ml twice each day increasing to 5ml 3 or 4 times each day if needed; 6 to 12 years, adult dose. Infatabs: under 6 years of age, half of 1 tablet 2, 3 or 4 times each day; 7 to 12 years, 1 tablet 2, 3 or 4 times each day. *Special care*: pregnancy, breast-feeding, liver disease. Adequate intake of vitamin D is necessary and drug should be stopped gradually. *Possible interaction*: isoniazid, sulthiame, anticoagulants of the coumarin group, chloramphenicol, oral contraceptives, doxycycline. *Side effects*: upset stomach, lack of sleep, allergic effects, blood changes, unsteadiness, swelling of gums and lymph glands; in young persons there may be unusual growth of hair (hirsutism) and motor activity. Rapid abnormal eye movements (nystagmus) may occur and drug should be withdrawn in the event of skin rash. *Manufacturer*: Parke-Davis.

EPANUTIN PARENTERAL

Description: an anticonvulsant and class I antiarrhythmic preparation available in ampoules for injection containing 50mg phenytoin sodium per ml. *Used for*: status epilepticus (an emergency situation in which a patient suffers continuous epileptic seizures without regaining consciousness in between. If the convulsions are not halted, the person suffers irreversible brain damage and may die). Also used for prevention of seizures during neurosurgical operations and for heart arrhythmias, particularly those caused by digitalis. *Dosage*: adults, status epilepticus, 150–250mg by slow intravenous injection followed by 100–150mg after half an hour if needed. Heart arrhythmias, 3.5–5mg/kg body weight in first instance, by intravenous injection, the rate of which should not be greater than 50mg per minute. This can be repeated once if required. Children for status epilepticus only, dose in proportion to that for a 70kg adult, reduced accordingly. *Special care*: pregnant women, breast-feeding mothers, ECG and close monitoring need; resuscitation equipment should be on hand. *Avoid use*: patients with heart block. *Possible interaction*: isoniazid, sulthiame, anticoagulants of the coumarin group, chloramphenicol, oral contraceptives, doxycycline. *Side effects*: upset stomach, lack of sleep, allergic effects, blood changes, unsteadiness, swelling of gums and lymph glands; in young persons there may be unusual growth of hair (hirsutism) and motor activity. Rapid abnormal eye movements (nystagmus) may occur and drug should be withdrawn in the event of skin rash. *Manufacturer*: Parke-Davis.

EPILIM

Description: an anticonvulsant and carboxylic acid derivative, sodium valproate, available as lilac, enteric-coated tablets containing 200mg or 500mg. **EPILIM CRUSHABLE** white, scored tablets(100mg); EPILIM SYRUP (red) contains 200mg per 5ml; **EPILIM LIQUID** (sugar-free, red) contains 200mg per 5ml; **EPILIM CHRONO** sustained-release tablets are lilac-coloured and contain 200mg, 300mg and 500mg as valproate and valproic acid. **EPILIM INTRAVE-NOUS** contains 400mg powder in vial for reconstitution and injection. *Dosage*: adults, 600mg each day in 2 divided doses in first instance, then gradually increasing after intervals of 3 days by 200mg until optimum control dose is achieved. Usual maintenance dose is in the order of 1–2g each day with a maximum of 2.5g. Children, less than 20kg body weight, 20mg/kg each day at first; over 20kg, 400mg each day at first. Both in divided doses and both gradually increased until optimum control dose is achieved. Epilim Intravenous (for patients not able to take the oral preparations), adults, 400–800mg each day by slow intravenous injection or infusion with a maximum dose of 2.5g. Children, 20–30mg/kg body weight by slow intravenous injection or infusion. *Special care*: pregnant women, children with brain damage, mental retardation or congenital metabolic disorders accompanying severe epilepsy. Patients should be monitored for signs of liver failure and liver function tests should be carried out. Patients having urine tests for diabetes may show false positives for ketones. *Avoid use*: patients with liver disorders. *Possible interaction*: other anticonvulsant drugs, anticoagulants, antidepressants. *Side effects*: liver failure, oedema, pancreatitis, gain in weight, loss of hair, blood changes, effects on nervous system. *Manufacturer*: Sanofi Winthrop.

EPOGAM

Description: a fatty acid preparation in the form of gelatin caspules containing 40mg gamolenic acid and marked Epogam 240. Also, **EPOGAM PAEDI-ATRIC**, gelatin capsules containing 80mg and marked EPOGAM 60. *Used for*: relief of eczema. *Dosage*: Capsules are snipped open and contents poured onto food, in drink, or swallowed directly. Adults 4 to 6 capsules twice each day. Epogram paediatric, 2 to 3 capsules each day. Children, over 1 year, 2 to 4 Epogram 240 capsules or 1 to 2 Epogram Paediatric capsules, both twice each day. *Special care*: patients with epilepsy. *Avoid use*: children under 1 year. *Side effects*: headache, nausea. *Manufacturer*: Searle.

EPPY

Description: a sympathomimetic preparation available in the form of eye drops containing 1% adrenaline. *Used for*: glaucoma (primary open angle and secondary). *Dosage*: adults, 1 drop once or twice each day. *Avoid use*: children, patients with narrow angle glaucoma or aphakia (absence of all or part of the lens of the eye, usually because it has been surgically removed, e.g. to treat cataracts). *Possible interaction*: TCADs, MAOIs. *Side effects*: headache, pain in region of eyes and redness due to increased blood flow (hyperaemia), melanosis; rarely, systemic effects. *Manufacturer*: Chauvin.

EPREX

Description: a preparation of synthesized human erythropoietin, a glycoprotein hormone, produced by some kidney cells and released into the blood in conditions in which there is a lack of oxygen reaching the tissues. This increases the rate of production of red blood cells (erythropoiesis) which are responsible for transporting oxygen in the circulation. Eprex is produced in vials or prefilled syringes as a medium for injection and containing epoetin alfa solution. *Used for*: anaemia which accompanies chronic renal failure in both dialysis and non-dialysis patients. *Dosage*: adults, dialysis patients, (following dialysis), 50iu/kg body weight 3 times each week at first by intravenous or subcutaneous injection. Non-dialysis patients, same dose by subcutaneous injection. Dose increased and adjusted depending upon response and haemoglobin level required. Children, 50iu/kg body weight 3 times each week after dialysis, in first instance. Dose is then adjusted according to patient's condition. *Special care*: pregnancy, liver failure, hypertension, ischaemic vascular disease, history of epilepsy. Haemoglobin levels, blood pressure, electrolyte levels and blood count require consistent monitoring. Iron supplements may be needed and treatment for any other causes of anaemia; diet and dialysis treatment may need to be altered. *Avoid use*: hypertension which is uncontrolled. *Possible interaction*: cyclosporin. *Side effects*: headache, rise in blood pressure, feverish flu-like symptoms, skin reactions, seizures, thrombosis. *Manufacturer*: Janssen-Cilag.

EQUAGESIC^{CD}

Description: a compound analgesic preparation which is a controlled drug and combines an opiate, muscle relaxant and salicylate. Three layered pink, white, yellow tablets contain 75mg ethoheptazine citrate, 150mg meprobamate and 250mg aspirin and are marked WYETH on the yellow surface. *Used for*: relief of severe muscle and bone pain. *Dosage*: adults, 2 tablets 3 or 4 times each day. *Special care*: for short-term use only; special care in elderly persons, those suffering from depression or at risk of suicide. Patients with heart failure, liver disease, history of epilepsy. *Avoid use*: pregnancy, breast-feeding, children, kidney disease, porphyria, peptic ulcer, alcoholism, haemophilia, allergy to aspirin or other anti-inflammatory drugs. *Possible interaction*: anticoagulants, antidiabetic drugs, alcohol, central nervous system sedatives, uricosurics (drugs which lower uric acid levels). *Side efects*: blood changes, giddiness, nausea, sleepiness, rash, ataxia. *Manufacturer*: Wyeth.

EQUANIL^{CD}

Description: a carbamate tranquillizer which acts as an anxiolytic and a controlled drug. It is available in the form of white, scored tablets of 2 different strengths containing 200mg or 400mg of meprobamate. Both are marked E and WYETH. *Used for*: short-term relief of anxiety and muscular tension. *Dosage*: adults, 400mg 3 times each day at at night; elderly persons, 200mg 3 times each day. *Special care*: pregnancy, breast-feeding, liver or kidney disease, history of depression, epilepsy. Drug should be stopped gradually. *Avoid use*: children, patients suffering from alcoholism or acute intermittent porphyria. *Possible interaction*: CNS depressants, phenytoin, TCADs, rifampicin, alcohol, anticoagulants of the coumarin type, phenothiazines, griseofulvin, oral contraceptives. *Side effects*: addiction may occur and ability to perform skilled tasks such as driving impaired. Gastro-intestinal upset, hypotension, disturbance to central nervous system and excitement, feeling of "pins and needles" (paraesthesia), blood disorders, low blood pressure, allergic reactions. *Manufacturer*: Wyeth.

ERADACIN

Description: a 4-quinolone antibiotic preparation produced in the form of yellow/red capsules containing 150mg acrosoxacin. *Used for*: treatment of acute gonorrhoea. *Dosage*: adults, 1 dose of 2 tablets each day. *Special care*: pregnant women, patients with liver or kidney disease. *Avoid use*: children. *Side effects*: drowsiness, headaches, giddiness, gastro-intestinal upset. *Manufacturer*: Sanofi Winthrop.

ERVEVAX

Description: a form of live attenuated virus of Wistar RA27/3 used as a vaccine against Rubella (German measles). It is produced as pink pellets in vials, along with diluent, for reconstitution and injection. *Used for*: immunization against Rubella. *Dosage*: 0.5ml by intravenous, intramuscular or subcutaneous injection. *Avoid use*: pregnancy, severe fever, altered immunity due to malignant diseases including leukaemia and lymphoma. *Possible interaction*: other live vaccines (with the exception of polio vaccine taken by mouth), transfusions, cytotoxic drugs, immunoglobulins, corticosteroids, irradiation. *Side effects*: pains in joints, rash, feverishness, lymphadenopathy (a disease of lymph vessels and nodes). *Manufacturer*: SmithKline Beecham.

ERYMAX

Description: an antibiotic preparation of the macrolide, erythromycin, produced as small enteric-coated pellets contained in clear/orange capsules (250mg strength). *Used for*: infections sensitive to erythromycin especially in patients with penicillin hypersensitivity. These include legionnaire's disease, campylobacter enteritis, syphilis, chronic prostatitis, pneumonia, non-gonococcal urethritis and acne. Also used as a preventative against whooping cough and diphtheria. *Dosage*: adults, for most infections, 250mg at 6-hour intervals or 500mg every 12 hours taken before or with food. For acne, 1 tablet twice each day for 1 month, then 1 tablet daily as maintenance dose. Children, infections, 30–50mg/kg body weight each day in divided doses at 6-hour intervals or twice daily. *Special care*: patients with liver disease. *Possible interaction*: digoxin, astemizole, anticoagulants taken by mouth, terfenadine, carbamazepine, theophylline. *Side effects*: allergic reactions, gastro-intestinal upset, cholestatic jaundice. *Manufacturer*: Elan.

ERYTHROCIN

Description: an antibiotic preparation of the macrolide, erythromycin, produced in the form of oblong, white, film-coated tablets, containing 250mg and 500mg (as stearate), all marked with company symbol. *Used for*: infections sensitive to erythromycin especially in patients with penicillin hypersensitivity. Acne. *Dosage*: adults, 1–2g each day in divided doses. *Special care*: patients with liver disease. *Avoid use*: children. *Possible interaction*: digoxin, anticoagulants taken by mouth, astemizole, theophylline, terfenadine, carbamazepine. *Side effects*: allergic reactions, gastro-intestinal upset, cholestatic jaundice. *Manufacturer*: Abbott.

ERYTHROMID

Description: an antibiotic preparation of the macrolide, erythromycin, produced in the form of enteric-coated and film-coated orange tablets containing 250mg. Also, **ERYTHROMID DS®** enteric-coated and film-coated orange tablets containing 500mg. *Used for*: infections sensitive to erythromycin especially in patients with penicillin hypersensitivity. Acne. *Dosage*: adults, 1–2g each day in divided doses with a maximum of 4g in exceptionally severe cases of infection. Children over 8 years, same as adult dose. *Special care*: patients with liver disease. *Avoid use*: children under 8 years of age. *Possible interaction*: digoxin, oral anticoagulants, astemizole, theophylline, terfenadine, carbamazepine. *Side effects*: allergic reactions, gastro-intestinal upset, cholestatic jaundice. *Manufacturer*: Abbott.

ERYTHOPED A

Description: an antibiotic preparation of the macrolide, erythromycin (as ethyl succinate), produced as oval, film-coated yellow tablets (500mg); ERYTHROPED A sachets contain 1g in the form of granules. **ERYTHROPED SACHETS** contain 250mg; **ERYTHROPED SUSPENSION** contains 250mg per 5ml solution. **ERYTHROPED SUGAR-FREE SUSPENSION** contains 125mg per 5ml. **ERYTHROPED FORTE** available as 500mg per 5ml suspension or as granules in sachet. **ERYTHROPED P.I. SUGAR-FREE SUSPENSION** contains 125mg per 5ml solution. *Used for*: infections sensitive to erythromycin especially in patients with penicillin hypersensitivity. Acne. *Dosage*: adults, 1g twice each day. Children under 2 years, 250mg; 2 to 8 years, 500mg; over 8 years, 1g. All twice daily. *Special care*: patients with liver disease. *Possible interaction*: digoxin, oral anticoagulants, astemizole, theophylline, terfenadine, carbamazepine. *Side effects*: allergic reactions, gastro-intestinal upset, cholestatic jaundice. *Manufacturer*: Abbott.

ESIDREX

Description: a proprietary thiazide diuretic preparation produced in the form of white scored tablets containing 25mg and 50mg of hydrochlorthiazide, and marked CIBA and UT. *Used for*: oedema and hypertension. *Dosage*: 25–100mg each morning after breakfast as a single dose, in first instance. Dose is then reduced to 25–50mg taken on alternate days. *Special care*: pregnancy, breast-feeding, elderly persons, diabetes, kidney or liver disease, gout, cirrhosis of the liver, SLE. Monitoring of electrolytes, glucose and fluid levels should be carried out. *Avoid use*: patients with serious kidney or liver failure, sensitivity to sulphonamide drugs, Addison's disease, hypercalcaemia. *Possible interaction*: NSAIDs, alcohol, opioid and barbiturate drugs, antidiabetic preparations, corticosteroids, cardiac glycosides, lithium, carbenoxolone, tubocurarine. *Side effects*: disturbance of metabolism and electrolyte levels, sensitivity to light, blood changes, rash, gastro-intestinal upset, pancreatitis, anorexia, giddiness, impotence. *Manufacturer*: CIBA.

ESKAZOLE

Description: an anthelmintic preparation designed to act against the larval stages of 2 species of small parasitic tapeworms, *Echinococcus granulosus* and *Echinococcus multilocularis*. It is produced in the form of oblong, orange, scored tablets marked SKF, containing 400mg algendazole. *Used for*: hydatid cysts. *Dosage*: adults over 60kg body weight 800mg each day for 28 days in divided doses, followed by 14 tablet-free days. There should be a maximum of 3 cycles of treatment. *Special care*: blood counts and liver function tests should be carried out. *Avoid use*: children, adults under 60kg bodyweight, women should use non-hormonal methods of contraception during treatment and for 1 month afterwards. *Possible interaction*: oral contraceptives, theophylline, anticoagulants, hypoglycaemics taken orally. *Side effects*: changes in blood and liver enzymes, headache, rash, giddiness, fever, hair loss. Any advere side effects should be reported. *Manufacturer*: SmithKline Beecham.

ESTRACOMBI

Description: a combined oestrogen, progestogen preparation in the form of patches containing either 50 g oestradiol per 24 hours, or 50 g oestradiol and 250 g norethisterone acetate per 24 hours, marked CGDWD and CGFNF respectively. *Used for*: hormone replacement therapy for menopausal women. Prevention of osteoporosis after the menopause. *Dosage*: oestradiol only patch is applied to hairless skin below waist twice each week for 2 weeks, followed by the combined patch twice weekly for 2 weeks. The patches are changed every 3 to 4 days and placed on a different area of skin each time. *Special care*: patients with a history, or considered to be at risk, of thrombosis, those with liver disease. Liver function should be monitored and breasts and pelvic organs examined periodically during the period of therapy. Women with any of the following require particularly careful monitoring: diabetes, fibroids in uterus, multiple

sclerosis, hypertension, tetany, epilepsy, porphyria, gallstones, migraine, otosclerosis, history of breast cancer. *Avoid use*: pregnancy, breast-feeding, thrombosis or thromboembolic disorders, serious heart, kidney or liver disease, endometriosis or vaginal bleeding which is undiagnosed, hormone-dependent
cancers such as breast or uterine carcinoma, Dublin-Johnson or Rotor syndrome. *Possible interaction*: drugs which induce liver enzymes. *Side effects*: enlargement of and soreness in breasts, breakthrough bleeding, vomiting, nausea, gastro-intestinal disturbance, gain in weight, dizziness, headache. Withdraw
immediately if frequent severe headaches or migraines occur, disordered vision, pregnancy, rise in blood pressure, signs of thromboembolism, jaundice.
Stop before planned surgery. *Manufacturer*: CIBA.

ESTRACYT

Description: a preparation of a sex hormone used to treat cancer, which is an
oestrogenic alkylating agent, produced in the form of off-white capsules containing 140mg estramustine phosphate (as disodium salt). *Used for*: prostatic
cancer. *Dosage*: adults, 4 capsules each day in divided doses taken 1 hour before meals or 2 hours afterwards, in first instance. Dose is then adjusted according to response of patient's conditioin with an average between 1 and 10
capsules each day. Capsules must not be taken with milk or dairy products.
Special care: bone marrow disorder. *Avoid use*: patients with serious heart or
liver disease or peptic ulcer. *Possible interaction*: milk and dairy products. *Side
effects*: enlargement of breasts, toxic effects on heart, disturbance of liver function, gastro-intestinal upset. *Manufacturer*: Pharmacia & Upjohn.

ESTRADERM

Description: an oestrogen patch containing either 25, 50 or 100 g oestradiol.
Used for: hormone replacement therapy in menopausal women. Prevention of
osteoporosis following menopause. *Dosage*: for oestrogen replacement; 1 patch
is applied to hairless skin below waist and replaced every 3 or 4 days at a different site. The 50 g patch is used for prevention of osteoporosis. *Special care*:
patients with a history, or at risk, of thrombosis, those with liver disease. Liver
function should be monitored and breasts and pelvic organs examined periodically during the period of therapy. Women with any of the following require
particularly careful monitoring: diabetes, fibroids in uterus, multiple sclerosis,
hypertension, tetany, epilepsy, porphyria, gallstones, migraine, otosclerosis (an
hereditary rare disorder of the inner ear), history of breast cancer. *Avoid use*:
pregnant women, breast-feeding mothers, thrombosis or thromboembolic disorders, serious heart, kidney or liver disease, endometriosis or vaginal bleeding
which is undiagnosed, hormone-dependent cancers such as breast or uterine
carcinoma, Dublin-Johnson or Rotor syndrome. *Possible interaction*: drugs
which induce liver enzymes. *Side effects*: enlargement of and soreness in breasts,
breakthrough bleeding, vomiting, nausea, gastro-intestinal disturbance, gain
in weight, dizziness, headache. Withdraw immediately if frequent, severe head-

aches or migraines occur, disordered vision, pregnancy, rise in blood pressure, signs of thromboembolism, jaundice. Stop before planned surgery. *Manufacturer*: CIBA.

ESTRADURIN

Description: a preparation of a sex hormone used to treat cancer and local anaesthetic. It is produced as a powder in vials for reconstitution and injection and contains 80mg polyoestradiol phosphate and 5mg mepivacaine. *Used for*: prostate cancer. *Dosage*: adults, 80–160mg every 4 weeks given by deep intramuscular injection. Maintenance dose in order of 40–80mg. *Side effects*: enlargement of breasts, impotence, oedema, heart disease and thromboembolism, jaundice, nausea. *Manufacturer*: Pharmacia & Upjohn.

ESTRAPAK

Description: a combined oestrogen/progestogen preparation available as a patch containing 50 g oestradiol per 24 hours, and as red tablets, marked DG and LK, containing 1mg norethisterone acetate. *Used for*: hormone replacement therapy for menopausal women. Prevention of osteoporosis after the menopause. *Dosage*: apply patch to hairless skin below waist and replace with new patch in different site every 3 to 4 days. Take 1 tablet each day starting on 15th day through to 26th day of each period of 28 days of oestrogen replacement therapy. Therapy should begin within 5 days of the start of the period if this is present. *Special care*: patients with a history, or considered to be at risk, of thrombosis, those with liver disease. Liver function should be monitored and breasts and pelvic organs examined periodically during the period of therapy. Women with any of the following require particularly careful monitoring: diabetes, fibroids in uterus, multiple sclerosis, hypertension, tetany, epilepsy, porphyria, gallstones, migraine, otosclerosis, history of breast cancer. *Avoid use*: pregnancy, breast-feeding, thrombosis or thromboembolic disorders, serious heart, kidney or liver disease, endometriosis or vaginal bleeding which is undiagnosed, hormone-dependent cancers such as breast or uterine carcinoma, Dublin-Johnson or Rotor syndrome. *Possible interaction*: drugs which induce liver enzymes. *Side effects*: enlargement of and soreness in breasts, breakthrough bleeding, vomiting, nausea, gastro-intestinal disturbance, gain in weight, dizziness, headache. Withdraw immediately if frequent, severe headaches or migraines occur, disordered vision, pregnancy, rise in blood pressure, signs of thromboembolism, jaundice. Stop before planned surgery. *Manufacturer*: CIBA.

ETHMOZINE

Description: a class I antiarrhythmic preparation, moracizine hydrochloride, available in the form of white, film-coated tablets of different strengths. Round tablets contain 200mg; oval tablets contain 250mg and capsule-shaped tablets contain 300mg. All are marked ROBERTS and with name and strength. *Used for*: ventricular arrhythmias (arising in the ventricles of the heart). *Dosage*:

adults, 200–300mg at 8-hour intervals which may be increased, if required, by 150mg per day every 3 days to a maximum daily dose of 900mg. *Special care*: pregnancy, liver or kidney disease, congestive heart failure, sick sinus syndrome. Therapy should be started in hospital and electrolyte levels stabilized before beginning. ECG should be monitored. *Avoid use*: breast-feeding, children, patients with heart block, heart shock, recent myocardial infarction. *Possible interaction*: cimetidine, theophylline, digoxin. *Side effects*: gastro-intestinal upset, chest, muscle and bone pains, disturbance of sleep, blurring of vision, sweating, dry mouth, nervousness, giddiness. If unexplained liver disorder, withdraw drug. *Manufacturer*: Monmouth.

EUDEMINE

Description: an antihypertensive (vaso-dilator) and hyperglycaemic produced in ampoules for injection to treat hypertension and as tablets for hypoglycaemia. Ampoules contain 15mg diazoxide/ml and white, sugar-coated tablets contain 50mg diazoxide. *Used for*: serious hypertension, especially arising from kidney disease, hypertensive crisis, intractable hypoglycaemia. *Dosage*: adults, for hypertension, 300mg by fast, intravenous injection while patient is lying down. Children, 5mg/kg body weight by fast intravenous injection. Adults and children, for hypoglycaemia, 5mg/kg body weight each day at first in 2 or 3 divided doses. Afterwards, adjust according to response. *Special care*: pregnancy, serious kidney, heart or cerebral disease, kidney failure, low blood protein levels. Regular checks on blood count, blood pressure, blood glucose levels are required and also monitoring of development and growth in children. *Possible interaction*: anticoagulants of coumarin type, other antihypertensives, diuretics. *Side effects*: hyperglycaemia, nausea, imbalance electrolyte and fluid levels, tachycardia, vomiting, arrhythmias, orthostatic hypotension (low blood pressure when person is standing), delay in onset of labour, possible coma. *Manufacutrer*: Link.

EUGLUCON

Description: an oral hypoglycaemic preparation, glibenclamide, in the form of white tablets of 2 strengths. Tablets marked EU and 2.5 contain 2.5mg and scored, oblong tablets, marked EU-BM, contain 5mg. Glibenclamide belongs to a group of antidiabetic agents called sulphonylureas which enhance the effects of insulin and stimulate its secretion from cells in the pancreas. *Used for*: diabetes which develops in adults (maturity-onset or non-insulin dependent type II diabetes). *Dosage*: adults, 5mg each day at first, taken at breakfast time, increasing if required by 2.5mg each day at intervals of 1 week. The maximum daily dose is 15mg. *Special care*: elderly persons or patients with kidney failure. *Avoid use*: pregnancy, breast-feeding, some other types of diabetes (including juvenile, unstable-brittle and growth-onset), patients with infections, hormonal disorders, serious kidney or liver disease, stress, undergoing surgery, ketoacidosis (accumulation of ketones in the body characterized by "pear drops" smell on breath and resulting from diabetes mellitus). *Possible interaction*: chloramphenicol, diuretics, anticoagulants taken by mouth, glucagon, chlorpropamide, metiformin, aspirin, MAOIs, oral contraceptives, corticotrophin, corticosteroids, alcohol, phenylbutazone, cyclophosphamide, rifampicin, bezafibrate, diuretics, anticoagulants taken orally. *Side effects*: allergic reactions including skin rash. *Manufacturer*: Hoechst.

EUGYNON 30

Description: a combined oestrogen/progestogen and contraceptive produced in the form of white, sugar-coated tablets containing 30 g ethinyloestradiol and 250 g levonorgestrel. *Used for*: oral contraception. *Dosage*: 1 tablet each day for 21 days starting on first day of period followed by 7 tablet-free days. *Special care*: hypertension, severe kidney disease, dialysis, Raynaud's disease, diabetes, multiple sclerosis, asthma, varicose veins, elevated levels of prolactin (a hormone) in the blood (hyperprolactaemia). Risk of thrombosis increases with smoking, age and obesity. Blood pressure, breasts and pelvic organs should be checked during period of treatment. *Avoid use*: pregnancy, heart and circulatory diseases, angina, sickle cell anaemia, pulmonary hypertension. Also hormone-dependent cancers, otosclerosis, undiagnosed vaginal bleeding, chorea, liver disease, history of cholestatic jaundice of pregnancy, infectious hepatitis, Dublin-Johnson syndrome, Rotor syndrome, recent trophoblastic disease. *Possible interaction*: phenytoin, carbamazepine, tetracyclines, primidone, chloral hydrate, glutehimide, rifampicin, griseofulvin, dichloralphenazone, ethosuximide, barbiturates. *Side effects*: feeling of bloatedness due to fluid retention, leg pains, breast enlargement, muscular cramps, weight gain, breakthrough bleeding, depression, vaginal discharge, loss of libido, nausea, brown patches on skin (chloasma). Stop drug immediately if frequent, severe headaches occur or signs of thromboses, rise in blood pressure. Drug should be discontinued before major planned surgery. *Manufacturer*: Schering H.C.

EUMOVATE

Description: a moderately potent topical steroid in the form of cream and ointment containing 0.05% clobetasone butyrate. *Used for*: dermatitis, eczema and skin conditions responsive to steroids. *Dosage*: apply thinly to affected area up to 4 times each day. *Special care*: should not be used on face or on children for more than 5 days. Should be stopped gradually. *Avoid use*: prolonged or extensive use especially pregnant women or continual use as a preventative. Should not be used to treat acne, leg ulcers, scabies, peri-oral dermatitis, tuberculous skin conditions, skin disorders caused by viruses, ringworm, any untreated bacterial or fungal skin infections. *Side effects*: thinning of skin, adrenal gland suppression, hair growth, Cushingoid type symptoms (Cushing's syndrome). *Manufacturer*: Glaxo Wellcome.

EUMOVATE EYEDROPS

Description: Moderately potent steroid eyedrops containing 0.1% clobetasone butyrate. Also EUMOVATE-N which additionally contains an antibiotic (0.5% neomycin sulphate as eyedrops). *Used for*: drops containing clobetasone butyrate only are used for non-infected inflammatory conditions of the eye. Eumovate-N drops are used for infected inflammatory conditions of the eye. *Dosage*: 1 or 2 drops 4 times each day with more severe infections requiring more frequent application every 1 or 2 hours. *Special care*: do not use for prolonged periods especially pregnant women and young children. *Avoid use*: patients with soft contact lenses, those with tuberculous, fungal or viral infections, glaucoma, dendritic ulcer, infections containing pus. *Side effects*: thinning of cornea, cataracts, rise in pressure within eye, fungal infection, sensitization (patient becomes hypersensitive to drug). *Manufacturer*: Cusi.

EVOREL

Description: an oestrogen patch containing 50 g oestradiol per 24 hours. *Used for*: hormone replacement therapy in menopausal women. *Dosage*: apply patch to hairless area of skin below waist and change for a new patch in a different site after 3 or 4 days. Women who have not had a hysterectomy should also receive a progestogen preparation for 12 out of each 28 day period of treatment. *Special care*: patients with history of or considered to be at risk of thrombosis, those with liver disease. Careful monitoring of women with any of the following is required: fibroids in uterus, otosclerosis, porphyria, tetany, epilepsy, gallstones, migraine, multiple sclerosis, hypertension, diabetes. Regular examination of pelvic organs and breasts required during course of therapy, especially in women with family history of breast cancer. *Avoid use*: pregnancy, breast-feeding, women with breast cancer or other cancers which are hormone-dependent, e.g. of genital tract; serious heart, liver or kidney disease, endometriosis, thrombosis, Dublin-Johnson or Rotor syndrome, undiagnosed vaginal bleeding. *Possible interaction*: drugs which induce liver enzymes. *Side effects*: enlargement and tenderness of breasts, nausea and vomiting, weight gain, breakthrough bleeding, gastro-intestinal upset, headache, giddiness. Withdraw drug immediately if any sign of thrombosis, rise in blood pressure, severe and frequent headaches, migraines, disturbance of vision, jaundice, pregnancy. Stop before planned surgery. *Manufacturer*: Janssen-Cilag.

EXELDERM

Description: an antifungal preparation, an imidazole, produced in the form of a cream containing 1% sulconazole nitrate. *Used for*: fungal skin and nail infections. *Dosage*: massage in twice each day and continue for 2 to 3 weeks after symptoms have disappeared. *Avoid use*: contact with eyes. *Side effects*: skin irritation—stop use. *Manufacturer*: Zeneca.

EXIREL

Description: a bronchodilator selective β_2-agonist produced in the form of capsules. Olive/turquoise capsules contain 10mg pirbuterol (as hydrochloride) and beige/turquoise capsules contain 15mg. All are marked with strength, 3M and MXR. Also, **EXIREL INHALER** containing 0.2mg pirbuterol (as acetate) per metered dose delivered by aerosol inhaler. *Used for*: bronchial spasm in asthma, emphysema and bronchitis. *Dosage*: adults, tablets, 10–15mg 3 or 4 times each day with a maximum dose of 60mg. Inhaler, relief of acute attack, 1 or 2 puffs in 1 dose; prevention, 2 puffs 3 or 4 times each day with a maximum of 12 puffs in 24 hours. *Special care*: pregnant women, patients with weak hearts, heart arrhythmias, hypertension, angina, hyperthyroidism. *Avoid use*: children. *Possible interaction*: sympathomimetics. *Side effects*: dilation of peripheral blood vessels, headache, nervousness, tremor. *Manufacturer*: 3M Health Care.

EXOCIN

Description: a 4-quinolone antibiotic preparation produced in the form of eyedrops containing 0.3% olfloxacin. *Used for*: bacterial eye infections. *Dosage*: 1 or 2 drops every 2 to 4 hours into eye during first 2 days of treatment. Then reduce to 1 or 2 drops 4 times daily. Use for a maximum period of 10 days. *Special care*: pregnancy, breast-feeding. *Avoid use*: patients with soft contact lenses. *Side effects*: short-lived eye irritation, rarely headache, dizzines, nausea, numbness. *Manufacturer*: Allergan.

EXOSURF NEONATAL

Description: a preparation which acts as a lung surfactant produced as a powder in vials (with diluent) for reconstitution. The powder contains 108mg colfosceril palmitate. *Used for*: newborn babies suffering from respiratory distress syndrome who are receiving mechanical ventilation. *Dosage*: 67.5mg/kg body weight by means of endotracheal tube; may be repeated after 12 hours. *Special care*: for use in babies of a weight greater than 700g; must be continually monitored due to risk of too much oxygen entering blood. *Side effects*: tube may become blocked by mucous secretions; risk of pulmonary haemorrhage. *Manufacturer*: Glaxo Wellcome.

EYE-CROM

Description: an anti-inflammatory preparation in the form of eye drops containing 2% sodium cromoglycate. *Used for*: allergic conjunctivitis. *Dosage*: 1 or 2 drops into eye up to 4 times each day continuing after symptoms have disappeared. *Avoid use*: patients with soft contact lenses. *Side effects*: passing stinging or burning in eye. *Manufacturer*: Norton.

F

FABROL

Description: a mucolytic preparation produced in the form of granules in sachets for dissolving in water containing 200mg acetylcysteine. It is for cystic fibrosis patients with accompanying abdominal complications. *Used for*: bronchitis and infections of the respiratory tract in which a lot of mucus is produced; abdominal problems in cystic fibrosis. *Dosage*: respiratory diseases, 3 sachets daily in divided doses; cystic fibrosis, normally 1 or 2 sachets 3 times each day. Children, respiratory diseases, under 2 years, 1 sachet each day; 2 to 6 years, 1 sachet twice each day; over 6 years, as adult dose. Cystic fibrosis, under 2 years, half to 1 sachet 3 times each day; 2 to 6 years, 1 or 2 sachets 3 times each day. *Special care*: patients with diabetes. *Side effects*: headache, skin rash, vomiting and nausea, gastro-intestinal upset, tinnitus; rarely bronchospasm, anaphylactic reactions (notify Committee on Safety of Medicines). *Manufacturer*: Zyma.

FAMVIR

Description: a preparation which interferes with the manufacture of DNA within cells infected by a virus and is a nucleoside analogue produced in the form of white, film-coated tablets containing 250mg famciclovir. The tablets are marked with the strength and name. *Used for*: infections caused by herpes zoster virus. *Dosage*: adults, 1 tablet 3 times each day for 1 week. *Special care*: kidney disease. *Avoid use*: children, pregnancy breast-feeding mothers. *Side effects*: nausea, headache. *Manufacturer*: Smith Kline Beecham.

FANSIDAR

Description: a compound antimalarial preparation, combining a sulphonamide with a diaminopyrimidine drug, produced in the form of quarter-scored white tablets containing 500mg sulfadoxine and 25mg pyrimethamine. The tablets are marked with a hexagon and ROCHE. *Used for*: treatment and prevention of malaria (caused by *Plasmodium falciparum*), especially where the disease does not respond to chloroquine. *Dosage*: for prevention, adults and children over fourteen years, 1 tablet taken weekly; for treatment, adults and children over fourteen years, 2 to 3 tablets as a single dose. Children, for prevention, under 4 years of age quarter of adult dose; 4 to 8 years, half adult dose; 9 to fourteen years threequarters adult dose. For treatment, under 4 years of age, half tablet; 4 to 6 years, 1 tablet; 7 to 9 years, 1 and a half tablets; 10 to fourteen years, 2 tablets. All ages take tablets as a single dose. *Special care*: patients should avoid being out in the sun and regular blood checks are required during long-term preventative treatment. *Avoid use*: pregnancy, breast-feeding, new-born babies, patients with serious kidney or liver disease, blood changes or a sensitivity to sulphonamide drugs. *Possible interaction*: folate inhibitors. *Side effects*: discontinue therapy if pharyngitis (inflammation of pharynx) or pruritis occur. Gastro-intestinal upset, blood changes, skin rash. More rarely, allergic skin conditions. *Manufacturer*: Roche.

FARLUTAL

Description: an anticancer drug which is a synthetic version of the female sex hormone, progestogen. It is produced in the form of a suspension in vials for injection, containing 200mg medroxyprogesterone acetate per ml and also in tablets of 3 strengths. White tablets contain 100mg; white scored tablets contain 250mg. Both are marked with tablet strength. White, scored, elongated tablets contain 500mg and are marked FCE 500. *Used for*: cancer of breast, endometrium (womb), kidney cells and prostate gland. *Dosage*: adults, tablets, breast cancer, 1–1.5g each day; kidney or prostate cancer, 100–500mg each day. *Special care*: patients suffering from epilepsy, diabetes, kidney or heart disease, asthma, migraine. *Avoid use*: children, pregnant women, patients with thromboembolism, liver disease, thrombophlebitis (inflamed veins), hypercalcaemia. *Side effects*: abnormal menstruation, abnormal production of breast milk, corticoid symptoms. *Manufacturer*: Pharmacia & Upjohn.

FASIGYN

Description: an antibacterial preparation which is a nitroimidazole drug effective against certain anaerobic bacteria. It is produced in the form of white, film-coated tablets containing 500mg tinidazole. *Used for*: treatment of infections caused by anaerobic bacteria and prevention of such during surgery. Particular sites of such infections are the mouth, gut and vagina (purulent gingivitis, pelvic inflammatory disease, non-specific vaginitis). *Dosage*: adults, prevention of infection, 4 tablets taken as 1 dose; treatment, 4 tablets taken as 1 dose at first followed by 2 each day for 5 to 6 days. *Special care*: pregnancy, breast-feeding. *Avoid use*: children, patients with blood changes or neurological disorders. *Possible interaction*: alcohol. *Side effects*: unpleasant taste in mouth and furring of tongue, gastro-intestinal upset, nettle rash (urticaria), disturbance of central nervous system, dark-coloured urine, angioneurotic oedema. Rarely, nerve damage and leucopenia if drug is taken long-term. *Manufacturer*: Pfizer.

FAVERIN

Description: an antidepressant drug, fluvoxamine, of a type known as 5HT reuptake inhibitors. Faverin is produced in the form of yellow, enteric-coated tablets of 2 strengths containing 50mg, marked DUPHAR and 291, or 100g, marked DUPHAR and 313. *Used for*: depression. *Dosage*: adults, 100mg taken at night in first instance with a normal maintenance dose in the order of 100–

200mg each day in divided doses. The maximum dose is 300mg each day. *Special care*: pregnancy, breast-feeding, kidney or liver disease or history of epilepsy. *Avoid use*: children. *Possible interaction*: alcohol, benzodiazepines, tryptophan, MAOIs, lithium, carbamazepine, propanolol, phenytoin, theophylline, tricyclic antidepressants. *Side effects*: gastro-intestinal upset, nausea, diarrhoea, vomiting, nervousness, sleepiness, anorexia, convulsions, tremor. *Manufacturer*: Solvay.

FELDENE

Description: a proprietary NSAID and oxicam, piroxicam, which is produced in a number of different forms. Feldene Capsules: blue/maroon capsules, marked FEL 10 and Pfizer, contain 10mg; maroon capsules, marked FEL 20 and Pfizer, contain 20mg. **FELDENE DISPERSIBLE**: scored, white tablets containing either 10mg or 20mg and marked FEL 10 and Pfizer or FEL 20 and Pfizer respectively. Higher strength tablets are oblong in shape. **FELDENE MELT**: fast dissolving, off-white coloured tablets containing 20mg; **FELDENE SUPPOSITORIES** contain 20mg; **FELDENE INTRAMUSCULAR INJECTION**: solution in ampoules containing 20mg per ml. **FELDENE GEL**: a topical gel containing 0.5% piroxicam. *Used for*: arthritic diseases including juvenile arthritis, gout, rheumatoid arthritis, ankylosing spondylitis, osteoarthritis and other skeletal and muscle diosrders. *Dosage*: adults, preparations taken by mouth or suppositories depending upon condition being treated, but about 20–40mg each day (Melt tablets are dissolved on tongue and dispersible tablets dissolved in water or swallowed whole). Injection, used for acute attacks, 1 dose of 20–40mg by deep intramuscular injection into buttock. Then tablets should be taken for maintenance. Feldene Gel is for use by adults only in patients with tendinitis, musculoskeletal injuries or joint problems. 3cm gel is applied to affected area 3 or 4 times each day for 4 weeks. Children over 6 years of age, for juvenile arthritis only, usually dispersible tablets, under 15kg of body weight, 5mg; 16–25kg of body weight, 10mg; 26–45kg body weight, 15mg; over 45kg body weight, 20mg. All are daily doses. Injection and gel are not for use in children. *Special care*: eldery, heart failure, liver or kidney disease. Feldene gel should not be applied to broken or infected skin or eyes, and mucous membranes should be avoided. *Avoid use*: pregnancy, breast-feeding, patients with allergy to NSAID or aspirin, peptic ulcers, history of ulcers, anal inflammation (use suppositories). *Possible interaction*: other NSAIDs, lithium, anticoagulants, hypoglycaemics. *Side effects*: gastro-intestinal upset, oedema, central nervous system disturbance, malaise, tinnitus, inflammation at injection site. Gel may cause skin irritation, rash and itching. *Manufacturer*: Pfizer.

FEMODENE

Description: a combined oestrogen/progestogen hormonal oral contraceptive in the form of white, sugar-coated tablets containing 30 g ethinyloestradiol and 75 g gestodene. *Used for*: oral contraception. *Dosage*: 1 tablet daily, beginning on day 1 of period, for 21 days followed by 7 tablet-free days. *Special care*: hypertension, severe kidney disease receiving dialysis, Raynaud's disease, diabetes, multiple sclerosis, asthma, varicose veins, elevated levels of prolactin (a hormone) in the blood (hyperprolactaemia). Risk of thrombosis increases with smoking, age and obesity. Blood pressure, breasts and pelvic organs should be checked during period of treatment. *Avoid use*: pregnancy, heart and circulatory diseases, angina, sickle cell anaemia, pulmonary hypertension. Also hormone-dependent cancers, undiagnosed vaginal bleeding, chorea, liver disease, history of cholestatic jaundice of pregnancy, infectious hepatitis, Dublin-Johnson syndrome, Rotor syndrome, recent trophoblasic disease. *Possible interaction*: phenytoin, carbamazepine, tetracyclines, primidone, chloral hydrate, glutehimide, rifampicin, griseofulvin, dichloralphenazone, ethosuximide, barbiturates. *Side effects*: feeling of bloatedness due to fluid retention, leg pains, breast enlargement, muscular cramps, weight gain, breakthrough bleeding, depression, vaginal discharge, loss of libido, nausea, brown patches on skin (chloasma). Stop drug immediately if frequent, severe headaches occur or signs of thromboses, rise in blood pressure. Drug should be discontinued before major planned surgery. *Manufacturer*: Schering H.C.

FEMODENE E.D.

Description: a combined oestrogen/progestogen hormonal oral contraceptive preparation consisting of 21 white, sugar-coated tablets containing 30µg ethinyloestradiol and 75µg gestodene and 7 white, sugar-coated placebo tablets containing lactose. *Used for*: oral contraception. *Dosage*: 1 tablet daily starting on first day of period with numbered tablet from red part of pack. Tablets are taken each day without a break, either hormonal or placebo depending upon the time in the cycle. *Special care*: hypertension, severe kidney disease receiving dialysis, Raynaud's disease, diabetes, multiple sclerosis, asthma, varicose veins, elevated levels of prolactin (a hormone) in the blood (hyperprolactaemia). Risk of thrombosis increases with smoking, age and obesity. Blood pressure, breasts and pelvic organs should be checked during period of treatment. *Avoid use*: pregnancy, heart and circulatory diseases, angina, sickle cell anaemia, pulmonary hypertension. Also hormone-dependent cancers, otosclerosis, undiagnosed vaginal bleeding, chorea, liver disease, history of cholestatic jaundice of pregnancy, infectious hepatitis, Dublin-Johnson syndrome, Rotor syndrome, recent trophoblasic disease. *Possible interaction*: phenytoin, carbamazepine, tetracyclines, primidone, chloral hydrate, glutehimide, rifampicin, griseofulvin, dichloralphenazone, ethosuximide, barbiturates. *Side effects*: feeling of bloatedness due to fluid retention, leg pains, breast enlargement, muscular cramps, weight gain, breakthrough bleeding, depression, vaginal discharge, loss of libido, nausea, brown patches on skin (chloasma). Stop drug immediately if frequent, severe headaches occur or signs of thromboses, rise in blood pressure. Drug should be discontinued before major planned surgery. *Manufacturer*: Schering H.C.

FEMULEN

Description: a hormonal preparation which is a progestogen only contraceptive in the form of white tablets containing 500µg ethinodiol diacetate marked with manufacturer's name. *Used for*: oral contraception. *Dosage*: 1 tablet at same time each day starting on first day of period and continuing without a break. *Special care*: patients with history of, or considered to be at risk of thrombosis, hypertension, cysts on ovaries, hormone dependent cancer, liver disease. Blood pressure, breasts and pelvic organs should be checked regularly during the course of treatment. *Avoid use*: pregnancy, previous ectopic pregnancy, history of heart or arterial disease or stroke, liver tumour, recent trophoblastic cancer, undiagnosed vaginal bleeding. *Possible interaction*: meprobamate, chloral hydrate, ethosuximide, barbiturates, carbamazepine, chlorpromazine, griseofulvin, dichloralphenazone, pyrimidone, rifampicin, phenytoin, glutethimide. *Side effects*: headache, breast tenderness, ovarian cysts, acne, disruption to normal pattern of menstrual bleeding, acne. Discontinue immediately if jaundice, signs of thrombosis or thrombophlebitis occur. *Manufacturer*: Searle.

FENBID SPANSULE

Description: a proprietary NSAID which is a propionic acid produced in the form of sustained-release spansules. Maroon/pink capsules contain off-white pellets consisting of 300mg ibuprofen. *Used for*: pain and arthritic conditions including ankylosing spondylitis, rheumatoid arthritis, osteoarthritis and other disorders of the skeleton and joints. *Dosage*: 2 capsules twice each day at first increasing to 3 capsules twice daily if required. The maintenance dose is in the order of 1 or 2 capsules twice each day. *Special care*: pregnancy, breast-feeding, elderly, asthma, disease of the gastro-intestinal tract, heart, liver or kidney disorders. Patients taking the drug long-term require careful monitoring. *Avoid use*: children, patients with allergy to aspirin or other anti-inflammatory drugs, peptic ulcer. *Possible interaction*: thiazide diuretics, quinolones, anticoagulant drugs. *Side effects*: rash, gastro-intestinal upset and possibly bleeding, thrombocytopenia (If a patient contracts aseptic meningitis, it must be reported to the Committee on the Safety of Medicines). *Manufacturer*: Goldshield.

FENOPRON

Description: a proprietary NSAID and propionic acid, fenoprofen (as calcium salt), produced in the form of tablets of 2 different strengths. Oval-shaped, orange tablets, coded DISTA 4019, contain 300mg ; oblong-shaped orange tablets coded DISTA 4021, contain 600mg. *Used for*: pain and arthritic conditions including ankylosing spondylitis, rheumatoid arthritis and osteoarthritis. *Dosage*: 300–600mg 3 to 4 times daily with a maximum daily dose of 3g. *Special care*: pregnancy, breast-feeding, elderly, liver or kidney disease, heart failure, asthma, a history of disorders involving gastro-intestinal bleeding. Patients taking the drug long-term should receive careful monitoring. *Avoid use*: children, patients with ulcers, allergy to aspirin or anti-inflammatory drugs, serious kidney disorders. *Possible interaction*: aspirin, quinolones, loop diuretics, anticoagulants, hydantoins, phenobarbitone, sulphonylureas. *Side effects*: allergic responses, intolerance of gastro-intestinal tract, blood changes, kidney and liver disorders. *Manufacturers*: Novex.

FENTAZIN

Description: a potent antipsychotic preparation and group III phenothiazine (a piperazine), produced as tablets of 2 strengths. White, sugar-coated tablets, coded 1C, contain 2mg perphenazine; white, sugar-coated tablets coded 2C contain 4mg. *Used for*: various serious psychiatric disorders including schizophrenia, psychoses, anxiety, nervous stress, vomiting and nausea. *Dosage*: adults, 12mg each day in divided doses with a maximum of 24mg daily; elderly persons, quarter to half the full dose. *Special care*: pregnancy, breast-feeding, epilepsy, glaucoma, Parkinson's disease, liver disease, hypothyroidism, myasthenia gravis, cardiovascular disease, phaeochromocytoma, enlarged prostate gland. *Avoid use*: children, patients with depressed bone marrow or in comatose states. *Possible interaction*: alcohol, anti-arrhythmic drugs, anaesthetics, antidepressants, antacids, rifampicin, sulphonylureas, antihypertensives, antiepileptic and antidiabetic drugs. *Side effects*: allergic responses, effects on liver and jaundice, changes in menstruation, breasts, weight gain, impotence, effects on heart rhythm (tachycardia), blurred vision, dry mouth, difficulty with urination, blocked nose, constipation, drowsiness, pallor, apathy, insomnia, hypotension, convulsions, effects on eyes and skin colouration with higher doses. *Manufacturer*: Forley.

FERFOLIC SV

Description: a combined mineral and vitamin preparation with a haematinic (iron) and vitamin B component. It is produced in the form of pink, sugar-coated tablets containing 4mg folic acid, 250mg ferrous gluconate and 10mg ascorbic acid. *Used for*: anaemias and conditions characterized by deficiency of iron and folic acid. Also used as a preventative to reduce the risk of neural tube defects in a foetus, when a mother known to be at risk is planning a pregnancy. *Dosage*: adults, for deficiency, 1 tablet 3 times each day. Prevention of neural tube defects, 1 tablet each day when conception is planned and continuing during first 3 months of pregnancy. *Avoid use*: children, patients with megaloblastic anaemia. *Possible interaction*: tetracycline antibiotics. *Side effects*: constipation, nausea. *Manufacturer*: Sinclair.

FERTIRAL

Description: a hormonal preparation of gonadotrophin-releasing hormone, produced in the form of a solution in ampoules for infusion containing 500 micrograms gonadorelin per ml. *Used for*: amenorrhoea and certain types of infertility in women. *Dosage*: determined individually. *Special care*: maximum period of treatment is 6 months and should be discontinued in the event of pregnancy. *Avoid use*: patients with cysts in the ovaries or lining of the womb.

Side effects: headache, nausea, abdominal pain, pain at infusion site, menorrhagia (abnormally long or heavy menstrual periods). *Manufacturer*: Hoechst.

FILAIR

Description: an anti-inflammatory corticosteroid preparation containing 50 or 100 g beclomethasone dipropionate delivered by metered dose aerosol. Also, **FILAIR FORTE** containing 250 g. *Used for*: reversible obstructive airways disease (asthma). *Dosage*: adults, 100 g, 3 or 4 times each day or 200 g twice each day. In extremely severe conditions 600–800 g in divided doses, with a maximum of 1mg, may be taken. Filair Forte, 500 g twice each day or 250 g 4 times each day. Children, Filair only, 50–100 g 2, 3 or 4 times each day. *Special care*: pregnancy, history of or active pulmonary tuberculosis, those transferring from other (systemic) steroid drugs. *Side effects*: hoarse voice, candidiasis (yeast-like fungal infection) of throat and mouth. *Manufacturer*: 3M Health Care.

FLAGYL

Description: an antibacterial preparation and nitroimidazoles, which is effective against anaerobic bacteria and certain other infective organisms. It is produced in a variety of forms: Flagyl tablets, off-white, film-coated tablets contain 200mg and 400mg metronidazole, the higher strength being capsule-shaped. Both are marked with strength and tablet name. **FLAGYL-S SUSPENSION** contains 200mg metronidazole (as benzoate) per 5ml liquid. **FLAGYL SUPPOSITORIES** contain 500mg and 1g metronidazole. **FLAGYL COMPAK** consists of fourteen off-white, film-coated, capsule-shaped tablets containing 400mg metronidazole, marked with name and strength and also fourteen pale yellow coloured pessaries containing 100,000 units nystatin. **FLAGYL INTRAVENOUS INFUSION** contains 5mg metronidazole per ml in ampoules for intravenous infusion. *Used for*: infections caused by anaerobic bacteria, amoebic dysentery, abscess of liver, trichomoniasis (of urogenital tract), vaginosis of bacterial origin, dental infections and severe ulcerative gingivitis. Prevention of infection before surgery. *Dosage*: depending upon condition being treated, adults, in the order of 400mg–1g every 8 hours in first instance, then reduced doses. Period of treatment is usually 1 week. Children receive reduced doses usually in the order of 7.5mg/kg body weight. In cases of vaginosis, sexual partner should also receive therapy at same time. *Special care*: pregnancy, breastfeeding, patients with disorders of central nervous system, hepatic encephalopathy (a liver disease in which toxic substances normally removed by the liver interfere with the function of the brain). *Possible interaction*: phenobarbitone, alcohol, lithium, anticoagulant drugs taken orally. *Side effects*: central nervous system effects, dark coloured urine, unpleasant taste in mouth and furring of tongue, gastro-intestinal upset, rash, angioneurotic oedema, leucopenia. Longterm therapy may cause neuropathy (nerve disorders) and epileptic-type fits. *Manufacturer*: R.P.R.

FLAMAZINE

Description: an antibacterial cream containing 1% silver sulphadiazine. *Used for*: burns, skin wounds, pressure sores, infected leg ulcers, areas where skin has been removed for grafting. *Dosage*: apply a layer of cream 3–5mm thick beneath dressing which should be changed daily for burns and 3 times each week for ulcers. *Special care*: patients with liver or kidney disorders. *Avoid use*: pregnancy, newborn babies. *Possible interaction*: wound-cleaning agents with enzyme action, phenytoin, hypoglycaemic drugs taken orally, sulphonamides. *Manufacturer*: S.& N.

FLAXEDIL

Description: a muscle relaxant produced as a solution in ampoules for injection, containing 40mg gallamine triethiodide per ml. *Used for*: to produce paralysis during surgical operations after the patient has become unconscious and for seriously ill patients receiving prolonged artificial ventilation in intensive care. *Dosage*: given by intravenous injection. Adults, 80–120mg and then 20–40mg as needed. Child, 1.5mg/kg body weight; newborn baby, 600 g/kg body weight. *Special care*: kidney disorder. *Avoid use*: serious kidney disease. *Possible interaction*: some antiarrhythmic drugs, some antibacterial drugs, propranolol, verapamil, nifedipine, some cholinergics, magnesium salts, lithium. *Side effects*: tachycardia. *Manufacturer*: Rhône-Poulenc Rorer.

FLEMOXIN

Description: an antibiotic preparation which is a broad-spectrum penicillin. Flemoxin is produced as white, scored, dissolvable tablets of 2 strengths containing 375mg (marked gbr 183) and 750mg (marked gbr 185) amoxycillin (as trihydrate). *Used for*: soft tissue, respiratory tract, urinary tract and ear, nose and throat infections. *Dosage*: depending upon type of infection; adults in the order of 375mg–3g, usually twice each day. Tablets may be dissolved in water or swallowed whole. Children, 2–5 years of age, 750mg twice each day; 5 to 10 years, half adult dose; over 10 years, adult dose. *Special care*: patients with lymphatic leukaemia, glandular fever. *Side effects*: allergic reactions, rash, gastrointestinal upset. *Manufacturer*: Paines and Byrne.

FLEXIN CONTINUS

Description: a NSAID available as continuous-release tablets of thee strengths, all of which are capsule-shaped and marked with strength and 1C. Green, red and yellow tablets contain 25mg, 50mg and 75mg indomethacin respectively. *Used for*: arthritic disorders of joints and skeleton including osteoarthritis, ankylosing spondylitis, rheumatoid arthritis, degenerative disease of the hip joint, other musculo-skeletal and back disorders which cause pain, dysmenorrhoea (period pain). *Dosage*: adults, 25–200mg each day in 1 or 2 divided doses taken with food, milk or antacid preparation. *Special care*: elderly persons, patients with heart failure, liver or kidney disease, disorders of the central nervous system. Those taking the drug long-term require careful monitoring and eye tests. *Avoid use*: pregnancy, breast-feeding, allergy to aspirin or anti-inflammatory drug, defects in blood coagulation, stomach ulcer or ulcer of gastrointestinal lesions. *Possible interaction*: corticosteroids, ß-blockers, quinolones, diuretics, methotrexate, salicylates, lithium, probenecid, anticoagulants. *Side effects*: rash, blood changes, effects on central nervous system, giddiness, visual disturbance, corneal deposits, blood in urine, adverse kidney effects (nephrotoxicity), tinnitus, inflammation of small blood vessels (angitis). Drug should be discontinued if recurring headaches or gastro-intestinal bleeding occur. *Manufacturer*: Napp.

FLIXONASE

Description: a corticosteroid nasal spray 50µg fluticasone propionate per metered dose. *Used for*: prevention and treatment of allergic rhinitis (hay fever), nasal congestion. *Dosage*: adults, 2 sprays into each nostril in the morning, with a maximum of 4 sprays into both nostrils daily. Children, over 4 years of age, 1 spray (maximum of 2) into each nostril daily. *Special care*: pregnancy, breast-feeding, transferring from other (systemic) steroid drugs taken orally. *Avoid use*: children under 4 years of age. *Side effects*: nosebleed, irritation of nose, interference with sense of taste and smell. *Manufacturer*: A & H.

FLIXOTIDE

Description: a corticosteroid preparation containing fluticasone propionate for use with diskhaler and inhaler. 50, 100, 250 and 500µg fluticasone propionate disks are for use with breath-operated diskhaler delivery system. Also, 25, 50, 125 and 250µg fluticasone propionate per dose are for use with metered dose aerosol delivery system. *Used for*: prevention of bronchial asthma. *Dosage*: adults, 100–1000µg twice each day; children over 4 years of age, 50–100µg twice each day. *Special care*: pregnancy, transferring from other (systemic) steroid drugs taken orally, those with history of or with active tuberculosis. *Avoid use*: children under 4 years of age. *Side effects*: candidiasis (a yeast-like fungal infection) of throat and mouth, hoarseness, occasional unexplained bronchospasm. *Manufacturer*: A & H.

FLOLAN

Description: an anticoagulant prostaglandin preparation produced in the form of a powder containing 500µg epoprostenol (as sodium salt) with a diluent for reconstitution and infusion. *Used for*: prevention of blood clotting during and following heart surgery; kidney dialysis (with heparin). *Dosage*: according to manufacturer's literature. *Special care*: if being given with heparin in kidney dialysis, anticoagulant monitoring must be carried out. Must be given by continuous intravenous infusion. *Side effects*: vasodilation, flushing, hypotension, headache, pallor, bradycardia, sweating. *Manufacturer*: Glaxo Wellcome.

FLORINEF

Description: a corticosteroid mineralocorticoid preparation produced in the form of scored, pink tablets coded 429 and marked SQUIBB, containing 0.1mg fludrocortisone acetate. Mineralocorticoids regulate the salt/water balance in the body. *Used for*: treatment of salt-losing adrenogenital syndrome and to partially replace hormones in Addison's disease. *Dosage*: adults, 0.05–3mg each day; children, according to body weight, age and condition being treated. *Special care*: pregnancy, hypertension, epilepsy, kidney inflammation (nephritis, glomerulonephritis), diabetes, inflamed veins, stomach ulcer. Patients with glaucoma, secondary cancers, osteoporosis, liver cirrhosis, tuberculosis and other bacterial, viral or fungal infections, recent surgical bowel anastomoses, those suffering from psychoses or stress. Contact wtht chicken pox should be avoided and medical advice sought in the event of this occurring. Withdraw drug gradually. *Possible interaction*: anticoagulants taken orally, diuretics, ephedrine, phenytoin, cardiac glycosides, NSAIDs, phenobarbitone, hypoglycaemics, rifampicin, anticholinesterases. *Side effects*: fluid retention, hypertension, weakness in muscles, loss of potassium, Cushingoid changes (as in Cushing's syndrome). *Manufacturer*: Squibb.

FLOXAPEN

Description: a penicillinase-resistant form of penicillin. (Penicillinase is an enzyme produced by some bacteria that renders penicillin inactive, hence the infection being treated will be resistant to the antibiotic). Floxapen is produced in several forms: black/caramel-coloured capsules of 2 strengths containing 250mg and 500mg flucloxacillin sodium, each marked with strength and name. FLOXAPEN SYRUP contains 125mg flucloxacillin (as magnesium salt) per 5ml, supplied as powder for reconstitution with water to make 100ml. FLOXAPEN SYRUP FORTE contains 250mg per 5ml, supplied as powder to make 100ml. FLOXAPEN INJECTION is supplied as powder in vials for reconstitution at strengths of 250mg, 500mg and 1g flucloxacillin (as sodium salt). *Used for*: ear, nose, throat, soft tisssue, skin infections and other infections including those caused by staphylococci bacteria resistant to penicillin. *Dosage*: capsules and syrup, 250mg 4 times each day taken 1 hour to half an hour before meals. Injection, 250mg–1g given intravenously 4 times each day. Children, capsules, syrup and injection, age 2 years and under, quarter of adult dose; age 2 to 10 years, half adult dose; over 10 years, adult dose. *Avoid use*: allergy to penicillin. *Side effects*: gastro-intestinal upset, allergic responses, rarely cholestatic jaundice. *Manufacturer*: Beecham.

FLUANXOL

Description: an antidepressant preparation and a thioxanthene, available as red, sugar-coated tablets of 2 strengths, containing 0.5mg and 1mg of flupenthixol (as dihydrochloride), both marked LUNDBECK. *Used for*: short-term treatment of depression which may be accompanied by symptoms of anxiety. *Dosage*: adults, 1–2mg as a single dose taken in the morning with a maximum daily amount of 3mg in divided doses. Elderly persons, 0.5mg as a single morning dose with a daily maximum of 2g in divided doses. *Special care*: patients with serious heart, circulatory, liver or kidney disease, arteriosclerosis, Parkinsonism, elderly persons in confused states. *Avoid use*: children, overactive, excitable persons, those with very severe depression. *Possible interaction*: other antidepressants, central nervous system sedatives, antihypertensives, anticonvulsants, levodopa, alcohol, antidiabetic drugs. *Side effects*: dry mouth, blocked nose, visual disturbances, muscular spasms and Parkinsonism-like symptoms, hypotension, tiredness and lethargy. Weight gain, sleepiness, constipation, difficulty passing urine, enlargement of breasts and abnormal production of milk, dermatitis, blood changes, tachycardia and effects on ECG, jaundice, fits. *Manufacturer*: Lundbeck.

FLUVIRIN

Description: a vaccine against influenza containing inactivated surface antigens of 3 strains of influenza virus produced in the form of 15 s of each strain per 0.5ml solution in pre-filled syringes. *Used for*: immunization against influenza. *Dosage*: adults, 0.5ml by intramuscular or deep subcutaneous injection. Children over 4 years of age, 0.5ml followed by a further 0.5ml after 1 month to 6 weeks. *Special care*: pregnant women. *Avoid use*: children under 4 years of age, patients with allergy to chicken or egg protein (as vaccines are cultivated on these). *Side effects*: feverishness, headache, malaise, soreness at injection site, all uncommon and transient. *Manufacturer*: Evans.

FLUZONE

Description: a vaccine against influenza containing inactivated split virion of 3 strains of influenza virus. Produced in the form of pre-filled syringes containing 15µs of each strain per 0.5ml. *Used for*: immunization against influenza. *Dosage*: adults, 0.5ml by subcutaneous or intramuscular injection; children 6 months to 3 years, 0.25ml followed by further 0.25ml afer 1 month; 3 years to 12 years, 0.5ml followed by further 0.5ml after 1 month; over thirteen years as adult. *Avoid use*: patients with feverish illness, those with allergy to egg protein. *Side effects*: feverishness, headache, malaise, soreness at injection site (of transient nature). *Manufacturer*: Pasteur Vaccines..

FML

Description: an anti-inflammatory corticosteroid in the form of eyedrops containing 0.1% fluorometholone. Also FML NEO corticosteroid and aminoglycoside eyedrops containing 0.1% fluorometholone and 0.5% neomycin sulphate. *Used for*: FML—eye inflammation in which there is an absence of infection. FML Neo—eye inflammation in which infection is present. *Dosage*: adults, 1 to 2 drops 2, 3 or 4 times daily directly into eye; children over 2 years of age, as adult dose. *Special care*: glaucoma; prolonged use in young children or pregnant women. *Avoid use*: infections with tuberculous, viral or fungal origin and those in which pus is present; soft contact lenses. *Side effects:* rise in pressure within eye, thinning of cornea, secondary fungal infection, cataract. *Manufacturer*: Allergan.

FOLICIN

Description: a haematinic and mineral supplement available in the form of white, sugar-coated tablets containing 2.5mg folic acid, 2.5mg manganese sulphate and 200mg dried ferrous sulphate (equivalent to 60mg iron). *Used for*: prevention and treatment of anaemia in pregnant women. *Dosage*: adults, 1 to 2 tablets each day. *Avoid use*: patients with megaloblastic anaemia. *Possible interaction*: levodopa, tetracyclines. *Side effects*: constipation, nausea. *Manufacturer*: Link.

FORCEVAL

Description: a preparation containing minerals, trace elements and vitamins produced in the form of brown/red gelatin capsules marked 6377 and FORCEVAL. Also, **FORCEVAL JUNIOR** available as oval brown gelatin capsules marked 571 and FORCEVAL. *Used for*: a dietary supplement to prevent and treat mineral and vitamin deficiencies in patients unable to obtain adequate amounts from food alone. May be used, for example, in patients recuperating from serious illness or surgery, and those on special controlled diets or who have intolerance to foods. *Dosage*: 1 capsule daily; children, Forceval Junior only, over 5 years of age, 2 capsules each day. *Avoid use*: children under 5 years, patients with disorders of iron absorption and storage (haemochromatosis) or with hypercalcaemia. *Possible interaction*: tetracyclines, anticoagulant drugs, phenytoin. *Manufacturer*: Unigreg.

FORTAGESIC^{CD}

Description: a controlled drug combining a narcotic analgesic with paracetamol, which has analgesic and antipyretic properties (reduces fever). It is produced in the form of white tablets, marked with name and symbol, containing 15mg pentazocine (as hydrochloride) and 500mg paracetamol. Pentazocine is a moderately potent analgesic and is less likely to cause addiction than some other narcotic drugs. *Used for*: pain caused by disorders of bone and muscle. *Dosage*: 2 tablets up to 4 times each day; children over 7 years, 1 tablet every 3 to 4 hours with a maximum of 4 in 24 hours. *Special care*: pregnancy, liver, kidney or respiratory diseases, porphyria. *Avoid use*: patients with brain injury or disease, raised intracranial pressure or who are narcotic dependent. *Possible interaction*: alcohol, other narcotic drugs, MAOIs. *Side effects*: nausea, dizziness, sedation, drug-induced symptoms of psychosis. *Manufacturer*: Sanofi Winthrop.

FORTRAL^{CD}

Description: a narcotic antagonist and controlled drug, produced in a variety of forms. White, film-coated tablets contain 25mg pentazocine hydrochloride, marked with symbol and name. **FORTRAL CAPSULES** marked FORTRAL 50 and coloured yellow/grey, contain 50mg. **FORTRAL INJECTION** contain 30mg pentazocine (as acetate) per ml in ampoules. **FORTRAL SUPPOSITORIES** contain 50mg. *Used for*: relief of pain. *Dosage*: adults, tablets or capsules, 25–100mg after meals every 3 to 4 hours; injection, 30–60mg by intravenous, intramuscular or subcutaneous injection every 3 to 4 hours; suppositories, 1 when required with a maximum of 4 in 24 hours. Children, tablets or capsules, 6 to 12 years, 25mg every 3 to 4 hours. Injection, children 1 to 12 years, either a maximum of 1mg/kg body weight as single dose by subcutaneous or intramuscular injection, or 0.5mg/kg body weight given intravenously as single dose. *Special care*: pregnancy, liver, kidney or respiratory diseases. *Avoid use*: children under 1 year of age, patients with brain injury or disease, raised intracranial pressure, narcotic dependent or who have porphyria. *Possible interaction*: other narcotic drugs, alcohol, MAOIs. *Side effects*: nausea, dizziness, sedation, drug-induced symptoms of psychosis. *Manufacturer*: Sterwin.

FORTUM

Description: a cephalosporin antibiotic preparation produced in the form of powder in vials for reconstitution and injection, containing 250mg 500mg, 1g, 2g and 3g ceftazidime (as pentahydrate). *Used for*: urinary and gastro-intestinal tract infections, infections of ear, nose and throat, joints, bones, soft tissues, skin, meningitis, septicaemia and infections in patients who are immunocompromised. *Dosage*: adults, 1g every 8 hours or 2g at 12 hour intervals. If infection is extremely severe, 2g every 8 to 12 hours. Single doses above 1g should be given intravenously, lower doses by intravenous injection or infusion or intramuscularly. Children, 2 months and under, 25–60mg/kg body weight in 2 divided doses each day; over 2 months, 30–100mg/kg body weight each day in 2 or 3 divided doses. A dose of up to 150mg/kg body weight may be given in cases of meningitis or if immuno-compromised. In children, the intravenous route should be used. Elderly persons, a maximum dose of 3g each day depending upon type and severity of infection. *Special care*: pregnant women, patients with allergy to penicillin (about 10% of whom are also allergic to cephalosporins), kidney disease. *Possible interaction*: loop diuretics, aminoglycosides. *Side effects*: gastro-intestinal upset, pain at injection site, blood changes involving white blood cells, candidiasis (infection caused by yeast-like fungus), allergic reactions, positive Coombs test, rise in level of blood urea and liver enzymes. *Manufacturer*: Glaxo Wellcome.

FOSCAVIR

Description: an antiviral preparation containing 24mg foscarnet sodium hexahydrate per ml produced as bottles of isotonic infusion. *Used for*: life-threatening infections of viral origin particularly those of the eyes in patients with AIDS (cytomegalovirus retinitis). *Dosage*: adults, 20mg/kg body weight by intravenous infusion over half an hour, then 21–200mg/kg body weight each day for 2 to 3 weeks. (Dose depending upon kidney function). *Special care*: patients with kidney disease, hypocalcaemia. Blood tests are required during therapy and patient should receive adequate fluids. *Avoid use*: patients with severe kidney disease, pregnancy, breast-feeding. *Side effects*: rash, nausea, headache, vomiting, tiredness, disturbance of kidney function including kidney failure, decreased haemoglobin and calcium levels. Rarely, convulsions, inflamed veins, hypoglycaemia. *Manufacturer*: Astra.

FRAGMIN

Description: an anticoagulant preparation which is a low molecular weight heparin produced as a solution in ampoules for injection and which contain 2500 units or 10,000 units dalteparin sodium per ml. **FRAGMIN PRE-FILLED SYRINGES** contain 2500 units or 5000 units dalteparin sodium per 0.2ml. *Used for*: prevention of thrombosis during and after surgery and clotting in extracorporeal circulation during dialysis treatment. *Dosage*: dependent upon condition being treated (i.e. surgery or dialysis) and if patient is at high or low risk of bleeding (dialysis). *Special care*: pregnancy, breast-feeding, liver disease, those at high risk of bleeding or in whom therapeutic effects of drug occur in narrow dose range. Careful monitoring and blood checks required. *Possible interaction*: cardiac glycosides, other anticoagulant and antiplatelet drugs, indomethacin, tetracyclines, probencid, antihistamines, dextran, sulphinpyrazone, aspirin, ethacrynic acid, vitamin K antagonists, cytostatics, dipyradamole, cardiac glycosides. *Side effects*: bleeding if dose is high. *Manufacturer*: Pharmacia & Upjohn.

FRISIUM

Description: an anxiolytic and anticonvulsant which is a long-acting benzodiazepine produced in the form of blue capsules containing 10mg clobazum and marked FRISIUM. *Used for*: anxiety and tense and agitated states; additional therapy in the treatment of epilepsy. *Dosage*: adults, 20–30mg each day in divided dose or as single bedtime dose with a maximum of 60mg daily. Elderly persons, 20 mg each day. Children, age 3 to 12 years, half adult dose. *Special care*: pregnancy, women in labour, breast-feeding, elderl, liver or kidney disease. Short-term use and withdraw gradually. *Avoid use*: patients with breathing difficulties, lung diseases and respiratory depression, those suffering from phobic, psychotic or obsessional psychiatric illnesses. Children under 3 years. *Possible interaction*: other central nervous system depressant drugs, anticonvulsants, alcohol. *Side effects*: gastro-intestinal upset, light-headedness, disturbance of vision, vertigo, sleepiness, hypotension, confusion, rash, urine retention, reduced libido, ataxia. Rarely there may be blood changes and jaundice. Performance of skilled tasks and judgement is impaired, risk of dependence with higher doses and longer term therapy. *Manufacturer*: Hoechst.

FROBEN

Description: an analgesic preparation which is a proprionic acid produced in the form of tablets of 2 strengths. Yellow, sugar-coated tablets contain 50mg and 100mg flurbiprofen, marked F50 and F100 respectively. Also **FROBEN SR** which are yellow, sustained-release capsules marked FSR containing 200mg flurbiprofen. **FROBEN SUPPOSITORIES** contain 100mg flurbiprofen *Used for*: pain including dysmenorrhoea (period pain) (Froben tablets); musculoskeletal diseases, osteoarthritis and ankylosing spondylitis (Froben SR and Suppositories). *Dosage*: adults, tablets, 100–200mg each day in divided doses with a maximum daily dose of 300mg. SR Capsules, 1 each day after evening meal. Suppositories, 150mg—200mg each day as divided doses with a daily maximum of 300mg. *Special care*: pregnancy, breast-feeding, elderly, liver or kidney disease, heart failure, asthma. Those taking the drug long-term require careful monitoring. *Avoid use*: children, patients with allergy to aspirin or anti-inflammatory drugs, those with stomach ulcer or gastro-intestinal bleeding. *Possible interaction*: anticoagulant drugs, frusemide, quinolones. *Side effects*: rash, intolerance of gastro-intestinal system, rarely thrombocytopenia, jaundice. *Manufacturer*: Knoll.

FRU-CO

Description: a potassium-sparing and loop diuretic produced in the form of scored, orange tablets containing 40mg frusemide amd 5mg amiloride hydrochloride (co-amilofuse), marked FRO-CO. *Used for*: oedema accompanying kidney or liver disease, heart failure. *Dosage*: adults, 1 or 2 tablets taken in the morning. *Special care*: pregnancy, breast-feeding, elderly, liver or kidney disease, enlarged prostate gland, difficulty in urination, gout, diabetes, acidosis. *Avoid use*: children, hyperkalaemia, coma resulting from cirrhosis of the liver, progressive kidney failure. *Possible interaction*: other potassium-sparing diuretics and potassium supplements, hypoglycaemics, aminoglycosides, cephalosporins, lithium, antihypertensives, digitalis, NSAIDs, non-depolarizing muscle relaxants (anaesthetics), ACE inhibitors. *Side effects*: rash, gastrointestinal upset, malaise; rarely, blood changes. *Manufacturer*: Baker Norton.

FRUMIL

Description: a preparation which is a loop and potassium-sparing diuretic produced in the form of scored, orange tablets containing 40mg frusemide and 5mg amiloride hydrochloride (co-amilofruse) marked FRUMIL. Also **FRUMIL LS**, orange tablets containing 20mg frusemide and 2.5mg amiloride hydrochloride, marked LS. **FRUMIL FORTE**, orange scored tablets containing 80mg frusemide and 10mg amiloride hydrochloride, marked DS. *Used for*: oedema accompanying kidney or liver disease and heart failure. *Dosage*: adults, Frumil tablets, 1 or 2 taken in morning; Frumil LS and Frumil Forte, 1 tablet taken in morning. *Special care*: elderly, liver or kidney disease, enlarged prostate gland, difficulty in urination, gout, diabetes, acidosis. *Avoid use*: children, pregnancy, breast-feeding, hyperkalaemia, coma resulting from cirrhosis of the liver, progressive kidney failure. *Possible interaction*: other potassium-sparing diuretics and potassium supplements, ACE inhibitors, hypoglycaemics, antihypertensives, non-depolarizing muscle relaxants (anaesthetics), cardiac glycosides, NSAIDs, aminoglycosides, lithium, cephalosporins. *Side effects*: rash, gastro-intestinal upset, malaise; rarely, blood changes. *Manufacturer*: R.P.R.

FRUSENE

Description: a potassium-sparing and loop diuretic produced in the form of scored yellow tablets containing 40mg frusemide and 50mg triamterene. *Used for*: oedema accompanying liver or heart disease, congestive heart failure. *Dosage*: adults, half to 2 tablets each day with a daily maximum of 6 (in divided doses). *Special care*: pregnancy, breast-feeding mothers, gout, enlarged prostate gland, difficulty in urination, acidosis, liver or kidney disease, diabetes. *Avoid use*: children, patients with coma resulting from liver cirrhosis, hyperkalaemia, progressive kidney failure. *Possible interaction*: other potassium-sparing diuretics and potassium supplements, aminoglycosides, cardiac glycosides, neuromuscular blocking drugs, lithium, theophylline, NSAIDs, cephalosporins. *Side effects*: rash, gastro-intestinal upset, malaise; rarely, blood changes. *Manufacturer*: Orion.

FUCIBET

Description: a potent steroid and antibacterial agent in the form of a cream containing 0.1% betmethasone valerate and 2% fusidic acid. *Used for*: eczema in which bacterial infection is likely to be present. *Dosage*: apply thinly 2 or 3 times each day to affected skin and reduce dose when condition improves. *Special care*: short-term use only (maximum of few weeks when lower potency substitute should be tried, if needed), withdraw gradually. *Avoid use*: children, extensive or longer-term use in pregnant women, infections due to ringworm, virus, tuberculosis, untreated bacterial and fungal infections, leg ulcers, scabies, acne. *Side effects*: adrenal gland suppression, skin thinning, abnormal hair growth, skin changes as in Cushing's syndrome. *Manufacturer*: Leo.

FUCIDIN H

Description: an antibacterial agent and mildly potent corticosteroid. It is available as ointment, cream or gel, all containing 2% sodium fusidate and 1% hydrocortisone. *Used for*: dermatitis in which bacterial infection is likely to be present. *Dosage*: apply thinly 2 or 3 times each day to affected skin and reduce dose when condition improves. *Special care*: limit use in children or on face to a maximum period of 5 days. *Avoid use*: extensive or long-term use especially in pregnant women, infections due to ringworm, virus, tuberculosis, untreated bacterial and fungal infections, leg ulcers, scabies, acne. *Side effects*: adrenal gland suppression, skin thinning, abnormal hair growth, skin changes as in Cushing's syndrome. *Manufacturer*: Leo.

FUCITHALMIC

Description: an antibacterial preparation produced in the form of an eye gel which becomes liquid when in contact with eye, containing 1% fusidic acid. *Used for*: conjunctivitis where bacteria, especially staphylococci, are cause of infection. *Dosage*: apply 1 drop into eye twice each day. *Side effects*: allergic reaction, local irritation of short-lived nature. *Manufacturer*: Leo.

FULCIN

Description: an antifungal preparation produced in the form of tablets of 2 strengths and as a solution. Scored, white tablets, marked ICI, contain 125mg and 500mg griseofulvin. **FULCIN SUSPENSION** contains 125mg griseofulvin per 5ml of suspension. *Used for*: fungal infections of scalp, skin and nails where ointments and creams have been ineffective or are not considered to be appropriate. *Dosage*: adults, 125mg 4 times each day or a single dose of 500mg. Children, 10mg/kg body weight in divided doses or as a single dose. *Avoid use*: pregnancy, serious liver disease or porphyria. *Possible interaction*: oral contraceptives, alcohol, barbiturates, anticoagulants of the coumarin group. *Side effects*: allergic responses and rash, sensitivity to light, headache, stomach upset, blood changes involving white blood cells; rarely, a collagen disease. *Manufacturer*: Zeneca.

FUNGILIN

Description: an antifungal preparation and polyene antibiotic, amphotericin, effective against filamentous and yeast-like fungi and which does not produce drug resistance. Fungilin is produced in the form of scored brown tablets containing 100mg and marked SQUIBB 430. **FUNGILIN SUSPENSION** coloured yellow and containing 100mg per ml of solution. **FUNGILIN LOZENGES** coloured yellow containing 10mg and marked SQUIBB 929. *Used for*: candidiasis of the intestine, vagina and skin (thrush) and prevention of infection. Lozenges are used for mouth infections. *Dosage*: adults, 1 to 2 tablets or 1–2ml suspension each day; lozenges, 1 dissolved slowly in mouth 4 to 8 times each day. Children, suspension, 1ml 4 times each day. *Side effects*: gastro-intestinal upset if dose is high. *Manufacturer*: Squibb.

FUNGIZONE

Description: an antifungal preparation and polyene antibiotic, effective against filamentous and yeast-like fungi and which does not produce drug resistance. It is produced as a powder in vials for reconstitution and injection containing 50mg amphotericin sodium desoxycholate complex. *Used for*: serious, life-threatening systemic fungal infections. *Dosage*: by intravenous infusion, 250µs/kg body weight each day increasing to 1mg in cases of severe infection, if drug is tolerated. Maximum dose is 1.5mg/kg body weight each day or every other day. *Special care*: produces toxic side effects when given in this way, hence patients require close monitoring of liver and kidney function, blood counts, electrolyte levels in blood plasma. *Special care*: pregnancy, breast-feeding. Change injection site frequently. *Side effects*: irritation at injection site, rash, vomiting, diarrhoea, nausea, headache, abdominal pain, anorexia, pain in muscles and joints, fever, adverse effects on liver, kidneys, heart, nerves, convulsions, loss of hearing, anaphylactic-type allergic reactions. *Manufacturer*: Squibb.

FURADANTIN

Description: an antibacterial preparation which is of a type known as nitofurans (synthetic antibiotic drugs). It is produced in the form of scored, yellow pentagonal-shaped tablets of 2 strengths containing 50mg and 100mg nitrofurantoin both marked with strength and name. Also **FURADANTIN SUSPENSION** containing 25mg nitrofurantoin per 5ml suspension. *Used for*: treatment and prevention of genital and urinary tract infections, (e.g. in patient undergoing surgery or exploratory procedure), pyelitis. *Dosage*: adults, depending upon condition being treated, in the order of 50–100mg 4 times each day for 1 week (or once a day at bedtime if for prevention of infection on longer term basis). Children, age 3 months to 10 years, in the order of 3mg/kg body weight 4 times each day for 1 week or 1mg/kg once daily if for prevention. Over 10 years, same as adult. *Special care*: children under 3 months, breast-feeding, elderly, patients with diabetes, vitamin B deficiency or who are debilitated, anaemia, imbalance of electrolyte (salt) levels. Patients should receive monitoring of liver and lung function if undergoing long-term treatment. *Avoid use*: women at end of pregnancy, kidney disorder, anuria or oliguria. *Possible interaction*: probenecid, quinolones, magnesium trisilicate, sulphinpyrazone. *Side effects*: gastro-intestinal upset, blood changes, allergic reactions. Drug should be stopped immediately if signs of peripheral nerve damage, lung disorder, breakdown of red blood cells (haemolysis), hepatitis occur. *Manufacturer*: Procter & Gamble.

FYBOGEL MEBEVERINE

Description: a bulking agent and antispasmodic preparation, produced in the form of effervescent granules in sachets for dissolving in water, containing 135mg mebeverine hydrochloride, 3.5g ispaghula husk. *Used for*: irritable bowel syndrome, diverticular disease, constipation due to insufficient dietary fibre. *Dosage*: adults, 1 sachet every morning and evening half an hour before meals in water. Additional sachet before midday meal may also be taken. *Avoid use*: patients with intestinal obstruction, serious heart, circulatory and kidney disorders. *Manufacturer*: Reckitt and Colman.

G

GALENAMET

Description: a preparation that is an H_2-receptor antagonist which acts to reduce the secretion of stomach acid, thereby promoting the healing of ulcers. It is available in tablets of 3 strengths containing 200mg, 400mg and 800mg cimetidine. *Used for*: gastro-intestinal ulcers, Zollinger-Ellison syndrome, reflux oesophagitis. *Dosage*: for ulcers, 400mg twice each day morning and night, or 800mg taken at night; occasionally, 400mg 4 times each day may be required with an absolute maximum of 2.4g daily in divided doses (in rare cases of stress ulceration). Zollinger-Ellison syndrome and reflux oesophagitis 400mg 4 times each day. Children, 20–30mg/kg body weight each day in divided doses. *Special care*: pregnancy, breast-feeding, liver or kidney disease. *Possible interaction*: phenytoin, warfarin, theophylline, some antidepressants, sulphonylureas, carbamazepine, some antifungal drugs, quinine, chloroquine, some antipsychotic drugs, benzodiazepines, ß-blockers, calcium channel blockers, cyclosporin, fluorouracil, flosequinan. *Side effects*: rash, dizziness, fatigue, headache, confusion, change in bowel habit, lowered blood count, liver effects, allergic responses, bradycardia, pancreatitis, nephritis (inflammation in kidney), gynaecomastia, heart block. All are rare, but have been reported and may be more likely with higher doses. *Manufacturer*: Galen.

GALENAMOX

Description: an antibiotic preparation of amoxycillin, a broad-spectrum penicillin but one which is inactivated by the penicillinase enzymes produced by some bacteria. Hence some infections do not respond as the bacteria causing them are resistant. Galenamox is available in the form of capsules of 2 strengths containing 250mg and 500mg amoxycillin (as trihydrate). Also as **GALEN-AMOX SUSPENSION** containing 125mg or 250mg per 5ml solution. *Used for*: middle ear infections, secondary infections in chronic bronchitis, urinary tract infections, gonorrhoea, typhoid fever, prevention of endocarditis. *Dosage*: depending upon type of infection but in the order of 250mg–500mg every 8 hours with higher doses of 3g every 12 hours sometimes being required. Children, depending upon condition being treated but in the order of 125mg–250mg every 8 hours (up to 10 years of age). Higher doses may sometimes be needed. *Manufacturer*: Galen.

GAMANIL

Description: a TCAD preparation available as scored, maroon-coloured, film-coated tablets containing 70mg lofepramine (as hydrochloride). *Used for*: depression. *Dosage*: adults, 1 tablet in morning and either 1 or 2 at night. Reduced doses for elderly patients. *Special care*: elderly, breast-feeding, glaucoma, urinary retention, hyperthyroidism, diabetes, adrenal gland tumour, epilepsy, certain psychiatric disorders or at risk of suicide. Regular blood tests should be carried out. *Avoid use*: pregnancy, heart block, heart attack, serious liver disease. *Possible interaction*: other antidepressants, antihypertensives, barbiturates, alcohol, MAOIs, cimetidine, local anaesthetics containing noradrenaline or adrenaline, oestrogens. *Side effects*: blurred vision, hypotension, sweating, anxiety, dizziness, sleeplessness, ataxia, muscle weakness, drowsiness, palpitations, dry mouth, tachycardia, constipation, gastro-intestinal upset, weight changes, allergic responses including skin rash, blood changes, loss of libido or impotence, enlargement of breasts, abnormal milk production, jaundice. Also psychiatric effects especailly in the elderly. *Manufacturer*: Merck.

GAMMABULIN

Description: a preparation of 16% human normal immunoglobulin (HNIG) as a solution for intramuscular injection. *Used for*: immunization against hepatitis A, measles, rubella in pregnant women, antibody deficiency syndrome. *Dosage*: prevention of hepatitis A, adults and children, 0.02–0.04ml/kg body weight and possibly 0.06–0.12ml/kg body weight if risk is great. Prevention of measles, 0.2ml/kg body weight. Prevention of rubella in pregnant women, 20ml. All given by intramuscular injection. *Possible interaction*: live vaccines. *Manufacturer*: Immuno.

GANDA

Description: an adrenergic neurone blocker with a sympathomimetic produced in the form of drops to reduce pressure within the eye. It is available in 2 strengths: GANDA 1 + 0.2 contains 1% guanethidine monosulphate and 0.2% adrenaline; GANDA 3 + 0.5 contains 3% guanethidine monosulphate and 0.5% adrenaline. *Used for*: glaucoma. *Dosage*: 1 drop into eye once or twice each day. *Special care*: examination of eye for signs of damage to cornea and conjunctiva is required during long-term therapy, and drops should be withdrawn if this occurs. *Avoid use*: narrow angle glaucoma, aphakia (a condition in which all or part of the lens of the eye is absent, usually due to surgical removal of a cataract). *Possible interaction*: MAOIs. *Side effects*: headache, discomfort in eye, skin reactions, melanosis (over-production of the pigment melanin), initial rise in pressure within eye; rarely, other whole body (systemic) effects. *Manufacturer*: Chauvin.

GARAMYCIN

Description: an antibiotic preparation available in the form of drops containing 0.3% gentamicin (as sulphate). *Used for*: external ear and eye infections. *Dosage*: 3 to 4 drops 3 to 4 times each day. *Special care*: patients with perforated ear drum (if being used to treat ear infections). *Avoid use*: infections of viral, tuberculous or fungal origin or in which pus is present. *Side effects*: superinfection, possible mild irritation of short-lived duration, blurred vision (eye infections). *Manufacturer*: Schering-Plough.

GASTROBID CONTINUS

Description: an antidopaminergic preparation used to treat gastro-intestinal upset and available as white, sustained-release tablets containing 15mg metoclopramide hydrochloride marked with strength and NAPP. *Used for*: hiatus hernia, reflux oesophagitis (where there is a backflow of acid stomach juice) duodenitis and gastritis (inflammation of duodenum and stomach), dyspepsia. Also, nausea and vomiting including that which may result from chemotherapy for cancer. *Dosage*: adults over 20 years of age, 1 tablet twice each day. *Special care*: pregnancy, breast-feeding, kidney disease. *Avoid use*: children and young adults under 20 years, recent surgery of gastro-intestinal tract, those with breast cancer which is prolactin-dependent or phaeochromocytoma. *Possible interaction*: anticholinergic drugs, butyrophenones, phenothiazines. *Side effects*: elevated prolactin levels in blood, extrapyramidal responses (concerned with reflex muscle movements of a stereotyped nature, e.g. knee jerk). *Manufacturer*: Napp.

GASTROMAX

Description: an antidopaminergic preparation used to treat gastro-intestinal upset and available as yellow/orange sustained-release capsules containing 30mg metoclopramide hydrochloride. *Used for*: gastro-intestinal disturbance and upset, nausea and vomiting including that which may be drug-induced (cancer chemotherapy). *Dosage*: adults over 20 years of age and elderly persons, 1 tablet each day taken before a meal. *Special care*: elderly persons and patients with kidney disease. *Avoid use*: children and young adults under 20 years of age, pregnancy, breast-feeding, phaeochromocytoma. *Possible interaction*: anticholinergic drugs, butyrophenones, phenothiazines. *Side effects*: raised prolactin levels in blood, extrapyramidal responses (concerned with reflex muscle movements of a stereotyped nature, e.g. knee jerk). *Manufacturer*: Pfizer.

GASTROZEPIN

Description: an anticholinergic preparation (a selective antimuscarine drug) which acts to reduce the production and secretion of acid stomach juices. It is produced in the form of scored white tablets containing 50mg pirenzepine marked G over 50 and with manufacturer's logo. *Used for*: stomach and duodenal ulcers. *Dosage*: adults, 1 tablet twice each day taken thirty minutes before meals for a period of 1 month to 6 weeks. Maximum of 3 tablets each day in divided doses. *Special care*: kidney disease. *Avoid use*: children, pregnancy, closed angle glaucoma, enlarged prostate gland, paralytic ileus (a condition in which there is a reduction or absence of movement along the gastro-intestinal tract, which may result from a number of different causes), pyloric stenosis. *Side ef-*

fects: disturbance of vision and dry mouth; rarely, blood changes. *Manufacturer*: Boots.

GENOTROPIN

Description: a preparation of the synthetic human growth hormone, somatotropin, produced as a powder containing 4 units in vials (along with ampoules of solution for reconstitution). Various other preparations are available, e.g. **GENOTROPIN MULTIDOSE, GENOTROPIN CARTRIDGES, GENOTROPIN KABIVIAL MULTIDOSE** and **GENOTROPIN KABIQUICK**. *Used for*: children in whom growth is stunted due to absence or reduced amount of pituitary growth hormone, Turner's syndrome. *Dosage*: growth hormone deficiency, usual dose in the order of 0.5–0.7 units/kg body weight each week by subcutaneous injection. Turner's syndrome, 1 unit/kg body weight each week by subcutaneous injection. *Special care*: patients with diabetes mellitus. *Avoid use*: patients with closed epiphyses. *Manufacturer*: Pharmacia & Upjohn.

GENTICIN

Description: an antibiotic and aminoglycoside preparation in the form of drops containing 0.3% gentamicin (as sulphate). *Used for*: ear and eye bacterial infections. *Dosage*: ear, 2, 3 or 4 drops 3 or 4 times each day; eye, 1 to 3 drops 3 or 4 times each day. *Special care*: with ear infections in patients with perforated eardrum. *Side effects*: superinfection (secondary infection); eye infections, slight irritation of eye which is short-lived, blurring of vision. *Manufacturer*: Roche.

GENTISONE HC

Description: a compound antibiotic and corticosteroid in the form of eardrops containing 0.3% gentamicin (as sulphate) and 1% hydrocortisone acetate. *Used for*: external and middle ear infections. *Dosage*: 2 to 4 drops placed in ear 3 or 4 times each day and at bedtime. As an alternative, wicks dipped in the solution may be placed in the ear to deliver the dose. *Special care*: pregnancy, limit use in young children, patients with perforated eardrum. *Side effects*: superinfection (secondary infection). *Manufacturer*: Roche.

GESTANIN

Description: a hormonal preparation of a progestogen produced in the form of white tablets containing 5mg allyloestrenol and coded ORGANON and GK4. *Used for*: recurrent or threatened miscarriage, threatened premature labour. *Dosage*: recurrent miscarriage, 1 tablet 3 times each day as soon as there is confirmation of the pregnancy continuing until 1 month beyond the end of the risk period; threatened premature labour, up to 8 tablets each day according to response. *Avoid use*: patients with liver disease. *Side effects*: nausea. *Manufacturer*: Organon.

GESTONE

Description: a hormonal preparation of a progestogen produced in ampoules for injection in 2 strengths, containing 25mg and 50mg progesterone/ml. Also, as 2ml ampoules containing 100mg progesterone. *Used for*: maintenace of pregnancy in early stages in women with history of spontaneous abortion. *Dosage*: adults, 25–100mg each day by deep intramuscular injection from fifteenth day of pregnancy to eighth to sixteenth week. *Special care*: patients with migraine, epilepsy, diabetes. *Avoid use*: patients with breast cancer, history of thrombosis, liver disease, vaginal bleeding which is undiagnosed. *Manufacturer*: Ferring.

GLAUCOL

Description: a ß-blocker produced in the form of an eye solution in single dose vials of 2 strengths containing 0.25% and 0.5% timolol (as maleate). *Used for*: open angle glaucoma, secondary glaucoma, hypertension within the eye. *Dosage*: adults, 1 drop of lower strength solution twice each day increasing to higher strength if necessary. *Special care*: pregnancy, breast-feeding, elderly. Withdraw drops gradually. *Avoid use*: patients with heart block, bradycardia, asthma, history of obstructive lung disease. *Possible interaction*: antihypertensive drugs, adrenaline, verapamil. *Side effects*: irritation of eye, absorption into blood may cause other systemic (whole body) ß-blocker side effects, e.g. disturbance of sleep, cold hands and feet, fatigue on exercise, bradycardia, gastro-intestinal upset, heart failure, bronchospasm. *Manufacturer*: Baker Norton.

GLIBENESE

Description: a sulphonylurea drug produced in the form of scored, oblong, white tablets containing 5mg glipizide and marked Pfizer and GBS/5. *Used for*: maturity-onset diabetes. *Dosage*: adults, 2.5mg–5mg each day taken either before breakfast or lunch. Dose may be increased if required by 2.5–5mg daily every third, fourth or fifth day with a maximum of 40mg each day. Doses in excess of 15mg daily should be taken before meals as divided doses. Usual maintenance dose is in the order of 2.5–30mg depending upon response. *Special care*: elderly, kidney failure. *Avoid use*: children, pregnancy, breast-feeding, other forms of diabetes including unstable brittle diabetes, growth-onset diabetes, juvenile diabetes, ketoacidosis (an accumulation of ketones within the body due to diabetes), infections, serious kidney or liver disease. Also, patients suffering from stress, infections or undergoing suregery. *Possible interaction*: sulphonamides, anticoagulants taken orally, corticotrophin, corticosteroids, aspirin, rifampicin, glucagon, oral contraceptives, MAOIs, alcohol, chloramphenicol, ß-blockers, clofibrate, bezafibrate, diuretics, chloropropamide, metformin, acetohexamide. *Side effects*: allergic reactions, skin rash. *Manufacturer*: Pfizer.

GLUCAGON

Description: a hyperglycaemic preparation produced as a powder in vials along with diluent for reconstitution and injection. Glucagon is produced by Lilly as

1.09mg glucagon hydrochloride and by Novo as 1mg glucagon hydrochloride. *Used for*: patients in whom blood sugar level has fallen to seriously low levels (e.g. diabetics taking insulin) and who have become unconscious. *Dosage*: 0.5mg–1mg by intravenous, intramuscular or subcutaneous injection in patients who cannot be roused enough to take glucose or sucrose by mouth. If patient still does not wake up, an intravenous dose of glucose should be given. *Special care*: pregnancy, breast-feeding. *Avoid use*: phaeochromocytoma, pancreatic tumours (glucagonoma or insulinoma). *Possible interaction*: warfarin. *Side effects*: gastrointestinal upset, diarrhoea, nausea, vomiting, allergic responses, hypokalaemia. *Manufacturer*: Lilly and Novo.

GLUCOBAY

Description: an oral hypoglycaemic preparation which acts to inhibit the activity of the digestive enzyme, alpha-glucosidase, which breaks down carbohydrates. It is produced in the form of off-white tablets of 2 strengths containing 50mg and 100mg acarbose and marked G50 or G100 respectively and with Bayer logo. *Used for*: additional therapy (or on its own) in diabetes which is non-insulin dependent and is not completely controlled by diet or oral hypoglycaemics. *Dosage*: adults, 50mg 3 times each day at first for 6 to 8 weeks increasing to 100mg 3 times daily if required. The maximum dose is 200mg 3 times each day. *Special care*: with maximum dose, the level of liver enzyme, hepatic transaminase, should be carefully monitored. Also monitor patients receiving hypoglycaemics. *Avoid use*: pregnancy, breast-feeding, various disorders of the gastro-intestinal tract including inflammation of the bowel, obstruction of intestine, ulceration of colon, disorders of absorption. *Possible interaction*: pancreatic enzymes, adsorbent agents, cholestyramine, neomycin. *Side effects*: flatulence, feeling of bloatedness, diarrhoea, pain in abdomen. *Manufacturer*: Bayer.

GLUCOPHAGE

Description: a biguanide antidiabetic drug in white, film-coated tablets of 2 strengths (500mg and 850mg of metformin hydrochloride) and marked with strength and GL. *Used for*: additional therapy with sulphonylureas in maturity-onset diabetes, or on its own. Also, as additional therapy in insulin-dependent diabetes, particularly in overweight patients. *Dosage*: 500mg twice each day initially or 850mg taken with meals. Dose may be gradually increased to a daily maximum of 3g and then should be reduced for maintenance. Normal maintenance dose is three 500mg or two 850mg doses each day. *Special care*: elderly, kidney failure. *Avoid use*: pregnancy, breast-feeding, other forms of diabetes including growth-onset, juvenile, unstable brittle diabetes, ketoacidosis (excess amount of ketones in body), infections, hormonal disorders, stress, serious kidney or liver disease, patients undergoing surgery. *Possible interaction*: MAOIs, sulphonamides, oral anticoagulants, corticotrophin, corticosteroids, aspirin, rifampicin, glucagon, oral contraceptives, alcohol, chloramphenicol, ß-blockers, clofibrate, bezafibrate, diuretics, chloropropamide, metformin, acetohexamide. *Side effects*: allergic reactions, skin rash. *Manufacturer*: Lipha.

GLURENORM

Description: sulphonylurea available as scored, white tablets containing 30mg gliquidone and marked G. *Used for*: maturity-onset diabetes. *Dosage*: in the order of 45–600mg each day in divided doses before meals. Maximum dose is 180mg each day. *Special care*: elderly persons, patients with kidney failure. *Avoid use*: pregnancy, breast-feeding, other forms of diabetes including growth-onset, juvenile, unstable brittle diabetes, ketoacidosis (excess amount of ketones in body as a result of diabetes detected by smell of acetone on breath), infections, hormonal disorders, stress, serious kidney or liver disease, patients undergoing surgery. *Possible interaction*: MAOIs, sulphonamides, anticoagulants taken by mouth, corticotrophin, corticosteroids, aspirin, rifampicin, glucagon, oral contraceptives, alcohol, chloramphenicol, ß-blockers, clofibrate, bezafibrate, diuretics, chloropropamide, metformin, acetohexamide. *Side effects*: allergic reactions, skin rash. *Manufacturer*: Sanofi Winthrop.

GLYPRESSIN

Description: a vasopressin analogue, produced as a powder in vials containing 1mg terlipressin, along with diluent for reconstitution and injection. *Used for*: bleeding varicose veins in the oesophagus. *Dosage*: adults, 2mg given by intravenous bolus injection (a dose given all at once) followed by further 1 or 2mg doses 4, 5 or 6 hours later for a maximum period of 72 hours. *Special care*: patients with various heart conditions including weak heart, arrhythmias, and also serious atherosclerosis or hypertension. Blood levels of electrolytes (salts), fluid balance and blood pressure require careful monitoring. *Avoid use*: pregnancy. *Side effects*: hypertension, paleness, headache, cramps in abdomen. *Manufacturer*: Ferring.

GONADOTROPHIN L.H.

Description: a hormonal preparation available as a powder in ampoules, with solvent for reconstitution and injection. It is available at various strengths containing 500 units, 1000 units and 5000 units of chorionic gonadotrophin. *Used for*: in males, delayed puberty, failure of the testes to descend into the scrotum (cryptorchidism), a reduced amount of spermatozoa in the semen (oligospermia), a cause of infertility. In females, infertility caused by a lack of ovulation. *Dosage*: boys, 7 to 10 years, 500 units 3 times each week given by injection for a period of 6 to 10 weeks. Adults, as directed by physician. Women, 10,000 units by injection in middle of monthly cycle following therapy to stimulate maturation of ovarian follicles. *Special care*: heart or kidney disease, asthma, migraine or epilepsy. *Side effects*: fatigue, headache, oedema, allergic reactions; young boys may become sexually precocious. *Manufacturer*: Paines and Byrne.

GOPTEN

Description: an antihypertensive preparation and ACE inhibitor available as capsules of 3 strengths. Yellow/red, orange/red and red/red capsules contain 0.5mg, 1mg and 2mg trandolapril respectively. *Used for*: hypertension. *Dosage*: adults, 0.5mg once each day in first instance, then doubling at 2 to 4 week intervals. The maximum single dose is 4mg each day with a maintenance dose of 1–2mg once daily. *Special care*: any diuretics should be stopped 2 or 3 days before treatment begins. Special care in patients udergoing anaesthesia or surgery, those with congestive heart failure, liver or kidney disease, having kidney dialysis. Kidney function should be monitored before starting and during therapy. *Avoid use*: children, pregnancy, breast-feeding, obstruction of heart outflow or aortic stenosis. Those with angioneurotic oedema, caused by previous treatment with ACE inhibitors. *Possible interaction*: NSAIDs, potassium-sparing diuretics. *Side effects*: headache, cough, rash, giddiness, weakness, palpitations, hypotension. Rarely there may be depression of bone marrow, blood changes (agranulocytosis—characterized by serious deficiency of certain white blood cells), angioneurotic oedema. *Manufacturer*: Knoll.

GRANEODIN

Description: a broad-spectrum aminoglycoside antibiotic preparation available as an ointment containing 0.25% neomycin sulphate and 0.025% gramicidin. *Used for*: minor bacterial infections of the skin and prevention of infection during minor surgery. *Dosage*: apply ointment to affected area 2, 3 or 4 times daily. *Special care*: dressings should not be used and ointment is not suitable for large areas of damaged skin. *Avoid use*: persistent, more deep-rooted infections. *Side effects*: toxic effects on tissues and organs, sensitization. *Manufacturer*: Squibb.

GRANOCYTE

Description: a drug containing recombinant granulocyte stimulating factor produced as a powder in vials, along with solution, for reconstitution and injection. It contains 263µg lenograstim (recombinant human granulocyte-colony stimulating factor). *Used for*: neutropenia in patients who have had bone marrow transplants, or cytotoxic cancer chemotherapy. *Dosage*: adults, bone marrow transplant patients, 150 micrograms/m^2 body surface by subcutaenous infusion over half-hour period each day. Therapy should begin the day after transplantation and continue until conditon improves, for a maximum period of 28 days. Cancer therapy, 150 micrograms/m^2 body surface each day by subcutaneous injection, starting the day after chemotherapy has finished. Continue until condition improves for a maximum period of 28 days. Children over 2 years, same as adult dose. *Special care*: pregnancy, breast-feeding, precancerous myeloid (bone marrow) conditions, serious kidney or liver disease. Regular blood counts and checks should be carried out. *Avoid use*: children under 2 years of age, patients with myeloid growths. *Side effects*: pain at injection site and in bones. *Manufacturer*: Chugai Pharma UK Limted/Rhône-Poulenc Rorer Limited.

GREGODERM

Description: an antibacterial, antifungal and mildly potent steroid preparation available in the form of an ointment containing 2,720 units neomycin sulphate, 100,000 units nystatin, 100,000 units polymixin B sulphate and 10mg hydrocortisone/g. *Used for*: inflammation of the skin where infection is also present, psoriasis, itching in anal and urogenital areas. *Dosage*: apply ointment 2 or 3 times each day to affected area. *Special care*: use should be limited in children, infants and on face to a maximum period of 5 days. Should be gradually withdrawn after longer-term use. *Avoid use*: extensive or long-term use in pregnancy or for prevention of skin conditions. Patients with acne, or skin infections with tuberculous or viral origin, leg ulcers, ringworm, scabies, dermatitis in region of mouth, any untreated bacterial or fungal infections. *Side effects*: skin thinning, suppression of adrenal glands, abnorml hair growth, changes as in Cushing's syndrome. *Manufacturer*: Unigreg.

GRISOVIN

Description: an antifungal preparation available in the form of white, film-coated tablets of 2 strengths containing 125mg and 500mg griseofulvin both marked with name, strength and manufacturer's name. *Used for*: fungal infections of nails, skin and scalp, especially those not suitable for treatment with topical preparations. *Dosage*: adults, 500mg–1g each day in divided doses after meals. Dose should not fall below 10mg/kg body weight. Children, 10mg/kg body weight each day as divided doses. *Special care*: pregnancy, long-term use. *Avoid use*: patients with serious liver disease, porphyria, SLE (a rare collagen disease). *Possible interaction*: anticoagulants of the coumarin type, oral contraceptives, alcohol, barbiturates. *Manufacturer*: Glaxo Wellcome.

GYNO-DAKTARIN 1

Description: an antifungal and antibacterial preparation, miconazole nitrate, produced in a variety of forms: white, soft vaginal capsules contain 1200mg ; **GYNO-DAKTARIN PESSARIES** contain 100mg per pessary; **GYNO-DAKTARIN COMBIPAK** consists of 14 pessaries plus cream; **GYNO-DAKTARIN CREAM** contains 2% per 78g with applicator. *Used for*: candidiasis (thrush) of the vagina or vulva. *Dosage*: adults, capsules, 1 at night, inserted into vagina as single dose. Pessaries, 1 inserted twice each day for 7 days. Combipak, 1 pessary and 1 application of cream inserted twice each day. Cream, 1 applicatorful of cream inserted twice each day for 7 days. Male sexual partner should also apply cream twice daily for 7 days. *Side effects*: slight burning or discomfort of short-lived nature. *Manufacturer*: Janssen-Cilag.

GYNO-PEVARYL 1

Description: an antifungal preparation available as vaginal pessaries or cream or a combination of both, all containing econazole nitrate. **GYNO-PEVARYL PESSARIES** contain 150mg; **GYNO-PEVARYL CREAM** contains 1% in 15g. Also available, **GYNO-PEVARYL 1 COMBIPAK** (1 pessary and 15g cream); **GYNO-PEVARYL COMBIPAK** (3 pessaries, 15g cream). *Used for*: vulvitis (inflammation of vulva), vaginitis (inflammation of vagina), treatment of sexual partner in order to prevent reinfection. *Dosage*: adults, pessaries, 1 inserted at night as single dose or for 3 consecutive nights; cream, apply twice each day for 2 weeks. *Side effects*: slight burning or discomfort of short-lived nature. *Manufacturer*: Cilag.

H

HAELAN

Description: a moderately potent steroid preparation available as cream and ointment containing 0.0125% flurandrenolone. Also, **HAELAN C** (combining the steroid with an antibacterial/antifungal agent), which also contains 3% clioquinol as cream and ointment. **HAELAN TAPE** is a clear, adhesive polythene film impregnated with 4µg/cm². *Used for*: inflammatory skin conditions which are responsive to steroids. Haelan C is used when infection is present. *Dosage*: cream or ointment, apply 2 or 3 times each day to clean skin. Tape, apply to affected area and leave in place for 12 hours. *Special care*: Haelan C may stain clothing and skin; use in children or on face should be limited to a maximum period of 5 days. Short-term use and withdraw slowly if use has been more prolonged. *Avoid use*: extensive or prolonged use in pregnancy or continuous use as preventative measure, patients with untreated bacterial or fungal infections, acne, leg ulcers, scabies, skin disease of tuberculous or viral origin, ringworm, dermatitis in area of mouth. (Haelan C is, however, used for some infected conditions). *Side effects*: adrenal gland suppression, skin thinning, abnormal hair growth, skin changes as in Cushing's syndrome. *Manufacturer*: Novex.

HALCIDERM

Description: a very potent topical steroid preparation available in the form of a cream containing 0.1% halcinomide. *Used for*: inflammatory skin conditions responsive to steroids. *Dosage*: apply to affected area 2 or 3 times each day. *Special care*: should not be used for more than 5 days, short-term use only and a milder substitute should be tried as soon as possible. *Avoid use*: children, extensive or prolonged use, especially in pregnancy or as a preventative measure. Avoid use in patients with untreated bacterial or fungal infections, acne, leg ulcers, scabies, skin disease of tuberculous or viral origin, ringworm, dermatitis in area of mouth. *Side effects*: adrenal gland suppression, skin thinning, abnormal hair growth, skin changes as in Cushing's syndrome. *Manufacturer*: Squibb.

HALDOL DECANOATE

Description: an antipsychotic drug, haloperidol (as decanoate), which is a depot butyrophenone available in ampoules for injection at 2 strengths containing 50mg/ml and 100mg/ml. Also, **HALDOL TABLETS** of 2 strengths, blue, coded H5, containing 5mg and yellow, coded H10, containing 10mg. Both are marked Janssen and also scored. **HALDOL ORAL LIQUID** containing 2mg/ml and 10mg/ml and **HALDOL INJECTION** containing 5mg/ml. *Used for*: Haldol decanoate, long-term sedative treatment for various forms of psychiatric illness including psychoses, schizophrenia, disturbed behaviour. Other preparations: mania, schizophrenia, psychoses, symptoms precipitated by alcohol withdrawal; delirium tremens. Also used as pre-anaesthetic sedative for anxiety, vomiting and nausea and disturbed behaviour in children. *Dosage*: Haldol decanoate, adults only, usual dose in order of 50mg–300mg by deep intramuscular injection once each month. Other oral preparations, adults, 0.5mg–5mg 2 or 3 times each day depending upon condition being treated. Dose may be gradually increased if needed to a daily maximum of 200mg and then should be reduced for maintenance. Haldol injection, for psychoses, 2–30mg by intramuscular injection followed by further dose of 5mg at 1 to 8 hour intervals until condition improves. Children, oral preparations, 0.05mg/kg body weight each day in 2 divided doses. *Special care*: pregnancy, breast-feeding, serious heart and circulatory disease, kidney or liver failure, Parkinsonism, epilepsy. *Avoid use*: patients in states of coma. *Possible interaction*: rifampicin, carbamazepine, lithium, alcohol. *Side effects*: hypotension, pallor, drowsiness, tachycardia, palpitations, nightmares, hypothermia, disturbance of sleep, depression, dry mouth, blocked nose, difficulty in urination, blurring of vision, changes in menstruation, breasts and weight, blood changes, ECG and EEG changes, jaundice, skin reactions. *Manufacturer*: Janssen-Cilag.

HALFAN

Description: an antimalarial preparation which is a phenanthrene drug, produced in the form of scored, capsule-shaped, white tablets, marked HALFAN, containing 250mg halofantrine hydrochloride. *Used for*: treatment of malaria caused by *Plasmodium vivax* and *Plasmodium falciparum*. *Dosage*: adults, 6 tablets taken at 6 hour intervals in 3 divided doses. The dose is repeated 1 week later in patients who are not immune. Tablets should not be taken with meals. Children, over 37kg in weight, same as adult. *Special care*: women who may become pregnant, patients with malarial complications or malaria affecting the brain. *Avoid use*: pregnancy, breast-feeding, children under 37kg in weight, patients with some forms of heart disease. Not to be used as a preventative for malaria. *Possible interaction*: TCADs, antiarrhythmic drugs, astemizole, neuroleptic drugs, terfenadine, chloroquine, quinine, mefloquine. *Side effects*: heart arrhythmia, pain in abdomen, gastro-intestinal upset, a short-lived rise in transaminase enzymes in the blood. *Manufacturer*: S.K. & F.

HAMARIN

Description: a xanthine oxidase inhibitor produced in the form of scored, white tablets containing 300mg allopurinol and marked with name, strength and triangle symbol. Allopurinol acts on the enzyme xanthine oxidase which converts the substances xanthine and hypoxanthine into uric acid. Hence the levels of uric acid in the blood are reduced and there is less likelihood of an attack of gout. *Used for*: treatment of gout, prevention of stones formed from uric acid or calcium oxalate. *Dosage*: adults, usual single dose in the order of 100mg–300mg each day increasing for prevention to a maintenance dose in the range 200–600mg daily. *Special care*: pregnancy, elderly, liver or kidney disease. When treatment starts, an anti-inflammatory drug or colchicine should be taken for 4 weeks and the patient should drink plenty of fluids. *Avoid use*: children, acute gout. *Possible interaction*: chloropamide, azanthioprine, mercatopurine, anticoagulant drugs. *Side effects*: acute gout, nausea, drug should be stopped in the event of skin rash occurring. *Manufacturer*: Roche.

HARMOGEN

Description: a hormonal oestrogen preparation produced in the form of long, peach-coloured, scored tablets containing 1.5mg piperazine oestrone sulphate and marked LV. *Used for*: hormonal replacement therapy in menopausal women and prevention of osteoporosis following menopause. *Dosage*: adults, 1 to 2 tablets each day, along with a progestogen preparation for the last 10 to 13 days of each 28 day cycle in women who have not had a hysterectomy. *Special care*: patients considered to be at risk of thrombosis or with liver disease. Women with any of the following disorders should be carefully monitored: fibroids in the womb, multiple sclerosis, diabetes, tetany, porphyria, epilepsy, liver disease, hypertension, migraine, otosclerosis, gallstones. Breasts, pelvic organs and blood pressure should be checked at regular intervals during the course of treatment. *Avoid use*: pregnancy, breast-feeding, women with conditions which might lead to thrombosis, thrombophlebitis, serious heart, kidney or liver disease, breast cancer, oestrogen-dependent cancers including those of reproductive system, endometriosis, vaginal bleeding which is undiagnosed. *Possible interaction*: drugs which induce liver enzymes. *Side effects*: tenderness and enlargement of breasts, weight gain, breakthrough bleeding, giddiness, vomiting and nausea, gastro-intestinal upset. Treatment should be halted immediately if severe headaches occur, disturbance of vision, hypertension or any indications of thrombosis, jaundice. Also, in the event of pregnancy and 6 weeks before planned surgery. *Manufacturer*: Pharmacia & Upjohn.

HAVRIX MONODOSE

Description: a preparation of inactivated hepatitis A virus HM available in pre-filled syringes containing 1440 ELISA units/ml adsorbed on aluminium hydroxide. **HAVRIX ORIGINAL**, pre-filled 1ml syringes containing 720 ELISA units/ml of hepatitis A virus HM 175 strain adsorbed on aluminium hydroxide. Also, **HAVRIX JUNIOR**, pre-filled 0.5ml syringes containing 720 ELISA units/ml of hepatitis A virus HM 175 strain adsorbed on aluminium hydroxide. *Used for*: immunization against hepatitis A virus. *Dosage*: adults and children age 16 and over, Havrix Monodose, primary immunization, 1 intramuscular injection of 1ml followed by repeated dose 6 to 12 months later. Havrix original, primary immunization, 1 intramuscular injection of 1ml followed by repeated doses after 2 to 4 weeks and 6 to 12 months. Children under 16 years, Havrix junior only, age 1 to 15 years, primary immunization, 0.5ml by intramuscular injection followed by repeated doses 2 to 4 weeks and 6 to 12 months later. *Special care*: pregnancy, breast-feeding, infections, dialysis or with lowered immunity. Patients with bleeding disorders may need subcutaneous injection. *Avoid use*: patients with severe fever, children under 1 year. *Possible interaction*: nausea, fatigue, malaise, soreness and skin reactions at injection site, appetite loss. *Manufacturer*: Smith Kline Beecham.

HEMABATE

Description: a prostaglandin preparation produced in ampoules for injection containing 250µg carboprost as trometamol salt/ml. *Used for*: haemorrhage following childbirth in patients who have not responded to other drugs (oxytocin and ergometrine). *Dosage*: 1 deep intramuscular injection of 250 micrograms which may be repeated after 1½ hours. If condition is very severe, repeat dose can be given after 15 minutes. Maximum total dose is 12mg. *Special care*: patients with hypertension, hypotension, history of glaucoma or hypertension in eye, diabetes, asthma, jaundice, epilepsy, previous uterine injury (high doses may cause rupture of uterus). *Avoid use*: patients with heart, liver, kidney or lung disease, pelvic inflammatory disease. *Side effects*: gastro-intestinal upset, vomiting, nausea, diarrhoea, flushing, high temperature (hyperthermia), bronchospasm. Rarely, chills, headache, fluid in lungs, sweating, giddiness, pain and skin changes at injection site. *Manufacturer*: Pharmacia & Upjohn.

HEMINEVRIN

Description: a hypnotic, sedative preparation produced in the form of capsules and as a syrup. Grey-brown capsules contain 192mg chlormethiazole in miglyol, 1 capsule being equivalent to 5ml of syrup. Syrup contains 250mg chlormethiazole edisylate/5ml. *Used for*: insomnia in elderly persons, short-lived therapy only. Sedation in elderly patients with senile psychosis, anxiety, confusion, disturbance of sleep, tension, alcohol withdrawal. *Dosage*: adults, capsules, 2 at bedtime or 1 three times each day for sedation. Syrup, 10ml in drink at bedtime or three 5ml doses through day for sedation. For alcohol withdrawal symptoms, 3 capsules 4 times each day reducing over 6 days to nil. *Special care*: lung, liver or kidney disease. *Avoid use*: breast-feeding, children, serious lung disease. *Possible interaction*: other central nervous system sedatives, alcohol. *Side effects*: blocked and sore nose, sore eyes, gastro-intestinal upset, sedation, judgement and performance of skilled tasks (e.g. driving) is impaired, confusion, agitation, anaphylactic type allergic reactions. *Manufacturer*: Astra.

HEMINEVRIN I-V INFUSION

Description: an anticonvulsant sedative preparation in solution for infusion containing 8mg chlormethiazole edisylate/ml. *Used for*: status epilepticus (a life-threatening condition characterized by continuous convulsions which can cause irreversible brain damage and a dangerous imbalance in the level of salts in the body), pre-eclamptic toxaemia (an abnormal condition which may arise in pregnancy). *Dosage*: adults, 60 drops per minute until patient is sedated and then 10–15 drops per minute. Status epiiepticus, 40–100ml over a period of 5 to 10 minutes, all by rapid infusion. Children, status epilepticus, 80µg/kg body weight (0.01ml) per minute at first, with increase if required every 2 to 4 hours until condition is under control. Then dose is gradually reduced unless seizures recur. *Special care*: patients with lung disorder or history of obstructive lung disease. *Avoid use*: breast-feeding, patients with severe lung disorders. *Possible interaction*: central nervous system, sedatives, alcohol. *Side effects*: blocked and sore nose, sore eyes, sedation, confusion, agitation, gastro-intestinal upset. Judgement and the ability to perform skilled tasks is impaired. *Manufacturer*: Astra.

HERPID

Description: an antiviral preparation available as a solution containing 5% idoxuridine in dimethyl sulphoxide. *Used for*: skin infections caused by *Herpes zoster* and *Herpes simplex*. *Dosage*: adults, apply solution (with applicator brush) 4 times each day for a period of 4 days. *Avoid use*: pregnancy, breast-feeding. *Manufacturer*: Yamanouchi.

HIBTITER

Description: a preparation of inactivated surface antigen consisting of polysaccharide from the capsule of *H. influenzae* type B joined to diphtheria protein. *Used for*: immunization against meningitis, epiglottitis and other diseases caused by *H. influenzae* type B. *Dosage*: children only, aged 2 months to 1 year, 3 intramuscular injections of 0.5ml at 4 week intervals, normally along with diphtheria, tetanus, polio immunization. *Special care*: same vaccine must be used throughout course of immunization. *Avoid use*: children with acute infections. *Side effects*: possible skin reaction (reddening) at injection site. *Manufacturer*: Wyeth.

HONVAN

Description: a hormonal oestrogen preparation available in ampoules for injection and also in the form of tablets, both containing tetrasodium fosfesterol which is converted to stilboestrol by enzyme activity. The ampoules contain 276mg tetrasodium fosfesterol/5ml and white tablets contain 100mg. *Used for*: cancer of the prostate gland. *Dosage*: adults, injection, 552–1104mg by slow intravenous injection daily for a minimum of 5 days. Then 276mg 1 to 4 times each week for maintenance. Tablets, for maintenance, 100–200mg 3 times each day then reducing to 100–300mg in divided doses as daily dose. *Special care*: patients with liver disease. *Side effects*: thrombosis, oedema, nausea, gynaecomastia, impotence, pain in perineal area. *Manufacturer*: Asta Medica.

HORMONIN

Description: a hormonal oestrogen preparation available in the form of scored, pink tablets containing 0.27mg oestriol, 1.4mg oestrone and 0.6mg oestradiol. *Used for*: hormone replacement therapy in women with menopausal symptoms, prevention of osteoporosis after menopause. *Dosage*: 1 to 2 tablets each day, with a progestogen for last 12 or 13 days of 28 day cycle unless patient has had a hysterectomy. *Special care*: women at risk of thrombosis or with liver disorder—liver function should be monitored. Women with any of the following should also receive careful monitoring: otosclerosis, porphyria, fibroids in the uterus, epilepsy, migraine, multiple sclerosis, diabetes, hypertension, tetany, gallstones. Blood pressure, pelvic organs and breasts should be checked regularly during the course of treatment. *Avoid use*: pregnancy, breast-feeding, breast cancer, cancer of reproductive system or any hormone-dependent cancer, serious heart, liver or kidney disease, any conditions likely to lead to thrombosis, Rotor or Dublin-Johnson syndrome, endometriosis or vaginal bleeding of unknown cause. *Possible interaction*: drugs which induce liver enzymes. *Side effects*: breast enlargement and soreness, weight gain, nausea, vomiting, gastrointestinal upset, headache, giddiness, breakthrough bleeding. *Manufacturer*: Shire.

HUMATROPE

Description: a synthetic growth hormone available as powder in ampoules, with diluent for reconstitution and injection, containing 4 units or 16 units of somatropin (rbe). *Used for*: failure of growth in children due to lack of growth hormone, Turner's syndrome. *Dosage*: children, deficiency of growth hormone, either 0.07 units/kg body-weight each day or 0.16 units/kg body-weight 3 times each week, all by intramuscular or subcutaneous injection. Turner's syndrome, 0.8–0.9 units/kg body-weight each week in 6 or 7 doses given by intramuscular or subcutaneous injection. *Special care*: children with diabetes, intracranial lesion (damaged tissue within cranium), a deficiency of ACTH (adrenocorticotrophic hormone—an adrenal gland hormone). Thyroid function should be monitored during the course of therapy. *Avoid use*: patients with tumour, fused epiphyses, pregnancy, breast-feeding. *Manufacturer*: Lilly.

HUMEGON

Description: a combined preparation of human menopausal gonadotrophins (HMG) available as powder in ampoules with solvent in 2 strengths. 75 units HMG (equivalent to 75 units of follicle-stimulating hormone (FSH) and 75 units luteinizing hormone (LH)) and 150 units HMG (equivalent to 150 units FSH and 150 units LH). *Used for*: male and female infertility due to a lack of gonadotrophin resulting in insufficient stimulation of the gonads (sex organs). Also, for stimulation of ovaries to produce excess eggs for IVF (*in vitro* fertilization). *Dosage*: males and females, by intramuscular injection, according to individual's requirements as directed by physician. *Special care*: males and females, exclude all other causes of infertility. Females, monitor size of ovaries and levels of oestrogen during the course of therapy. *Avoid use*: tumours of the pituitary gland, testes and ovaries. *Side effects*: skin rashes, risk of miscarriage and multiple pregnancy. *Manufacturer*: Organon.

HYDERGINE

Description: a cerebral activator-ergot alkaloid available as scored, white tablets containing 1.5mg or 4.5mg codergocrine mesylate both marked with strength and name. *Used for*: additional therapy in the treatment of moderate dementia in elderly persons. *Dosage*: adults, 4.5mg each day. *Special care*: severe bradycardia. *Avoid use*: children. *Side effects*: blocked nose, rash, flushing, headache, pain in abdomen, giddiness, hypotension, when rising from lying down (postural hypotension). *Manufacturer*: Sandoz. HYDREA *Description*: a DNA reactive cytotoxic drug available as pink/green capsules containing 500mg hydroxyurea marked SQUIBB and 830. *Used for*: treatment of chronic myeloid leukaemia. *Dosage*: 20–30mg/kg body weight each day or 80mg/kg body weight every third day. *Side effects*: nausea, vomiting, skin rashes, bone marrow suppression. *Manufacturer*: Squibb.

HYDRENOX

Description: a thiazide diuretic preparation as scored white tablets containing 50mg hydroflumethazide marked H inside a hexagon shape. *Used for*: hypertension, oedema. *Dosage*: adults, for oedema, 50–200mg as a single dose taken in the morning, in first instance, then reducing to a 25mg–50mg maintenance dose taken on alternate days. For hypertension, 25mg–50mg each day. Children, 1mg/kg body weight each day. *Special care*: pregnancy, breast-feeding, elderly, kidney or liver disease, liver cirrhosis, SLE, diabetes, gout. Glucose, fluid and electrolyte (salt) levels should be monitored during therapy. *Avoid use*: patients with hypercalcaemia, serious kidney or liver disease, a sensitivity to sulphonamide drugs, Addison's disease. *Possible interaction*: NSAIDs, barbiturates, alcohol, opiod drugs. Cardiac glycosides, lithium, carbenoxolone, corticosteroids, tubocurarine. *Side effects*: gastro-intestinal upset, blood changes, sensitivity to light, disturbance of electrolyte balance and metabolism, skin rash, pancreatitis, anorexia, dizziness, impotence. *Manufacturer*: Knoll.

HYDROCAL

Description: a topical, mildly potent corticosteroid preparation available as cream or ointment containing 1% hydrocortisone acetate and calamine. *Used for*: irritated skin conditions responsive to steroids. *Dosage*: apply to affected skin 2 or 3 times each day. *Special care*: use in children or on face should be limited to a period not exceeding 5 days. Stop gradually if preparation has been used for a long period. *Avoid use*: extensive or long-term use, especially in pregnant women or for prevention of skin conditions. Patients with bacterial or fungal infections which are untreated. Skin disease of viral or tuberculous origin or due to ringworm, acne, dermatitis in mouth area, leg ulcers, scabies. *Side effects*: thinning of skin, suppression of adrenal glands, abnormal hair growth, skin changes as in Cushing's syndrome. *Manufacturer*: Bioglan.

HYDROCORTISTAB CREAM

Description: a mildly potent topical steroid preparation available as cream or ointment containing 1% hydro-cortisone acetate. *Used for*: irritated skin conditions responsive to steroids. *Dosage*: apply thinly to affected skin 2 or 3 times each day. *Special care*: use in children or on face should be limited to a period not exceeding 5 days. Stop gradually if preparation has been used for a long period. *Avoid use*: extensive or long-term use, especially in pregnant women or for prevention of skin conditions. Patients with bacterial or fungal infections which are untreated. Skin disease of viral or tuberculous origin or due to ringworm, acne, dermatitis in mouth area, leg ulcers, scabies. *Side effects*: thinning of skin, suppression of adrenal glands, abnormal hair growth, skin changes as in Cushing's syndrome. *Manufacturer*: Boots.

HYDROCORTISTAB TABLETS

Description: a corticosteroid (gluco-corticoid and mineralocorticosteroid) preparation available as scored, white tablets containing 20mg hydrocortisone. Also **HYDROCORTISTABL INJECTION** available in ampoules containing 25mg hydrocortisone acetate/ml. *Used for*: tablets, hormone replacement therapy, emergency treatment or asthma attack, anaphylaxis, allergic drug response, serum sickness, angioneurotic oedema. Injection, directly into joints in rheumatic diseases and soft tissue injuries. *Dosage*: adults, tablets, replacement therapy, 20–30mg each day; emergency treatment, as directed by physician according to patient's condition. Injection, 5–50mg each day directly into joint with a maximum of 3 injections daily. Children, tablets, replacement therapy, 10–30mg each day in divided doses; emergency treatment as directed by physician according to patient's condition. Injection, 5–30mg each day directly into joint with a maximum of 3 injections daily. *Special care*: pregnancy, hyperthyroidism, liver cirrhosis, inflammation in kidneys (glomerulonephritis, nephritis), inflammation of veins, peptic ulcer, hypertension. Also, diabetes, recent surgical anastomoses of gastro-intestinal tract, epilepsy, osteoporosis, infectious diseases characterized by skin rash, other infections, tuberculosis, those of fungal or viral origin. Patients with psychoses or suffering from stress. Drug should be gradually withdrawn and patients in contact with *Herpes zoster* virus or chicken pox should seek medical advice and treatment. *Possible interaction*: anticoagulants taken orally, diuretics, NSAIDs, cardiac glycosides, anticholinesterases, rifampicin, hypoglycaemics, phenytoin, ephedrine, phenobarbitone. *Side effects*: peptic ulcer, skin changes, osteoporosis, depression and euphoria, hyperglycaemia. *Manufacturer*: Knoll.

HYDROCORTISYL

Description: a mildly potent topical steroid preparation available as cream or ointment containing 1% hydrocortisone acetate. *Used for*: irritated skin conditions responsive to steroids. *Dosage*: apply thinly to affected skin 2 or 3 times each day. *Special care*: use in children or on face should be limited to a period not exceeding 5 days. Stop gradually if preparation has been used for a long period. *Avoid use*: extensive or long-term use, especially in pregnant women or for prevention of skin conditions. Patients with bacterial or fungal infections which are untreated. Skin disease of viral or tuberculous origin or due to ringworm, acne, dermatitis in mouth area, leg ulcers, scabies. *Side effects*: thinning of skin, suppression of adrenal glands, abnormal hair growth, skin changes as in Cushing's syndrome. *Manufacturer*: Hoechst.

HYDROCORTONE

Description: a corticosteroid (gluco-corticoid and mineralocorticoid) available as quarter-scored, white tablets containing 10mg or 20mg hydro-cortisone and coded MSD 619, MSD 625 respectively. *Used for*: hormone replacement therapy due to reduced production of hormones from the adrenal cortex (adrenal glands). *Dosage*: 20–30mg each day in divided doses or as directed by physician. *Special care*: pregnancy, hyperthyroidism, liver cirrhosis, inflammation in kidneys (glomerulonephritis, nephritis), thrombophlebitis, peptic ulcer, hypertension. Also, diabetes, recent surgical anastomoses of gastro-intestinal tract, epilepsy, osteoporosis, infectious diseases characterized by skin rash, other infections, tuberculosis, those of fungal or viral origin. Patients with psychoses or suffering from stress. Drug should be gradually withdrawn and patients in contact with *Herpes zoster* virus or chicken pox should seek medical advice and treatment. *Possible interaction*: anticoagulants taken orally, diuretics, NSAIDs, cardiac glycosides, anticholinesterases, rifampicin, hypoglycaemics, phenytoin, ephedrine, phenobarbitone. *Side effects*: peptic ulcer, skin changes as in Cushing's syndrome, osteoporosis, depression and euphoria, hyperglycaemia. *Manufacturer*: M.S.D.

HYDROMET

Description: a compound antihypertensive preparation combining a central alpha-agonist and thiazide diuretic. It is available as pink, film-coated tablets containing 250mg methydopa and 15mg hydrochlorothiazide, marked MSD

423. *Used for*: hypertension. *Dosage*: adults, 1 tablet twice each day at first gradually increasing at intervals of 2 days. The maximum daily dose is 12 tablets. *Special care*: pregnancy, breast-feeding, diabetes, kidney or liver disease, gout, history of liver disease, haemolytic anaemia, undergoing anaesthesia. A potassium supplement may be needed. *Avoid use*: patients with serious liver disease, severe kidney failure, phaeochromocytoma, depression. *Possible interaction*: antidiabetic substances, TCADs, ACTH (adreno-corticotrophic hormone), corticosteroids, MAOIs, tubocurarine, sympathomimetics, phenothiazines, digitalis, lithium. *Side effects*: blocked nose, dry mouth, gastro-intestinal upset, headache, blood changes, sedation, depression, weakness, bradycardia. *Manufacturer*: M.S.D.

HYDROSALURIC

Description: a thiazide diuretic preparation available as scored, white tablets of 2 strengths containing 25mg and 50mg of hydrochlorthiazide and marked MSD 42 and MSD 105 respectively. *Used for*: hypertension, oedema. *Dosage*: adults, oedema, 25mg–100mg once or twice each day or when needed with a maximum daily dose of 200mg. Hypertension, 25–50mg as a single or divided dose each day at first, then adjusting but with a maximum daily dose of 100mg. Children, 6 months and under, 3.5mg/kg body weight each day; 6 months to 2 years, 12.5–37.5mg each day; 2 to 12 years, 27.5–100mg each day. All are in 2 divided doses. *Special care*: pregnancy, liver or kidney disease, gout, electrolyte (salts) imbalance, SLE, diabetes. Patients may also require a potassium supplement. *Avoid use*: breast-feeding mothers, patients with serious liver or kidney disease, anuria, hypercalcaemia, Addison's disease. *Possible interaction*: NSAIDs, anti-hypertensives, central nervous system depressants, muscle relaxants, corticosteroids, ACE inhibitors, digitalis, lithium. *Side effects*: blood changes, fatigue, sensitivity to light, gout, hypokalaemia. *Manufacturer*: M.S.D.

HYGROTON

Description: a proprietary, thiazide-like diuretic preparation produced in the form of scored, pale yellow tablets containing 50mg chlorthalidone marked GEIGY and coded ZA. *Used for*: hypertension, oedema. *Dosage*: adults, hypertension, 25mg–50mg each day as a single dose with breakfast. Oedema, 50mg each day or 100–200mg every other day reducing to a maintenance dose in the order of 50–100mg 3 times each week. Children, up to 2mg/kg body weight each day. *Special care*: pregnancy, breast-feeding, elderly, kidney or liver disease, liver cirrhosis, SLE, gout, diabetes. Glucose, fluid and electrolyte (salts) levels should be carefully monitored during the course of therapy. *Avoid use*: patients with serious kidney or liver failure, sensitivity to sulphonamide drugs, hypercalcaemia, Addison's disease. *Possible interaction*: NSAIDs, barbiturates, antidiabetic substances, corticosteroids, alcohol, tubocurarine, opiods, carbenoxolone, lithium, cardiac glycosides. *Side effects*: gastro-intestinal upset, blood changes, skin rash, upset of electrolyte balance and metabolism, sensitivity to light, anorexia, impotence, disturbance of vision, pancreatitis, dizziness. *Manufacturer*: Geigy.

HYPNOMIDATE

Description: a reparation which induces general anaesthesia produced in ampoules for injection containing 2mg etomidate/ml. Also, **HYPNOMIDATE CONCENTRATE** containing 125mg etomidate/ml (diluted before use). *Used for*: induction of general anaesthesia. *Dosage*: by slow intravenous injection, 100–300 g/kg body weight/minute, dose depending upon patient's condition. *Special care*: best used following premedication. *Avoid use*: porphyria. *Possible interaction*: anxiolytics, hypnotics, antidepressants, anti-hypertensives, antipsychotics, calcium-channel blockers, ß-blockers. *Side effects*: muscle movement and pain with injection (lessened with premedication). Repeated doses may cause adrenal gland suppression. *Manufacturer*: Janssen-Cilag.

HYPNOVEL

Description: a benzodiazepine drug which has hypnotic, anxiolytic effects, available as a solution in ampoules for injection containing 10mg midazolam/ml. *Used for*: sedation in patients undergoing minor surgery, those in intensive care, premedication in patients who are to receive general anaesthesia, induction of anaesthesia. *Dosage*: adults, for sedation, 2mg (1–1.5mg in elderly persons) given by intravenous injection over thirty seconds. Then 0.5–1mg at 2 minute intervals if needed. Usual dose range is in the order of 2.5–7.5mg (1–2mg in elderly persons). Sedation of intensive care patients, 30–300 g/kg body weight by intravenous infusion over 5 minutes followed by 30–200 g/kg body weight every hour. Reduced doses may be indicated, especially if another drug (opioid analgesic) is also being given. Premedication, 70–100 g/kg body weight 1 hour to half an hour before general anaesthetic, given by intramuscular injection. Usual dose is in the order of 5mg (2.5mg in elderly persons). *Special care*: breastfeeding, elderly, liver or kidney disease, lung disorders, myasthenia gravis, personality disorder. If use has been prolonged (as with intensive care patients) the drug should be gradually withdrawn. *Avoid use*: patients with serious lung disorders, depressed respiration or in the last 3 months of pregnancy. *Possible interaction*: central nervous system depressants, cimetidine, alcohol, erythromycin, anticonvulsant drugs. *Side effects*: pain at injection site, dizziness, headache, circulatory changes, temporary halt in breathing (apnoea), hiccoughs. *Manufacturer*: Roche.

HYPOVASE

Description: an antihypertensive preparation which is a selective alpha$_1$-blocker. It is produced as tablets of various strengths all containing prazosin hydrochloride. White 500µg tablets marked Pfizer; scored, orange 1mg tablets marked HYP/1; scored, white 2mg tablets marked HYP/2; scored, white 5mg tablets marked HYP/5 and Pfizer. *Used for*: congestive heart failure, hypertension, Raynaud's disease, additional therapy in the treatment of urinary tract obstruction when the cause is benign enlargement of the prostate gland. *Dosage*: adults, congestive heart failure, 500µg in first instance increasing to 1mg 3 or 4 times each day. Then a usual maintenance dose in the order of 4–20mg in divided doses. Hypertension, 500µg as evening dose at first, followed by 500µg 2 or 3 times each day for a period of 3 days to 1 week. Then, 1mg 2 or 3 times each day for 3 days to 1 week. The dose may be further increased gradually as required with a daily maximum of 20mg. Raynaud's disease, 500µg twice each day at first, then a maintenance dose of 1 or 2mg twice each day. Additional therapy in urine obstruction, 500µg twice each day at first increasing to a maintenance dose of 2mg twice each day. *Special care*: heart failure, patients suffering from congestive heart failure caused by stenosis; urinary tract obstruction, patients liable to fainting during urination. *Possible interaction*: other anti-hypertensive drugs. *Side effects*: dry mouth, dizziness on rising from lying down, sudden short-lived loss of consciousness, weariness, skin rash, blurring of vision. *Manufacturer*: Invicta.

HYTRIN and HYTRIN BPH

Description: an antihypertensive preparation which is a selective alpha$_1$-blocker produced as tablets of 4 different strengths, all containing terazosin (as hydrochloride). White 1mg, yellow 2mg, brown 5mg and blue 10mg tablets are all marked with triangle-shaped symbols and logo. *Used for*: hypertension, urine obstruction caused by benign enlargement of prostate gland. *Dosage*: 1mg taken at bedtime at first then gradually increased at weekly intervals. The usual maintenance dose is in the order of 2–10mg taken once each day. *Special care*: in patients liable to fainting. *Possible interaction*: other anti-hypertensive drugs. *Side effects*: initial dose may cause fainting, hypotension on rising from lying down, dizziness, weariness, fluid retention and swelling of lower limbs. *Manufacturer*: Abbott.

IDOXENE

Description: an antiviral preparation available as an eye ointment containing 0.5% idoxuridine. *Used for*: herpetic keratitis (an inflammation and infection of the cornea caused by *Herpes simplex* virus). *Dosage*: apply 4 times each day and at bedtime and continue for 3 to 5 days after condition has cleared. Maximum period of treatment is 3 weeks. *Special care*: pregnancy. *Possible interaction*: boric acid, corticosteroids. *Side effects*: local irritation in eye and pain, swelling due to oedema. *Manufacturer*: Spodefell.

IDURIDIN

Description: an antiviral skin preparation available as a solution with applicator in 2 strengths, containing 5% and 40% idoxuridine, both in dimethyl sulphoxide. *Used for*: viral skin infections caused by *Herpes zoster* and *Herpes simplex*. *Dosage*: adults and children over 12 years, apply 5% solution to infected area 4 times daily for 4 days. For severe *Herpes zoster* infections (shingles) only, the 40% solution should be used, applied on lint and changed every 24 hours, for a period of 4 days. *Special care*: preparation may stain clothing. *Avoid use*: children under 12 years, pregnancy, breast-feeding. *Manufacturer*: Ferring.

ILOSONE

Description: a macrolide antibiotic preparation available as red/ivory capsules containing 250mg erythromycin estolate and marked DISTA. Also **ILOSONE TABLETS**, oblong, pink, containing 500mg; **ILOSONE SUSPENSION** contains 125mg erythromycin estolate/5ml; **ILOSONE SUSPENSION FORTE** contains 250mg/5ml. *Used for*: respiratory and urinary tract infections, soft tissue, skin, dental infections, infections of the middle ear, acne. *Dosage*: adults, 250mg every 6 hours with a maximum of 4g each day. Children 20–50mg/kg body weight each day in divided doses. *Avoid use*: patients with liver disease or disorder, history of jaundice. *Possible interaction*: anticoagulants taken orally, probenecid, carbamazepine, ergotamine, cyclosporin, lincomycin, theophylline, dihydroergotamine, alfentanil, clindamycin, triazolam, bromocriptine, digoxin. *Side effects*: gastro-intestinal upset, allergic responses, cholestatic jaundice. *Manufacturer*: Novex.

ILUBE

Description: a lubricant eye preparation available in the form of drops containing 5% acetylcysteine and 0.35% hypromellose. *Used for*: dry eyes caused by insufficient secretion of tears or abnormal mucus production. *Dosage*: 1 or 2 drops into affected eye 3 or 4 times each day. *Avoid use*: patients with soft contact lenses. *Manufacturer*: Cusi.

IMDUR

Description: an antianginal nitrate preparation available in the form of scored oval, yellow, film-coated, sustained-release tablets containing 60mg isosorbide mononitrate marked A/ID. *Used for*: prevention of angina. *Dosage*: adults, 1 tablet each day taken in the morning increasing to 2 daily if necessary, as a single dose. If headache occurs, reduce to half a tablet each day. *Avoid use*: children. *Side effects*: nausea, headache, dizziness. *Manufacturer*: Astra.

IMIGRAN

Description: a preparation which is a seratonin agonist available as capsule-shaped, white, film-coated tablets containing 100mg sumatriptan (as succinate), marked with name and company. Also, **IMIGRAM SUBJECT INJECTION**, pre-filled syringes containing 6mg sumatriptan/0.5ml with auto-injector. *Used for*: acute attacks of migraine which may be accompanied by aura. *Dosage*: tablets, 1 tablet as soon as possible after attack starts which may be repeated if condition improves, but should not exceed 3 tablets in 24 hours. If migraine does not respond in first instance, a repeat dose should not be taken. Injection, 6mg by subcutaneous injection as soon as possible after attack begins which may be repeated after 1 hour if condition improves. The maximum dose is 12mg in 24 hours. *Special care*: pregnancy, breast-feeding, liver, kidney or heart disease, indications of coronary artery disease; persons who have misused other migraine preparations. Patients should exercise care if driving or operating machinery. *Avoid use*: children, elderly persons, patients with history of heart attack, heart spasm, uncontrolled hypertension, heart disease, Prinzmetal's angina. *Possible interaction*: ergotamine, 5-HT re-uptake inhibitors (an antidepressant group), lithium, MAOIs. *Side effects*: blood pressure rise, pain at injection site, tiredness, feeling of heaviness and pressure, dizziness, sleepiness, slight disturbance of liver function. Drug should be withdrawn if there is pain in chest or throat and cause investigated. *Manufacturer*: Glaxo Wellcome.

IMMUKIN

Description: a preparation of recombinant human interferon gamma-Ib available as a solution for injection in vials for injection at a strength of 200 micrograms/ml. *Used for*: additional treatment (with antibiotics) to lessen the incidence of serious infections acquired by patients with chronic granulomatous disease (any 1 of a number of diseases giving rise to masses of granulation tissue, known as granulomata, e.g. tuberculosis and leprosy). *Dosage*: adults and children with body surface area exceeding 0.5m^2, 50µg/m^2 by subcutaneous injection 3 times each week. Children with body surface area less than 0.5m^2, 1.5µg/kg body weight 3 times each week. *Special care*: patients with serious liver or kidney disease, heart disease (congestive heart failure, arrhythmia, ischaemic heart disease), seizures, central nervous system disorders. Blood, liver and kidney function tests and urine analysis must be carried out during the course of therapy. *Avoid use*: children under 6 months. *Possible interaction*: alcohol. *Side effects*: headache, chills, pain, fever, rash, nausea and vomiting, pain at injection site, ability to perform skilled tasks, e.g. driving and operating machinery may be impaired. *Manufacturer*: Boehringer-Ingelheim.

IMUNOVIR

Description: an antiviral preparation and immunopotentiator produced in the form of white tablets containing 500mg inosine pranobex. *Used for*: infections of mucous membranes and skin caused by *Herpes simplex* virus, (type I and/or II) e.g. genital warts, subacute inflammation of the brain. *Dosage*: *Herpes simplex* infections, 1g 4 times each day for 1 to 2 weeks; inflammation of the brain, 50–100mg/kg body weight each day in divided doses. *Special care*: patients with abnormally high blood levels of uric acid (hyperuricaemia), gout, kidney disease. *Avoid use*: children. *Side effects*: raised uric acid levels. *Manufacturer*: Nycomed.

IMURAN

Description: a cytotoxic immunosuppressant preparation, azathioprine, produced in the form of film-coated tablets of 2 strengths. Orange tablets (25mg) are marked Imuran 25; yellow tablets (50mg) are marked Imuran 50. Also, IMURAN INJECTION containing 50mg azathioprine (as sodium salt) produced as powder in vials for reconstitution. *Used for*: to suppress organ or tissue rejection following transplant operations; some diseases of the auto-immune system especially when treatment with corticosteroids alone has proved to be inadequate. *Dosage*: tablets and/or injection, prevention of rejection of transplant, usually up to 5mg/kg body weight at first and then a maintenance dose in the order of 1–4mg/kg body weight each day. Auto-immune diseases, up to 3mg/kg body weight each day at first reducing to 1–3mg/kg body weight daily as maintenance dose. *Special care*: the injection is an irritant and hence should only be used if tablets cannot be taken. Special care in pregnant women, patients should avoid excessive exposure to sun, persons with kidney or liver disease or suffering from infections. Blood counts and other monitoring for toxic effects should be carried out. *Possible interaction*: skin rashes, bone marrow suppression, gastro-intestinal upset, toxic effects on liver. *Manufacturer*: Glaxo Wellcome.

INDERAL

Description: a preparation which is a non-cardioselective ß-blocker produced as pink, film-coated tablets containing 10mg, 40mg and 80mg propanolol hydrochloride all marked with name, strength and ICI. Also, INDERAL INJECTION containing 1mg/ml in ampoules for injection. *Used for*: heart arrhythmias, prevention of second heart attack, angina, enlarged and weakened heart muscle. Fallot's tetralogy (a congenital defect of the heart), phaeochromocytoma, situational and generalized anxiety. *Dosage*: heart attack, 40mg 4 times each day for 2 or 3 days starting from 5 to 21 days after first attack. Then a maintenance dose of 80mg twice each day. Arrhythmias, 10–40mg 3 or 4 times each day. Angina, 40mg 2 or 3 times each day at first increasing at weekly intervals if required to a usual dose in the order of 120–240mg daily. Hypertension, 80mg twice each day at first increasing at weekly intervals if required to usual dose in the order of 160–320mg daily. Phaeochromocytoma, 60mg each day taken along with an alpha-blocker for 3 days before operation for removal. If tumour is inoperable, a 30mg daily dose should be taken. Situational anxiety, 40mg twice each day, generalized anxiety, the same dose by increasing to 3 times each day if needed. Children, arrhythmias, 0.25–0.5mg/kg body weight 3 to 4 times each day. Fallot's tetralogy, up to 1mg/kg body weight 3 or 4 times each day. Phaeochromocytoma, 0.25–0.5mg/kg body weight 3 or 4 times each day. *Spe-

cial care: pregnancy, breast-feeding, patients underoing planned surgery, those with liver or kidney disease, diabetes, metabolic acidosis. Patients with weak hearts may require diuretics and digitalis. Drug should be gradually withdrawn. *Avoid use*: patients with history of bronchospasm, obstructive airways disease, heart block, heart shock, disease of peripheral arteries, sinus bradycardia, uncompensated heart failure. *Possible interaction*: sympathomimetics, cimetidine, heart depressant anaesthetics, indomethacin, clonidine withdrawal, hypoglycaemics, class I antiarrhythmics, ergotamine, verapamil, reserpine, antihypertensives. *Side effects*: bradycardia, cold hands and feet, tiredness with exercise, gastro-intestinal upset, disturbance of sleep, bronchospasm, heart failure. Drug should be gradually withdrawn if skin rash or dry eyes occur. *Manufacturer*: Zeneca.

INDERAL LA

Description: an antianginal, antihypertensive and anxiolytic preparation which is a non-cardioselective ß-blocker. It is produced as pink/purple sustained-release capsules containing 160mg propanolol hydrochloride marked ICI and INDERAL LA. Also, **HALF-INDERAL LA**, pink/purple sustained-release capsules containing 80mg propanolol hydrochloride marked ICI and HALF-INDERAL LA. *Used for*: angina, hypertension, additional therapy in thyrotoxicosis, also treatment of symptoms of anxiety. *Dosage*: angina, 80mg or 160mg each day with a maximum daily dose of 240mg. Hypertension, 160mg each day at first increasing by 80mg gradually if needed until condition is controlled. Thyrotoxicosis, 80mg or 160mg each day with a maximum daily dose of 240mg. Situational anxiety, 80mg each day, generalized anxiety, 80–160mg each day. *Special care*: pregnancy, breast-feeding, patients undergoing planned surgery, liver or kidney disease, diabetes, metabolic acidosis. Patients with weak hearts may require diuretics and digitalis. Drug should be gradually withdrawn. *Avoid use*: children, patients with history of bronchospasm, obstructive airways disease, heart block, heart shock, disease of peripheral arteries, sinus bradycardia, uncompensated heart failure. *Possible interaction*: sympathomimetics, cimetidine, heart depressant anaesthetics, indomethacin, clonidine withdrawal, hypoglycaemics, class I antiarrhythmics, ergotamine, verapamil, reserpine, antihypertensives. *Side effects*: bradycardia, cold hands and feet, tiredness with exercise, gastro-intestinal upset, disturbance of sleep, bronchospasm, heart failure. Drug should be gradually withdrawn if skin rash or dry eyes occur. *Manufacturer*: Zeneca.

INDERETIC

Description: an antihypertensive preparation combining a non-cardioselective ß-blocker and thiazide diuretic, available as white capsules containing 80mg propanolol hydrochloride and 2.5mg bendrofluazide. *Used for*: hypertension. *Dosage*: adults, 1 tablet twice each day. *Special care*: pregnancy, breast-feeding, patients undergoing general anaesthesia or planned surgery, liver or kidney disease, gout, diabetes, metabolic acidosis. Patients with weak hearts may require diuretics and digitalis. Potassium supplements may be needed and patient's electrolyte levels should be monitored. *Avoid use*: children, patients with heart block, heart shock, sinus bradycardia, peripheral disease of the arteries, sick sinus syndrome, uncompensated heart failure, obstruction of heart outflow, aortic stenosis (narrrowing of aorta). Those with history of breathing difficulties, bronchospasm, obstructive airways disease. *Possible interaction*: sympathomimetics, class I antiarrhythmics, indomethacin, cimetidine, clonidine withdrawal, antihypertensives, ergot alkaloids, heart depressant anaesthetics, depressants, reserpine, hypoglycaemics. Digitalis, potassium-sparing diuretics, potassium supplements, lithium. *Side effects*: bradycardia, cold hands and feet, fatigue on exertion, disturbance of sleep, gastro-intestinal upset, heart failure, bronchospasm. Blood changes, sensitivity to light, gout, muscular weakness. *Manufacturer*: Zeneca.

INDEREX

Description: an antihypertensive preparation which combines a non-cardioselective ß-blocker and thiazide diuretic. It is available as grey/pink sustained-release capsules containing 160mg propanolol and 80mg bendrofluazide marked ICI and Inderex. *Used for*: hypertension. *Dosage*: adults, 1 twice each day. *Special care*: pregnancy, breast-feeding, patients undergoing general anaesthesia or planned surgery, liver or kidney disease, gout, diabetes, metabolic acidosis. Patients with weak hearts may require diuretics and digitalis. Potassium supplements may be needed and patient's electrolyte levels should be monitored. *Avoid use*: children, patients with heart block, heart shock, sinus bradycardia, peripheral disease of the arteries, sick sinus syndrome, uncompensated heart failure, obstruction of heart outflow, aortic stenosis (narrrowing of aorta). Those with history of breathing difficulties, bronchospasm, obstructive airways disease. *Possible interaction*: sympathomimetics, class I antiarrhythmics, indomethacin, cimetidine, clonidine withdrawal, antihypertensives, ergot alkaloids, heart depressant anaesthetics, central nervous system depressants, reserpine, hypoglycaemics. Digitalis, potassium-sparing diuretics, potassium supplements, lithium. *Side effects*: bradycardia, cold hands and feet, fatigue on exertion, disturbance of sleep, gastro-intestinal upset, heart failure, bronchospasm. Blood changes, sensitivity to light, gout, muscular weakness. *Manufacturer*: Zeneca.

INDOCID

Description: an NSAID and indole available in a variety of forms: capsules are ivory-coloured and contain 25mg and 50mg indomethacin both marked with name and strength. **INDOCID SUSPENSION** contains 25mg/5ml; **INDOCID SUPPOSITORIES** contain 100mg indomethacin. **INDOCID-R** are blue/yellow sustained-release capsules containing 75mg indomethacin marked INDOCID-R 693. *Used for*: diseases of skeleton and joints including ankylosing spondylitis, osteoarthritis, lumbago, rheumatoid arthritis, degenerative disease of hip joint, acute joint disorders, acute gout (except Indocid-R). Also, dysmenorrhoea. *Dosage*: adults, capsules and suspension, 50–200mg each day in divided doses with meals. Indocid-R, 1 tablet once or twice each day, suppositories, 1 at night and 1 in the morning if needed. *Special care*: elderly persons, patients with heart failure, disorders of central nervous system, liver or kidney disease. Patients taking drug long-term should receive careful monitoring. *Avoid use*: children, pregnancy, breast-feeding, history of gastro-intestinal ulcer or peptic ulcer, allergy to anti-inflammatory drug or aspirin, angioneurotic oedema, recent proctitis (inflammation of the rectum and anus). *Possible interaction*: methotrexate, anticoagulants, corticosteroids, quinolones, probenecid, aminoglycosides, salicylates, ß-blockers, lithium, diuretics. *Side effects*: blood changes, effects on central nervous system, gastro-intestinal intolerance, disturbance of vision and corneal deposits. If recurring headaches or gastro-intestinal bleeding occur, drug should be withdrawn. Eye tests should be carried out during the course of long-term therapy. *Manufacturer*: Morson.

INDOCID PDA

Description: a prostaglandin synthetase inhibitor produced as a powder in vials for reconstitution and injection containing 1mg indomethacin (as sodium trihydrate). *Used for*: patent ductus arteriosus (PDA) in premature babies (a condition in which there is a connection between the aorta and pulmonary artery, the ductus arteriosus, which normally closes after birth). *Dosage*: 3 intravenous injections, at intervals of 12 to 24 hours depending upon baby's age, condition and urinary output. *Special care*: kidney function and plasma levels of electrolytes should be monitored. *Avoid use*: babies with serious kidney disorders, untreated infection, bleeding, disorders of blood coagulation. *Possible interaction*: frusemide, aminoglycosides, digitalis. *Side effects*: bleeding, disturbance in urine production, elevated creatine levels in blood, imbalance in electrolyte (salts) levels. If liver disease develops, drug should be withdrawn. *Manufacturer*: Morson.

INDOMOD

Description: an NSAID Indole preparation available in the form of capsules of 2 strengths containing enteric-coated, continuous-release pellets. Orange capsules, marked AB27, contain 25mg and brown capsules, marked AB26, contain 75mg indomethacin respectively. *Used for*: joint and bone disorders, including ankylosing spondylitis, rheumatoid arthritis, osteoarthritis, tenosynovitis, tendinitis, bursitis, gout. *Dosage*: adults, 50–75mg as single or 2 doses each day increasing once a week by 25 or 50mg to a maximum daily dose of 200mg. *Special care*: elderly persons, patients with heart failure, liver or kidney disease, disorders of central nervous systen. Patients taking drug long-term require careful monitoring and eye tests. *Avoid use*: pregnancy, breast-feeding, history of ulcers or active ulcer, allergy to NSAID or aspirin. *Possible interaction*:

salicylates, proben-ecid, ß-blockers, corticosteroids, lithium, diuretics, quinolones, anticoagulants. *Side effects*: disturbance of vision, deposits in cornea; if recurrent headaches or gastro-intestinal bleeding occur, drug should be withdrawn. *Manufacturer*: Pharmacia & Upjohn.

INFLUVAC

Description: a preparation of inactivated surface antigen obtained from 4 strains of influenza virus. It is produced in pre-filled syringes containing 15µg of each strain of influenza virus/0.5ml suspension. *Dosage*: adults, 0.5ml by deep subcutaneous or intramuscular injection. Children, aged 4 to 13 years, 0.5ml then repeated dose 4 to 6 weeks later. *Avoid use*: children under 4 years, patients with allergy to poultry, eggs or feathers, (chick embryos used to culture virus strains). Patients with feverish conditions. *Side effects*: tiredness, headache, feverishness, pain at injection site. *Manufacturer*: Solvay.

INNOHEP

Description: an anticoagulant preparation which is a low molecular weight heparin produced as solutions in ampoules or pre-filled syringes for injection. Syringes contain 3500 units activity of anti-factor Xa tinzaparin/0.3ml. Ampoules contain 5000 units activity of anti-factor Xa tinzaparin/0.5ml. *Used for*: prevention of thrombosis in patients having orthopaedic or general surgical operations. *Dosage*: orthopaedic surgery, 50 units/kg body weight 2 hours before operation by subcutaneous injection then same dose once each day for next 7 to 10 days. General surgery, 3500 units 2 hours before operation by subcutaneous injection then same dose once each day for next 7 to 10 days. *Special care*: pregnancy, breast-feeding, asthma, severe liver or kidney disease. *Avoid use*: children, patients liable to bleeding, active peptic ulcer, serious hypertension which is uncontrolled, septic endocarditis. *Possible interaction*: drugs which affect blood coagulation or platelets. *Side effects*: risk of haemorrhage, slight bruising, skin rash, blood changes, short-lived rise in liver enzymes. *Manufacturer*: Leo.

INNOVACE

Description: an antihypertensive preparation which is an ACE inhibitor produced as tablets of different strengths, all marked INNOVACE and containing enalapril maleate: white, round 2.5mg tablets; white, scored 5mg tablets; red, triangular 10mg tablets; peach, triangular 20mg tablets. *Used for*: congestive heart failure, with digitalis and potassium-sparing diuretics. Prevention of heart attack and progression of disease in left ventricle of heart. *Dosage*: adults, 2.5mg once each day at first increasing to a usual maintenance dose in the order of 20mg, maximum is 40mg. Treatment should normally begin in hospital and diuretics discontinued or reduced before therapy starts. *Special care*: breast-feeding, patients undergoing anaesthesia, those with kidney disease and hypertension associated with this, patients have kidney dialysis, serious congestive heart failure. Kidney function should be monitored during course of therapy.

Avoid use: children, pregnancy, patients with obstruction to outflow of heart or aortic stenosis (narrowing of aorta). *Possible interaction*: potassium supplements or potassium-sparing diuretics, other antihypertensives, lithium. *Side effects*: tiredness, headache, dizziness, cough, gastro-intestinal upset, oedema, hypotension. *Manufacturer*: M.S.D.

INNOZIDE

Description: an antihypertensive preparation combining an ACE inhibitor and thiazide diuretic produced in the form of scored, yellow tablets containing 20mg enalapril maleate and 12.5mg hydrochlorthiazide marked MSD 718. *Used for*: mild to moderate hypotension in patients who have become accustomed to the same components taken individually. *Dosage*: adults, 1 tablet each day with a maximum of 2 if needed. *Special care*: breast-feeding, electrolytes (salts) or fluid imbalance, kidney or liver disease, heart disease or disease of the blood vessels of the brain. Patients receiving kidney dialysis, suffering from gout, diabetes or undergoing anaesthesia. *Avoid use*: children, pregnancy, angio-neurotic oedema resulting from previous treatment with ACE inhibitor, anuria. *Possible interaction*: hypoglycaemics, tubocurarine, corticosteroids, potassium supplements, potassium-sparing diuretics, NSAIDs, central nervous system depressants, lithium. *Side effects*: cough, tiredness, headache, skin rash, hypotension, pain in chest, dizziness, weakness, kidney failure, impotence, angioneurotic oedema. *Manufacturer*: M.S.D.

INSTILLAGEL

Description: a disinfectant and local anaesthetic preparation produced as a gel in disposable syringes. It contains 2% lignocaine hydrochloride, 0.25% chlorhexidine gluconate, 0.06% methyl hydroxybenzoate, 0.025% propyl hydroxybenzoate. *Used for*: catheter disinfection and lubrication during insertion and as local anaesthetic. *Dosage*: 6–11ml into urethra. *Special care*: those with serious, local haemorrhage. *Manufacturer*: CliniMed.

INTAL SYNCRONER

Description: a bronchodilator and NSAID, sodium cromoglycate, produced in a variety of different forms: **INTAL METERED DOSE AEROSOL** with spacer device, delivers 5mg/dose. **INTAL IHHALER** also delivers 53mg/dose and is a metered dose aerosol. **INTAL SPINCAP**, clear yellow spincaps contain 20mg and are marked INTAL P and FISONS. **INTAL NEBULIZER SOLUTION** contains 10mg/2ml in ampoules for use with nebulizer. **INTAL FISONAIRE**, a metered dose aerosol with spacer device within chamber delivering 5mg/dose. *Used for*: prevention of bronchial asthma. *Dosage*: adults and children, inhaler, 2 puffs 4 times each day reducing to 1 puff for maintenance. Spincaps, 4 each day in spinhaler taken at regular times. Nebulizer, 20mg 4 to 6 times each day continuously. *Side effects*: irritated throat, short-lived cough; rarely, bronchospasm. *Manufacturer*: R.P.R.

INTRAVAL SODIUM

Description: a general anaesthetic preparation produced as a powder for recon-stitution containing 0.5 and 2.5g thiopentone sodium. *Used for*: induction of general anaesthesia. *Dosage*: (in fit persons who have received premedication), 100–150mg over 10 to 15 seconds by intravenous injection; may be repeated after half a minute if required. Or, up to 4mg/kg body weight may be given. Children, 2–7mg/kg body weight. *Special care*: depression of respiration and heart may occur if dose is too high. *Possible interaction*: alcohol. *Side effects*: sedative effects and slow metabolism for up to 24 hours. Ability to perform skilled tasks, e.g. driving, may be impaired. *Manufacturer*: R.P.R..

INTRON A

Description: a single-subtype recombinant interferon preparation produced as a powder in vials with solution for reconstitution and injection, in different strengths of 1, 3, 5, 10, 25 and 30 megaunits interferon alfa-2b (rbe). *Used for*: leukaemia, maintenance of remission in multiple myeloma, non-Hodgkins lym-phoma, AIDS-related Kaposi's sarcoma. *Dosage*: according to individual need as directed by physician. *Avoid use*: pregnant women. *Possible interaction*: theo-phylline. *Side effects*: weariness, depression, influenza-like symptoms, bone marrow suppression, rash; seizures and coma (with higher doses especially in elderly persons). *Manufacturer*: Schering-Plough.

INTROPIN

Description: a potent sympathomimetic drug which is an intropic agent pro-duced in ampoules for injection containing 40mg dopamine hydrochloride/ml. *Used for*: cardiogenic shock following heart attack and heart failure in cardiac surgery. *Dosage*: 2–5µg/kg body-weight/minute by intravenous infusion but dose is critical. *Special care*: hypovalaemia (abnormally low volume of circulating blood) should be corrected. *Avoid use*: patients with phaeochromocytoma, fast arrhythmia. *Possible interaction*: antidepressants. *Side effects*: tachycardia, hypo and hypertension, constriction of peripheral blood vessels, vomiting and nau-sea. *Manufacturer*: DuPont.

IODOFLEX

Description: a preparation which is absorbent and antibacterial available as a paste with removable gauze, containing cadexomer iodine. *Used for*: chronic leg ulcers. *Dosage*: adults and children over 2 years, apply up to 50g to ulcer and cover with additional dressing; renew when dressing is saturated or 3 times each week. Dose should not exceed 150g in any week and use should be re-stricted to a period of 3 months. *Special care*: patients with disorders of the thyroid gland. *Avoid use*: children under 2 years, pregnancy, breast-feeding, patients with thyroid disorders (Grave's disease, Hashimoto's thyroiditis, non-toxic nodular goitre). *Possible interaction*: sulphafurazoles, lithium, sulphony-lureas. *Manufacturer*: Perstop.

IODOSORB

Description: an adsorbent and antibacterial available as a powder in sachets containing cadexomer iodine. Also **IODOSORB OINTMENT** containing cadexomer iodine. *Used for*: leg ulcers, bedsores and moist wounds. *Dosage*: adults, apply a layer at least 3mm thick and cover with sterile dressing. Change when dressing is saturated. Ointment, (for chronic leg ulcers), as above but no more than 150g should be used in any 1 week and course of therapy should not exceed 3 months. *Special care*: patients with disorders of the thyroid gland. *Avoid use*: children, pregnancy, breast-feeding, patients with thyroid disorders (Grave's disease, Hashimoto's thyroiditis, non-toxic nodular goitre). *Possible interaction*: sulphafurazoles, lithium, sulphonylureas. *Manufacturer*: Perstop.

IONAMIN^{CD}

Description: a central nervous system stimulant which acts as an appetite-suppressant. It is available as sustained-release capsules of 2 strengths: yellow/grey containing 15mg phentermine as resin complex and yellow, containing 30mg phentermine as resin complex. Both are marked with name and strength. *Used for*: obesity. *Dosage*: adults, 15–30mg each day before breakfast. *Special care*: angina, hypertension, heart arrhythmias. For short-term use only. *Avoid use*: children, pregnancy, breast-feeding, hyperthyroidism, serious hypertension, arteriosclerosis. Those with history of drug or alcohol abuse or psychiatric illnesses. *Possible interaction*: methyldopa, sympathomimetics, guanethidine, MAOIs, psychotropic drugs. *Side effects*: drug dependence and tolerance, dry mouth, rise in blood pressure, agitation and nervousness, palpitations, psychiatric disturbances. *Manufacturer*: Torbet.

IOPIDINE

Description: an eye solution which is an alpha$_2$-agonist available in single dose (0.25ml) ampoules containing 1.15% apraclonidine hydrochloride. *Used for*: control and prevention of any rise in pressure within the eye following anterior segment laser surgery. *Dosage*: 1 drop into eye 1 hour before laser treatment and 1 drop immediately after surgery is completed. *Special care*: pregnancy, breast-feeding, serious heart and circulatory disease, hypertension, history of fainting. If there is a great reduction in the pressure within the eye, this should receive careful monitoring. *Avoid use*: children. *Possible interaction*: MAOIs, sympathomimetics, TCADs. *Side effects*: blanching of conjunctiva of eye and retraction of eyelids, dilation of pupil. Possible effects on heart and circulation due to absorption of drug. *Manufacturer*: Alcon.

IPRAL

Description: a sulphonamide antibiotic preparation which is a folic acid inhibitor available as white tablets containing 100mg and 200mg trimethoprim, marked SQUIBB 513 and SQUIBB 514 respectively. *Used for*: prevention and treatment of infections of the urinary tract; treatment of respiratory tract infections. *Dosage*: adults, treatment, 200mg twice each day; prevention of urinary tract infections, 100mg taken at night. Children, over 6 years of age, 100mg twice each day. *Special care*: patients with kidney disorder or folate deficiency. Regular blood tests are required during long-term treatment. *Avoid use*: children under 6 years, pregnancy, serious kidney disease. *Side effects*: gastro-intestinal upset, skin reactions, folate deficiency if drug is taken long-term. *Manufacutrer*: Squibb.

ISMELIN

Description: an antihypertensive preparation, guanethidine sulphate, which is an adrenergic neurone blocker, available as white tablets containing 10mg and pink tablets containing 25mg. Both are marked with strength and name. Also **ISMELIN INJECTION** containing 10mg/ml in ampoules. *Used for*: hypertension. *Dosage*: adults, 10mg each day at first increasing by 10mg once a week if needed to a usual dose in the order of 25–50mg. *Special care*: pregnancy, kidney disease, asthma, peptic ulcer, arteriosclerosis, anaesthesia. *Avoid use*: patients with heart or kidney failure, phaeochromocytoma. *Possible interaction*: sympathomimetics, MAOIs, hypoglycaemics, digitalis, contraceptive pill, TCADs, antiarrhythmics, antipsychotics, other anti-hypertensives. *Side effects*: blocked nose, blood changes, oedema, failure to reach sexual climax (males), bradycardia, diarrhoea, hypotension when rising from lying down. *Manufacturer*: Ciba.

ISOPTO ATROPINE

Description: lubricant and anticholinergic eyedrops containing 1% atropine sulphate and 0.5% hypromellose. *Used for*: to produce long-lasting mydriasis (the drug is mydriatic)—fixed dilation of the pupil of the eye, and cycloplegia (cycloplegic)—paralysis of the ciliary muscles. This is in order to allow detailed examination of the eye to be carried out. *Dosage*: adults, for uveitis (inflammation of the uveal tract), 1 drop 3 times each day; for refraction, 1 to 2 drops 1 hour before eye is examined. Children, uveitis, 1 drop 3 times each day; refraction, 1 drop twice each day for 1 to 2 days before eye is examined. *Special care*: infants, pressure should be applied over lachrymal (tear) sac for 1 minute. *Avoid use*: patients with soft contact lenses, narrow angle glaucoma. *Side effects*: dry mouth, sensitivity to light, stinging in eye, blurring of vision, headache, tachycardia. Also changes in behaviour and psychotic responses. *Manufacturer*: Alcon.

ISOPTO CARBACHOL

Description: lubricant and cholinergic eyedrops containing 3% carbachol and 1% hypromellose. *Used for*: glaucoma. *Dosage*: adults, 2 drops 3 times each day. *Avoid use*: children, patients with severe iritis (inflammation of the iris), abrasion of the cornea, wearing soft contact lenses. *Manufacturer*: Alcon.

ISOPTO CARPINE

Description: lubricant and cholinergic eyedrops available at different strengths containing 0.5%, 1%, 2%, 3% and 4% pilocarpine all with 0.5% hypromellose. *Used for*: glaucoma. *Dosage*: adults, 2 drops 3 times each day. *Avoid use*: children, patients with severe iritis (inflammation of the iris), wearing soft contact lenses. *Manufacturer*: Alcon.

ISOTREX

Description: a topical preparation of vitamin A derivative available as a gel containing 0.05% isotretinoin. *Used for*: acne vulgaris. *Dosage*: apply thinly once or twice each day for at least 6 to 8 weeks. *Special care*: avoid mucous membranes, mouth, angles of nose, eyes, damaged or sunburnt areas. Ultraviolet light should be avoided. *Avoid use*: pregnancy, breast-feeding, family history or history of epithelioma of skin (abnormal growth which may or may not be malignant). *Possible interaction*: keratolytics. *Side effects*: local skin irritation. *Manufacturer*: Stiefel.

ISTIN

Description: an antianginal and anti-hypertensive preparation which is a class II calcium antagonist. It is available as 5mg and 10mg white tablets containing amlodipine besylate, marked Pfizer and ITN 5 and ITN 10 respectively. *Used for*: angina in myocardial ischaemia, hypertension. *Dosage*: adults, 5mg once each day; maximum dose, 10mg daily. *Special care*: pregnancy, breast-feeding, children, liver disease. *Side effects*: oedema, headache, dizziness, tiredness, nausea, flushing. *Manufacturer*: Pfizer.

J

JECTOFER

Description: a haematinic compound available in ampoules for injection containing iron sorbitol and citric acid (equivalent to 50mg of iron/ml). *Used for*: anaemia caused by iron deficiency. *Dosage*: adults and children over 3kg in weight by intramuscular injection as a single dose. The maximum dose for each injection is 100mg. *Avoid use*: patients with certain other types of anaemia (hypoplastic or aplastic), seriously damaged kidney or liver, acute leukaemia. *Side effects*: heart arrhythmias. *Manufacturer*: Astra.

JEXIN

Description: a non-depolarizing (or competitive) muscle relaxant preparation used in anaesthesia produced in ampoules for injection containing 10mg tubocurarine chloride/ml. *Used for*: production of muscle relaxation during surgery and for patients in intensive care units receiving long-term assisted ventilation. *Dosage*: adults, 15–30mg by intravenous injection at first then 5–10mg as needed. Children, 300–500µg/kg body weight at first, then 60–100µg/kg, as needed. Newborn babies, 200–250µg/kg body weight at first then 40–50µg/kg, as needed. *Special care*: kidney disease or damage, those in whom hypotension would be undesirable. *Avoid use*: patients with myasthenia gravis. *Possible interaction*: aminoglycosides, clindamycin, azlocillin, colistin, verapamil, nifedipine, cholinergics, magnesium salts. *Side effects*: short-lived hypotension, skin rash. *Manufacturer*: Evans.

JUNIFEN

Description: an NSAID produced as a sugar-free, orange-flavoured suspension containing 100mg ibuprofen/5ml. *Used for*: relief of pain and reduction of fever in children. *Dosage*: children, 1 to 2 years, 2.5ml; 3 to 7 years, 5ml; 8 to 12 years, 10ml. All given 3 to 4 times each day. *Special care*: pregnancy, breast-feeding, patients with liver, kidney or heart disease or damage, asthma, gastro-intestinal disease, patients receiving long-term therapy require careful monitoring. *Avoid use*: children under 1 year and those less than 7kg body weight, allergy to aspirin or NSAID, peptic ulcer. *Possible interaction*: thiazide diuretics, anticoagulants, quinolones. *Side effects*: rash, thrombocytopenia, gastro-intestinal upset or haemorrhage. *Manufacturer*: Boots.

K

KABIGLOBULIN

Description: a preparation of human normal immunoglobulin (HNIG) available as a 16% solution in ampoules for injection. *Used for*: prevention of hepatitis A infection, prevention of measles, prevention of rubella in pregnancy, burns, antibody deficiency conditions. *Dosage*: prevention of hepatitis A, adults and children, usual dose 0.02ml 0 0.04ml/kg body weight or 0.06–0.12 ml if risk is greater. Prevention of measles, 0.02ml/kg body weight or 0.04ml/kg body weight to allow mild attack. Rubella in pregnancy, adults, 20ml to prevent clinical attack. All doses given by intramuscular injection. *Possible interaction*: live vaccines. *Manufacturer*: Pharmacia & Upjohn.

KABIKINASE

Description: a fibrinolytic preparation available as a powder in vials for reconstitution and injection in 3 strengths, containing 250,000 units, 750,000 units and 1.5 million units streptokinase. *Used for*: to disperse blood clots in life-threatening conditions as in pulmonary embolism, heart atack, deep vein thrombosis, arterial thromboembolism, clots during haemodialysis (kidney dialysis). *Dosage*: adults, up to 600,000 units given over thirty minutes by intravascular route (into blood vessel), in first instance. Maintenance dose, 100,000 units every hour for 3 to 6 days. Heart attack, 1.5 million units by intravenous infusion over 1 hour then 150mg of aspirin each day for a minimum of 4 weeks. Children, 1300–1400 units/kg body weight each hour for 3 to 6 days. Other conditions may require different doses. *Special care*: patients with pancreatitis, ensure no pre-existing clot which on dissolution might cause embolism. Special care with follow-on anticoagulant therapy. *Avoid use*: pregnancy, patients with recent haemorrhage, surgery or injury, bleeding disorders. Also coagulation disorders, serious hypertension, streptococcal infections, serious liver or kidney damage or disease, peptic ulcer, endocarditis caused by bacteria. Patients with known allergy to streptokinase or who have received treatment with this or anistreplase during the previous 5 days to 6 months. *Possible interaction*: drugs acting on blood platelets, anticoagulants. *Side effects*: haemorrhage, fever, hypotension, heart arrhythmias; rarely, anaphylaxis (shock). *Manufacturer*: Pharmacia & Upjohn.

KALSPARE

Description: a compound diuretic preparation with thiazide-like activity and also potassium-sparing, available in the form of film-coated orange tablets, containing 50mg chlorthalidone and 50mg triamterene, scored on 1 side and marked A on the other. *Used for*: hypertension, oedema. *Dosage*: adults, hypertension, 1 tablet every morning increasing to 2 as single daily dose if required. Oedema, 1 tablet every morning increasing to 2 daily as single dose if condition has not improved after 7 days. *Special care*: pregnancy, breast-feeding, liver or kidney disease or damage, diabetes, gout, acidosis. *Avoid use*: patients with serious or worsening kidney failure, anuria, hyperkalaemia. *Possible interaction*: potassium-sparing diuretics, potassium supplements, ACE inhibitors, lithium, antihypertensives, digitalis. *Side effects*: sensitivity to light, cramps, skin rash, blood changes, gout. *Manufacturer*: Dominion.

KALTEN

Description: a compound hypertensive preparation combining a cardio-selective ß-blocker, thiazide and potassium-sparing diuretic. It is available as cream/red capsules containing 50mg atenolol, 25mg hydrochlorothiazide and 2.5mg amiloride hydrochloride marked with logo and KALTEN. *Used for*: hypertension. *Dosage*: adults, 1 tablet each day. *Special care*: pregnancy, breast-feeding, general anaesthesia, liver or kidney disease, diabetes, gout, metabolic acidosis. Patients with weak hearts may require treatment with diuretics and digitalis. *Avoid use*: obstructive airways disease or history of bronchospasm, heart block, heart shock, heart failure, disease of peripheral arteries, sick sinus syndrome, serious or worsening kidney failure, anuria. *Possible interaction*: sympathomimetics, heart depressant anaesthetics, central nervous system depressants, ergotamine, class I antiarrhythmics, indomethacin, verapamil, hypoglycaemics, clonidine withdrawal, reserpine, cimetidine, clonidine withdrawal. Potassium supplements, potassium-sparing diuretics, digitalis, lithium. *Side effects*: gastrointestinal upset, cold hands and feet, disturbance of sleep, fatigue on exertion, bronchospasm, bradycardia. Sensitivity to light, gout, blood changes, muscle weakness. If unexplained skin rash or dry eyes occur, therapy should be stopped. Withdraw drug gradually. *Manufacturer*: Zeneca.

KANNASYN

Description: a broad-spectrum aminoglycoside antibiotic preparation available as a powder in vials for reconstitution and injection containing 1g kanamycin (as acid sulphate). *Used for*: serious infections such as meningitis and septicaemia, especially where there is resistance to other antibiotics. *Dosage*: adults, 1g by intramuscular injections each day in 2, 3 or 4 divided doses for a maximum period of 6 days. Children, 15mg/kg body weight by intramuscular injections in 2, 3 or 4 divided doses each day for a maximum period of 6 days. *Special care*: patients with kidney disorders, Parkinsonism, myasthenia gravis; careful control of blood levels and dosage is required. *Avoid use*: pregnancy, breastfeeding. *Possible interaction*: anaesthetics, frusemide, neuromuscular blocking drugs, ethacrynic acid. *Side effects*: damage to hearing and balance, harmful effects on kidneys. *Manufacturer*: Sanofi Swinthrop.

KAPAKE

Description: a compound analgesic preparation available in the form of scored, white oval tablets containing 500mg paracetamol and 30mg codeine phosphate, marked KAPAKE. *Used for*: severe pain. *Dosage*: adults, 1 or 2 tablets every 4 hours with a maximum of 8 in 24 hours. *Special care*: elderly, kidney or liver disease, inflammation or obstruction of the bowel, enlargement of the prostate gland, Addison's disease, hypothyroidism. *Avoid use*: children, pregnancy, breastfeeding, breathing difficulties, obstructive airways disease, raised pressure inside cranium, alcoholism. *Possible interaction*: MAOIs, central nervous system depressants. *Side effects*: drug dependence and tolerance, dry mouth, dizziness, nausea, blurring of vision, constipation, nausea, sleepiness. *Manufacturer*: Galen.

KEFADOL

Description: a cephalosporin antibiotic preparation available as a powder in vials for reconstitution and injection containing 1g cefamandole (as nafate). *Used for*: life-threatening, severe infections. *Dosage*: adults, 500mg–2g given by intramuscular or intravenous injection every 4 to 8 hours with a maximum dose of 12g every 24 hours. Children over 1 month, 50—100mg/kg body weight each day every 4 to 8 hours, with a maximum dose of 150mg/kg body weight daily. *Special care*: patients with kidney disease or sensitivity to penicillin. *Avoid use*: children under 1 month. *Possible interaction*: aminoglycosides, loop diuretics. *Side effects*: gastro-intestinal upset, blood changes (reduction in levels of white blood cells), thrombocytopenia. Also, allergic reactions, rise in level of blood urea and liver enzymes, cholestatic jaundice, short-lived hepatitis, positive Coomb's test (a test for rhesus antibodies). *Manufacturer*: Dista.

KEFLEX

Description: a cephalosporin antibiotic preparation, cephalexin monohydrate, produced in a number of different forms. White/dark green capsules contain 250mg , and dark green/pale green capsules contain 500mg coded LILLY H69 and LILLY H71 respectively. **KEFLEX TABLETS**, peach-coloured containing 250mg coded LILLY U57 and peach, oval tablets containing 500mg coded LILLY U49. Also, **KEFLEX SUSPENSION** in 2 strengths containing 125mg and 250mg/5ml solution. *Used for*: urinary tract infections, inflammation of middle ear, infections of respiratory tract, skin, bone, soft tissue. Also dental infections. *Dosage*: adults, 1–4g each day in divided doses. Children, 25–50mg/kg body weight each day in divided doses. *Special care*: patients with kidney disorder and allergy to penicillins. *Possible interaction*: loop diuretics. *Side effects*: gastro-intestinal upset, allergic reactions. *Manufacturer*: Lilly.

KEFZOL

Description: a cephalosporin antibiotic preparation available as a powder in vials for reconstitution and injection, at 2 strengths, containing 500mg and 1g cephazolin (as salt). *Used for*: septicaemia, endocarditis, skin, soft tissue, respiratory, urinary tract infections. *Dosage*: adults, 500mg–1g every 6 to 8 hours by intramuscular or intravenous injection. Children, over 1 month in age, 25–50mg/kg body weight each day by intramuscular or intravenous injection in divided doses. *Special care*: kidney disease or disorder, hypersensitivity to beta-lactam antibiotics. In beta-haemolytic infections, treatment should be given for a minimum period of 10 days. *Avoid use*: children under 1 month. *Possible interaction*: aminoglycosides, loop diuretics, probenecid. *Side effects*: gastro-intestinal upset, blood changes involving white blood cells, candidosis (thrush), pain at injection site, seizures. A rise in levels of blood urea and liver enzymes, positive Coomb's test (a test for rhesus antibodies). *Manufacturer*: Lilly.

KELFIZINE W

Description: a sulphonamide antibiotic preparation available as white tablets containing 2g sulfametopyrazine, marked weekly dose on 1 side and name on the reverse. *Used for*: treatment and prevention of chronic bronchitis, urinary tract infections. *Dosage*: adults, 1 tablet each week. *Special care*: patients with kidney or liver disease or damage. Persons taking drug over long period should receive regular blood checks. *Avoid use*: children, women in late pregnancy, nursing mothers. *Possible interaction*: hypoglycaemics taken orally, folate antagonists. *Side effects*: gastro-intestinal upset, skin rashes, haemolytic anaemia, inflammation of the tongue, blood changes if taken long-term. *Manufacturer*: Pharmacia & Upjohn.

KELOCYANOR

Description: a chelating agent (1 which binds to a metal) available as a solution in ampoules for injection containing 1.5% dicobalt edetate in glucose. *Used for*: as an antidote in patients with cyanide poisoning. *Dosage*: adults and children, 20ml (300mg) by intravenous injection over 1 minute followed straight away by 50ml dextrose intravenous infusion 50%. Both may be repeated once or twice as required. *Side effects*: tachycardia, vomiting, short-lived hypotension, toxic effects from cobalt. *Manufacturer*: Lipha.

KEMADRIN

Description: an anticholinergic preparation available as scored white tablets containing 5mg procyclidine hydrochloride marked WELLCOME S3A. Also, **KEMADRIN INJECTION** available as 2ml ampoules containing 2mg procyclidine hydrchloride. *Used for*: Parkinsonism, especially drug-induced symptoms. *Dosage*: adults, 2.5mg 3 times each day after meals, in first instance, then increasing every second or third day by 2.5–5mg. The usual maximum daily dose is 30mg. Injection, 10–20mg each day by intramusucular or intravenous injection. *Special care*: heart disease, enlarged prostate gland, obstruction of gastro-intestinal tract, narrow angle glaucoma. Drug should be gradually withdrawn. *Avoid use*: children, patients with tardive dyskinesia (a movement disorder especially affecting elderly people). *Possible interaction*: antihistamines, phenothiazines, antidepressants. *Side effects*: anticholinergic side effects, confusion with higher doses. *Manufacturer*: Glaxo Wellcome.

KEMICETINE SUCCINATE

Description: a chloramphenicol antibiotic available as a powder in vials for re-constitution and injection containing 1g chloramphenicol (as sodium succinate). *Used for*: serious, life-threatening infections including *H. influenzae*, meningitis and typhoid. *Dosage*: adults, 1g by intravenous injection every 6 to 8 hours. Children, newborn babies, 25mg/kg body weight each day; others, 50mg/kg body weight daily. All given intravenously every 6 hours in divided doses. *Special care*: patients with liver or kidney disease or damage. *Possible interaction*: hypoglycaemics, anticoagulants, phenytoin. *Side effects*: gastro-intestinal upset, dry mouth, disturbance of vision, rash, Grey syndrome in babies. Drug causes serious blood changes such as aplastic anaemia and is reserved for use in conditions in which no effective alternative is available, and patient's life is at risk. Regular blood tests should be performed. *Manufacturer*: Pharmacia & Upjohn.

KENALOG

Description: an anti-inflammatory corticosteroid (glucocorticoid) preparation available in pre-filled syringes and vials for injection, containing 40mg triamcinolone acetonide/ml. *Used for*: pain in joints, stiffness and swelling due to rheumatoid arthritis, osteoarthritis. Inflammation of connective tissue (bursa) around joint (bursitis), tendon sheath (tenosynovitis), inflammation of the elbow joint (epicondylitis). Also used for collagen disorders, deficiency of hormones of adrenal cortex, serious dermatitis, allergic disorders. *Dosage*: adults by intramuscular injection, 40mg by deep injection into gluteal muscle; further doses according to patient's condition. For allergic states, e.g. hay fever, 40–100mg as single dose. Joint disorders, 5–40mg by intra-articular injection (directly into joint) according to joint size. Maximum dose if more than one joint is being treated is 80mg. Children, age 6 to 12 years, in proportion to adult dose according to age, severity of condition, bodyweight and joint size. *Special care*: pregnancy, inflammation of kidneys, osteoporosis, infections, viral or fungal conditions, tuberculosis, diabetes. Also, glaucoma, recent surgical anastomoses, thrombophlebitis, epilepsy, liver cirrhosis, hypertension, hyperthyroidism. Patients with osteoporosis, secondary cancers, disease characterized by skin rash (exanthematous disease) e.g. measles, psychoses, suffering from stress. Patients should avoid contact with *Herpes zoster* virus or chicken pox and should seek medical help if inadvertently exposed. Drug should be gradually withdrawn. *Avoid use*: children under 6 years. *Possible interaction*: cardiac glycosides, NSAIDs, phenytoin, anticoagulants taken orally, anticholinesterases, phenobarbitone, hypoglycaemics, rifampicin, ephedrine, diuretics. *Side effects*: skin changes as in Cushing's syndrome, peptic ulcer, osteoporosis, hyperglycaemia, euphoria and depression. *Manufacturer*: Squibb.

KERLONE

Description: an antihypertensive preparation which is a cardioselective ß-blocker available as scored, white, film-coated tablets containing 20mg betaxolol hydrochloride marked KE 20. *Used for*: hypertension. *Dosage*: adults, 1 tablet each day, (half for elderly persons in first instance). *Special care*: pregnancy, breast-feeding, diabetes, liver or kidney disease, metabolic acidosis, undergoing general anaesthesia. Drug should be gradually withdrawn. Patients with weak hearts may require digitalis and diuretic treatment. *Avoid use*: children, patients with history of bronchospasm, obstructive airways disease, heart block, heart failure, heart shock, peripheral disease of the arteries, sick sinus syndrome. *Possible interaction*: CNS depressants, indomethacin, clonidine withdrawal, ergotamine, sympathomimetics, class I antiarrhythmics, cimetidine, verapamil, other antihypertensives, reserpine, hypoglycaemics. *Side effects*: bradycardia, cold hands and feet, fatigue on exertion, disturbance of sleep, gastro-intestinal upset, bronchospasm, heart failure. Withdraw if dry eyes or skin rash occur. *Manufacturer*: Lorex.

KETALAR

Description: a general anaesthetic available as a solution in vials for injection at strengths of 10mg, 50mg and 100mg/ml, containing ketamine (as hydrochloride). *Used for*: induction and maintenance of general anaesthesia especially in children requiring repeated anaesthesia. *Dosage*: by intravenous injection or infusion depending upon period of time for which general anaesthesia is required. *Avoid use*: patients prone to hallucination, those with hypertension. *Possible interaction*: ACE inhibitors, TCADs, antipsychotics, ß-blockers, antihypertensives, anxiolytics and hypnotics. *Side effects*: hallucinations (but incidence is reduced if used with diazepam and is less of a problem in children), possible tachycardia and rise in arterial blood pressure. Relatively slow recovery time. *Manufacturer*: Parke-Davis.

KETOVITE

Description: a multivitamin preparation available as yellow, sugar-free tablets containing 1mg thiamine hydrochloride, 0.5mg acetomenaphthone, 1mg riboflavine, 0.33mg pyridoxine hydrochloride, 3.3mg nicotinamide, 16.6mg ascorbic acid, 50mg inositol, 1.16mg calcium pantothenate, 0.25mg folic acid, 0.17mg biotin, 5mg tocopheryl acetate. Also **KETOVITE LIQUID**, a pink, sugar-free vitamin supplement, containing 150mg choline chloride, 12.5 micrograms cyanocobalamin, 400 units vitamin D, 2500 units vitamin A, all/5ml. *Used for*: dietary supplement for patients on synthetic diets due to disorders of amino acid or carbohydrate metabolism. *Dosage*: 1 tablet 3 times each day and 5ml of solution once daily. *Possible interaction*: levodopa. Manufacturer: Paines and Byrne.

KINIDIN DURULES

Description: a class I antiarrhythmic preparation available as white, sustained-release tablets containing 250mg quinidine bisulphate. *Used for*: disorders of heart rhythm including types of tachycardia, atrial fibrillation and extrasystoles. *Dosage*: adults, 1 tablet each day at first increasing to 2 to 5 daily. *Special care*: patients with tachycardia, hypotension, hypokalaemia, congestive heart failure. *Avoid use*: children, pregnancy, heart block, myasthenia gravis, inflammation or damage of heart muscle, uncompensated heart failure, toxic effects of digitalis. *Possible interaction*: digitalis, cimetidine, anticoagulants taken orally, vasodilators, non-depolarizing substances, antihypertensives. *Side effects*: hepatitis, allergic responses, cinchonism (a condition resulting from overdose of quinine and quinidine characterized by ringing in the ears, deafness, headache, brain congestion). *Manufacturer*: Astra.

KLARICID

Description: a macrolide antibiotic preparation, available in a variety of forms: oval, yellow, film-coated tablets containing 250mg clarithromycin marked with logo; **KLARICID PAEDIATRIC SUSPENSION** containing 125mg/5ml solution; **KLARICID INTRAVENOUS INJECTION** containing 500mg clarithromycin as powder in vials for reconstitution. *Used for*: infections of respiratory tract, middle ear, soft tissue and skin. *Dosage*: adults, and children over 12 years, tablets, 1 twice each day for 1 week; serious infections, 2 tablets daily for up to 2 weeks. Injection, 1g by intravenous infusion in 2 divided doses each day for 5 days. Children, use paediatric suspension under 1 year, 7.5mg/kg body weight, 1 to 2 years, 2.5ml; 3 to 6 years, 5ml; 7 to 9 years, 7.5ml; 10 to 12 years, 10ml. All twice each day in divided doses. *Special care*: pregnancy, breast-feeding, liver or kidney disease. *Possible interaction*: anticoagulants taken by mouth, carbamazepine, theophylline, terfenadine, digoxin. *Side effects*: gastro-intestinal upset, vomiting, diarrhoea, nausea, pain in abdomen, short-lived central nervous system effects, headache, skin rash, pain and skin reactions at injection site. *Manufacturer*: Abbott.

KONAKION

Description: a vitamin A derivative available as a solution in ampoules for injection containing 1mg phytomenadione/0.5ml, and as white, sugar-coated tablets containing 10mg phytomenadione. *Used for*: hypoprothrombinaemia (an abnormally low level of prothrombin clotting factor II in the blood, characterized by bleeding and loss of blood clotting ability). Also, haemorrhagic disease of the newborn (a bleeding disorder of newborn infants caused by vitamin K deficiency). *Dosage*: adults, 10–20mg by intramuscular or slow intravenous injection, or as tablets. The maximum dose is 40mg in 24 hours. Newborn babies, 1mg given intramuscularly; babies over 3 months, 5–10mg each day. *Side effects*: sweating, flushing, lack of oxygen in blood (cyanosis) causing bluish tinge to skin and mucous membranes. Symptoms of analphylaxis may occur with injection. *Manufacturer*: Roche.

KYTRIL

Description: an anti-emetic preparation which is a $5HT_3$-antagonist that acts to block vomiting and nausea reflexes which occur when $5HT_3$ receptors in the gut are stimulated. It is available as triangular, white, film-coated tablets containing 1mg granisetron as hydrochloride. Also, KYTRIL INJECTION available as a solution in ampoules containing 1mg/ml. *Used for*: prevention and treatment of vomiting and nausea caused by cytotoxic drug therapy. *Dosage*: 1 tablet 1 hour before chemotherapy begins followed by 1 every 12 hours. Injection, 3mg diluted in 20–50ml infusion fluid given over 5 minutes by intravenous route. Can be repeated if required at 10 minute intervals with a maximum dose of 9mg in 24 hours. *Special care*: pregnant women, patients with obstruction of intestine. *Avoid use*: children, breast-feeding. *Side effects*: constipation, headache, short-lived rise in level of liver enzymes. *Manufacturer*: Smith Kline Beecham.

L

LACTITOL

Description: an osmotic laxative, lactitol monohydrate (10g) as powder in a sachet. *Used for*: constipation, acute or chronic portal systemic encephalopathy, PSE (hepatic coma-toxic waste not neutralized in the liver, reaching the brain or substances required for brain function not synthesized in the liver). *Dosage*: 1 sachet mixed with food or drink morning or evening. For constipation, adults, 2 sachets reducing to 1 daily; children 1 to 6 years, quarter to half sachet; 6 to 12 years half to 1 sachet; 12 to 16 years, 1 to 2 sachets; all daily. Not for children under 12 months. For PSE, 0.5–0.7g/kg weight per day in 3 divided doses with meals. *Special care*: pregnancy. Maintain fluid intake and monitor electrolyte in long-term treatment of elderly or debilitated. *Avoid use*: obstruction of intestine, galactosaemia (accumulation of galactose in the blood in children who cannot utilize this sugar due to inborn lack of the appropriate enzyme). *Possible interaction*: antacids, neomycin for those with PSE. *Side effects*: flatulence, bloating, gastro-intestinal discomfort, chronic itching around the anus. *Manufacturer*: Zyma.

LAMICTAL

Description: a triazine, lamotrigine, available as yellow tablets of strength 25mg, 50mg and 100mg marked with name and strength. *Used for*: anticonvulsant. *Dosage*: 50mg daily for 2 weeks, then 50mg twice daily for 2 weeks increasing to maintenance dose of 200–400mg daily in 2 divided doses. If sodium valproate is being taken, 25mg on alternate days for 2 weeks then 25mg daily for 2 weeks up to a maintenance dose of 100–200mg daily in 1 or 2 doses. Not recommended for children or the elderly. *Special care*: pregnancy, lactation. Monitor liver, kidney and clotting in patients developing fever, flu, rash, drowsiness or deterioration of seizure control. Withdraw gradually over 2 weeks. *Avoid use*: liver or kidney disease. *Possible interaction*: sodium valproate, primidone, phenobarbitone, phenytoin, carbamazepine. *Side effects*: dizziness, blurred vision, headache, drowsiness, gastro-intestinal upsets, rash, Stevens-Johnson syndrome, angioneurotic oedema. *Manufacturer*: Glaxo Wellcome.

LAMISIL

Description: an allylamine antifungal, terbinafine hydrochloride, as white 250mg tablets marked LAMISIL. *Used for*: fungal infections of skin and nails. *Dosage*: 1 daily for 2 to 6 weeks (athlete's foot); groin infection, 2 to 4 weeks; body infection 4 weeks and 6 to 12 weeks for nail infections. Not for children. Also

LAMISIL CREAM, a 1% cream. *Used for*: fungal and yeast infections of the skin. *Dosage*: apply to infected area 1 or 2 times per day for 1 to 2 weeks. Not for children. *Special care*: pregnancy, lactation, chronic liver disorder, impaired kidney function. *Possible interaction*: any drug affecting liver enzymes. *Side effects*: headache, myalgia, arthralgia, allergic skin reaction, gastro-intestinal upset. *Manufacturer*: Sandoz.

LAMPRENE

Description: a phenazine, clofazimine, available as 100mg strength in brown gelatin capsules marked GEIGY AND GM. *Used for*: leprosy. *Dosage*: as advised, but often as part of a 3-drug treatment when 300mg once a month given by the physician and 50mg daily, self-administered. Treatment may be prolonged (over 2 years). *Special care*: pregnancy, lactation, diarrhoea, abdominal pain, liver or kidney disease. *Side effects*: dry skin, pruritis, discolouration of hair, skin and secretions, gastro-intestinal upsets. Dosage can be reduced accordingly. *Manufacturer*: Geigy.

LANOXIN

Description: a cardiac glycoside, digoxin, available as 250 g white tablet marked WELLCOME Y3B. Also **LANOXIN-PF**, 62.5 g blue tablet marked WELLCOME USA, **LANOXIN-PG ELIXIR**, 50 g/ml and **LANOXIN INJECTION**, 250 g/ml digoxin in 2ml ampoules. *Used for*: digitalis treatment, especially congestive heart failure. *Dosage*: maintenance dose: adults, 125–750 g daily; elderly, 62.5–250 g daily; for children, see literature. *Special care*: acute myocardial infarction, atrio-ventricular block, thyroid disorder, severe lung disease, kidney impairment. *Avoid use*: hypercalcaemia, ventricular tachycardia, hypertrophic obstructive cardiomyopathy. *Possible interaction*: calcium tablets or injections, cardiac glycosides, potassium-depleting agents, lithium, quinidine, antacids, antibiotics. *Side effects*: changes in heart rhythm, gastro intestinal upsets, visual disturbances. *Manufacturer*: Glaxo Wellcome.

LANVIS

Description: a cytotoxic preparation of thioguanine available as 40mg yellow tablets marked WELLCOME U3B. *Used for*: treatment of acute leukaemias. *Dosage*: 2–2.5mg/kg daily at the outset. *Special care*: interference with production of red blood cells in the bone marrow, causing some loss of immunity to infection. Monitor blood regularly. *Side effects*: nausea, vomiting, gastro-intestinal upsets, hair loss. *Manufacturer*: Glaxo Wellcome.

LARGACTIL

Description: a group I phenothiazine, chlorpromazine hydrochloride available in 10, 25, 50 and 100mg white tablets marked with LG and strength. Also, **LARGACTIL SYRUP** (25mg/5ml), **LARGACTIL FORTE SUSPENSION**, chlorpromazine carbonate equivalent to 100mg chlorpromazine hydrochloride per 5ml and **LARGACTIL INJECTION**, 25mg/ml chlorpromazine hydrochloride in 2ml ampoules. *Used for*: disturbances of the CNS that require sedation, schizophrenia, nausea and vomiting (of terminal illness), induction of hypothermia, mood disorders. *Dosage*: 25mg 3 times per day, increasing by 25mg per day. Maintenance dose 75–300mg daily. See literature for children. Injection: 25–50mg by deep intramuscular injection in a single dose. Can be repeated after 6 to 8 hours; to be followed by oral therapy as soon as possible. *Special care*: pregnancy, lactation. Children: use in severe cases only. *Avoid use*: heart failure, epilepsy, Parkinsonism, liver or kidney disorder, hypothyroidism, elderly, glaucoma, enlarged prostate, unconscious patients, depression of bone marrow function. *Possible interaction*: depressants of the CNS, alcohol, antidepressants, anticonvulsants, antidiabetics, levodopa, analgesics, antihypertensives. *Side effects*: muscle spasms (eye, neck, back, face), restlessness, rigidity and tremor, tardive dyskinesia (repetitious muscular movements), dry mouth, blocked nose, difficulty in passing urine, tachycardia, blurred vision, hypotension, constipation, weight gain, impotence, galactorrhoea, gynaecomastia, amenorrhoea, blood and skin changes, lethargy, fatigue, ECG irregularities. *Manufacturer*: Rhône-Poulenc Rorer.

LARIAM

Description: a 4-aminoquinolone, mefloquine hydrochloride, as 250mg white tablets. *Used for*: treatment and prevention of malaria. *Dosage*: prevention: 1 tablet weekly; children, 15–19kg quarter tablet; 20–30kg, half tablet; 31–45kg three-quarters tablet. Not recommended under 15kg. For visits up to 3 weeks, dose to be taken weekly on the same day for a minimum of 6 weeks starting 1 week before departure and continuing for 4 weeks after return. For stays over 3 weeks, weekly dose on the same day during the stay starting 1 week before and continuing for 4 weeks after return. Do not use for more than 3 months. For treatment dosages, see literature. *Special care*: patients with heart conduction disorders. Women must use reliable contraception during and for 3 months after the stay. *Avoid use*: liver or kidney damage, pregnancy, lactation, history of convulsions or psychiatric disorders. *Possible interaction*: sodium valproate; typhoid vaccination, delay use for at least 12 hours after quinine. *Side effects*: in treatment: dizziness, nausea, vomiting, appetite loss, gastro-intestinal upset. *Manufacturer*: Roche.

LARODOPA

Description: the dopamine precursor, levodopa, as 500mg white tablets marked ROCHE in a hexagon. *Used for*: Parkinsonism. *Dosage*: over 25 years, 125mg twice daily after food increasing after 1 week to 125mg 4 to 5 times per day and further at weekly intervals by 375mg daily, the total in 4 or 5 divided doses. Maintenance dose of 2.5–8g. Not recommended for anyone under 25. *Special care*: cardiovascular, liver, kidney, lung or endocrine disease, glaucoma, pregnancy, peptic ulcer. Monitor blood, and liver, kidney and cardiovascular function. *Avoid use*: glaucoma, severe psychoses, history of malignant melanoma. *Possible interaction*: MAOIs, antihypertensives, sympathomimetics, pyridoxine, ferrous sulphate. *Side effects*: anorexia, nausea, vomiting, involuntary movements, heart and CNS disturbances, urine discolouration, low blood pressure when standing up. *Manufacturer*: Cambridge.

LASIKAL

Description: a loop diuretic and potassium supplement comprising 20mg frusemide and 750mg potassium chloride in a sustained release matrix, forming a white/yellow two-layered tablet marked LK. *Used for*: oedema with the need of a potassium supplement. *Dosage*: 2 daily as 1 morning dose increasing to 4 if necessary (in 2 divided doses) or reducing to 1 daily. *Special care*: diabetes, enlarged prostate or impaired urination, liver or kidney disease, pregnancy, lactation, gout. *Avoid use*: Addison's disease, hyperkalaemia, cirrhosis of the liver. *Possible interaction*: digitalis, lithium, NSAIDs, aminoglycosides, antihypertensives, cephalosporins, potassium-sparing diuretics. *Side effects*: rash, gout, gastro-intestinal upset. Discontinue if ulceration or obstruction of small bowel occurs. *Manufacturer*: Hoechst.

LASILACTONE

Description: a loop and potassium-sparing diuretic consisting of 20mg frusemide and 50mg spironolactone in a blue/white capsule. *Used for*: oedema that has not responded to other therapy, hypertension of certain types. *Dosage*: 1 to 4 daily, not recommended for children. *Special care*: liver or kidney disease, impaired urination, enlarged prostate, diabetes, pregnancy, lactation, gout. Not to be used long-term for young patients. *Avoid use*: kidney failure, liver cirrhosis, hyperkalaemia, Addison's disease. *Possible interaction*: potassium supplements, potassium-sparing diuretics, antihypertensives, lithium, digitalis, ACE inhibitors, NSAIDs, cephalosporins, aminoglycosides. *Side effects*: rash, gout, blood changes, gynaecomastia, gastro-intestinal upsets. *Manufacturer*: Hoechst.

LASIX

Description: a loop diuretic, frusemide, available as 20mg white tablets marked DLF and 40mg white tablets marked DLI, both also marked with manufacturer's symbol. *Used for*: oedema, mild to moderate hypertension. *Dosage*: 20–80mg in 1 dose daily or every other day. Children 1–3mg/kg per day. Also **LASIX 500**, 500mg frusemide in yellow tablet form marked with the manufacturer's symbol and DIX on the reverse. *Used for*: acute or chronic kidney insufficiency (used under hospital supervision). *Dosage*: see literature. Also **LASIX PAEDIATRIC LIQUID**, 1mg/ml frusemide. *Dosage*: 1–3mg/kg daily. Also, **LASIX INJECTION**, 10mg/ml frusemide in 2, 5 and 25ml ampoules. *Dosage*: 20–50mg intramuscularly or slow intravenous injection. Children, 0.5–1.5mg/kg daily. *Special care*: gout, diabetes, enlarged prostate, liver or kidney disease, impaired urination, pregnancy, lactation. Potassium supplements may be necessary. *Avoid* *use*: liver cirrhosis. *Possible interaction*: NSAIDs, antihypertensives, cephalo-sporins, aminoglycosides, lithium, digitalis. *Side effects*: gout, rash, gastro-intestinal upset. *Manufacturer*: Hoechst.

LASIX + K

Description: A loop diuretic and potassium supplement, frusemide, available in 40mg white tablets marked with the manufacturer's symbol and DLI on the reverse; and 750mg potassium chloride as pale yellow sustained-release tablets. *Used for*: diuretic therapy where potassium is required. *Dosage*: 1 frusemide tablet in the morning, and 1 potassium chloride tablet at midday and in the evening. Not for children. *Special care*: liver or kidney disease, diabetes, gout, enlarged prostrate (prostatic hypertrophy) or impaired urination, pregnancy, lactation. *Avoid use*: liver cirrhosis, Addison's disease, hyperkalaemia. *Possible interaction*: NSAIDs, cephalosporins, antihypertensives, digitalis, lithium, aminoglycosides, potassium-sparing diuretics. *Side effects*: rash, gout, gastro-intestinal upset. Discontinue if ulceration or obstruction of small bowel occurs. *Manufacturer*: Hoechst.

LASORIDE

Description: a loop and potassium-sparing diuretic comprising 40mg frusemide and 5mg amiloride hydrochloride in yellow tablets. *Used for*: rapid diuretic treatment and conservation of potassium. *Dosage*: 1 to 2 tablets in the morning, adjust for elderly. Not for children. *Special care*: enlarged prostate, impaired urination, diabetes, gout, pregnancy, lactation, elderly. Electrolyte and fluid levels should be checked regularly. *Avoid use*: liver cirrhosis, kidney failure, Addison's disease, hyperkalaemia, electrolyte imbalance. *Possible interaction*: NSAIDs, digitalis, antidiabetic drugs, antihypertensives, lithium, ototoxic or nephrotoxic antibiotics, potassium supplements, potassium-sparing diuretics, certain muscle relaxants. *Side effects*: gastro-intestinal upset, itching, blood changes, malaise, reduced alertness, calcium loss. Occasionally minor mental disturbances, pancreatitis, altered liver function. *Manufacturer*: Hoechst.

LEDCLAIR

Description: a chelating agent, sodium calcium edetate as 200mg/ml in 5ml ampoules. *Used for*: treatment of poisoning with lead and other heavy metals. *Dosage*: up to 40mg/kg twice daily by intravenous drip or intramuscular injection for adults and children. To diagnose poisoning, 25mg/kg intramuscularly 3 times per day. See literature in both cases. *Special care*: impaired kidney function. *Side effects*: nausea, cramp, kidney damage on overdosage. *Manufacturer*: Sinclair.

LEDERCORT

Description: a glucocorticoid, triamcinolone, in strengths of 2mg (blue, oblong tablet marked LL11) and 4mg (white, oblong tablet marked LL 9352). *Used for*: rheumatoid arthritis, allergies. *Dosage*: 2–24mg daily but see literature. *Special care*: thrombophlebitis, psychoses, recent intestinal anastomoses, chronic nephritis, certain cancers, osteoporosis, peptic ulcer, skin eruption/rash related to a disease, viral, fungal or active infections, tuberculosis. Hypertension, glaucoma, epilepsy, acute glomerulonephritis (inflammation of kidney glomerulus), diabetes, cirrhosis, hypothyroidism, pregnancy, stress. To be withdrawn gradually. *Possible interaction*: NSAIDs, oral anticoagulants, phenytoin, ephedrine, phenobarbitone, rifampicin, diuretics, cardiac glycosides, anticholinesterases, hypoglycaemics. *Side effects*: osteoporosis, depression, euphoria, hyperglycaemia, peptic ulcers, Cushingoid changes. Also available as triamcinolone acetonide, 0.1% cream. *Used for*: inflamed skin disorders. *Dosage*: use sparingly 3 or 4 times per day. *Special care*: maximum 5 days use on face or for children. Withdraw gradually. *Avoid use*: acne, scabies, leg ulcers, peri-oral dermatitis; tuberculous, viral skin or ringworm infections, untreated bacterial or fungal infections. Do not use extensively or for a prolonged period in pregnancy. *Side effects*: skin striae and atrophy, Cushingoid changes (see Cushing's syndrome), adrenal gland suppression, telangiectasia (collections of distended blood capillaries). *Manufacturer*: Lederle.

LEDERFEN

Description: propionic acid as fenbufen in light blue tablet marked LEDERFEN (300mg), and light blue oblong tablet marked LEDERFEN 450 (450mg). Also, **LEDERFEN CAPSULES**, 300mg fenbufen in dark blue capsules marked LEDERFEN. *Used for*: osteoarthritis, rheumatoid arthritis, ankylosing spondylitis and acute muscle/bone disorders. *Dosage*: 300mg in the morning with 600mg at night, or 450mg twice daily. Not for children. Also **LEDERFEN F**, fenbufen as white effervescent tablets (450mg). *Dosage*: 1 dissolved in water, twice per day. Not for children. *Special care*: heart failure, kidney or liver disease, pregnancy, lactation, elderly. Monitor those on long-term treatment. *Avoid use*: active peptic ulcers or history of gastro-intestinal lesions, allergy induced by aspirin or anti-inflammatory drug. *Possible interaction*: anticoagulants, salicylates, quinolones. *Side effects*: gastro-intestinal intolerance, rash. *Manufacturer*: Wyeth.

LEDERFOLIN

Description: folinic acid (as calcium folinate), 350mg strength, powder in a vial. Also, LEDERFOLIN SOLUTION as 10mg/ml in a 35ml ampoule. *Used for*: alongside 5-fluorouracil in treatment of advanced colorectal cancer. *Dosage*: see literature. *Special care*: toxicity of 5-fluorouracil increased. *Manufacturer*: Wyethe.

LEDERMYCIN

Description: a tetracycline, demeclocycline hydrochloride available as dark red/light red capsules marked LEDERLE 9123 (150mg strength). *Used for*: respiratory and soft tissue infections. *Dosage*: 300mg twice per day or150mg 4 times. Not for children. *Special care*: liver and kidney disease. *Avoid use*: pregnancy, lactation. *Possible interaction*: milk, mineral supplements, antacids, oral contraceptives. *Side effects*: sensitivity to light, gastro-intestinal upset, further infections. *Manufacturer*: Wyeth.

LEDERSPAN 20mg

Description: a glucocorticoid, triamcinolone hexacetonide in vials, 20mg/ml. *Used for*: local inflammation of joints and soft tissues in arthritis, tendinitis and bursitis (inflammation of the connective tissue surrounding a joint). *Dosage*: 2–30mg depending upon condition and size of joint or synovial space at 3 to 4 weekly intervals. Also LEDERSPAN 5mg *Description*: triamcinolone hexacetonide in a vial (5mg/ml). *Used for*: skin conditions. *Dosage*: 0.5mg (or less) per square inch of affected skin. *Special care*: thrombophlebitis, psychoses, recent intestinal anastomoses, chronic nephritis, certain cancers, osteoporosis, peptic ulcer, skin eruption/rash related to a disease, viral, fungal or active infections, tuberculosis. Hypertension, glaucoma, epilepsy, acute glomerulonephritis (inflammation of kidney glomerulus), diabetes, cirrhosis, hypothyroidism, pregnancy, stress. To be withdrawn gradually. *Possible interaction*: NSAIDs, oral anticoagulants, phenytoin, ephedrine, phenobarbitone, rifampicin, diuretics, cardiac glycosides, anticholinesterases, hypoglycaemics. *Side effects*: osteoporosis, depression, euphoria, hyperglycaemia, peptic ulcers, Cushingoid changes. *Manufacturer*: Wyeth.

LENTARON

Description: an aromatase inhibitor, formestane, available as a powder (250mg strength) in a vial with 2ml diluent. *Used for*: advanced stages of breast cancer occurring after the menopause. *Dosage*: 250mg intramuscularly every 2 weeks in gluteal muscle (buttock). Site of injection alternated. *Special care*: avoid making injection into vein or sciatic nerve. *Avoid use*: pregnancy, lactation, pre-menopausal women. *Side effects*: pain and irritation at site of injection, vaginal bleeding or irritation, hot flushes, arthralgia, pelvic or muscular cramps, oedema, thrombophlebitis, sore throat, upset in the CNS or gastro-intestinal tract. *Manufacturer*: Ciba.

LENTIZOL

Description: a tricyclic antidepressant, amitriptyline hydrochloride available as sustained-release pink capsules (25mg) or pink/red capsules (50mg) both with white pellets and marked with LENTIZOL and the capsule strength. *Used for*: treatment of depression when sedation is required. *Dosage*: 50–100mg at night, up to a maximum of 200mg per day. Elderly, 25–75mg daily. Not for children. *Special care*: liver disorders, hyperthyroidism, glaucoma, lactation, epilepsy, diabetes, adrenal tumour, heart disease, urine retention. Psychotic or suicidal patients. *Avoid use*: heart block, heart attacks, severe liver disease, pregnancy.

Possible interaction: MAOIs (or within 14 days of their use), alcohol, anti-depressants, barbiturates, anticholinergics, local anaesthetics that contain adrenaline or noradrenaline, oestrogens, cimetidine, antihypertensives. *Side effects*: constipation, urine retention, dry mouth, blurred vision, palpitations, tachycardia, nervousness, drowsiness, insomnia. Changes in weight, blood and blood sugar, jaundice, skin reactions, weakness, ataxia, hypotension, sweating, altered libido, gynaecomastia, galactorrhoea. *Manufacturer*: Parke-Davis.

LESCOL

Description: a suppressant of cholesterol production and sodium salt of fluvastatin available as red-brown/pale yellow (20mg strength) or red-brown/orange-yellow (40mg strength) capsules, marked with XU, the strength and the company logo. *Used for*: hypercholesterolaemia (high blood cholesterol levels) for patients where levels cannot be controlled by diet. *Dosage*: over 18 years, 20–40mg once per day in the evening. Adjust to response, monitor lipid levels. Not for children. *Special care*: history of liver disease, or high alcohol intake (test liver function), myalgias or muscle weakness particularly with fever or if generally unwell. Any condition predisposing to rhabdomyolysis. *Avoid use*: kidney or liver disease, pregnancy, lactation. *Possible interaction*: immunosuppressive drugs, rifampicin, erythromycin, nicotinic acid, gemfibrozil. *Side effects*: flatulence, abdominal pain, sinusitis, insomnia, nausea, dyspepsia, hypoaesthesia (some loss of sense of touch), infection of the urinary tract, disorders of the teeth. *Manufacturer*: Sandoz.

LEUCOMAX

Description: a recombinant human granulocyte macrophage-colony stimulating factor (GM-CSF) available as molgramostim in the form of powder in vials. There are 3 strengths: 150, 300 and 700 g (equivalent to 1.67, 3.33 and 7.77 million-unit). *Used for*: reduction in neutropenia and therefore risk of infection associated with cytotoxic chemotherapy, speeding up bone marrow recovery after transplantation of same, neutropenia in patients on gamciclovir in AIDS-related cytomegalovirus retinitis. *Dosage*: chemotherapy, 60,000–110,000 units/kg/day (by subcutaneous injection) for 7 to 10 days commencing 24 hours after last chemotherapy; bone marrow transplantation, 110,000 units/kg/day (by intravenous infusion) commencing 24 hours after transplantation and until white cell count is at required level (maximum 30 days treatment); in ganciclovir treatment, 60,000 units/kg/day by subcutaneous injection for 5 days, then adjust to response. *Special care*: full blood monitoring necessary, monitor those with lung disease, pregnancy and lactation, history of autoimmune disease. Not recommended for those under 18 years. *Avoid use*: bone marrow cancer. *Side effects*: anorexia, nausea, vomiting, diarrhoea, shortness of breath, weakness, rash, rigors, fever, muscle and bone pains, local reaction at site of injection. Anaphylaxis, cardiac failure, convulsions, hypotension, heartbeat abnormalities, pericarditis, pulmonary oedema. *Manufacturer*: Sandoz/Schering Plough.

LEUKERAN

Description: an alkylating agent and cytotoxic drug, chlorambucil, available as yellow tablets (2 and 5mg strengths), marked WELLCOME C2A and H2A respectively. *Used for*: ovarian cancer, Hodgkin's disease, chronic lymphocytic leukaemia. *Dosage*: 100–200 g/kg daily for 4 to 8 weeks, but see literature. *Special care*: kidney disease. *Avoid use*: porphyria. *Side effects*: bone marrow suppression, rashes. *Manufacturer*: Glaxo Wellcome.

LEVOPHED

Description: a vasoconstrictor and sympathomimetic amine, noradrenaline (as the acid tartrate) as 1mg/ml, in ampoules for dilution. Also, LEVOPHED SPECIAL, 0.1mg/ml. *Used for*: cardiac arrest, acute hypotension. *Dosage*: intravenous infusion of 8µg/ml at a rate of 2.3ml/minute initially, adjusted to the response. By intracardiac or rapid intravenous injection, 0.5–0.75ml of a solution with 200µg/ml . *Special care*: extravasation at site of injection (escape of fluid, e.g. blood into tissues) may cause localized necrosis. *Avoid use:* pregnancy, myocardial infarction. *Possible interaction*: anaesthetics, tricyclics, ß-blockers, dopexamine. *Side effects*: headache, uneven heartbeat. *Manufacturer*: Sanofi Winthrop.

LEXOTAN

Description: an anxiolytic benzodiazepine for intermediate-acting use, bromazepam, available as lilac and pink tablets (1.5mg and 3mg strengths respectively) marked with L and the strength. *Used for*: short-term treatment of severe or disabling anxiety, with or without insomnia. *Dosage*: 3–18mg per day (elderly, 1.5–9mg) in divided doses. Not for children. *Special care*: chronic kidney or liver disease or lung insufficiency, pregnancy, labour, lactation, elderly. May impair judgement. Avoid long-term use and withdraw gradually. *Avoid use*: acute lung disorders, depression of respiration, phobias, chronic psychosis. *Possible interaction*: anticonvulsants, alcohol, depressants of the CNS. *Side effects*: gastro-intestinal upset, vertigo, ataxia, confusion, drowsiness, lightheadedness, hypotension, skin reactions and visual changes, urine retention, changes in libido. Dependence a risk with high doses and long treatment. *Manufacturer*: Roche.

LEXPEC

Description: a haematinic (haemoglobin-increasing drug), folic acid, available as a syrup containing 2.5mg/5ml. *Used for*: megaloblasic anaemia caused by a deficiency of folic acid. *Dosage*: 20–40 ml per day for 14 days, then 5–20ml per day. Children, 10–30ml per day. Also, **LEXPEC WITH IRON**, a combination of folic acid (2.5mg) with ferric ammonium citrate (400mg)/5ml of syrup; and **LEXPEC WITH IRON-M**, 0.5mg folic acid and 400mg of ferric ammonium citrate/5ml of syrup. *Used for*: anaemia during pregnancy caused by iron and folic acid deficiency. *Dosage*: 5–10ml per day before food for the pregnancy and

1 month after. *Avoid use*: megaloblastic anaemia due to vitamin B_{12} deficiency. *Possible interaction*: tetracyclines. *Side effects*: nausea, constipation, discolouration of teeth (syrup should be drunk through a straw). *Manufacturer*: Rosemont.

LI-LIQUID

Description: Lithium salt (the citrate) available as a sugar-free liquid in concentrations of 5.4mmol and 10.8mmol/5ml. *Used for*: mania, hypomania (excitable, hyperactive and irritable), self-mutilation, extreme mood changes. *Dosage*: 10.8–32.4mmol per day initially in 2 divided doses. Lithium levels in serum to be maintained, see literature. *Special care*: start treatment in hospital and maintain salt and fluid levels. Record kidney, heart and thyroid functions. *Avoid use*: Addison's disease, pregnancy, lactation, hypothyroidism, kidney or heart insufficiency, sodium imbalance. *Possible interaction*: NSAIDs, phenytoin, diuretics, carbamazepine, diazepam, flupenthixol, methyldopa, haloperidol, tetracyclines, metoclopramide. *Side effects*: hand tremor, weak muscles, diarrhoea, nausea, oedema, weight gain, disturbances to CNS and in ECG, skin changes, polyuria, polydipsia, hypo- or hyperthyroidism. *Manufacturer*: Rosemont.

LIBRIUM

Description: a long-acting benzodiazepine, chlordiazepoxide, available in 3 strengths: 5mg (yellow-green tablets), 10mg (light blue-green) and 25mg (dark blue-green), all marked with LIB and the strength. Also, LIBRIUM CAPSULES, as green-yellow (5mg) and green/black (10mg) capsules marked with LIB and the strength. *Used for*: treatment of severe anxiety over the short-term, with or without insomnia, symptoms of acute alcohol withdrawal. *Dosage*: 30mg per day initially to a maximum of 100mg. For insomnia, 10–30mg at bedtime. For alcohol withdrawal, 25–100mg repeated in 2 to 4 hours if necessary. Elderly, 5mg per day to begin with. Not for children. *Special care*: chronic kidney or liver disease or lung insufficiency, pregnancy, labour, lactation, the elderly. May impair judgement. Avoid long-term use and withdraw gradually. *Avoid use*: acute lung disorders, depression of respiration, phobias, chronic psychosis. *Possible interaction*: anticonvulsants, alcohol, depressants of the CNS. *Side effects*: gastro-intestinal upset, vertigo, ataxia, confusion, drowsiness, light-headedness, hypotension, skin reactions and visual changes, urine retention, changes in libido. Dependence a risk with high doses and long treatment. *Manufacturer*: Roche.

LIMCLAIR

Description: a chelating agent, trisodium edetate, available in ampoules (strength 200mg/ml). *Used for*: parathyroidism, digitalis arrhythmia, hypercalcaemia, corneal opacities. *Dosage*: up to 70mg/kg daily by slow intravenous infusion, but see literature. For children, up to 60mg/kg daily by same means. *Special care*: tuberculosis. *Avoid use*: kidney disease. *Manufacturer*: Sinclair.

LINGRAINE

Description: an ergot-derived alkaloid ergotamine tartrate available as green tablets, strength 2mg. *Used for*: migraine and headache. *Dosage*: 1 under the tongue at the start of the attack, repeat 30–60 minutes later if required; maximum 3 in 24 hours and 6 in 1 week. Not for children. *Avoid use*: liver or kidney disease, severe hypertension, sepsis; coronary, peripheral or occlusive vascular disease; pregnancy, lactation, porphyria, hyperthyroidism. *Possible interaction*: ß-blockers, erythromycin. *Side effects*: leg cramps, stomach pain, nausea. *Manufacturer*: Sanofi Winthrop.

LIORESAL

Description: a gamma-amino-butyric acid (GABA) derivative, baclofen, available as a white tablet (strength 10mg), marked CG and KJ. Also LIORESAL LIQUID, a sugar-free liquid containing 5mg/5ml. *Used for*: muscle relaxant, for cerebral palsy, meningitis, spasticity of voluntary muscle due to cerebrovascular accidents, multiple sclerosis, spinal lesions. *Dosage*: 5mg 3 times per day to begin with, increasing by 5mg 3 times per day at intervals of 3 days. Maximum 100mg per day. For children, see the literature. *Special care*: epilepsy, pregnancy, cerebrovascular accidents, the elderly, psychosis, hypertonic (abnormally increased tone or strength) bladder sphincter, liver or kidney disorders, defective respiration. Withdraw gradually. *Avoid use*: peptic ulcer. *Possible interactions*: lithium, antihypertensives, tricyclic antidepressants, depressants of the CNS, alcohol, fentanyl, levodopa, carbidopa, ibuprofen. *Side effects*: sedation and drowsiness, nausea, disturbances of the central nervous system, muscle fatigue, hypotension, disturbance of the heart, lung or circulatory system, frequent and painful urination (dysuria). *Manufacturer*: Ciba.

LIPANTIL

Description: an isobutyric acid derivative, fenofibrate, for lowering of lipids. Available as a white capsule, 100mg strength. *Used for*: certain types of hyperlipidaemia (high levels of fat in the blood) resistant to the influence of diet. *Dosage*: 3 tablets per day initially, in divided doses with food. 2 to 4 tablets per day for maintenance. For children, 5mg/kg body weight/day. *Special care*: in cases of kidney impairment. *Avoid use*: severe liver or kidney disorder, pregnancy, lactation, disease of the gall bladder. *Possible interaction*: oral hypoglycaemics, anticoagulants, phenylbutazone. *Side effects*: headache, tiredness, vertigo, gastro-intestinal upsets, rashes. *Manufacturer*: Fournier.

LIPOSTAT

Description: a preparation of pravastratin (as the sodium salt) available as pink oblong tablets in 10 and 20mg strengths, marked with the company name and 154 or 178. *Used for*: hypercholesterolaemia (high levels of blood cholesterol) which does not respond to other treatments (levels above 7.8mmol/l of cholesterol). *Dosage*: 10mg at night to begin with, adjusting to the response at intervals of 4 weeks. Usually 10–40mg as 1 dose, daily, at night. Not for children. *Special care*: history of liver disease. Liver function tests to be undertaken during treatment. *Avoid use*: pregnancy, lactation, liver disease. *Possible interaction*: gemfibrozil and similar derivatives of isobutyric acid, to be taken 1 hour before or 4 hours after colestipolor cholestyramine. *Side effects*: muscle pain, headache, rashes, nausea, vomiting, tiredness, diarrhoea, chest pains not related to the heart. *Manufacturer*: Squibb.

LISKONUM

Description: a sedative, available as white, oblong, controlled-release tablets containing 450mg lithium carbonate (equivalent to 12.2mmol of lithium ions, Li⁺). *Used for*: acute mania, hypomania, prevention of the recurrence of manic depression. *Dosage*: blood lithium levels to be kept in the range 0.8–1.5mmol/l (for mania or hypomania) and 0.5–1.0mmol/l for prevention. Not for children. *Special care*: commence treatment in hospital, salt and fluid intake to be kept up. Thyroid and kidney functions to be checked. Any symptoms of intoxication should be reported. *Avoid use*: pregnancy, lactation, Addison's disease, kidney or heart disease, hypothyroidism, sodium imbalance. *Possible interaction*: NSAIDs, diuretics, flupenthixol, fluoxetine, methyldopa, carbamazepine, fluvoxamine, haloperidol, phenytoin, metoclopramide. *Side effects*: muscle weakness, hand tremor, diarrhoea, nausea, disturbances to heart and brain, oedema, weight gain, hypo- or hyperthyroidism, intense thirst, frequent urination, changes in kidney, skin reactions. *Manufacturer*: Smith, Kline & French.

LITAREX

Description: a white, oval, controlled-release tablet containing 564mg lithium citrate (equivalent to 6mmol of lithium ions, Li⁺). *Used for*: acute mania, prevention of recurrence of emotional disorders. *Dosage*: 1 morning and evening to begin with. Blood lithium level should then be kept in the range 0.8–1.0mmol/l. *Special care*: commence treatment in hospital, salt and fluid intake to be kept up. Thyroid and kidney functions should be checked. Any symptoms of intoxication should be reported. *Avoid use*: pregnancy, lactation, Addison's disease, kidney or cardiovascular disease, the elderly, hypothyroidism, conditions altering sodium balance. *Possible interaction*: NSAIDs, diuretics, flupenthixol, methyldopa, carbamazepine, haloperidol, phenytoin, antidepressants, metoclopramide. *Side effects*: muscle weakness, diarrhoea, nausea, hand tremor, heart and brain disturbances, oedema, weight gain, hypo- or hyperthyroidism, intense thirst, frequent urination, skin reactions. *Manufacturer*: Dumex.

LIVIAL

Description: a white tablet containing 2.5mg tibolone (a gonadomimetic), marked MK2, ORGANON and *. *Used for*: vasomotor symptoms (affecting blood vessel constriction or dilatation) associated with menopause. *Dosage*: a tablet daily for a minimum of 3 months. *Special care*: kidney disorder or history of same, migraine, diabetes, epilepsy, high blood cholesterol levels. Menstrual bleeding may occur irregularly if started within 1 year of last period. Treatment to be stopped if liver disorder, cholestatic jaundice or thromboembolic disorders occur. *Avoid use*: undiagnosed vaginal bleeding, hormone-dependent tumours, pregnancy, lactation, severe liver disease, cardio- or cerebrovascular disorder. *Possible interaction*: carbamazepine, phenytoin, anticoagulants, rifampicin. *Side effects*: headache, dizziness, vaginal bleeding, bodyweight changes, seborrhoeic dermatitis (eczema associated with oil-sebum-secreting glands), abnormal liver function, gastro-intestinal upset, hair growth, oedema in front of the tibia. *Manufacturer*: Organon.

LOBAK

Description: a muscle relaxant and analgesic, comprising 100mg chlormezanone and 450mg paracetamol available as white tablets marked LOBAK. *Used for*: relief of painful muscle spasms. *Dosage*: 1 or 2 three times per day, up to a maximum of 8. Half dose for the elderly not recommended for children. *Special care*: pregnancy, lactation, kidney or liver disease. *Avoid use*: porphyria. *Possible interaction*: MAOIs, depressants of the central nervous system, alcohol. *Side effects*: dizziness, drowsiness, reduced alertness, dry mouth, rash, jaundice. *Manufacturer*: Sanofi Winthrop.

LOCABIOTAL

Description: an antibiotic and anti-inflammatory, fusafungine available as a metered dose aerosol (125 g per dose). *Used for*: inflammation and infection of the upper respiratory tract. *Dosage*: 5 oral sprays or 3 sprays in each nostril, 5 times per day. Children: over 12 years, 4 oral sprays 3 times per day or 3 sprays in each nostril 5 times per day; 6 to 12 years, 3 oral sprays 3 times per day or 2 sprays in each nostril 5 times per day; 3 to 5 years, 2 oral sprays 3 times per day or 1 spray in each nostril 5 times per day. Not recommended for children under 3 years. *Manufacturer*: Servier.

LOCERYL

Description: an antifungal cream, containing 0.25% amorolfine hydrochloride. *Used for*: microscopic fungal or ringworm skin infestation. *Dosage*: apply daily in the evening, usually for 2 to 3 weeks. Continue for 3 to 5 days after cure. Not for children. Also, **LOCERYL LACQUER**, 5% amorolfine hydrochloride as a lacquer. *Used for*: microscopic fungal, yeast and mould nail infestation. *Dosage*: apply once or twice per week; review every 3 months. Not for children. *Special care*: do not allow to come into contact with eyes, ears or mucous membranes. *Avoid use*: pregnancy, lactation. *Side effects*: sometimes pruritus (itching), temporary burning sensation. *Manufacturer*: Roche.

LOCOID

Description: a strong steroid, hydrocortisone 17-butyrate, as a 0.1% cream and ointment. *Used for*: eczema, psoriasis, skin disorders. *Dosage*: apply 2 or 3 times per day. Also, **LOCOID LIPOCREAM**, 0.1% hydrocortisone 17-butyrate in a base containing 70% oil. *Used for*: skin disorders. *Dosage*: apply 2 or 3 times per day. Also **LOCOID SCALP LOTION**, 0.1% hydrocortisone 17-butyrate in an alcoholic solution. *Used for*: seborrhoea of the scalp. *Dosage*: apply twice daily. Also, **LOCOID C**, a strong steroid 0.1% hydrocortisone 17-butyrate with an antifungal and antibacterial, 3% chlorquinaldol, available as cream and ointment. *Used for*: eczema, psoriasis, and skin disorders when there is also infection. *Dosage*: apply 2 to 4 times per day. *Special care*: maximum 5 days use on face, withdraw gradually after prolonged use. *Avoid use*: acne, dermatitis around the mouth, leg ulcers, scabies, viral skin disease, ringworm or tubercular infection, untreated infections caused by fungi or bacteria. Avoid prolonged or extensive use during pregnancy. Children. *Side effects*: suppression of adrenal glands, skin striae and atrophy, telangiectasia (multiple telangiectases—collections of distended blood capillaries), Cushingoid changes. *Manufacturer*: Yamanouchi.

LOCORTEN-VIOFORM

Description: an antibacterial and corti-costeroid, comprising 1% clioquinol and 0.02% flumethasone pivalate, as drops. *Used for*: inflammation of the outer ear where there may be secondary infection. *Dosage*: 2 to 3 drops twice daily for 7 to 10 days for all but children under 2 years of age. *Special care*: lactation. *Avoid use*: primary infections of the outer ear, perforated eardrum. *Side effects*: skin irritation, discolouration of hair. *Manufacturer*: Novartis Consumer.

LODINE

Description: a NSAID, pyranocarboxylate, available as 200mg etodolac in dark grey/light grey capsules with 2 red bands and marked LODINE 200, and 300mg etodolac in light grey capsules with 2 red bands and marked LODINE 300. Also, **LODINE TABLETS**, 200mg etodolac in brown, film-coated tablets marked LODINE 200. *Used for*: osteoarthrosis, rheumatoid arthritis. *Dosage*: 200 or 300mg twice per day, or 400 or 600mg as 1 dose if response is better. Maximum daily dose of 600mg. Not for children. Also, **LODINE SR**, 600mg etodolac as grey, sustained-release tablets, marked LODINE and SR 600. *Dosage*: 1 daily. Not for children. *Special care*: liver, kidney or heart disorder, heart failure, elderly. Monitor those on long-term treatment. *Avoid use*: active or history of peptic ulcer, history of gastro-intestinal bleeding, aspirin or anti-inflammatory induced allergy, pregnancy, lactation. *Possible interaction*: hypoglycaemics, anticoagulants, quinolones. *Side effects*: gastro-intestinal upset or bleeding, nausea, epigastric (upper central abdomen) pain, headache, dizziness, nephritis, rash, tinnitus, angioneurotic oedema. *Manufacturer*: Monmouth.

LOESTRIN 20

Description: an oestrogen/progestogen, ethinyloestradiol (20mg) with norethisterone acetate (1.5mg) in green tablets. Also **LOESTRIN 30**, which contains

30mg ethinyloestradiol. *Used for*: oral contraception. *Dosage*: 1 tablet daily for 21 days, commencing on the fifth day of menstruation, then 7 days without tablets. *Special care*: hypertension, Raynaud's disease (reduced blood supply to an organ of the body's extremities), asthma, severe depression, diabetes, varicose veins, multiple sclerosis, chronic kidney disease, kidney dialysis. Blood pressure, breasts and pelvic organs to be checked regularly; smoking not advised. *Avoid use*: history of heart disease, infectious hepatitis, sickle cell anaemia, porphyria, liver tumour, undiagnosed vaginal bleeding, pregnancy, hormone-dependent cancer, haemolytic uraemic syndrome (rare kidney disorder), chorea, otosclerosis. *Possible interaction*: barbiturates, tetracyclines, griseofulvin, rifampicin, primidone, phenytoin, chloral hydrate, ethosuximide, carbamazepine, glutethimide, dichloralphenazone. *Side effects*: fluid retention and bloating, leg cramps/pains, breast enlargement, headaches, nausea, loss of libido, weight gain, vaginal discharge, cervical erosion (alteration of epithelial cells), chloasma (pigmentation of nose, cheeks or forehead), breakthrough bleeding (bleeding between periods). *Manufacturer*: Parke-Davis.

LOGIPARIN

Description: an anticoagulant, and low molecular weight heparin (LMWH), tinzaparin sodium available as 11,700 units of anti-Factor Xa (a blood coagulation factor) per ml in syringes. *Used for*: prevention of thromboembolism during general or orthopaedic surgery. *Dosage*: general surgery—3,500 units injected subcutaneously 2 hours before an operation then 3,500 per day for 7 to 10 days. Orthopaedic surgery—2,500 units (body weight under 60kg), 3,500 units (60–80kg), 4,500 units (over 80kg), all injected subcutaneously before the operation and repeated once daily for a further 7 to 10 days. Not for children. *Special care*: pregnancy, lactation, asthma, severe liver or kidney disorder. *Avoid use*: tendency to haemorrhage, peptic ulcer, severe hypertension, endocarditis. *Possible interaction*: drugs that affect coagulation or platelet function. *Side effects*: increased risk of haemmorhage, bruising, skin rashes, thrombocytopenia, temporary increase in liver enzymes. *Manufacturer*: Novo Nordisk.

LOGYNON

Description: an oestrogen/progestogen contraceptive comprising ethinyloestradiol and levonorgestrel in the combinations: 30μg/50μg (6 brown tablets), 40μg/75μg (5 white tablets), 30μg/125μg (10 ochre tablets). *Used for*: oral contraception. *Dosage*: 1 tablet daily for 21 days starting on the first day of menstruation, then 7 days without tablets. *Special care*: hypertension, Raynaud's disease (reduced blood supply to an organ of the body's extremities), asthma, severe depression, diabetes, varicose veins, multiple sclerosis, chronic kidney disease, kidney dialysis. Blood pressure, breasts and pelvic organs to be checked regularly; smoking not advised. *Avoid use*: history of heart disease, infectious hepatitis, sickle cell anaemia, porphyria, liver tumour, undiagnosed vaginal bleeding, pregnancy, hormone-dependent cancer, haemolytic uraemic syndrome (rare kidney disorder), chorea, otosclerosis. *Possible interaction*: barbiturates, tetracyclines, griseofulvin, rifampicin, primidone, phenytoin, chloral hydrate, ethosuximide, carbamazepine, glutethimide, dichloralphenazone. *Side effects*: fluid retention and bloating, leg cramps/pains, breast enlargement, depression, headaches, nausea, loss of libido, weight gain, vaginal discharge, cervical erosion (alteration of epithelial cells), chloasma (pigmentation of nose, cheeks or forehead), breakthrough bleeding (bleeding between periods). *Manufacturer*: Schering H.C.

LOGYNON ED

Description: an oestrogen/progestogen contraceptive comprising ethinyl-oestradiol and levonorgestrel in the combinations: 30µg/50µg (6 brown tablets), 40µg/75µg (5 white tablets), 30µg/125µg (10 ochre tablets) plus 7 white tablets containing inert lactose. *Used for*: oral contraception. *Dosage*: 1 tablet daily for 28 days starting on the first day of the cycle. *Special care*: hypertension, Raynaud's disease (reduced blood supply to an organ of the body's extremities), asthma, severe depression, diabetes, varicose veins, multiple sclerosis, chronic kidney disease, kidney dialysis. Blood pressure, breasts and pelvic organs to be checked regularly; smoking not advised. *Avoid use*: history of heart disease, infectious hepatitis, sickle cell anaemia, porphyria, liver tumour, undiagnosed vaginal bleeding, pregnancy, hormone-dependent cancer, haemolytic uraemic syndrome (rare kidney disorder), chorea, otosclerosis. *Possible interaction*: barbiturates, tetracyclines, griseofulvin, rifampicin, primidone, phenytoin, chloral hydrate, ethosuximide, carbamazepine, glutethimide, dichloralphenazone. *Side effects*: fluid retention and bloating, leg cramps/pains, breast enlargement, depression, headaches, nausea, loss of libido, weight gain, vaginal discharge, cervical erosion (alteration of epithelial cells), chloasma (pigmentation of nose, cheeks or forehead), breakthrough bleeding (bleeding between periods). *Manufacturer*: Schering H.C.

LOMOTIL

Description: an opiate and anticholinergic, diphenoxylate hydrochloride (2.5mg) and atropine sulphate (25µg) in a white tablet marked SEARLE. Also, LOMOTIL LIQUID (5ml is equivalent to 1 tablet). *Used for*: diarrhoea. *Dosage*: 4 tablets or 20ml to begin with then half this dose every 6 hours until control is achieved. Children: 13 to 16 years, 2 tablets or 10ml 3 times per day; 9 to 12 years, 1 tablet or 5ml 4 times per day; 4 to 8 years, 1 tablet or 5ml 3 times daily. Not recommended below 4 years. *Special care*: pregnancy, lactation, liver disorder, do not start if there is severe dehydration or imbalance of electrolytes. *Avoid use*: acute ulcerative colitis, obstruction in the intestines, jaundice, pseudomembranous colitis (a severe form of colitis). *Possible interaction*: depressants of the CNS, MAOIs. *Side effects*: allergic reactions, gastro-intestinal upset, disturbances of the CNS, anticholinergic effects. *Manufacturer*: Searle.

LONITEN

Description: a vasodilator and antihypertensive, minoxidil, available as white tablets (2.5mg, 5mg and 10mg) marked with the tablet strength and on the reverse with U. *Used for*: severe hypertension. *Dosage*: 5mg per day initially in 1 or 2 divided doses, increasing at intervals of 3 days, to 10mg and thereafter by increases of 10mg daily to a maximum of 50mg. Children: 0.2mg/kg to begin with daily in 1 or 2 divided doses, increasing by 0.1–0.2mg/kg at intervals of 3 days to a maximum of 1mg/kg body weight daily. *Special care*: heart attack. Antihypertensives (other than diuretics and ß-blockers) should be withdrawn gradually before starting treatment. Diuretics and sympathetic suppressants to be given at the same time. *Avoid use*: phaeochromocytoma. *Side effects*: oedema, tachycardia, hair-growth. *Manufacturer*: Pharmacia & Upjohn.

LOPID

Description: an isobutyric acid derivative, gemfibrozil, available as white/maroon capsules (300mg strength) marked LOPID 300. Also LOPOID TABLETS, 600mg gemfibrozil in white oval tablets marked LOPID. *Used for*: prevention of coronary heart disease through lowering high levels of cholesterol or other fats in the blood. *Dosage*: 600mg twice per day to a maximum of 1500mg per day. *Special care*: blood count, liver function and lipid profile tests before treatment and blood counts over the first year of treatment. Annual check on eyes, period check on serum lipids. To be stopped in cases of persistent abnormal liver function. *Avoid use*: gallstones, alcoholism, pregnancy, lactation, liver disorder. *Possible interaction*: anticoagulants, simvastatin, pravastatin. *Side effects*: headache, dizziness, blurred vision, muscle pain, painful extremities, skin rash, impotence, gastro-intestinal upset. *Manufacturer*: Parke-Davis.

LOPRAZOLAM

Description: an intermediate-acting benzodiazepine hypnotic, loprazolam mesylate, available in 1mg tablets. *Used for*: treatment of insomnia or waking at night over the short-term. *Dosage*: 1 or 2 at bedtime; up to 1 for the elderly. Not for children. *Special care*: chronic kidney or liver disease, lung insufficiency, pregnancy, labour, lactation, elderly. May cause impaired judgement. Avoid prolonged use and withdraw gradually. *Avoid use*: acute lung disease, psychotic, phobic or obsessional states, depression of respiration. *Possible interaction*: depressants of the CNS, alcohol, anticonvulsants. *Side effects*: ataxia, confusion, light-headedness, drowsiness, gastro-intestinal upset, changes in vision and libido, skin rash, hypotension, retention of urine. Dependence risk increases with prolonged treatment or higher dosages. *Manufacturer*: Roussel.

LOPRESOR

Description: a ß-blocker, metoprolol tartrate, available as pink tablets (50mg strength) and light blue tablets (100mg strength), marked GEIGY. *Used for*: prevention of mortality after myocardial infarction (MI), arrhythmias. *Dosage*:

see literature for initial dosage after MI, 200mg per day for maintenance. Arrhythmias, 50mg twice or 3 times per day to a daily maximum of 300mg. *Also used for*: angina. *Dosage*: 50–100mg 2 or 3 times per day. Also **LOPRESOR SR**, 200mg metoprolol tartrate in a yellow, sustained-release capsule-shaped tablet marked CG/CG and CDC/CDC on the reverse. *Dosage*: 1 per day; up to 2, once per day if necessary. *Also used for*: hypertension, additional therapy in thyrotoxicosis. *Dosage*: hypertension, 100mg daily to begin with increasing if necessary to 200mg in 1 or 2 divided doses. Thyrotoxicosis, 50mg, 4 times per day. Or 1 tablet of Lopresor SR in the morning. *Also used for*: migraine. *Dosage*: 100–200mg per day in divided doses. *Special care*: history of bronchospasm and certain ß-blockers, diabetes, liver or kidney disease, pregnancy, lactation, general anaesthesia. Withdraw gradually. Not for children. *Avoid use*: heart block or failure, slow heart rate (bradycardia), sick sinus syndrome (associated with sinus node disorder), certain ß-blockers, severe peripheral arterial disease. *Possible interaction*: verapamil, hypoglycaemics, reserpine, clonidine withdrawal, some antiarrhythmics and anaesthetics, antihypertensives, depressants of the CNS, cimetidine, indomethacin, sympathomimetics. *Side effects*: bradycardia, cold hands and feet, disturbance to sleep, heart failure, gastro-intestinal upset, tiredness on exertion, bronchospasm. *Manufacturer*: Geigy.

LOPRESORETIC

Description: a ß-blocker and thiazide diuretic, metoprolol tartrate (100mg) and chlorthalidone (12.5mg), available as an off-white tablet marked GEIGY 56. *Used for*: hypertension. *Dosage*: 1 daily to begin with in the morning increasing if required to 3 or 4 per day in single or divided doses. Not for children. *Special care*: history of bronchospasm and certain ß-blockers, diabetes, liver or kidney disease, pregnancy, lactation, general anaesthesia, gout, check electrolyte levels, K⁺ supplements may be required depending on the case. Withdraw gradually. Not for children. *Avoid use*: heart block or failure, slow heart rate (bradycardia), sick sinus syndrome (associated with sinus node disorder), certain ß-blockers, severe peripheral arterial disease, pregnancy, lactation, severe kidney failure, anuria, hepatic cornea. *Possible interaction*: verapamil, hypoglycaemics, reserpine, clonidine withdrawal, some antiarrhythmics and anaesthetics, antihypertensives, depressants of the CNS, cimetidine, indomethacin, sympathomimetics, lithium, potassium supplements with potassium-sparing diuretics, digitalis. *Side effects*: bradycardia, cold hands and feet, disturbance to sleep, heart failure, gastro-intestinal upset, tiredness on exertion, bronchospasm, gout, weakness, blood disorders, sensitivity to light. *Manufacturer*: Geigy.

LORAZEPAM

Description: an intermediate-acting benzodiazepine, lorazepam, available in tablets strength 1mg. *Used for*: moderate to severe anxiety. *Dosage*: 1–4mg per day in divided doses, elderly 0.5–2mg. Not for children. *Special care*: chronic liver or kidney disease, chronic lung disease, pregnancy, labour, lactation, elderly. May impair judgement. Withdraw gradually and avoid prolonged use. *Avoid use*: depression of respiration, acute lung disease; psychotic, phobic or obsessional states. *Possible interaction*: anticonvulsants, depressants of the CNS, alcohol. *Side effects*: ataxia, confusion, light-headedness, drowsiness, hypotension, gastro-intestinal upsets, disturbances in vision and libido, skin rashes, retention of urine, vertigo. Sometimes jaundice or blood disorders. *Manufacturer*: available from Wyeth.

LORMETAZEPAM

Description: an intermediate-acting benzodiazepine, lormetazepam, available in 0.5mg and 1mg tablets. *Used for*: insomnia. *Dosage*: 1mg at bedtime elderly 0.5mg. Not for children. *Special care*: chronic liver or kidney disease, chronic lung disease, pregnancy, labour, lactation, elderly. May impair judgement. Withdraw gradually and avoid prolonged use. *Avoid use*: depression of respiration, acute lung disease; psychotic, phobic or obsessional states. *Possible interaction*: anticonvulsants, depressants of the CNS, alcohol. *Side effects*: ataxia, confusion, light-headedness, drowsiness, hypotension, gastro-intestinal upsets, disturbances in vision and libido, skin rashes, retention of urine, vertigo. Sometimes jaundice or blood disorders. *Manufacturer*: available from APS, Cox, Wyeth.

LORON

Description: a diphosphonate, sodium clodronate, available in ampoules as a solution of 30mg/ml. *Used for*: hypercalcaemia induced by tumour. *Dosage*: 300mg per day initially, by slow intravenous infusion, for a maximum of 10 days. For maintenance use tablets or capsules. Not for children. Also **LORON TABLETS**, containing 520mg sodium clodronate and in white oblong tablets marked BM E9. *Dosage*: 2 to 4 tablets per day in 1, or 2 divided doses 1 hour before or after food. Maximum usage, 6 months. Not for children. Also, **LORON CAPSULES**, 400mg sodium clodronate, in white capsules marked BM B7. *Dosage*: 4 to 8 capsules per day in 1, or 2 divided doses 1 hour before or after food for a maximum period of 6 months. Not for children. *Special care*: kidney function, serum calcium and phosphate to be monitored. *Avoid use*: pregnancy, lactation, kidney failure, inflammation of the intestines. *Possible interaction*: antacids, mineral supplements, other diphosphonates. *Side effects*: gastro-intestinal upset. Sometimes allergic reactions, hypocalcaemia. Temporary proteinuria. *Manufacturer*: B.M.UK.

LOSEC

Description: a proton pump inhibitor (limits gastric H⁺), omeprazole, available in pink/brown capsules (20mg) marked A/OM and 20, and brown capsules (40mg) both of which contain enteric-coated granules. *Used for*: reflux oesophagitis, duodenal and benign gastic ulcers, Zollinger-Ellison (ZE) syndrome. *Dosage*: reflux oesophagitis: 20mg per day for 4 weeks, plus a further 4 to 8 weeks if necessary. In unresponsive (refractory) cases, 40mg once per day. 20mg daily for long-term treatment. Duodenal ulcer: 20mg per day for 8 weeks, and 40mg daily for long-term treatment. 20mg daily for long-term treatment. Gastric ulcer: 20mg per day for 8 weeks, increasing to 40mg for severe cases. Z-E syndrome: 60mg per day, modified according to response, maintenance 20–120mg daily (doses over 80mg in 2 divided doses). Not for children. *Special care*: for suspected gastric ulcer, malignancy must be excluded prior to treatment. *Avoid use*: pregnancy, lactation. *Possible interaction*: warfarin, digoxin, phenytoin, diazepam. *Side effects*: diarrhoea, headache, nausea, skin rashes, constipation. *Manufacturer*: Astra.

LOTRIDERM

Description: a potent steroid and antifungal agent, betamethasone dipropionate (0.05%) and clotrimazole (1%) available as a cream. *Used for*: short-term treatment fungal infections of the skin. *Dosage*: apply for 2 weeks, morning and evening (4 weeks for treatment of the feet). *Special care*: maximum 5 days use on face or for children, withdraw gradually after prolonged use. *Avoid use*: acne, dermatitis around the mouth, leg ulcers, scabies, viral skin disease, ringworm or tubercular infection, untreated infections caused by fungi or bacteria. Avoid prolonged or extensive use during pregnancy. Children. *Side effects*: irritation, localized mild burning sensation, hypersensitivity reactions. *Manufacturer*: Dominion.

LOXAPAC

Description: a dibenzoxapine, loxapine succinate, available in yellow/green (10mg), light green/dark green (25mg) and blue/dark green (50mg) capsules marked L2, L3 or L4 respectively. *Used for*: chronic and acute psychoses. *Dosage*: 20–50mg per day, to begin with, in 2 doses and increasing over 7 to 10 days to 60–100mg daily. Maximum, 250mg daily. Not for children. *Special care*: cardiovascular disease, epilepsy, urine retention, glaucoma, pregnancy, lactation. *Avoid use*: patients in a coma or depression induced by drugs. *Possible interaction*: anticholinergics, depressants of the CNS. *Side effects*: faintness, muscle twitches, weakness, dizziness, drowsiness, confusion, tachycardia, hyper- or hypotension, skin reactions, nausea, changes in ECG and eye, headache, vomiting, dyspnoea (shortness of breath), anticholinergic effects. *Manufacturer*: Wyeth.

LUDIOMIL

Description: a tetracyclic antidepressant, maprotiline hydrochloride, available as peach tablets (10mg, marked Co), greyish-red tablets (25mg, marked DP), light orange tablets (50mg, marked ER) and brown-orange tablets (75mg, marked FS). All are also marked CIBA. *Used for*: depression. *Dosage*: 25–75mg per day to start with in 1 or 3 divided doses, modifying after 1 or 2 weeks as required; maximum of 150mg daily. Elderly, 30mg once daily or 3 doses of

10mg per day. Not for children. *Special care*: pregnancy, lactation, elderly, cardiovascular disease, schizophrenia, hyperthyroidism. *Avoid use*: severe liver or
kidney disease, narrow-angle glaucoma, mania, history of epilepsy, urine retention, recent coronary thrombosis. *Possible interaction*: sympathomimetics,
barbiturates, MAOIs, antipsychotics, alcohol, antihypertensives, anaesthetics,
cimetidine, phenytoin, benzodiazepines. *Side effects*: skin rash, convulsions,
impaired reactions, anticholinergic effects. *Manufacturer*: Ciba.

LURSELLE

Description: a butylphenol, probucol, available as white tablets (250mg strength)
marked LURSELLE. *Used for*: treatment of high blood levels of protein-bound
lipids (hyper-lipoproteinaemia). *Dosage*: 2 tablets twice daily accompanying
the morning and evening meals. Not for children. *Special care*: heart disorders.
Monitor ECG before starting treatment. Stop treatment 6 months before a
planned pregnancy. *Avoid use*: pregnancy, lactation. *Side effects*: diarrhoea,
gastro-intestinal upset. *Manufacturer*: Merrell Dow.

LUSTRAL

Description: sertraline hydrochloride available as white, capsule-shaped tablets
in 50 and 100mg strengths and marked PFIZER with LTL-50 or LTL-100 respectively. *Used for*: depression and the prevention of relapse or further bouts
of depression. *Dosage*: 50mg per day at the start, with food, increasing by 50mg
if necessary, every 2 to 4 weeks to a daily maximum of 200mg. Maintenance is
usually 50–100mg per day. A dosage of 150mg or more should not be used for
more than 8 weeks. Not for children. *Special care*: pregnancy, lactation, unstable epilepsy, anyone undergoing electroconvulsive therapy. *Avoid use*: kidney or
liver disorders. *Possible interaction*: lithium, tryptophan, MAOIs. *Side effects*:
nausea, diarrhoea, tremor, increased sweating, dyspepsia, dry mouth, delay in
ejaculation. *Manufacturer*: Invicta.

M

MACROBID

Description: a preparation which is a nitrofuran antibacterial drug available as
yellow/blue modified-release capsules containing 100mg nitrofurantoin, marked
Eaton BID. *Used for*: infections of urinary tract, prevention of infection during surgical procedures on genital/urinary tract, pyelitis. *Dosage*: adults, treatment, 1 tablet twice each day with food; prevention of infection, 1 tablet twice
daily for 4 days starting on day of surgery. *Special care*: breast-feeding, patients

with diabetes, deficiency of vitamin B, debilitation, anaemia, imbalance in electrolyte (salts) levels. Elderly patients and those on long-term treatment require monitoring of liver, lung and nerve function. *Avoid use*: children, pregnant women at end of pregnancy, patients with kidney disease or damage or failure or reduction in ability to produce urine (anuria and oliguria). *Possible interaction*: probenecid, quinolones, magnesium trisilicate, sulphinpyrazone. *Side effects*: gastro-intestinal upset, blood changes, allergic responses, anorexia. Drug should be withdrawn if hepatitis, lung reactions, peripheral nerve damage or haemolysis occur. *Manufacturer*: Procter & Gamble.

MACRODANTIN

Description: an antibacterial nitrofuran drug available as white/yellow capsules containing 50mg nitrofurantoin, and yellow capsules containing 100mg nitrofurantoin. *Used for*: treatment and prevention of urinary tract infections (during surgical procedure), pyelitis. *Dosage*: adults and children over 10 years, treatment of acute infection, 50mg 4 times each day for 1 week; serious, recurring infection, 100mg 4 times each day for 1 week. Long-term suppression of infection, 50–100mg each day taken as single dose at bedtime. Prevention, 50mg 4 times each day for 4 days beginning on day of prcedure. Children, 3 months to 10 years, acute infection, 3mg/kg body weight in divided doses each day for 1 week. Suppression of infection, 1mg/kg body weight once each day. *Special care*: breast-feeding, patients who are debilitated, vitamin B deficiency, anaemia, imbalance in electrolyte (salts) levels, diabetes. Elderly patients and those on long-term treatment require regular monitoring of liver and lung function. *Avoid use*: pregnant women at end of pregnancy, patients with kidney disease or damage, anuria and oliguria. *Possible interaction*: probenecid, quinolones, sulphinpyrazone, magnesium trisilicate. *Side effects*: gastro-intestinal upset, allergic responses, blood changes, anorexia. Drug should be withdrawn if hepatitis, lung reactions, peripheral nerve damage or haemolysis occur. *Manufacturer*: Procter & Gamble.

MADOPAR

Description: a combined preparation of dopamine precursor (levodopa) and an enzyme which is a dopa decarboxylase inhibitor, benserazide (as hydrochloride), available as capsules of different strengths. '62.5' blue/grey capsles contain 50mg and 12.5mg respectively. '125' blue/pink capsules contain 100mg and 25mg. '250' blue/caramel capsules contain 200mg and 50mg. All capsules are marked ROCHE. Also, **MADOPAR DISPERSIBLE TABLETS**, white scored tablets of 2 different strengths: '62.5' contain 50mg and 12.5mg; '125' contain 100mg and 25mg. Tablets all marked with name and strength. Also, **MADOPAR CR** green/blue continuous-release capsules containing 100mg levodopa and 25mg benserazide (as hydrochloride), marked ROCHE. *Used for*: Parkinsonism. *Dosage*: adults over 25 years of age not already receiving levodopa, 1 '62.5' tablet 3 or 4 times each day at first taken after meals. Dose may be increased by

1 '125' tablet each day once or twice a week. Usual maintenance dose is in the order of 4 to 8 '125' tablets each day in divided doses. Elderly persons, 1 '62.5' once or twice each day with additional '62.5' tablet every third or fourth day if increase is required. Madopar continuous-release capsules: dose individually determined for each patient, usually 50% more than previous levodopa therapy. *Special care*: peptic ulcer, wide angle glaucoma, liver, kidney, heart, lung, circulatory diseases or endocrine (hormonal) disorders. Also, psychiatric disorders, soft bones (osteomalacia). Regular blood checks and monitoring of liver, kidney, heart and circulatory function should be carried out. *Avoid use*: children and young adults under 25 years of age, pregnancy, breast-feeding. Patients with history of malignant melanoma (tumours of melanocytes which form the skin pigment, melanin), narrow angle glaucoma, severe psychoses. *Possible interaction*: sympathomimetics, antihypertensives, other similar preparations, ferrous sulphate, MAOIs; antacids (Madopar CR). *Side effects*: heart and central nervous system disturbance, involuntary movements, hypotension when rising from lying down, anorexia, nausea, vomiting, discoloured urine. Rarely, haemolytic anaemia. *Manufacturer*: Roche.

MAGNAPEN

Description: a compound broad-spectrum penicillin and penicillinase-resistant (i.e. resistant to enzymes produced by some bacteria) preparation. It is available as turquoise/black capsules containing 250mg ampicillin and 250mg flucloxacillin and marked MAGNAPEN. Also, **MAGNAPEN SYRUP** containing 125mg ampicillin and 125mg flucloxacillin/5ml. **MAGNAPEN INJECTION** containing 500mg or 1g powder in vials for reconstitution and injection, both with equal quantities of ampicillin and flucloxacillin. *Used for*: severe and mixed infections where some penicillin-resistant (staphylococci) bacteria are present. *Dosage*: adults and children over 10, 1 capsule or 10ml syrup 4 times each day taken thirty minutes to 1 hour before meals. Injection, 500mg 4 times each day. Children, under 10 years, 5ml syrup 4 times each day thirty minutes to 1 hour before meals. Injection, under 2 years, quarter of adult dose; 2 to 10 years, half adult dose. *Special care*: patients with glandular fever (infectious mononucleosis). *Side effects*: gastro-intestinal upset, allergic reactions; rarely, cholestatic jaundice. *Manufacturer*: Beecham.

MALOPRIM

Description: a compound antimalarial preparation combining sulphone and diaminopyrimidine drugs, available as scored white tablets containing 100mg dapsone and 12.5mg pyrimethamine, marked WELLCOME H9A. *Used for*: prevention of malaria. *Dosage*: adults and children over 10 years, 1 tablet each week. Children, 5 to 10 years of age, 1 half tablet weekly. *Special care*: patient should continue to take tablets for 4 weeks after leaving area where malaria is present. Special care in breast-feeding mothers, pregnant women should take folate supplements, patients with liver or kidney disease. *Avoid use*: children under 5 years, patients with dermatitis herpetiformis (a type of dermatitis). *Possible interaction*: folate inhibitors. *Side effects*: severe haemolysis, skin sensitivity, blood disorders. *Manufacturer*: Glaxo Wellcome.

MANERIX

Description: an antidepressant preparation which is a reversible MAO-A inhibitor (monoamine oxidase A inhibitor) which acts to prevent the breakdown of this neuro-transmitter by enzyme, thereby prolonging its activity. It is available as scored, oblong, yellow, film-coated tablets containing 150mg moclobemide, marked ROCHE 150. *Used for*: severe depression. *Dosage*: adults, 2 tablets each day in divided doses (maximum of 4 daily) taken after meals. *Special care*: pregnancy, breast-feeding, serious liver disease, thyrotoxicosis. Also, patients with schizophrenia in which agitation is a predominant symptom. Some foods may need to be avoided. *Avoid use*: children, patients with phaeochromocytoma, severe confusional disorders. *Possible interaction*: morphine, cimetidine, some sympathomimetic amines, pethidine, fentanyl, some other antidepressants, codeine. *Side effects*: headache, giddiness, agitation and restlessness, confusion, nausea, disturbance of sleep. *Manufacturer*: Roche.

MAREVAN

Description: a coumarin anticoagulant preparation available as scored tablets of different strengths all containing warfarin sodium; brown 1mg tablets marked M1, blue 3mg tablets marked M3 and pink 5mg tablets marked M5. *Used for*: thromboembolic states. *Dosage*: adults, 10mg each day adjusted according to response. *Special care*: patients who are seriously ill, have kidney disease or disorder, hypertension, vitamin K deficiency, weight changes and elderly persons. *Avoid use*: pregnancy, within 24 hours of labour or surgery, reduced liver or kidney function, haemorrhage or bleeding disorders. *Possible interaction*: antibiotics, cimetidine, corticosteroids, hypoglycaemics taken orally, phenformin, sulphonamides, NSAIDs, quinidine, drugs have an effect on liver enzymes. *Side effects*: skin rash, diarrhoea, baldness. *Manufacturer*: Goldshield.

MARPLAN

Description: an antidepressant MAOI available as scored, pink tablets containing 10mg isocarboxazid, marked ROCHE. *Used for*: depression. *Dosage*: adults, 30mg each day at first reducing to a usual maintenance dose in the order of 10–20mg daily. Elderly persons, half adult dose. *Special care*: elderly persons and patients with epilepsy. *Avoid use*: children, patients with congestive heart failure, circulatory disease of arteries of brain (cerebral vascular disease), liver disease, phaeochromocytoma, blood changes, hyperthyroidism, heart disease. *Possible interaction*: anticholinergics, barbiturates, alcohol, hypoglycaemics, insulin, reserpine, guanethidine, methyldopa. Also sympathomimetic amines, especially ephedrine, amphetamine, levodopa, methylphenidate, phenylpropanolamine, fenfluramine. Also, pethidine, TCADs, narcotic analgesics. Many foods need to be avoided including: meat extracts (Bovril, Oxo), bananas, yeast extracts (Marmite), broad beans, foods made from textured vegetable proteins, alcohol, low alcohol drinks, pickled herrings, all foods that are not completely fresh. All these drugs and foods should be avoided for at least 14 days after treatment stops then tried cautiously. *Side effects*: allergic responses with certain foods, tiredness, muscle weakness, low blood pressure on rising, dizziness, swelling of ankles. Dry mouth, blurring of vision, gastro-intestinal upset, constipation, difficulty ir urination. Skin rashes, weight gain, blood changes, change in libido, jaundice. Sometimes psychiatric disturbances and confusion. *Manufacturer*: Cambridge.

MARVELON

Description: a combined oestrogen/progestogen oral contraceptive preparation available as white tablets containing 30mg ethinyloestradiol and 150 micrograms desogestrel, marked ORGANON, TR over 5 and with *. *Used for*: oral contraception. *Dosage*: 1 tablet each day for 21 days, starting on first or fifth day of monthly cycle, followed by 7 tablet-free days. *Special care*: patients with multiple sclerosis, serious kidney disease or kidney dialysis, asthma, Raynaud's disease, abnormally high levels of prolactin in the blood (hyperprolactinaemia), varicose veins, hypertension. Also, patients suffering from severe depression. Thrombosis risk increases with smoking, age and obesity. During the course of treatment, regular checks on blood pressure, pelvic organs and breasts should be carried out. *Avoid use*: pregnancy, those at risk of thrombosis, suffering from heart disease, pulmonary hypertension, angina, sickle cell anaemia. Also, undiagnosed vaginal bleeding, history of cholestatic jaundice during pregnancy, cancers which are hormone-dependent, infectious hepatitis, liver disorders. Also, porphyria, Dublin-Johnson and Rotor syndrome, otosclerosis, chorea, haemolytic uraemic syndrome, recent trophoblastic disease. *Possible interaction*: barbiturates, ethosuximide, glutethimide, rifampicin, phenytoin, tetracyclines, carbamazepine, chloral hydrate, griseofulvin, dichloralphenazone, primidone. *Side effects*: weight gain, breast enlargement, pains in legs, cramps, loss of sexual desire, headaches, depression, nausea, breakthrough bleeding, cervical erosion, vaginal discharge, brownish patches on skin (chloasma), oedema and bloatedness. *Manufacturer*: Organon.

MAXIDEX

Description: lubricant and corticosteroid eyedrops containing 0.5% hypromellose and 0.1% dexamethasone. *Used for*: inflammation of anterior segment of eye. *Dosage*: serious disease, 1 to 2 drops each hour, reducing dose as condition improves. For milder conditions, 1 or 2 drops 4, 5 or 6 times each day. *Special care*: long-term use by pregnant women and in babies. *Avoid use*: patients with glaucoma, suffering from tuberculous, viral or fungal infections or those producing pus; patients with soft contact lenses. *Side effects*: cataract, thinning of cornea, rise in pressure within eye, fungal infection. *Manufacturer*: Alcon.

MAXITROL

Description: a compound preparation in the form of eyedrops combining a corticosteroid, aminoglycoside, lubricant and peptide. It contains 0.1% dexamethasone, 0.35% neomycin sulphate, 0.5% hypromellose, 6000 units polymyxin B sulphate/ml. Also MAXITROL OINTMENT containing 0.1% dexamethasone, 0.35% neomycin sulphate, 6000 units polymixin B sulphate/gram. *Used for*: infected and inflamed conditions of the eye. *Dosage*: apply 3 or 4 times each day. *Special care*: long-term use by pregnant women or in babies. *Avoid use*: patients with glaucoma, suffering from tuberculous, viral or fungal infections or those producing pus; patients with soft contact lenses. *Side effects*: cataract, thinning of cornea, rise in pressure within eye, fungal infection. *Manufacturer*: Alcon.

MAXOLON

Description: an anti-emetic, antidopaminergic preparation, metoclopramide hydrochloride, which acts on the gastro-intestinal tract and is available in a number of different forms: white, scored tablets containing 10mg marked MAXOLON. **MAXOLON SYRUP** containing 5mg/5ml. **MAXOLON PAEDIATRIC LIQUID** containing 1mg/ml. **MAXOLON INJECTION** as a solution in ampoules for injection containing 10mg/2ml. **MAXOLON SR** clear capsules containing white, sustained-release granules at a strength of 15mg, marked MAXOLON SR 15. **MAXOLON HIGH DOSE** available as a solution in ampoules for injection containing 100mg/20ml. *Used for*: indigestion, gastro-intestinal disturbance, backflow of blood. Also, vomiting and nausea due to cytotoxic drug therapy, cobalt therapy, deep X-ray or post-operative sickness. *Dosage*: adults, over 20 years of age, 15mg twice each day with a daily maximum of 0.5mg/kg body weight. Children and young adults under 20 years, for vomiting caused by cancer chemotherapy or radiotherapy from 1 to 5mg, 2 or 3 times per day, depending upon body weight. *Special care*: pregnancy, breastfeeding, liver or kidney disease/damage, epilepsy. *Avoid use*: patients who have recently had operations on gastro-intestinal tract, phaeochromocytoma, breast cancer which is prolactin-dependent. *Possible interaction*: phenothiazines, anticholinergics, butyrophenones. *Side effects*: diarrhoea, raised levels of prolactin in blood, sleepiness, extrapyramidal reactions (involuntary muscle movements, changes in posture and muscle tone). *Manufacturer*: Monmouth.

MAXTREX

Description: a folic acid antagonist available as tablets of 2 strengths. Yellow tablets contain 2.5mg methotrexate and are marked M2.5 on 1 side and F on the other. Yellow, scored tablets contain 10mg and are marked M10. *Used for*: abnormal growths and serious psoriasis which has not been controlled by other treatments. *Dosage*: individually determined according to patient's condition and response. *Special care*: patients with gastro-intestinal diseases and disorders, liver or kidney disease or damage, low blood cell counts, psychiatric illness, elderly or young persons. Patients should be monitored for liver and kidney function and blood checks. *Avoid use*: pregnancy, breast-feeding, patients with serious liver or kidney disorder, abnormally low levels of white blood cells and platelets, severe anaemia. *Possible interaction*: alcohol, NSAIDs, live vaccines, drugs that bind to proteins, anticonvulsants, folic acid, etretinate. *Side effects*: gastro-intestinal upset, skin rashes, liver disorders, depression of bone marrow. *Manufacturer*: Pharmacia & Upjohn.

MEDIHALER-EPI

Description: a sympathomimetic preparation available as a metered dose aerosol delivering 0.28mg adrenaline acid tartrate per dose. *Used for*: additional treatment in anaphylaxis caused by sensitivity to insect stings or drugs. *Dosage*: adults, anaphylaxis only, at least 20 puffs. Children, 10–15 puffs. *Special care*: diabetes. *Avoid use*: patients with hyperthyroidism, serious heart disease, heart arrhythmias, hypertension. *Possible interaction*: sympathomimetics, TCADs, MAOIs. *Side effects*: palpitations, agitation, dry mouth, stomach pain. *Manufacturer*: 3M Health Care.

MEDIHALER-ERGOTAMINE

Description: an NSAID which is an ergot alkaloid available as a metered dose aerosol delivering 0.36mg ergotamine tartrate/metered dose. *Used for*: rapid treatment of migraine. *Dosage*: adults and children over 10, 1 dose repeated after 5 minutes if needed with a maximum of 6 doses in 24 hours and 15 in any 7 day period. *Avoid use*: pregnancy, breast-feeding, children under 10 years, patients with liver or kidney disorder, hypertension, heart disease or disease of peripheral arteries, sepsis. *Possible interaction*: ß-blockers, erythromycin. *Side effects*: muscle pain, nausea. *Manufacturer*: 3M Health Care.

MEDIHALER ISO

Description: a bronchodilator which is a non-selective ß-agonist available as a metered dose aerosol delivering 0.08mg isoprenaline sulphate per dose. Also, **MEDIHALER ISO FORTE** delivering 0.4mg isoprenaline sulphate per dose by metered dose aerosol. *Used for*: severe bronchitis and bronchial asthma. *Dosage*: adults, 1–3 puffs which may be repeated after half an hour if required. Maximum dose is 24 puffs in 24 hours. *Special care*: pregnancy, diabetes or hypertension. *Avoid use*: children, hyperthyroidism or severe coronary disease. *Possible interaction*: sympathomimetics, tricyclics, MAOIs. *Side effects*: palpitations, agitation, dry mouth. *Manufacturer*: 3M Health Care.

MEDRONE

Description: an anti-inflammatory, glucocorticoid corticosteroid available as tablets of different strengths, all containing methylprednisolone. Oval, pink, scored 2mg tablets marked UPJOHN; oval, white, scored 4mg tablets marked UPJOHN; white, scored 16mg tablets, marked UPJOHN 73; light-blue, scored 100mg tablets marked UPJOHN 3379. *Used for*: treatment/control of allergic and inflammatory disorders including dermatological, respiratory, neoplastic and collagen diseases and rheumatoid arthritis. *Dosage*: 2–40mg each day depending upon condition and response. *Special care*: pregnancy, active infections and those of fungal, viral or tuberculous origin, kidney inflammation, diseases characterized by skin rash, hypertension. Patients who have recently had surgical anastomoses of intestine, suffering from epilepsy, diabetes, liver cirrhosis, peptic ulcer, hyperthyroidism, secondary cancers. Patients suffering from stress or psychoses, contact with *Herpes zoster* or chicken pox should be avoided and medical treatment required if this occurs. *Possible interaction*: cardiac glycosides, phenytoin, rifampicin, NSAIDs, anti-cholinesterases, ephedrine, phenobarbitone, anticoagulants taken orally, diuretics, hypoglycaemics. *Side effects*: symptoms as in Cushing's syndrome, osteoporosis, peptic ulcer, hyperglycaemia, depression and euphoria. *Manufacturer*: Pharmacia & Upjohn.

MEFOXIN

Description: a cephalosporin antibiotic preparation available as a powder in vials for reconstitution and injection, in 2 strengths containing 1g or 2g cefoxitin. *Used for*: skin, soft tissue, respiratory tract infections, septicaemia and peritonitis. Prevention of infection in gynaecological and obstetric operations, treatment of post-operative infections. Gonorrhoea and urinary tract infections. *Dosage*: adults, 1–2g by intravenous or intramuscular injection at 8 hour intervals. Prevention of infection, 2g 30 minutes to 1 hour before surgery 10 every 6 hours post-operatively for 24 hours. Children, newborn babies up to 1 week, 20–40mg/kg body weight at 12 hour intervals. 1 week to 1 month of age, 20–40mg/kg at 8 hour intervals; 1 month and over, 20–40kg/kg at 6 to 8 hour intervals. Prevention of infection, newborn babies, 30–40mg/kg, 30 minutes to 1 hour before operation then every 8 to 12 hours post-operatively for 24 hours. Older babies and children, 30–40mg/kg at same times as in adults. *Special care*: pregnancy, breast-feeding, patients with allergy to penicillin, kidney disorder. *Possible interaction*: aminoglycosides, loop diuretics. *Side effects*: gastro-intestinal upset, blood changes, (reduction in levels of white blood cells and platelets), allergic reactions, pain at injection site, rise in levels of blood urea and liver enzymes. Positive Coomb's test (a test for detecting rhesus antibodies). *Manufacturer*: M.S.D.

MEGACE

Description: a hormonal progestogen preparation available as tablets of 2 strengths: scored, white tablets contain 40mg megestrol acetate marked 40; oval, off-white scored tablets contain 160mg marked 160. *Used for*: breast and endometrial cancer. *Dosage*: breast cancer, 160mg each day as single or divided doses. Endometrial cancer, 40–320mg each day in divided doses. All taken for at least 2 months. *Special care*: patients with inflamed veins (thrombophlebitis). *Avoid use*: pregnant women. *Side effects*: nausea, nettle rash (urticaria), gain in weight. *Manufacturer*: Bristol-Myers.

MELLERIL

Description: a phenothiazine group II antipsychotic drug available as white, film-coated tablets of different strengths containing 10mg, 25mg, 50mg and 100mg thioridazine hydrochloride respectively. All are marked with strength and MEL. Also, **MELLERIL SYRUP** containing 25mg/5ml. **MELLERIL SUSPENSION** in 2 strengths containing 25mg and 100mg thioridazine base/5ml. *Used for*: mania, schizophrenia, hypomania, additional short-term therapy in the treatment of psycho-neuroses. Symptoms of senility, disturbed behaviour and epilepsy in children. *Dosage*: depending upon severity and type of condition, in the order of 30–600mg each day. Children, 1 to 5 years, 1mg/kg body weight each day; over 5 years, 75–150mg/kg daily. Maximum dose in this age group is 300mg each day. *Special care*: myasthenia gravis, epilepsy, phaeochromocytoma, enlarged prostate gland, Parkinsonism, heart and circulatory diseases, glaucoma, liver or kidney disorders, respiratory diseases. *Avoid use*: pregnancy, breast-feeding, history of blood changes, coma, serious heart or circulatory diseases, severe depression, porphyria. *Possible interaction*: alcohol, antiarrhythmics, antacids, tricyclics, antimuscarines, calcium channel blockers, anxiolytics, lithium. *Side effects*: hypotension, changes in libido, apathy, depression, insomnia, dry mouth, blocked nose, effects on heart rhythm, disturbance of sleep, constipation, difficulty in passing urine. Blood changes, rashes, jaundice, effects on liver, menstrual changes, breast enlargement, weight gain, abnormal production of breast milk. Rarely, fits, blurring of vision due to deposition of pigment (higher doses). *Manufacturer*: Sandoz.

MENGIVAC (A + C)

Description: a vaccine preparation containing inactivated surface antigen of meningitis A and C. It is produced as a powder in vials, with diluent, containing 50 micrograms of both group A and group C polysaccharide antigens of *Neisseria meningitidis*. *Used for*: immunization against meningitis, types A and C. *Dosage*: adults and children over eighteen months, 0.5ml by deep subcutaneous or intramuscular injection. *Special care*: pregnancy, breast-feeding. *Avoid use*: patients with severe infections and feverish illnesses. *Possible interaction*: substances which suppress immune system. *Side effects*: local skin reactions, slight fever. *Manufacturer*: Merieux.

MENOPHASE

Description: a hormonal combined oestrogen/progestogen preparation available as tablets containing mestranol and norethisterone; 5 pink tablets contain 12.5µg mestranol; 8 orange tablets contain 25µg mestranol; 2 yellow tablets contain 50µg mestranol; 3 green tablets contain 25µg mestranol and 1mg norethisterone; 6 blue tablets contain 30µg mestranol and 1.5mg norethisterone; 4 lavender tablets contain 20µg mestranol and 750µg norethisterone. *Used for*: treatment of menopausal symptoms and prevention of osteoporosis following menopause. *Dosage*: 1 tablet each day starting on a Sunday with pink tablets and continuing in order, as indicated. Treatment should be continuous for 6 months to 1 year. *Special care*: patients with history of, or considered to be at risk of thrombosis. Women with any of the following should receive careful monitoring: epilepsy, gallstones, porphyria, multiple sclerosis, otosclerosis, diabetes, migraine, hypertension, tetany, fibroids in the uterus. Blood pressure, breasts and pelvic organs should be examined regularly during the course of treatment especially in women who may be at risk of breast cancer. *Avoid use*: pregnancy, breast-feeding, women with breast cancer, cancer of reproductive system or other hormonally dependent cancer. Women with inflammation of veins or other thromboembolic conditions, endometriosis, undiagnosed vaginal bleeding, serious liver, kidney or heart disease, Dublin-Johnson or Rotor syndromes. *Possible interaction*: drugs which induce liver enzymes. *Side effects*: soreness and enlargement of breasts, breakthrough bleeding, weight gain, gastrointestinal upset, dizziness, nausea, headache, vomiting. If frequent, severe, migraine-like headaches, distrubance of vision, rise in blood pressure, jaundice or indications of thrombosis occur, drug should immediately be withdrawn, and also in the event of pregnancy. Drug should be stopped 6 weeks before planned major surgery. *Manufacturer*: Syntex.

MENZOL

Description: an hormonal progestogen preparation available in the form of scored, white tablets containing 5mg norethisterone marked NE5, MENZOL 20-day. *Used for*: menstrual pain (dysmenorrhoea), menorrhagia, premenstrual syndrome (PMS). *Dosage*: 1 tablet 2 or 3 times each day (starting at different times in the monthly cycle depending upon condition being treated). Treatment usually continues for several cycles. *Special care*: patients with disturbance of liver function. *Avoid use*: pregnancy, severe disturbance of liver function, Dublin-Johnson or Rotor syndrome, history of jaundice during pregnancy, severe pruritus (itching) or herpes gestationus (a raised itchy rash which appears in the last 3 months of pregnancy). *Side effects*: weight gain, depression, headache, vomiting, breakthrough bleeding, nausea, oedema, masculinizing (androgenic) effects. *Manufacturer*: Schwarz.

MEPTID

Description: an analgesic preparation which is an opiate partial agonist available as film-coated orange tablets containing 200mg meptazinol marked MPL-023. Also, **MEPTID INJECTION** containing 100mg meptazinol as hydrochloride/ml. *Used for*: short-term relief of pain. *Dosage*: adults, 75–100mg by intramuscular injection or 50–100mg intravenously. May be repeated every 2 to 4 hours as required. Obstetric patients, 2mg/kg body weight given intramuscularly. *Special care*: patients with liver or kidney disease, serious breathing problems. *Avoid use*: children. *Side effects*: nausea, dizziness. *Manufacturer*: Monmouth.

MERBENTYL

Description: an anticholinergic preparation available as white tablets containing 10mg dicyclomine hydrochloride, marked M within 2 circles; white oval tablets containing 20mg, marked MERBENTYL 20. Also **MERBENTYL SYRUP** containing 10mg/5ml. *Used for*: spasm of stomach and gastro-intestinal tract. *Dosage*: adults, 10–20mg 3 times each day before or after meals. Children, 6 months to 2 years, 5–10mg 3 or 4 times each day fifteen minutes before food with a maximum of 40mg daily. Over 2 years, 10mg 3 times each day. *Special care*: enlarged prostate gland, glaucoma, reflux oesophagitis with hiatus hernia. *Avoid use*: children under 6 months of age. *Side effects*: thirst, dry mouth, dizziness. *Manufacturer*: Hoechst.

MERCILON

Description: an hormonal combinal oestrogen/progestogen preparation available as white tablets containing 20 g ethinyloestradiol and 150 g desogestrel, marked TR over 4. *Used for*: oral contraception. *Dosage*: 1 tablet each day for 21 days starting on first or fifth day of monthly cycle, followed by 7 tablet-free days. *Special care*: multiple sclerosis, serious kidney disease or kidney dialysis, asthma, Raynaud's disease, abnormally high levels of prolactin in the blood (hyperprolactinaemia), varicose veins, hypertension. Also, patients suffering from severe depression. Thrombosis risk increases with smoking, age and obesity. During the course of treatment, regular checks on blood pressure, pelvic organs and breasts should be carried out. *Avoid use*: pregnancy, those at risk of thrombosis, suffering from heart disease, pulmonary hypertension, angina, sickle cell anaemia. Also, undiagnosed vaginal bleeding, history of cholestatic jaundice during pregnancy, cancers which are hormone-dependent, infectious hepatitis, liver disorders. Also, porphyria, Dublin-Johnson and Rotor syndrome, otosclerosis, chorea, haemolytic uraemic syndrome, recent trophoblastic disease. *Possible interaction*: barbiturates, ethosuximide, glutethimide, rifampicin, phenytoin, tetracyclines, carbamazepine, chloral hydrate, griseofulvin, dichloralphenazone, primidone. *Side effects*: weight gain, breast enlargement, pains in legs and cramps, headaches, loss of sexual desire, depression, nausea, breakthrough bleeding, cervical erosion, brownish patches on skin (chloasma), vaginal discharge, oedema and bloatedness. *Manufacturer*: Organon.

MESTINON

Description: an anticholinesterase preparation which acts to inhibit the enzyme that breaks down acetylcholine so that the effects of the neurotransmitter are prolonged. It is produced in the form of white, quarter-scored tablets containing 60mg pyridostigmine bromide, marked ROCHE. *Used for*: myasthenia gravis, paralytic ileus. *Dosage*: myasthenia gravis, 5 to 20 tablets each day in divided doses; paralytic ileus, 1 to 4 tablets, as needed. Children, myasthenia gravis, under 6 years, 30mg at first, 6 to 12 years, 60mg at first. Both doses may be gradually increased by 15–30mg each day until condition is controlled. *Special care*: patients with epilepsy, Parkinsonism, asthma, recent heart attack, peptic ulcer, kidney disease, bradycardia, hypotension, abnormal overactivity of vagus nerve. *Avoid use*: patients with gastro-intestinal or urinary tract obstruction. *Possible interaction*: cyclopropane, depolarizing muscle relaxants, halothane. *Side effects*: over-production of saliva, nausea, diarrhoea, colic-type pain. *Manufacturer*: Roche.

METENIX

Description: a thiazide-like diuretic preparation available as blue tablets containing 5mg metolazone marked with strength and symbol. *Used for*: oedema, toxaemia of pregnancy, hypertension, ascites (collection of fluid in peritoneal cavity of the abdomen). *Dosage*: oedema, 5–10mg as a single daily dose with a maximum of 80mg each day; hypertension, 5mg each day at first reducing after 3 to 4 weeks to this dose taken every second day. *Special care*: pregnancy, breast-feeding, elderly, liver or kidney disease, cirrhosis of the liver, gout, diabetes, collagen disease. Fluid, electrolytes (salts), and glucose levels require monitoring during the course of therapy. *Avoid use*: children, hypercalcaemia, serious liver or kidney failure, allergy to sulphonamide drugs, Addison's disease. *Possible interaction*: NSAIDs, carben-oxolone, lithium, barbiturates, tubo-curarine, alcohol, cardiac glycosides, alcohol, corticosteroids, opioids. *Side effects*: gastro-intestinal disturbance, anorexia, sensitivity to light, disturbance of electrolyte balance and metabolism, pancreatitis, rash, impotence, blood changes, dizziness. *Manufacturer*: Hoechst.

METERFOLIC

Description: a haematinic and folic acid preparation available as grey, film-coated tablets containing ferrous fumarate (equivalent to 100mg iron) and 400µg folic acid, marked METERFOLIC. *Used for*: prevention of iron and folic acid deficiency during pregnancy. As a supplement taken when pregnancy is planned to prevent neural tube defects in foetus. *Dosage*: pregnant women, 1 tablet once or twice each day; prevention of neural tube defects, 1 tablet each day before conception and continuing for at least the first third of pregnancy. *Special care*: patients with history of peptic ulcer or haemolytic anaemia. *Avoid use*: patients with vitamin B_{12} deficiency. *Possible interaction*: tetracyclines. *Side effects*: constipation and nausea. *Manufacturer*: Sinclair.

METOPIRONE

Description: a diuretic preparation which is an aldosterone inhibitor. Used with glucocorticoids, it acts to eliminate fluid which has accumulated due to increased secretion of the mineralocorticoid hormone, aldosterone. It is produced as creams containing 250mg metyrapone, coded LN and CIBA. *Used for*: in addition to glucocorticoids to treat resistant oedema caused by excess secretion of aldosterone. Also, for Cushing's syndrome. *Dosage*: adults, resistant oedema, 250mg–6g each day; Cushing's syndrome, 2.5–4.5g each day as divided doses.

Special care: patients with decreased function of the pituitary gland. *Avoid use*: pregnancy, breast-feeding, children. *Side effects*: allergic responses, nausea, vomiting, hypotension. *Manufacturer*: Ciba.

METOSYN

Description: a potent topical steroid preparation available as cream and ointment containing 0.05% fluocinonide. Also, **METOSYN SCALP LOTION** containing 0.05% fluocinonide in an alcholic solution. *Used for*: inflamed and allergic skin conditions, those producing pus. *Dosage*: apply thinly each morning and night to affected area. *Special care*: short-term use only. *Avoid use*: children, long-term or extensive use especially in pregnant women, patients with untreated bacterial or fungal infections or skin infections of tuberculous or viral origin or due to ringworm. Also, patients with dermatitis in area of mouth, acne, leg ulcers or scabies. *Side effects*: suppression of adrenal glands, skin thinning, abnormal hair growth, changes as in Cushing's syndrome. *Manufacturer*: Zeneca.

METRODIN HIGH PURITY

Description: an hormonal gonadotrophin preparation available as freeze-dried powder in ampoules, with diluent, for reconstitution and injection, containing 75 units and 150 units urofolitrophin (follicle-stimulating hormone). *Used for*: absence or reduced ovulation caused by dysfunction of the hypothalamus, which regulates the hormonal output of the pituitary gland, in turn producing hormones which control the sex organs. Also, for superovulation in women having fertility treatment (IVF). *Dosage*: hypothalamic pituitary gland dysfunction, 75–150 units each day at first by subcutaneous or intramuscular injection. Subsequent treatment depends on response. Superovulation, 150–225 units each day. *Special care*: monitoring is essential hence treatment is usually under close medical supervision. Any hormonal disorders or brain lesions must be corrected before therapy starts. *Avoid use*: pregnant women. *Side effects*: allergic reactions, over-stimulation of ovaries which may lead to enlargement or rupture, multiple pregnancy. *Manufacturer*: Serono.

METROGEL

Description: a nitroimidazole antibiotic preparation available in the form of a gel, containing 0.75% metronidazole. *Used for*: inflammatory conditions relating to acne rosacea. *Dosage*: adults, apply thinly twice each day for 8 to 9 weeks. *Avoid use*: children, pregnant women. *Side effects*: local skin irritation. *Manufacturer*: Sandoz.

METROTOP

Description: an antibacterial preparation available in the form of a gel containing 0.8% metronidazol. *Used for*: to deodorize a tumour producing an unpleasant smell because of fungus infection. *Dosage*: apply to clean wound once or twice each day and cover. *Avoid use*: pregnancy, breast-feeding. *Side effects*: local skin irritation. *Manufacturer*: Seton.

MEXITIL

Description: a class I antiarrhythmic preparation, mexiletine hydrochloride, available in a variety of different forms. Purple/red capsules contain 50mg and red capsules contain 200mg both marked with strength and symbol. Also, **MEXITIL PERLONGETS**, red/turquoise sustained-release capsules contain 360mg. **MEXITIL INJECTION** contains 25mg/ml in ampoules for injection. *Used for*: arrhythmias originating from ventricles of heart. *Dosage*: capsules, 400–600mg at first then a further 200–250mg 2 hours later repeated 3 or 4 times each day. Perlongets, 1 capsule twice each day. *Special care*: hypotension, Parkinsonism, liver, kidney or heart failure, conduction defects of the heart, bradycardia. *Avoid use*: children. *Side effects*: effects on central nervous system, hypotension, gastro-intestinal upset. *Manufacturer*: Boehringer Ing.

MFV-JECT

Description: a preparation of inactivated material derived from 3 strains of influenza virus available in pre-filled syringes containing 15 micrograms of each type/5ml suspension. *Used for*: immunization against influenza. *Dosage*: adults, 0.5ml by intramuscular or deep subcutaneous injection. Children, 6 months to 3 years, 0.25ml repeated after 1 month to 6 weeks; 3 to 12 years, 0.5ml repeated after 1 month to 6 weeks. All given by intramuscular or deep subcutaneous injection. (Children who have been vaccinated before or infected with influenza require only 1 dose). *Avoid use*: patients with feverish illness, allergic to egg protein (used in culture of viruses). *Side effects*: malaise, fever. *Manufacturer*: Merieux.

MICROGYNON 30

Description: an hormonal oestrogen/progestogen combined preparation in the form of beige, sugar-coated tablets containing 30 g ethinyloestradiol and 150 g levonorgestrel. *Used for*: oral contraception. *Dosage*: 1 tablet each day starting on first day of period followed by 7 tablet-free days. *Special care*: patients with multiple sclerosis, serious kidney disease or kidney dialysis, asthma, Raynaud's disease, abnormally high levels of prolactin in the blood (hyperprolactinaemia), varicose veins, hypertension. Also, patients suffering from severe depression. Thrombosis risk increases with smoking, age and obesity. During the course of treatment, regular checks on blood pressure, pelvic organs and breasts should be carried out. *Avoid use*: pregnancy, those at risk of thrombosis, suffering from heart disease, pulmonary hypertension, angina, sickle cell anaemia. Also, undiagnosed vaginal bleeding, history of cholestatic jaundice during pregnancy, cancers which are hormone-dependent, infectious hepatitis, liver disorders. Also, porphyria, Dublin-Johnson and Rotor syndrome, otosclerosis, chorea, haemolytic uraemic syndrome, recent trophoblastic disease. *Possible interaction*: barbiturates, ethosuximide, glutethimide, rifampicin, phenytoin, tetracyclines, carbamazepine, chloral hydrate, griseofulvin, dichloralphenazone, primidone. *Side effects*: weight gain, breast enlargement, pains in legs and cramps, headaches, loss of sexual desire, depression, nausea, breakthrough bleeding, cervical erosion, vaginal discharge, brownish patches on skin (chloasma), oedema and bloatedness. *Manufacturer*: Schering H.C.

MICRONOR

Description: an hormonal progestogen available as white tablets containing 350μg norethisterone, marked C over 035. *Used for*: oral contraception. *Dosage*: 1 tablet at same time each day starting on first day of cycle and continuing without a break. *Special care*: history of or at risk of thrombosis or embolism, liver disease, cancer which is hormone-dependent, ovarian cysts, hypertension, migraine. Blood pressure, breasts and pelvic organs should be checked regularly during the course of treatment. *Avoid use*: pregnancy, patients who have previously had a stroke, poor circulation to heart leading to heart disease, diseased arteries, previous ectopic pregnancy. Also, undiagnosed vaginal bleeding, benign tumour (adenoma) of the liver derived from glandular tissue, recent trophoblastic disease. *Possible interaction*: chloral hydrate, barbiturates, meprobamate, phenytoin, rifampicin, carbamazepine, griseofulvin, primidone, glutethimide dichloralphenazone, chlorpromazine, ethosuximide. *Side effects*: changes in pattern of menstruation, headache, ovarian cysts, sore breasts, acne. *Manufacturer*: Janssen-Cilag.

MICROVAL

Description: an hormonal progestogen available in the form of white tablets containing 30μg levonorgestrel. *Used for*: oral contraception. *Dosage*: 1 tablet at same time each day starting of first day of monthly cycle and continuing without any break. *Special care*: history of or at risk of thrombosis or embolism, liver disease, cancer which is hormone-dependent, ovarian cysts, hypertension, migraine. Blood pressure, breasts and pelvic organs should be checked regularly during the course of treatment. *Avoid use*: pregnancy, patients who have previously had a stroke, poor circulation to heart leading to heart disease, diseased arteries, previous ectopic pregnancy. Also, women with undiagnosed vaginal bleeding, benign tumour (adenoma) of the liver derived from glandular tissue, recent trophoblastic disease. *Possible interaction*: chloral hydrate, barbiturates, meprobamate, phenytoin, rifampicin, carbamazepine, griseofulvin, primidone, glutethimide dichloralphenazone, chlorpromazine, ethosuximide. *Side effects*: changes in pattern of menstruation, headache, ovarian cysts, sore breasts, acne. *Manufacturer*: Wyeth.

MICTRAL

Description: a compound preparation combining a quinolone and alkalysing agent available as dissolvable granules in sachets, containing 660mg nalidixic acid, anhydrous citric acid, sodium bicarbonate and sodium citrate (equivalent to 4.1g citrate). *Used for*: cystitis and infections of lower urinary tract. *Dosage*: adults, 1 sachet in water taken 3 times daily in divided doses for a period of 3 days. *Special care*: pregnancy, breast-feeding, liver disease. Sunlight should be avoided. *Avoid use*: children, patients with kidney disorders, history of fits, porphyria. *Possible interaction*: antibacterials and anticoagulants. *Side effects*: sensitivity to light, gastro-intestinal upset, skin rashes, haemolytic anaemia, disturbance of vision, convulsions, blood changes. *Manufacturer*: Sanofi Winthrop.

MIDAMOR

Description: a potassium-sparing diuretic preparation available as diamond-shaped, yellow tablets containing 5mg amiloride hydrochloride marked MSD 92. *Used for*: used with other diuretics to save potassium. *Dosage*: 1 or 2 tablets each day with a daily maximum of 4. *Special care*: pregnancy, breast-feeding, kidney or liver disease, acidosis, gout, a tendency to hyperkalaemia due to diabetes. *Avoid use*: children, patients with serious or worsening kidney failure, hyperkalaemia, anuria. *Possible interaction*: ACE inhibitors, lithium, potassium-sparing diuretics, potassium supplements. *Side effects*: skin rash, gastro-intestinal upset. *Manufacturer*: Morson.

MIFEGYNE

Description: a preparation which is a progesterone antagonist available as bi-convex, cylindrical-shaped, yellow tablets containing 200mg mifepristone, marked with logo and 167 B. *Used for*: termination of early pregnancy, up to 63 days of gestation. *Dosage*: adults, 600mg as a single dose under close medical supervision. *Special care*: close observation required and patient may require further treatment to complete termination. Patients with obstructive airways disease or asthma, heart disease, replacement heart valves, kidney or liver disease, history of infected endocarditis. Patients should not take NSAIDs or aspirin for at least 12 days. *Avoid use*: women with more advanced pregnancy over 64 days, ectopic or suspected ectopic pregnancy, porphyria, haemorrhage or bleeding disorders, women who smoke aged over 35 years. Also, patients receiving anticoagulant therapy or who have had long-term treatment with corticosteroids. *Possible interaction*: aspirin, NSAIDs. *Side effects*: vomiting, nausea, vaginal bleeding which may be severe, fainting, malaise, womb and urinary tract infections, skin rashes. *Manufacturer*: Hoechst.

MIGRAVESS FORTE

Description: a compound preparation which is an anti-emetic and analgesic available in the form of effervescent, scored white tablets containing 5mg metoclopramide and 450mg aspirin marked F over F. Also, **MIGRAVESS EFFERVESCENT**, scored, white tablets containing 5mg metoclopramide and 325mg aspirin, marked M over M. *Used for*: relief of migraine. *Dosage*: adults, 2 tablets in water at start of migraine attack with a maximum daily dose of 6 tablets. Children, 12 to 15 years, half adult dose. *Special care*: pregnancy, liver or kidney disease, asthma. *Avoid use*: children under 12 years, patients with allergy to aspirin or NSAIDs, peptic ulcer, bleeding disorders. *Possible interaction*: anticoagulants, phenothiazines, uricosurics, anticholinergics, hypoglycaemics, butyrophenones. *Side effects*: sleepiness, extrapyramidal symptoms (characterized by involuntary and reflex muscle movements and changes in tone of muscles), diarrhoea, rise in levels of prolactin in blood. *Manufacturer*: Bayer.

MIGRIL

Description: a compound preparation combining an ergot alkaloid, antihistamine and xanthine produced as scored, white tablets containing 2mg ergotamine tartrate, 50mg cyclizine hydrochloride, 50mg caffeine hydrate, coded WELLCOME A4A. *Used for*: relief of migraine. *Dosage*: 1 at start of migraine attack followed by ½ to 1 tablet at 30 minute intervals. Maximum dose is 4 tablets for 1 migraine attack and 6 weekly. *Special care*: patients with hyperthyroidism, sepsis, anaemia. *Avoid use*: pregnancy, breast-feeding, children, patients with heart or circulatory disease, liver or kidney disorders, serious hypertension. *Possible interaction*: ß-blockers, central nervous system depressants, erythromycin. *Side effects*: sleepiness, rebound headache, pain in abdomen, dry mouth, peripheral ischaemia. *Manufacturer*: Glaxo Wellcome.

MILDISON LIPOCREAM

Description: a mildly potent topical steroid preparation available in the form of a cream containing 1% hydrocortisone. *Used for*: dermatitis and eczema. *Dosage*: apply to affected skin 2 or 3 times each day. *Special care*: use on face or in children should be limited to a maximum period of 5 days. Stop using gradually after longer-term use. *Avoid use*: long-term use or as a preventative especially by pregnant women, patients with untreated bacterial or fungal infections, skin infections of tuberculous or viral origin, scabies or ringworm. Also, leg ulcers, dermatitis in area of mouth, acne. *Side effects*: changes as in Cushing's syndrome, skin thinning, abnormal hair growth, suppression of adrenal glands. *Manufacturer*: Yamanouchi.

MINIHEP

Description: an anticoagulant preparation available as a solution in pre-filled syringes containing 5000 units sodium heparin/0.2ml. Also, **MINIHEP CALCIUM** solution in pre-filled syringes and ampoules containing 5000 units calcium heparin/0.2ml. Both are for subcutaneous injection only. *Used for*: pulmonary embolism and deep vein thrombosis. *Dosage*: 15,000 units every 12 hours; children 250 units/kg body weight 12 hourly. Both following on from first doses given by intravenous infusion or injection. *Special care*: pregnancy, kidney or liver disease. Drug should be withdrawn gradually if taken for more than 5 days. Platelet counts are required if taken for more than 5 days. *Avoid use*: bleeding disorders, haemophilia, serious hypertension, recent operation on eye or nervous system, cerebral aneurysm, serious liver disease, peptic ulcer, allergy to heparin, thrombocytopenia. *Possible interaction*: aspirin, dipyridamole, glyceryl trinitrate infusion. *Side effects*: allergic reactions, skin necrosis, osteoporosis (if taken long-term). Stop drug immediately if thrombocytopenia occurs. *Manufacturer*: Leo.

MINIMS AMETHOCAINE

Description: a topical anaesthetic preparation for the eye, in the form of drops in 2 strengths containing 0.5% or 1% amethocaine hydrochloride in single dose units. *Used for*: anaesthesia for eye during ophthalmic procedures. *Dosage*: adults and children, except newborn babies, 1 drop as required. *Special care*: protect eye. *Avoid use*: newborn babies. *Possible interaction*: sulphonamides. *Side effects*: short-lived burning sensation, dermatitis. *Manufacturer*: Chauvin.

MINIMS ATROPINE

Description: an anticholinergic preparation for the eye in the form of single-dose drops containing 1% atropine sulphate. *Used for*: to produce mydnasis (dilation of the pupil of the eye by contraction of certain muscles in the iris) and cytoplegia (paralysis of the muscles of accommodation in the eye along with relaxation of the ciliary muscle). This is to allow examination of eye. *Dosage*: adults and children, 1 drop as required. *Special care*: patients should not drive for 2 hours. *Avoid use*: patients with glaucoma. *Side effects*: contact dermatitis, occasionally toxic systemic reactions especially in elderly persons and children. Closed angle glaucoma is possible especially in elderly patients. *Manufacturer*: Chauvin.

MINIMS BENOXINATE

Description: a topical anaesthetic preparation for the eye produced in the form of single dose drops containing 0.4% oxybuprocaine hydrochloride. *Used for*: anaesthesia of eye during ophthalmic procedures. *Dosage*: 1 or more drops as needed. *Manufacturer*: Chauvin.

MINIMS CHLORAMPHENICOL

Description: a broad-spectrum antibiotic preparation produced in the form of single dose eyedrops containing 0.5% chloramphenicol. *Used for*: bacterial eye infections. *Dosage*: adults, 1 or more drops, as needed; children, 1 drop as needed. *Special care*: remove contact lenses. *Possible interaction*: chymotrypsin. *Side effects*: rarely, aplastic anaemia. Stop treatment immediately if local allergic reactions occur. *Manufacturer*: Chauvin.

MINIMS CYCLOPENTOLATE

Description: an anticholinergic eye preparation produced in the form of single dose eyedrops of 2 strengths containing 0.5% or 1% cyclopentolate hydrochloride. *Used for*: mydriasis (dilation of the pupil of the eye by contraction of certain muscles in the iris) and cytoplegia (paralysis of the muscles of accommodation within the eye along with relaxation of the ciliary muscle). This is in order to allow ophthalmic procedures to be carried out. *Dosage*: adults and children (except newborn babies), 1 or 2 drops as needed. *Special care*: patient with raised pressure within eye. *Avoid use*: patients with narrow angle glaucoma. *Side effects*: contact dermatitis, rarely toxic systemic effects especially in elderly and children, closed angle glaucoma is possible especially in elderly patients. *Manufacturer*: Chauvin.

MINIMS GENTAMICIN

Description: an antibiotic aminoglycoside preparation produced in the form of single dose eye drops containing 0.3% gentamicin as sulphate. *Used for*: bacterial infections of the eye. *Dosage*: 1 drop as required. *Manufacturer*: Chauvin.

MINIMS HOMATROPINE

Description: an anticholinergic eye preparation produced in the form of single dose drops containing 2% homatropine hydrobromide. *Used for*: to produce mydriasis (dilation of the pupil of the eye by contraction of certain muscles in the iris) and cytoplegia (paralysis of the muscles of accommodation in the eye along with relaxation of the ciliary muscle). *Used for*: narrow angle glaucoma. *Dosage*: adults and children, 1 or more drops as needed. *Special care*: patients should not drive for 2 hours. *Side effects*: contact dermatitis, possibly closed angle glaucoma in elderly patients. *Manufacturer*: Chauvin.

MINIMS LIGNOCAINE and FLUORESCEIN

Description: an eye preparation which is a local anaesthetic and stain available in the form of single dose eye drops containing 4% lignocaine hydrochloride and 0.25% fluorescein sodium. *Used for*: ophthalmic procedures. *Dosage*: adults and children, 1 or more drops as needed. *Manufacturer*: Chauvin.

MINIMS METIPRANOLOL

Description: a non-selective ß-blocker produced in the form of single dose eyedrops of 2 strengths containing 0.1% and 0.3% metipranolol. *Used for*: control of raised pressure within eye following surgery. Also, for chronic glaucoma in patients wearing soft contact lenses or who are allergic to preservatives. *Dosage*: glaucoma, 1 drop into eye twice each day. *Avoid use*: patients with obstructive airways disease, asthma, heart failure, bradycardia, heart block. *Possible interaction*: verapamil and possibly other drugs following systemic absorption. *Side effects*: dry eyes, allergic blepharoconjunctivitis (involving lining of eyelids). *Manufacturer*: Chauvin.

MINIMS NEOMYCIN

Description: an aminoglycoside broad-spectrum antibiotic preparation produced in the form of single dose eyedrops containing 0.5% neomycin sulphate. *Used for*: bacterial eye infections. *Dosage*: adults, 1 or more drops as needed. Children, 1 drop as needed. *Manufacturer*: Chauvin.

MINIMS PILOCARPINE

Description: a miotic preparation (one which causes contraction of the pupil) which is a cholinergic agonist and acts to cause constriction of the ciliary eye muscle. This helps to open drainage channels hence reducing pressure within the eye. It is produced as single dose eyedrops in 3 strengths containing 1%, 2% and 4% pilocarpine nitrate. *Used for*: emergency treatment of glaucoma. To reverse the effect of weak mydriatic drugs. *Dosage*: 1 drop every 5 minutes until the pupil is contracted. *Side effects*: headache, blurred vision, bradycardia, colic pains, sweating, over-production of saliva, bronchospasm may occur if systemic absorption (into body) of eyedrops occur. *Manufacturer*: Chauvin.

MINIMS PREDNISOLONE

Description: a corticosteroid preparation available as single dose eyedrops containing 0.5% prednisolone sodium. *Used for*: inflammation of the eye which is not infected. *Dosage*: adults and children, 1 or 2 drops every 1 or 2 hours then reduce frequency when condition improves. *Avoid use*: pregnancy, glaucoma or tuberculous, viral or fungal infections or those producing pus. Avoid long-term treatment in babies. *Side effects*: thinning of cornea, "steroid cataract" (especially prolonged use and higher doses), rise in pressure within eye, fungal infection. *Manufacturer*: Chauvin.

MINIMS TROPICAMIDE

Description: an anticholinergic preparation available as single dose eyedrops in 2 strengths containing 0.5% and 1% tropicamide. *Used for*: as a short-term mydriatic and cycloplegic drug. (A mydriatic produces mydriasis—dilation of the pupil of the eye by contraction of certain muscles in the iris. A cycloplegic produces cycloplegia—paralysis of the muscles of accommodation in the eye along with relaxation of the ciliary muscle). Enables ophthalmic examinations and procedures to be carried out. *Dosage*: adults and children, 1 or 2 drops every 5 minutes then repeated after 30 minutes if needed. *Special care*: in babies, pressure should be applied over the tear sac for 1 minute. Patients should not drive for 2 hours. *Avoid use*: patients with narrow angle glaucoma. *Side effects*: stinging on application which is short-lived. *Manufacturer*: Chauvin.

MINOCIN

Description: a tetracycline antibiotic available as film-coated orange tablets containing 100mg minocycline as hydrochloride, marked M over 100 on one side and LL on the other. Also, **MINOCIN MR**, yellow/brown modified-release capsules containing 100mg marked 8560 and Lederle. Also **MINOCIN 50**, beige, film-coated tablets containing 50mg marked M50 on one side and LL on the other. *Used for*: Minocin: ear, nose and throat, respiratory, soft tissue, skin and urinary tract infections. Minocin MR: acne. *Dosage*: adults, Minocin, 100mg twice each day; Minocin MR 1 each day swallowed whole; Minocin 50 1 tablet twice each day for at least 6 weeks. *Special care*: patients with liver disorder.

Avoid use: children, pregnancy, breast-feeding, kidney failure. *Possible interaction*: mineral supplements, antacids, penicillins. *Side effects*: gastro-intestinal upset, superinfections; rarely, disorders of balance, allergic responses. *Manufacturer*: Wyeth.

MINODIAB

Description: a sulphonylurea available as scored, white tablets of 2 strengths containing 2.5mg and 5mg glipizide. *Used for*: maturity-onset diabetes. *Dosage*: adults, 2.5mg or 5mg each day at first increasing by 2.5–5mg every week. The usual maintenance dose is 2.5–30mg each day, maximum 40mg. Doses higher than 15mg each day should be divided and taken about 15 minutes before meals. *Special care*: elderly, kidney failure. *Avoid use*: pregnancy, breast-feeding, children, patients with other types of diabetes (juvenile, unstable-brittle, growth-onset diabetes), serious liver or kidney diseases, hormonal disorders. Also patients with ketoacidosis, infections, stress, undergoing surgery. *Possible interaction*: anticoagulants taken orally, bezafibrate, aspirin, corticotrophin, corticosteroids, clofibrate, ß-blockers, alcohol, chlorpropamide, acetohexamide, melformin, MAOIs, oral contrraceptives, sulphonamides, glucagon, diuretics, phenylbutazone, chloramphenicol, cyclophosphamide, rifampicin. *Side effects*: allergic reactions including skin rash. *Manufacturer*: Pharmacia & Upjohn.

MINTEZOL

Description: an antihelmintic preparation used to treat infestation with various kinds of worm; available as scored, orange, chewable tablets containing 500mg thiabendazole. *Used for*: guinea worm, threadworm, hookworm, trichinosis, large roundworm, larva migrans, whipworm. *Dosage*: adults and children over 60kg body weight, 1.5g twice each day with meals. Less than 60kg, 25mg/kg twice each day with meals. *Special care*: patients with liver or kidney disorder. *Avoid use*: pregnancy, breast-feeding. *Possible interaction*: xanthine derivatives. *Side effects*: disturbances of vision and hearing, reduction in alertness, allergic reactions, liver damage, gastro-intestinal upset, hypotension, central nervous system disturbance, enuresis (incontinence, especially bedwetting). *Manufacturer*: M.S.D.

MINULET

Description: an hormonal combined oestrogen/progestogen preparation available as sugar-coated white tablets containing 30 g ethinyloestradiol and 75 g gestodene. *Used for*: oral contraception. Dosage: 1 tablet each day for 21 days beginning on first day of period followed by 7 tablet-free days. *Special care*: patients with multiple sclerosis, serious kidney disease, kidney dialysis, asthma, Raynaud's disease, abnormally high levels of prolactin in the blood (hyperprolactinaemia), varicose veins, hypertension. Also, patients suffering severe depression. Thrombosis risk increases with smoking, age and obesity. During the course of treatment, regular checks on blood pressure, pelvic organs and breasts should be carried out. *Avoid use*: pregnancy, patients considered to be at risk of thrombosis, suffering from heart disease, pulmonary hypertension, angina, sickle cell anaemia. Also, undiagnosed vaginal bleeding, history of cholestatic jaundice during pregnancy, cancers which are hormone-dependent, infectious hepatitis, liver disorders. Also, porphyria, Dublin-Johnson and Rotor syndrome, otosclerosis, chorea, haemolytic uraemic syndrome, recent trophoblastic disease. *Possible interaction*: barbiturates, ethosuximide, glutethimide, rifampicin, phenytoin, tetracyclines, carbamazepine, chloral hydrate, griseofulvin, dichloralphenazone, primidone. *Side effects*: weight gain, breast enlargement, pains in legs and cramps, headaches, loss of sexual desire, depression, nausea, breakthrough bleeding, cervical erosion, brownish patches on skin (chloasma), vaginal discharge, oedema and bloatedness. *Manufacturer*: Wyeth.

MITHRACIN

Description: a cytotoxic antibiotic preparation available as a powder in vials for reconstitution and injection containing 2.5mg plicamycin. *Used for*: hypercalcaemia due to malignancy. *Dosage*: 25μg/kg body 8 each day for 3 to 4 days repeated at minimum intervals of 1 week if necessary. Maintenance dose is 25μg/kg 1 to 3 times each week, all by intravenous infusion. *Special care*: patients with liver or kidney disease. *Side effects*: irritant to tissues, bone marrow suppression, vomiting, nausea, hair loss. *Manufacturer*: Pfizer.

MITOXANA

Description: an alkylating cytotoxic drug, available as powder in vials for reconstitution and injection in 2 strengths containing 1g and 2g ifosfamide. *Used for*: lymphomas, solid tumours, chronic lymphocytic leukaemia, usually given with mesna (*see* Uromitexan, a drug which lessens or prevents the toxic effects of ifosfamide on the bladder). *Dosage*: given intravenously as directed by physician. *Special care*: ensure plenty of fluids are taken—3 to 4 litres each day following injection. *Possible interaction*: warfarin. *Side effects*: bone marrow suppression, nausea, vomiting, hair loss, haemorrhagic cystitis (risk is reduced with increased fluid intake and mesna). *Manufacturer*: Asta Medica.

MIVACRON

Description: a short-acting, non-depolarizing muscle relaxant available in ampoules for injection containing 2mg mivacurium as chloride/ml. *Used for*: muscle paralysis during surgical operations. *Dosage*: adults, by intravenous injection, 70–150μg/kg body 8 at first then 100μg/kg every 15 minutes. By intravenous infusion, to maintain paralysis, 8–10μg/kg/minute, adjusted if needed to usual dose of 6–7μg/kg/minute. Children, intravenous injection, age 2 to 12 years, 100–200μg/kg at first then 100 g/kg every 6 to 7 minutes. Intravenous infusion, 10–15μg/kg/minute. *Special care*: patients with heart disease or asthma (slower injection rate required). *Avoid use*: patients with myasthenia gravis. *Possible interaction*: clindamycin, azlocillin, colistin, verapamil, nifedipine, dantrolene, ecothiopate, demacarium, neostigmine, pyridostiamine, magnesium salts. *Manufacturer*: Glaxo Wellcome.

MMR II

Description: a preparation of measles, mumps and rubella vaccine. It contains measles, mumps and rubella vaccine along with 0.25mg neomycin and is available as powder in vials, with diluent. *Used for*: immunization of children (and some adults) against measles, mumps and rubella. *Dosage*: children over 12 months, 0.5ml by subcutaneous or intramuscular injection. *Special care*: history of convulsions and feverishness, altered immunity states in whom fever is undesirable, patients who have had blood or plasma transfusion within last 3 months. *Avoid use*: pregnancy, women should avoid pregnancy for 3 months after vaccination. Acute feverish illnesses, thrombocytopenia, history of symptoms of anaphylaxis to eggs or neomycin (egg protein is used in culture of virus for vaccine). Do not give within 1 month of other live vaccines. *Possible interaction*: live vaccines. *Side effects*: allergic responses, fever, headache, malaise, skin rash. *Manufacturer*: Pasteur Merieux MSD.

MOBIFLEX

Description: an NSAID belonging to the Oxicam group available as film-coated, pentagonal brown tablets containing 20mg tenoxicam marked Mobiflex. Also, **MOBIFLEX MILK** granules in sachets containing 20mg; **MOBIFLEX EFFERVESCENT** tablets containing 20mg. **MOBIFLEX INJECTION** available as powder in vials for reconstitution containing 20mg. *Used for*: rheumatoid arthritis, osteoarthritis, treatment of soft tissue injuries, (short-term only). *Dosage*: 1 tablet or sachet in water each day; injection, 20mg by intravenous or intramuscular injection for first 1 or 2 days, then tablets or granules. *Special care*: elderly patients, those with liver or kidney disease or heart failure. *Avoid use*: pregnancy, children, inflammation of gastro-intestinal tract or bleeding, history of or actual peptic ulcer, allergy to NSAID or aspirin. *Possible interaction*: hypoglycaemics taken orally, lithium, anticoagulants, other NSAIDs. *Side effects*: headache, blood changes, skin rash, gastro-intestinal upset, rise in level of liver enzymes, oedema, distubance of vision. *Manufacturer*: Roche.

MODALIM

Description: an isobutyric acid derivative used to lower the levels of lipds (fats) in the blood. It is available as capsule-shaped, white, scored tablets containing 100mg ciprofibrate and marked MODALIM. *Used for*: hyperlipidaemias (elevated blood lipid levels) of types IIa, IIb, III and IV which cannot be controlled by diet alone. *Dosage*: adults, 1 or 2 tablets as a single daily dose. *Special care*: liver or kidney disease; live tests should be carried out during the course of treatment. *Avoid use*: pregnancy, breast-feeding, children, severe liver or kidney disease. *Possible interaction*: hypoglycaemics taken by mouth, oral contraceptives, anticoagulants. *Side effects*: vertigo, gastro-intestinal upset, loss of hair, impotence, muscle pain; rarely, sleepiness, dizziness. *Manufacturer*: Sanofi Winthrop.

MODECATE

Description: an antipsychotic preparation which is a depot phenothiazine group III, available in ampoules and disposable syringes containing 25mg fluphenazine decanoate/ml. Also **MODECATE CONCENTRATE** in ampoules containing 100mg/ml. *Used for*: maintenance of certain psychiatric illnesses especially schizophrenia. *Dosage*: adults, 12.5mg by deep intramuscular injection (into gluteal muscle) as first test dose in order to see if patient is liable to experience extrapyramidal (e.g. involuntary, reflex-type muscle movements) symptoms. Then, usual dose in the order of 12.5mg–100mg, according to response, every 2 to 5 weeks. Elderly receive lower initial test dose of 6.25mg. *Special care*: elderly, patients who exhibit extrapyramidal symptoms (reduce dose or use alternative drug), pregnancy, breast-feeding, patients wtih myasthenia gravis. Also heart disease, heart arrhythmias, epilepsy, liver or respiratory diseases, enlarged prostate gland, underactive thyroid gland, glaucoma, thyrotoxicosis. *Avoid use*: children, patients with phaeochromocytoma, liver or kidney failure, severe heart disease, severe atherosclerosis of cerebral arteries, coma. Also those suffering from severe depression. *Possible interaction*: alcohol, antacids, TCADs, antihypertensives, calcium-channel blockers, cimetidine. *Side effects*: extrapyramidal symptoms, effects on heart and heart rhythm, effects on central nervous system and EEG, sleepiness, apathy, depression, dry mouth, blocked nose, difficulty passing urine, constipation. Hormonal changes, effects on mestruation, enlargement of breasts, abnormal production of breast milk, impotence. Blood changes, skin rashes, jaundice, effects on liver. Effects on eyes, blurred vision, pigmentation of skin and eyes. *Manufacturer*: Sanofi Winthrop.

MODITEN

Description: an antipsychotic preparation which is a phenothiazine group III drug available as sugar-coated tablets in 3 strengths all containing fluphenazine hydrochloride; pink 1mg, yellow 2.5mg and white 5mg. *Used for*: schizophrenia, paranoia, mania, hypomania, short-term treatment of anxiety, agitation and disordered behaviour. *Dosage*: adults, schizophrenia and psychoses, 2.5mg–10mg as 2 or 3 divided doses each day with a maximum of 20mg. Anxiety and agitation, 1–2mg twice each day at first and then according to response. Elderly persons receive lower doses. *Special care*: patients who exhibit extrapyramidal reactions (e.g. involuntary reflex-type muscle movements) should receive lower doses or alternative drug; pregnancy, breast-feeding. Myasthenia gravis, enlarged prostate gland, thyrotoxicosis, heart disease, heart arrhythmias, epilepsy, liver or respiratory diseases, underactive thyroid gland, glaucoma. *Avoid use*: children, serious heart conditions, phaeochromocytoma, liver or kidney failure, severe atherosclerosis of cerebral arteries, coma. Also, patients who are severely depressed. *Possible interaction*: alcohol, antacids, TCADs, antihypertensives, calcium-channel blockers, cimetidine. *Side effects*: extrapyramidal symptoms, effects on heart and heart rhythm, effects on central nervous system and EEG, sleepiness, apathy, depression, dry mouth, blocked nose, difficulty passing urine, constipation. Hormonal changes, effects on mestruation, enlargement of breasts, abnormal production of breast milk, impotence. Blood changes, skin rashes, jaundice, effects on liver. Effects on eyes, blurred vision, pigmentation of skin and eyes. *Manufacturer*: Sanofi Winthrop.

MODRASONE

Description: a moderately potent topical steroid preparation available as cream and ointment containing 0.05% alclometasone diproprionate. *Used for*: skin conditions which respond to steroids. *Dosage*: apply thinly 2 or 3 times each day. *Special care*: do not use on face or in children for more than 5 days. Withdraw treatment gradually if use has been long-term. *Avoid use*: extensive or long-term use, especially pregnant women, or as a preventative. Patients with untreated fungal or bacterial infections, skin conditions with tuberculous or viral origin or ringworm. Also, patients with leg ulcers, acne, scabies, dermatitis in area of mouth. *Side effects*: changes as in Cushing's syndrome, skin thinning, suppression of adrenal glands, abnormal hair growth. *Manufacturer*: Dominion.

MODRENAL

Description: a preparation of a drug which inhibits the production of corticosteroid hormones by the adrenal glands. It is available as capsules of 2 strengths; black/pink capsules containing 60mg trilostane and yellow/pink capsules containing 120mg. Both are marked with the strength of the capsules. *Used for*: excessive activity of adrenal cortex resulting in excess hormone release as in primary aldosteronism (oversecretion of aldosterone, also called Conn's syndrome) and hypercortisolism. Also for breast cancer in post-menopausal women. *Dosage*: adults, 60mg 4 times each day at first then, according to response, adjusted to a usual daily dose in the order of 120mg–480mg as divided doses. The maximum is 960mg each day. Breast cancer, the initial dose is 240mg each day increasing by this amount at 3 day intervals to a maximum 960mg. Glucocorticoid treatment should be given at the same time in these patients. *Special care*: eliminate the presence of a tumour producing ACTH (adrenocorticotrophic hormone) before treatment begins, patients with kidney or liver disease, suffering from stress. Non-hormonal methods of contraception should be used. *Avoid use*: pregnancy, patients with serious liver or kidney disease. *Possible interaction*: aldosterone antagonists, potassium supplements, triamterene, amiloride. *Side effects*: nausea, diarrhoea, flushing, runny nose. *Manufacturer*: Wanskerne.

MODUCREN

Description: a compound antihypertensive preparation combining a non-cardioselective ß-blocker, a thiazide and potassium-sparing diuretic available as scored, blue tablets containing 25mg hydrochlorthiazide, 2.5mg amiloride hydrochloride and 10mg timolol maleate, marked MODUCREN. *Used for*: hypertension. *Dosage*: adults, 1 or 2 tablets as a single dose each day. *Special care*: pregnancy, breast-feeding, patients with weak hearts may require diuretics and digitalis, those with diabetes, undergoing general anaesthesia, kidney or liver disorders, gout. Electrolyte (salts) levels may need to be monitored. *Avoid use*: history of bronchospasm or obstructive airways disease, heart block, heart shock, uncompensated heart failure, disease of peripheral arteries, bradycardia. Patients with serious or worsening kidney failure or anuria. *Possible interaction*: sympathomimetics, class I antiarrhythmics, central nervous system depressants, clonidine withdrawal, ergot alkaloids, cardiac depressant anaesthetics, verapamil, reserpine, indomethacin, hypoglycaemics, cimetidine, other antihypertensives. Digitalis, potassium supplements, potassium-sparing diuretics, lithium. *Side effects*: cold hands and feet, disturbance of sleep, fatigue on exercise, bronchospasm, bradycardia, gastro-intestinal disturbances, heart failure, blood changes, gout, sensitivity to light, muscle weakness. If skin rash or dry eyes occur, withdraw drug gradually. *Manufacturer*: Morson.

MODURET 25

Description: a compound preparation combining a potassium-sparing and thiazide diuretic available as diamond-shaped, off-white tablets containing 2.5mg amiloride hydrochloride and 25mg hydrochlorothiazide, coded MSD 923. *Used for*: hypertension, congestive heart failure, liver cirrhosis (accompanied by an abnormal collection of fluid in the abdomen, ascites). *Dosage*: adults, 1 to 4 tablets each day in divided doses. *Special care*: patients with liver or kidney disorders, diabetes, acidosis and gout. *Avoid use*: children, pregnancy, breast-feeding, serious or worsening kidney failure, hyperkalaemia. *Possible interaction*: lithium, ACE inhibitors, potassium supplements and potassium-sparing diuretics, antihypertensives, digitalis. *Manufacturer*: DuPont.

MODURETIC

Description: a compound preparation combining a potassium-sparing and thiazide diuretic available in the form of diamond-shaped, scored, peach tablets containing 5mg amiloride hydrochloride and 50mg hydrochlorothiazide, marked NSD 917. Also, **MODURETIC SOLUTION** (in 5ml). *Used for*: hypertension, congestive heart failure, liver cirrhosis (accompanied by an abnormal collection of fluid in the abdomen, ascites). *Dosage*: 1 or 2 tablets or 5–10ml solution each day as single or divided doses. May be increased, if required, to a daily maximum of 4 tablets or 20ml. *Special care*: liver or kidney disorders, acidosis, gout, diabetes. *Avoid use*: children, pregnancy, breast-feeding, hyperkalaemia. *Possible interaction*: lithium, potassium-sparing diuretics, potassium supplements, antihypertensives, digitalis. *Side effects*: sensitivity to light, gout, rash, blood changes. *Manufacturer*: DuPont.

MOGADON

Description: a long-acting benzodiazepine preparation available as scored, white tablets containing 5mg nitrazepam marked with 2 "eyes" and ROCHE. *Used for*: insomnia, short-term only. *Dosage*: adults, 5–10mg, elderly persons, 2.5–5mg, with doses taken at bedtime. *Special care*: kidney or liver disorders, lung insufficiency, pregnancy, labour, breast-feeding. For short-term treatment as drug dependence and tolerance may develop. *Avoid use*: history of drug or alcohol abuse, serious lung insufficiency and depressed respiration. Suffering from psychoses, obsessional or phobic states. *Possible interaction*: CNS depressants, alcohol, anticonvulsants. *Side effects*: headache, drowsiness, loss of coordination (ataxia), confusion, hypotension, gastro-intestinal upset. Skin rash, retention of urine, changes in libido, vertigo, disturbance of vision. Rarely, jaundice and blood disorders. *Manufacturer*: Roche.

MOLIPAXIN

Description: an antidepressant preparation available in a variety of different forms, all containing trazodone hydrochloride. Pink, film-coated, scored tablets (150mg) are marked MOLIPAXIN 150. **MOLIPAXIN CAPSULES** are green/purple (50mg) marked with logo and R365B; fawn/purple (100mg) marked with logo and R365C. **MOLIPAXIN CR**, blue, octagonal-shaped sustained-release tablets (150mg) marked with strength and name. **MOLIPAXIN LIQUID** contains 50mg/5ml. *Used for*: depression which may be accompanied by anxiety. *Dosage*: 150mg each day as divided doses taken after meals or single night-time dose. After 1 week, dose may be increased to 300mg each day with a maximum of 600mg. Elderly persons, 100mg each day in divided doses after meals or as a single night-time dose. Maximum of 300mg each day. *Special care*: serious kidney or liver disease or epilepsy. *Avoid use*: children. *Possible interaction*: CNS depressants, clonidine, muscle relaxants, MAOIs, some anaesthetics. *Side effects*: dizziness, headache, drowsines. Discontinue if priapism (abnormal, persistent erection of penis, which is painful and not associated with sexual arousal) occurs. *Manufacturer*: Hoechst.

MONASPOR

Description: a cephalosporin antibiotic preparation available as powder in vials for reconstitution and injection containing 1g cefsulodin sodium. *Used for*: urinary tract, soft tissue, respiratory and some bone infections. Infections caused by the organism *Pseudomonas aerugginosa*. *Dosage*: adults, 1–4g daily in 2, 3 or 4 divided doses by intravenous or intramuscular injection. Children, 20–50mg/kg body weight each day by intravenous or intramuscular injection. *Special care*: pregnancy, patients allergic to penicillin, kidney failure. Tests of kidney function and blood counts should be carried out if taking drug long-term. *Possible interaction*: aminoglycosides, loop diuretics. *Side effects*: blood changes (abnormal reduction in number of blood platelets and white cells), gastro-intestinal upset, candidiasis (thrush), rise in level of blood urea and liver enzymes. Positive Coomb's test (a test for rhesus antibodies). *Manufacturer*: Ciba.

MONIT

Description: an antianginal nitrate preparation available as scored, white tablets containing 20mg isosorbide mononitrate marked STUART 20. Also, **MONIT LS**, white tablets containing 10mg and marked STUART 10; **MONIT SR**, white, sugar-coated sustained-release tablets containing 40mg. *Used for*: prevention of angina. *Dosage*: 1 tablet each day in the morning. *Avoid use*: children. *Side effects*: flushes, headache, dizziness. *Manufacturer*: Lorex.

MONOCLATE-P

Description: a preparation of freeze-dried coagulation factor VIII with antihaemophiliac activities of 250, 500 and 1000 units in vials for injection. *Used for*: treatment of haemophilia A. *Dosage*: by intravenous infusion according to body weight and severity of condition. *Special care*: in patients with blood groups A, B or AB there is a possibility of haemolysis after large or numerous doses. *Side effects*: allergic reactions, nausea, chills, pain at injection site. If more pronounced hypersensitivity reactions occur, discontinue treatment. *Manufacturer*: Centeon.

MONOCOR

Description: an antianginal and anti-hypertensive preparation which is a cardioselective ß-blocker available as pink, scored, film-coated tablets containing 5mg bisoprolol fumarate, marked 5 on one side and LL on the other. Also, white film-coated tablets containing 10mg, marked 10 on one side and LL on the other. *Used for*: angina and hypertension. *Dosage*: usual dose is 10mg once each day with a maximum of 20mg. *Special care*: pregnancy, breast-feeding, patients with weak hearts may require diuretics and digitalis. Also, liver or kidney disease, general anaesthesia, metabolic acidosis, diabetes. Drug should be gradually withdrawn. *Avoid use*: obstructive airways disease, history of bronchospasm, heart block, heart shock, uncompensated heart failure, sick sinus syndrome, disease of peripheral arteries, bradycardia. *Possible interaction*: CNS depressants, verapamil, indomethacin, reserpine, class I antiarrhythmics, hypoglycaemics, clonidine withdrawal, sympathomimetics, cardiac depressants anaesthetics, ergot alkaloids, antihypertensives. *Side effects*: gastro-intestinal upset, fatigue on exercise, cold hands and feet, disturbance of sleep, bronchospasm, bradycardia, heart failure. If skin rash or dry eyes occur, drug should be gradually withdrawn. *Manufacturer*: Wyeth.

MONONINE

Description: a preparation of freeze-dried human coagulation factor IX with slight antihaemophiliac activity. Available as 250, 500 and 1000 unit vials. *Used for*: haemophilia B. *Dosage*: by intravenous infusion depending on patient's weight and severity of bleeding. *Special care*: risk of thrombosis. *Avoid use*:

widespread coagulation within blood vessels. *Side effects*: allergic reactions, flushing, vomiting and nausea, headache, fever, chills, tingling sensation, tiredness. Possible thromboembolism. If hypersensitivity reactions occur, drug should be withdrawn. *Manufacturer*: Centeon.

MONOPARIN

Description: an anticoagulant preparation of heparin sodium available as 1000, 5000 and 25,000 units/ml in single dose ampoules. Also, MONOPARIN CA containing 25,000 units heparin calcium/ml. *Used for*: treatment of pulmonary embolism and deep vein thrombosis. *Dosage*: adults, initial loading dose of 5000 units (10,000 in severe conditions) by intravenous injection followed by continuous infusion at a rate of 1000–2000 units/hour. Or 15,000 units at 12 hour intervals may be given by subcutaneous injection. Small adult or child, lower initial dose then 15–25 units/kg body weight by intravenous infusion/hour or 250 units/kg by subcutaneous injection. *Special care*: pregnancy, liver or kidney disorders. If treatment period exceeds 5 days, platelet counts must be carried out. *Avoid use*: bleeding disorders or haemophilia, thrombocytopenia, serious liver disease, severe hypertension, peptic ulcer, cerebral aneurysm, recent surgery to central nervous system or eye. Known hypersensitivity to heparin. *Possible interaction*: aspirin, antiplatelet drugs, nitrates. *Side effects*: hypersensitivity responses, haemorrhage, osteoporosis (after long-term use), skin necrosis. Also, thrombocytopenia, in which case drug should be immediately withdrawn. *Manufacturer*: CP Pharmaceuticals.

MONOTRIM

Description: an antibacterial and folic acid inhibitor available in a variety of forms all containing trimethoprim. **MONOTRIM TABLETS** in 2 strengths, scored, white containing 100mg coded AE over 2; scored, white containing 200mg coded DE over 5, both marked with symbol. **MONOTRIM SUGAR-FREE SUSPENSION** containing 50mg/5ml. **MONOTRIM INJECTION** containing 20mg as lactate/ml. *Used for*: urinary tract infections and others sensitive to trimethoprim. *Dosage*: tablets or suspension, 200mg twice each day; injection, 200mg by intravenous injection or infusion every 12 hours. Children, tablets or suspension, age 6 weeks to 5 months, 25mg; 6 months to 5 years, 50mg; 6 to 12 years, 100mg. All doses twice each day. Injection, 8mg/kg body weight each day in 2 or 3 divided doses by intravenous injection or infusion. *Special care*: elderly, babies, folate deficiency or kidney disorders. During long-term treatment, regular blood tests should be carried out. *Avoid use*: pregnancy, serious kidney disease. *Possible interaction*: procainamide, warfarin, nicoumalone, sulphonylureas, phenytoin, maloprim, fansidar, methotrexate. *Side effects*: skin rashes, gastro-intestinal upset. *Manufacturer*: Solvay.

MONOZIDE 10

Description: a compound preparation combining a cardioselective ß-blocker and thiazide diuretic available as film-coated, white tablets containing 10mg bisoprolol fumerate and 6.25mg hydrochlorothiazide. *Used for*: hypertension. *Dosage*: adults, 1 tablet each day. *Special care*: pregnancy, breast-feeding, liver or kidney disease, diabetes, gout, metabolic acidosis. Patients with weak hearts may require digitalis and diuretics. Electrolyte (salts) levels require regular monitoring. Also, special care in patients undergoing general anaesthesia. *Avoid use*: children, obstructive airways disease, history of bronchospasm, uncompensated heart failure, heart block, heart shock, bradycardia, disease of peripheral arteries, sick sinus syndrome. Also, serious or worsening kidney failure, anuria. *Possible interaction*: CNS depressants, verapamil, indomethacin, class I antiarrhythmics, sympathomimetics, cardiac depressant anaesthetics, clonidine withdrawal, ergot alkaloids, reserpine, ergot alkaloids, hypoglycaemics, antihypertensives. Potassium supplements, potassium-sparing diuretics, lithium, digitalis. *Side effects*: cold hands and feet, disturbance of sleep, fatigue on exercise, gastro-intestinal upset, bradycardia, heart failure, bronchospasm, gout. Blood changes, muscle weakness, sensitivity to light. Drug should be gradually withdrawn if dry eyes or skin rash occur. *Manufacturer*: Wyeth.

MONURIL

Description: an antibacterial preparation available as granules in sachets containing 3g fosfomycin as trometamol. Also, **MONURIL PAEDIATRIC** containing 2g fosfomycin as trometamol as granules in sachets. *Used for*: lower urinary tract infections and prevention of infection during surgical procedures in this area. *Dosage*: adults, treatment, single 3g dose taken 1 to 2 hours after a meal or at night. Prevention, 3g taken 3 hours before procedure, dose is then repeated 24 hours afterwards. Children, treatment, age over 5 years, a single 2g dose taken 1 or 2 hours after a meal or at night. *Special care*: pregnancy, breast-feeding, elderly, kidney disease or disorder. *Avoid use*: children under 5 years, elderly people over 75 years, patients with serious kidney disease or disorder. *Possible interaction*: metoclopramide. *Side effects*: rash, gastro-intestinal upset. *Manufacturer*: Pharmax.

MOTENS

Description: an antihypertensive preparation which is a class II calcium antagonist available as white, film-coated tablets containing 2mg and 4mg lacidipine, marked 10L and 9L respectively, and with logo. *Used for*: hypertension. *Dosage*: adults, 2mg once each day as morning dose with breakfast. May be increased after 3 or 4 weeks to 6mg once each day if needed. The maintenance dose is 4mg once each day. Elderly, 2mg once each day increasing if needed to 4mg after 4 weeks. *Special care*: weak hearts, liver disease, disturbances of conduction (of electrical nerve impulses). *Avoid use*: children, pregnancy, breast-feeding. *Possible interaction*: cimetidine. *Side effects*: palpitations, flushing, headache, rash, oedema, polyuria, increase in amount of gum tissue. Drug should be withdrawn if chest pain occurs. *Manufacturer*: Boehringer Ingelheim.

MOTILIUM

Description: an antidopaminergic preparation available in a number of different forms all containing domperidone. Motilium Tablets are white, film-coated and contain 10mg, marked with the name. **MOTILIUM SUSPENSION** contains 1mg/ml solution; **MOTILIUM SUPPOSITORIES** contain 30mg. *Used for*: nausea and vomiting, indigestion (tablets). *Dosage*: tablets for indigestion, 10–20mg 2 or 3 times each day. For nausea and vomiting, 10–20mg as tablets or suspension or 1 or 2 suppositories, both every 4 to 8 hours. Children, for nausea and vomiting following cancer therapy only, 0.2–0.4mg/kg body weight as suspension every 4 to 8 hours, or 1 to 4 suppositories each day, dose determined by body weight. *Avoid use*: pregnancy. *Side effects*: extrapyramidal reactions (characterized by involuntary reflex muscle movements and spasms), skin rash, raised levels of prolactin in blood. *Manufacturer*: Sanofi Winthrop.

MOTIPRESS

Description: an anxiolytic and antidepressant combining a phenothiazine group III and TCAD available as triangular, sugar-coated yellow tablets containing 1.5mg fluphenazine hydrochloride and 30mg nortriptyline (as hydrochloride). *Used for*: anxiety and depression. *Dosage*: 1 tablet each day, preferably taken at bedtime. Maximum treatment period is 3 months. *Special care*: breast-feeding, epilepsy, disease of arteries of heart, glaucoma, liver disease, hyperthyroidism, tumours of adrenal glands. Patients with psychoses or at risk of suicide. *Avoid use*: pregnancy, damaged liver or kidneys, serious heart disorders, heart attack, heart block, blood changes, history of brain damage or grand mal epilepsy. *Possible interaction*: antidepressants, anticonvulsants, alcohol, within 2 weeks of taking MAOIs, barbiturates, adrenaline, noradrenaline, antihypertensives, anticholinergics, oestrogens, cimetidine. *Side effects*: sleepiness, vertigo, light-headedness, unsteadiness, disturbance of vision, rash, hypotension, gastro-intestinal upset, changes in libido, retention of urine. Allergic reactions, dry mouth, constipation, sweating, tachycardia, nervousness, heart arrhythmias. Impotence, effects on breasts, weight loss or gain. *Manufacturer*: Sanofi Winthrop.

MOTIVAL

Description: an anxiolytic and antidepressant preparation combining a phenothiazine group III and TCAD available as sugar-coated, pink, triangular-shaped tablets containing 0.5mg fluphenazine hydrochloride and 10mg nortriptyline as hydrochloride. *Used for*: anxiety and depression. *Dosage*: 1 tablet 3 times each day for a maximum period of 3 months. *Special care*: breast-feeding, epilepsy, disease of arteries of heart, glaucoma, liver disease, hyperthyroidism, tumours of adrenal glands. Patients with psychoses or at risk of suicide. *Avoid use*: pregnancy, damaged liver or kidneys, serious heart disorders, heart attack, heart block, blood changes, history of brain damage or grand mal epilepsy. *Possible interaction*: antidepressants, anticonvulsants, alcohol, within 2 weeks of taking MAOIs, barbiturates, adrenaline, noradrenaline, antihypertensives, anticholinergics, oestrogens, cimetidine. *Side effects*: sleepiness, vertigo, light-headedness, unsteadiness, disturbance of vision, rash, hypotension, gastro-intestinal upset, changes in libido, retention of urine. Allergic reactions, dry mouth, constipation, sweating, tachycardia, nervousness, heart arrhythmias. Impotence, effects on breasts, weight loss or gain. *Manufacturer*: Sanofi Winthrop.

MOTRIN

Description: an NSAID and proprionic acid, available in the form of film-coated tablets of 4 strengths. Red tablets contain 200mg ibuprofen; orange tablets contain 400mg; oval-shaped, peach-coloured tablets contain 600mg, all marked with a U. Orange, capsule-shaped tablets contain 800mg, marked with strength and name. *Used for*: pain, rheumatism and other bone and muscle disorders including osteoarthritis, rheumatoid arthritis and ankylosing spondylitis. *Dosage*: adults, 1200–1800mg each day in divided doses, the maximum being 2400mg daily. Children, 20mg/kg body weight each day with a maximum dose of 500mg for children weighing less than 30kg. For juvenile rheumatoid arthritis, 40mg/kg may be given. *Special care*: pregnancy, breast-feeding, elderly, liver or kidney disorders, heart disease, asthma, disease of gastro-intestinal tract. *Avoid use*: patients with known allergy to NSAID or aspirin, peptic ulcer. *Possible interaction*: thiazide diuretics, anticoagulants, quinolones. *Side effects*: rash, gastro-intestinal disorder or bleeding, thrombocytopenia. *Manufacturer*: Pharmacia & Upjohn.

MST CONTINUSCD

Description: an opiate preparation which is a controlled drug available as continuous-release film-coated tablets of different strengths, all containing morphine sulphate. White, 5mg; brown, 10mg; light green, 15mg; purple, 30mg; orange, 60mg; grey, 100mg; green, 200mg; tablets are all marked NAPP and with strength. Also, **CONTINUS SUSPENSION**, produced as granules in sachets for dissolving in water, to make raspberry-flavoured continuous-release suspension containing morphine (equivalent to morphine sulphate). Suspension is available in 20mg, 30mg, 60,mg, 100mg and 200mg strengths. *Used for*: long-term relief of severe pain when other drugs have proved inadequate. *Dosage*: 30mg every 12 hours at first, then adjusted to dose necessary to provide pain relief for 12 hours according to patient's response. Children, 0.2–0.8mg/kg body weight every 12 hours at first, then adjusted to dose necessary to provide pain relief for 12 hours. (Granules may be dissolved in water or mixed with food). *Special care*: elderly, liver or kidney disease; hypothyroidism (underactive thyroid gland). *Avoid use*: pregnant women, patients with severe liver disease, obstructive airways disease, depressed respiration. *Possible interaction*: central nervous system depressants, MAOIs. *Side effects*: nausea, constipation, vomiting, drug tolerance and dependence. *Manufacturer*: Napp.

MUCAINE

Description: a combined antacid and local anaesthetic preparation containing 10mg oxethazine, 4.75ml aluminium hydroxide gel and 100mg magnesium hydroxide/5ml suspension. *Used for*: hiatus hernia and oesophagitis. *Dosage*: adults, 10–20ml 3 times each day after meals and at night. *Avoid use*: children. *Manufacturer*: Wyeth.

MUCODYNE

Description: a mucolytic preparation available as a syrup containing 250mg carbocisteine/5ml. Also, **MUCODYNE CAPSULES**, yellow capsules containing 375mg carbocisteine marked MUCODYNE 375. **MUCODYNE PAEDIATRIC** contains 125mg carbocisteine/5ml as a syrup. *Used for*: copious, thick mucus, glue ear in children. *Dosage*: adults, 750mg, 3 times each day, reducing to 500mg. Children, syrup, aged 2 to 5 years, 2.5–5ml 4 times each day; 5 to 10 years, 10ml 3 times each day. *Special care*: pregnancy, history of peptic ulcer. *Avoid use*: children under 2 years, patients with peptic ulcer. *Side effects*: nausea, gastro-intestinal upset, rash. *Manufacturer*: R.P.R.

MULTILOAD

Description: an inter-uterine contraceptive device formed from copper wire on a polyethylene stem. Also, **MULTILOAD Cu 250 SHORT**, and **MULTILOAD Cu 375**. *Used for*: contraception. *Special care*: diabetes, anaemia, history of endocarditis or pelvic inflammatory disease, epilepsy, hypermenorrhoea (or menorrhagia, long or heavy menstrual periods). Examine after 3 months, then annually. *Avoid use*: pregnancy, past ectopic pregnancy, uterus disorders, infection of vagina or cervix, acute pelvic inflammatory diseases, cervical cancer, abnormal vaginal bleeding, endometrial disease, immunosuppressive therapy, copper allergy, cancer of the genitalia. *Possible interaction*: anticoagulants. *Side effects*: pain, pelvic infection, perforation of the uterus, abnormal bleeding. On insertion there may be attack of asthma or epilepsy, bradycardia, Remove if persistent bleeding or cramps, perforation of cervix or uterus, pregnancy, persistent pelvic infection. *Manufacturer*: Organon.

MULTIPARIN

Description: an anticoagulant preparation of heparin sodium available as 1000, 5000 and 25,000 units/ml in multidose vials. *Used for*: treatment of pulmonary embolism and deep vein thrombosis. *Dosage*: adults, initial loading dose of 5000 units (10,000 in severe conditions) by intravenous injection followed by continuous infusion at a rate of 1000–2000 units/hour. Or 15,000 units at 12 hour intervals may be given by subcutaneous injection. Small adult or child, lower initial dose then 15–25 units/kg body weight by intravenous infusion/hour or 250 units/kg by subcutaneous injection. *Special care*: pregnancy, liver or kidney disorders. If treatment period exceeds 5 days, platelet counts must be carried out. *Avoid use*: bleeding disorders or haemophilia, thrombocytopenia, serious liver disease, severe hypertension, peptic ulcer, cerebral aneurysm, having had recent surgery to central nervous system or eye. Known hypersensitivity to heparin. *Possible interaction*: aspirin, antiplatelet drugs, nitrates. *Side effects*: hypersensitivity responses, haemorrhage, osteoporosis (after long-term use), skin necrosis. Also, thrombocytopenia, in which case drug should be immediately withdrawn and, rarely, baldness. *Manufacturer*: CP Pharmaceuticals.

MUMPS VAX

Description: a preparation of mumps vaccine of live attenuated virus of the Jeryl Lynn strain available as powder in single dose vials with diluent, containing the virus and 0.25mg neomycin per dose. *Used for*: immunization against mumps for all ages over 1 year. *Dosage*: 1 dose of reconstituted vaccine by subcutaneous injection. *Avoid use*: children under 1 year, pregnant women, patients with infections, low levels of gammaglobulins in blood, severe egg allergy. *Possible interaction*: live vaccines, immunoglobulins, transfusions, cytotoxic drugs, radiation therapy, corticosteroids. *Manufacturer*: Pasteur Merieux MSD.

MYAMBUTOL

Description: an anti-tuberculous drug available as yellow tablets containing 100mg ethambutol and grey tablets containing 400mg ethambutol. *Used for*: treatment of tuberculosis along with other antituberculous drugs and prevention of tuberculosis. *Dosage*: prevention and treatment, 15mg/kg body weight each day as a single dose. Children, treatment, 25mg/kg each day for 60 days. Prevention, 15mg/kg each day as a single dose. *Special care*: breast-feeding, kidney disorders. Visual tests must be carried out. *Avoid use*: patients with inflammation of the optic nerve. *Side effects*: visual disturbances, blurred vision, distortion of colour vision—drug should be withdrawn. *Manufacturer*: Lederle.

MYCOBUTIN

Description: an antimycobacterial ansamycin drug available as brown/red capsules containing 150mg rifambutin. *Used for*: as sole therapy in prevention of monobacterial infections in immuno-compromised patients (whose immune system is not working properly). Additional treatment of mycobacterial infections. *Dosage*: prevention of mycobacterial infections, 2 tablets each day. As additional therapy in non-tuberculous mycobacterial disease, 3 to 4 tablets each day continuing for 6 months after infection has cleared. Pulmonary tuberculosis, 1 to 3 tablets each day as additional therapy for a minimum period of 6 months. *Special care*: severe liver or kidney failure. Blood checks and liver enzyme tests should be carried out. *Avoid use*: children, patients wearing soft contact lenses, pregnancy, breast-feeding. *Possible interaction*: triazole antifungal drugs, hypoglycaemics taken by mouth, oral contraceptives, cyclosporin, macrolides, anticoagulants, dapsone, zidovudine, digitalis, quinidine, analgesics, phenytoin, corticosteroids. *Side effects*: anaemia, leucopenia and thrombocytopenia, pain in muscles and joints, discolouration of urine, skin and bodily secretions. *Manufacterer*: Pharmacia & Upjohn.

MYDRIACYL

Description: an anticholinergic preparation available as eyedrops containing 0.5% and 1% tropicamide. *Used for*: to produce mydriasis (dilation of the pupil of the eye by contraction of certain muscles in the iris) and cytoplegia (paralysis of the muscles of accommodation in the eye along with relaxation of the ciliary muscle). *Dosage*: 1 or 2 drops of either strength at intervals between 1 and 5 minutes. *Special care*: patients in whom pressure within eye is not known. In infants, pressure should be applied over tear sac for 1 minute. *Avoid use*: patients wearing soft contact lenses, those with narrow angle glaucoma. *Side effects*: short-lived stinging, sensitivity to light, dry mouth, headache, tachycardia, blurred vision. Also, mental disturbances, behavioural changes, psychoses. *Manufactuer*: Alcon.

MYDRILATE

Description: an anticholinergic preparation available in the form of eyedrops in 2 strengths containing 0.5% and 1% cyclopentolate hydrochloride. *Used for*: refraction and uveitis (inflammation of the uveal tract which includes the choroid, iris and ciliary body, characterized by impaired vision and can cause blindness). *Dosage*: adults, refraction, 1 drop of solution of either strength repeated after 15 minutes if needed. Uveitis, 1 or 2 drops of either strength repeated as needed. Children, refraction, under 6 years, 1 or 2 drops of 1% solution; over 6 years, 1 drop of 1% solution. Uveitis, children over 3 months, same dose as adult. *Special care*: eye inflammation, raised pressure within eye. *Avoid use*: patients with glaucoma. *Side effects*: systemic toxic effects due to absorption of drops, especially elderly persons and children, contact dermatitis. *Manufacturer*: Boehringer Ingelheim.

MYLERAN

Description: an alkylating cytotoxic drug available as white tablets in 2 strengths containing 0.5mg and 2mg busulphan, coded F2A and K2A respectively, and WELLCOME. *Used for*: chronic myeloid leukaemia. *Dosage*: adults, to induce remission, 60μg/kg body weight each day with a maximum daily dose of 4mg. Maintenance dose is 0.5–2mg. *Special care*: pregnant women—patients should be treated in hospital. Frequent blood counts are required. *Avoid use*: patients with porphyria, children. *Possible interaction*: radiotherapy, other cytotoxic drugs. *Side effects*: severe bone marrow suppression, nausea, vomiting, hair loss, excessive pigmentation of skin. *Manufacturer*: Glaxo Wellcome.

MYOCRISIN

Description: a long-acting suppressive drug and gold salt available in ampoules for injection containing 10mg, 20mg and 50mg sodium aurothiomalate/0.5ml.

Used for: rheumatoid arthritis, juvenile arthritis. *Dosage*: initial test of 10mg by deep intramuscular injection followed by 50mg each week until condition improves. Children, initial test dose of one tenth to one fifth of ongoing dose which is 1mg/kg bodyweight weekly up to a maximum of 50mg. The interval between doses is gradually increased to 4 weeks depending on response. *Special care*: elderly, urine tests and blood counts are essential. Eczema, urticaria, colitis (inflamed bowel). No improvement can be expected in adults until 300mg–500mg has been given, and if condition has not changed after 1g total dose, drug should be withdrawn. *Avoid use*: pregnancy, breast-feeding, patients with history of blood changes, certain skin disorders, liver or kidney disease, porphyria. *Possible interaction*: phenylbutazone, penicillamine. *Side effects*: rash, eosinophilia (increased number of eosinophils (a type of white blood cells) in blood, an allergic response), albuminuria (presence of albumin in urine). Patients should report if itching (pruritis), bleeding gums, mouth ulcers, sore throat, sore tongue, diarrhoea, bruising, metallic taste in mouth or heavy menstrual bleeding occur. Also toxic effects on liver, cholestatic jaundice, baldness, lung fibrosis may occur. *Manufacturer*: R.P.R.

MYOTONINE

Description: a cholinergic preparation available as scored white tablets containing 10mg bethanechol chloride and white, cross-scored tablets containing 25mg bethanechol chloride. *Used for*: total or partial immobility of the bowel or stomach, large, abnormally extended colon, reflux oesophagitis, retention of urine. *Dosage*: adults, 10–25mg 3 to 4 times each day; children, reduced dose in proportion to that for 70kg adult. *Avoid use*: pregnancy, epilepsy, recent heart attack, serious hypotension, obstruction of urinary or gastro-intestinal tract, Parkinson's disease, severe bradycardia, asthma, hyperthyroidism, vagotonia (abnormal increase in the activity of the vagus nerve). *Side effects*: blurred vision, abdominal pains, nausea, frequency of urination, vomiting, sweating. *Manufacturer*: Glenwood.

MYSOLINE

Description: an anticonvulsant pyrimidinedone preparation available as scored, white tablets containing 250mg primidone, marked with 2 lines and ICI. Also, **MYSOLINE SUSPENSION** containing 250mg primidone/5ml. *Used for*: epilepsy. *Dosage*: 125mg taken at night in first instance increasing every 3 days by 125mg to 500mg each day. Then a further increase every third day of 250mg to a maximum dose of 1.5g daily. Children, same initial dose as adults but increasing by 125mg. Usual daily maintenance doses as follows: up to 2 years, 250–500mg; 2 to 5 years, 500–750mg; 6 to 9 years, 750mg–1g; 9 to 12 years, 750mg–1.5g. *Special care*: patients with kidney and liver disorders, serious lung insufficiency. *Avoid use*: pregnancy, breast-feeding, elderly, patients who are debilitated, porphyria, pain which is not controlled, history of drug or alcohol abuse. *Possible interaction*: CNS depressants, griseofulvin, alcohol, phenytoin, systemic steroids, chloramphenicol, rifampicin, metronidazole, anticoagulants of the coumarin type. *Side effects*: headache, respiratory depression, dizziness, unsteadiness, sleepiness, confusion, agitation, allergic responses, megaloblastic anaemia. Drug tolerance and dependence may occur. Drug is metabolized to phenobarbitone. *Manufacturer*: Zeneca.

MYSTECLIN

Description: a compound tetracycline and antifungal preparation available as sugar-coated orange tablets containing 250mg tetracycline hydrochloride and 250,000 units nystatin. *Used for*: injections and acne susceptible to tetracycline, particularly where candidiasis also occurs. *Dosage*: adults 1 or 2 tablets 4 times each day. *Special care*: liver or kidney disease. *Avoid use*: pregnancy, breast-feeding, children. *Possible interaction*: oral contraceptives, antacids, mineral supplements, milk, anticoagulants. *Side effects*: allergic responses, gastro-intestinal upset, superinfection. If rise in intracranial pressure occurs, drug should be withdrawn. *Manufacturer*: Squibb.

N

NACTON FORTE

Description: an anticholinergic, poldine methylsulphate, available as orange tablets (4mg strength), marked NACTON 4. *Used for*: peptic ulcer, acidity. *Dosage*: 4mg 3 times per day and at bedtime. Elderly, half dose. Not for children. Also NACTON, 2mg poldine methylsulphate as white tablets marked NACTON 2. *Dosage*: see literature. Not for children. *Special care*: glaucoma, tachycardia, difficulty in urinating. *Side effects*: anticholinergic effects *Manufacturer*: Pharmark.

NALCROM

Description: an anti-inflammatory non-steroid, sodium cromoglycate as clear capsules containing white powder (100mg) and marked FISONS and 101. *Used for*: food allergy. *Dosage*: 2 capsules 4 times per day before meals, maximum 40mg/kg per day. Children over 2 years, 1 capsule 4 times per day. Not recommended for children under 2. *Side effects*: rashes, joint pain, nausea. *Manufacturer*: R.P.R.

NALOREX

Description: a narcotic antagonist, naltrexone hydrochloride, available as mottled orange tablets (50mg strength) and marked DuPont and NTR. *Used for*: maintenance treatment for patients detoxified after opioid dependency. *Dosage*:

25mg daily to start with and then 50mg per day for at least 3 months. Treatment should be started in a drug addiction centre. Not for children. *Special care*: kidney or liver disorder. *Avoid use*: a current dependence on opiates, liver failure, acute hepatitis. *Side effects*: drowsiness, dizziness, cramps, vomiting, joint and muscle pains. *Manufacturer*: DuPont.

NAPRATEC

Description: an NSAID and propionic acid/prostaglandin analogue, available as naproxen, a yellow oblong tablet (500mg) marked Searle N500, and misoprostol, a white hexagonal tablet (200µg) marked Searle 1461. *Used for*: osteoarthritis, rheumatoid arthritis, ankylosing spondylitis where the stomach has to be protected against the medication. *Dosage*: 1 tablet of each drug taken twice daily with food. *Special care*: asthma, liver or kidney damage, elderly, disease of blood vesssels. Effective contraception must be used by women of child-bearing age. *Avoid use*: pregnancy, lactation, duodenal or gastric ulcer, allergy induced by aspirin or anti-inflammatory drugs. *Possible interaction*: diuretics, anticoagulants, sulphonylureas, quinolones, sulphonamides, hydantoins, lithium, ß-blockers, probenecid, methotrexate. *Side effects*: diarrhoea, abdominal pain, gastro-intestinal upset, vaginal bleeding, menorrhagia (long or heavy menstruation), rash, headache, urticaria, dizziness, tinnitus, vertigo, blood changes. *Manufacturer*: Searle.

NAPROSYN SR

Description: Propionic acid, naproxen (as the sodium salt) available as 500mg in white, capsule-shaped tablets marked 500. *Used for*: osteoarthritis, rheumatoid arthritis, ankylosing spondylitis, musculoskeletal disorders, acute gout. *Dosage*: 1 to 2 tablets once per day. Not for children. Also, **NAPROSYN EC**, naproxen as 250mg, 375mg and 500mg strength white tablets marked with tablet name, the strength and SYNTEX. **NAPROSYN TABLETS**, naproxen as 250mg (buff tablets), 375mg (pink tablets) and 500mg (buff tablets) marked with tablet name, strength and SYNTEX. **NAPROSYN SUSPENSION**, naproxen as 250mg per 10ml and **NAPROSYN GRANULES**, 500mg naproxen as peppermint-flavoured granules in a sachet. *Dosage*: 500–1000mg per day in 2 divided doses or as 1 dose morning or evening. For gout, 750mg to start with and then 250mg every 8 hours. For musculoskeletal disorders, 500mg to start with, then 250mg every 6 to 8 hours as necessary, no more than 1250mg per day after the first 24 hours. Children: for juvenile rheumatoid arthritis, 5 to 16 years, 10mg/kg body weight per day in 2 divided doses. Not for children under 5. Also, **NAPROSYN SUPPOSITORIES**, naproxen 500mg. *Dosage*: 1 at night with another in the morning (or 500mg by mouth) if necessary. *Special care*: liver or kidney damage, elderly, heart failure, asthma, pregnancy, lactation, a history of gastro-intestinal lesions. *Avoid use*: peptic ulcer, allergy caused by aspirin or anti-inflammatory drugs. *Possible interaction*: ACE inhibitors, ß-blockers, lithium, anticoagulants, quinolones, sulphonylureas, hydantoins, frusemide, methotrexate, probenecid. *Side effects*: headache, gastro-intestinal intolerance, rash, vertigo, blood changes, tinnitus. *Manufacturer*: Roche.

NARCAN

Description: a narcotic antagonist, nalo-xone hydrochloride, available as ampoules or pre-filled syringes (0.4mg/ml, 1mg/ml). *Used for*: diagnosis of opioid overdosage, reversal of opioid depression including that due to pentazocine and dextropropoxyphone. *Dosage*: 0.4–2mg by injection (intravenous, intramuscular or subcutaneous) every 2 to 3 minutes as necessary, or by intravenous infusion (see literature). Post-operative, 0.1–0.2mg intravenously as required. Children 10 g/kg by same means. Also, **NARCAN NEONATAL**, naloxone hydrochloride as 0.02mg/ml in 2ml ampoules. *Used for*: depression of neonatal respiration due to obstetric analgesia. *Dosage*: 10 g/kg by injection (intravenous, intramuscular or subcutaneous), repeated as required. *Special care*: pregnancy, opioid dependence. Patient should be monitored to determine whether repeat doses are needed. *Manufacturer*: DuPont.

NARDIL

Description: an antidepressant and MAOI, phenelzine sulphate, available as orange tablets (15mg strength). *Used for*: depression, phobias. *Dosage*: 1 tablet 3 times per day initially, reduced gradually for maintenance. Not for children. *Special care*: elderly, epilepsy. *Avoid use*: liver disease, blood changes, congestive heart failure, brain vascular disease, hyperthyroidism, phaeochromocytoma. *Possible interaction*: sympathomimetic amines (e.g. amphetamine and others), TCADs, pethidine and similar analgesics. The effect of barbiturates and alcohol, insulin, hypnotics may be enhanced and the side effects of anticholinergics may be enhanced or increased, antihypertensives. Avoid foods such as cheese, meat extracts (e.g. Oxo or Bovril), yeast extracts (e.g. Marmite), alcohol, broad beans, bananas, pickled herrings, vegetable proteins. Do not use any of these within 14 days of stopping the drug. *Side effects*: severe hypertension with certain foods (see above), dizziness, drowsiness, insomnia, weakness, fatigue, postural hypotension, constipation, dry mouth, gastro-intestinal upsets, difficulty in urinating, blurred vision, ankle oedema. Skin rashes, blood disorders, weight gain, jaundice, changes in libido. *Manufacturer*: Parke-Davis.

NARPHEN^{CD}

Description: an opiate, phenazocine hydrobromide available as white, scored tablets (strength 5mg) marked SNP/2. *Used for*: severe, prolonged pain including pancreatic and biliary pain. *Dosage*: 1 tablet every 4 to 6 hours, taken by mouth, or beneath the tongue, as necessary. Maximum single dose, 20mg. Not for children. *Special care*: hypothyroidism, chronic kidney or liver disease, elderly. In labour or during pregnancy. *Avoid use*: coma, epilepsy, acute alcoholism, breathing difficulty, blocked airways. *Possible interaction*: depressants of the central nervous system, MAOIs. *Side effects*: constipation, dizziness nausea. Danger of tolerance and dependence. *Manufacturer*: Napp.

NASEPTIN

Description: an antibacterial cream comprising chlorhexidine hydrochloride (0.1%) and neomycin sulphate (0.5%). *Used for*: staphylococcal infections of the nose. *Dosage*: small amounts to be applied into each nostril 2 to 4 times per day. *Special care*: prolonged use should be avoided. *Side effects*: sensitive skin. *Manufacturer*: Zeneca.

NATRILIX

Description: a vasorelaxant, indapamide hemihydrate, available as white, film-coated tablets (strength 2.5mg). *Used for*: hypertension. *Dosage*: 1 tablet in the morning. Not for children. *Special care*: pregnancy, severe kidney disease. *Avoid use*: lactation, severe liver disease. *Possible interaction*: corticosteroids, laxatives, lithium, cardiac glycosides, diuretics, anti-arrhythmics. *Side effects*: nausea, headache, hypokalaemia. *Manufacturer*: Servier.

NATULAN

Description: a cytostatic agent, procarbazine hydrochloride, available as yellow capsules (strength 50mg). *Used for*: Hodgkin's disease, advanced reticoloses (normally malignant overgrowths in the lymphatic or immune system), solid tumours that do not respond to other therapies. *Dosage*: see literature but likely to be 50mg per day to begin with, rising to 250–300mg per day in 50mg daily increments. Dose for maintenance (on remission), 50–150mg per day. *Special care*: induction therapy should commence in hospital. *Avoid use*: pregnancy, severe liver or kidney damage, severe leucopenia, thrombocytopenia. *Possible interaction*: alcohol, narcotics, barbiturates, phenothiazines, imipramine-type compounds. *Side effects*: nausea, loss of appetite, myelosuppression (reduction in the production of blood cells in the bone marrow). *Manufacturer*: Cambridge.

NAVIDREX

Description: a thiazide diuretic, cyclopenthiazide (0.5mg), available as white scored tablets marked CIBA and AO. *Used for*: oedema, heart failure, hypertension. *Dosage*: 0.25–1mg per day to a maximum of 1.5mg daily, but see manufacturer's literature. For children, contact the manufacturer. *Special care*: liver cirrhosis, liver or kidney disease, SLE, gout, the elderly, pregnancy, lactation. Electrolytes, glucose and fluids should be monitored. *Avoid use*: hypercalcaemia, Addison's disease, severe liver or kidney failure, if sensitive to sulphonamides. *Possible interaction*: corticosteroids, cardiac glycosides, lithium, carbenozolone, tubocurarine, antidiabetic drugs, NSAIDs, opioids, barbiturates, alcohol. *Side effects*: gastro-intestinal upset, anorexia, blood changes, rash, sensitivity to light, dizziness, pancreatitis, metabolic and electrolyte upset, impotence. *Manufacturer*: Ciba.

NAVISPARE

Description: a thiazide and potassium-sparing diuretic, cyclopenthiazide (0.25mg) with 2.5mg amiloride, available as yellow tablets marked CIBA and

RC. *Used for*: mild to moderate hypertension. *Dosage*: 1 or 2 tablets per day in the morning. Not for children. *Special care*: liver or kidney disease, diabetes, hyperlipidaemia, pregnancy, lactation, gout, respiratory or metabolic acidosis. *Avoid use*: severe kidney or liver failure, anuria, hyperkalaemia, Addison's disease, hypercalcaemia, hyponatiaemia (low blood sodium levels). *Possible interaction*: ACE inhibitors, other antihypertensives, lithium, digitalis, potassium supplements, potassium-sparing diuretics. *Side effects*: blood changes, gout, gastro-intestinal upset, fatigue, rash, sensitivity to light. *Manufacturer*: Ciba.

NAVOBAN

Description: a $5HT_3$-antagonist, tropisetron hydrochloride, which blocks vomiting reflexes, available as yellow/white capsules (5mg strength). Also, **NAVOBAN INJECTION**, containing 5mg/5ml in ampoules. *Used for*: chemotherapy-induced nausea and vomiting. *Dosage*: 5mg by intravenous injection of infusion before therapy and 1 capsule 1 hour before morning food, for 5 days. Not for children. *Special care*: uncontrolled hypertension. *Avoid use*: pregnancy, breast-feeding. *Possible interaction*: drugs that affect liver enzymes. *Side effects*: constipation, dizziness, headache, tiredness, stomach upset. *Manufacturer*: Sandoz.

NEBCIN

Description: an aminoglycoside, tabramycin sulphate, available as solution in vials containing 20, 40 or 80mg. *Used for*: infections of gastro-intestinal and respiratory tract, skin and soft tissue, CNS, urinary tract; septicaemia. *Dosage*: 3–5mg/kg per day by intramuscular injection, intravenous injection or infusion in 3 or 4 divided doses. Children: 6–7.5mg/kg daily in divided doses; babies up to 1 month, 4mg/kg per day in 2 doses. *Special care*: kidney damage; control dosage and blood levels. *Avoid use*: pregnancy, lactation. *Possible interaction*: loop diuretics, other aminoglycosides, neuromuscular blocking agents. *Side effects*: anaphylaxis, ototoxicity (affecting hearing and balance), nephrotoxicity, raised liver enzymes. *Manufacturer*: King.

NEGRAM

Description: a quinolone, nalidixic acid (500mg) available as light brown tablets marked NEGRAM with a symbol on the reverse. Also, **NEGRAM SUSPENSION**, containing 300mg/5ml as a suspension. *Used for*: infections of the grastro-intestinal tract by Gram-negative organisms. *Dosage*: 500mg–1g 4 times per day. Children up to 12 years, up to 50mg/kg per day. Not for children under 3 months. *Special care*: liver or kidney disease, lactation. Avoid sunlight. *Avoid use*: history of convulsions. *Possible interaction*: probenecid, anticoagulants. *Side effects*: rashes, blood changes, convulsions, disturbances in vision and stomach. *Manufacturer*: Sanofi Winthrop.

NEO-CORTEF

Description: an antibiotic and cortico-steroid comprising 0.5% neomycin in sulphate and 1.5% hydrocortisone acetate, as drops. *Used for*: otitis externa and eye inflammation. *Dosage*: 2 to 3 drops 4 times per day (otitis), 1 to 2 drops in each eye up to 6 times per day. Also, **NEO-CORTEF OINTMENT** *Dosage*: apply once or twice per day (otitis), apply 2 or 3 times per day or if drops are used during the day, use at night. *Special care*: prolonged use on infants or during pregnancy. *Avoid use*: perforated ear drum, glaucoma; fungal, viral, tuberculous or acute pus-containing infections. *Side effects*: sensitization, superinfection, cataract, rise in pressure within the eye. *Manufacturer*: Dominion.

NEO-CYTAMEN

Description: vitamin B_{12}, hydroxocobalamin, available as 1ml ampoules containing 1000µg per ml. *Used for*: megaloblastic anaemia, and other anaemias responsive to B_{12}, Leber's disease (a rare hereditary visual defect), tobacco amblyopia (reduced vision although eye structure appears normal). *Dosage*: 250–1000µg intramuscularly on alternate days for 7 to 14 days then 250µg once per week until blood count is normal. 1000µg every 2 to 3 months for maintenance. For amblyopia, see literature. *Possible interaction*: oral contraceptives, chloramphenicol. *Side effects*: some rare hypersensitivity reactions. *Manufacturer*: Evans.

NEO-MEDRONE CREAM

Description: a mild steroid and antibacterial, 0.25% methylprednisolone acetate and 0.5% neomycin sulphate, as a cream. *Used for*: allergic and inflammatory skin conditions where there is bacterial infection. *Dosage*: use 1 to 3 times per day. *Special care*: thrombophlebitis, psychoses, recent intestinal anastomoses, chronic nephritis, certain cancers, osteoporosis, peptic ulcer, skin eruption/rash related to a disease, viral, fungal or active infections, tuberculosis. Hypertension, glaucoma, epilepsy, acute glomerulonephritis (inflammation of kidney glomerulus), diabetes, cirrhosis, hypothyroidism, pregnancy, stress. To be withdrawn gradually. *Possible interaction*: NSAIDs, oral anticoagulants, phenytoin, ephedrine, phenobarbitone, rifampicin, diuretics, cardiac glycosides, anticholinesterases, hypoglycaemics. *Side effects*: osteoporosis, depression, euphoria, hyperglycaemia, peptic ulcers, Cushingoid changes. *Manufacturer*: Upjohn.

NEO-MERCAZOLE

Description: an antithyroid, carbimazole, available as pink tablets (strengths 5 and 20mg) marked BS with strength on the reverse. *Used for*: thyrotoxicosis. *Dosage*: 20–60mg per day initially in 2 or 3 divided doses until thyroid functions normally. 5–15mg per day for 6 to 18 months for maintenance, or maintain 20–60mg per day with 50–150 g supplemental thyroxine daily for 6 to 18 months. Children, 5–15mg per day in divided doses. *Special care*: pregnancy (but see literature). *Avoid use*: lactation, obstruction of the trachea. *Side effects*: arthralgia, headache, nausea, rashes. Depression of the bone marrow. Drug should be discontinued if there are mouth ulcers or a sore throat. *Manufacturer*: Roche.

NEO-NACLEX

Description: a thiazide, bendrofluazide (5mg), available as white, scored tablets marked NEO-NACLEX. *Used for*: hypertension, oedema. *Dosage*: 1 to 2 tablets once per day for oedema, ½ or 1 tablet for maintenance periodically. Hypertension, ½ to 2 once per day. Children, 50–100µg/kg body weight. *Special care*: cirrhosis of the liver, liver or kidney disease, diabetes, SLE, gout, pregnancy, breast-feeding, elderly. Monitor glucose, electrolytes and fluids. *Avoid use*: hypercalcaemia, severe liver or kidney failure, sensitivity to sulphonamides, Addison's disease. *Possible interaction*: lithium, cardiac glycosides, potassium-sparing diuretics, potassium supplements, corticosteroids, tubocurarine, NSAIDs, carbenoxolone, alcohol, opiods, barbiturates, antidiabetic drugs. *Side effects*: rash, blood changes, anorexia, dizziness, pancreatitis, gastro-intestinal upset, sensitivity to light, metabolic and electrolytes upsets. *Manufacturer*: Goldshield.

NEO-NACLEX-K

Description: a thiazide and potassium supplement, bendrofluazide (2.5mg) with 630mg potassium chloride in a slow-release, two-layer tablet, pink and white, marked NEO-NACLEX-K. *Used for*: hypertension and chronic oedema. *Dosage*: 1 to 4 per day (hypertension). 2 per day for oedema inreasing to 4 if required, maintenance 1 or 2 periodically. Not for children. *Special care*: liver cirrhosis, diabetes, liver or kidney disease, SLE, gout, elderly, pregnancy, lactation. Monitor glucose, fluid and electrolytes. *Avoid use*: hypercalcaemia, severe liver or kidney failure, Addison's disease, sensitivity to sulphonamides. *Possible interaction*: lithium, corticosteroids, cardiac glycosides, potassium supplements, potassium-sparing diuretics, NSAIDs, tubocurarine, carbenoxolone, alcohol, opioids, barbiturates, antidiabetic drugs. *Side effects*: rash, blood changes, gastrointestinal upsets, sensitivity to light, impotence, dizziness, pancreatitis, anorexia, upset to metabolism and electrolytes. Stop if signs of blockage or ulceration of small bowel occur. *Manufacturer*: Goldshield.

NEOCON 1/35

Description: an oestrogen/progestogen oral contraceptive containing 35µg ethinyloestradiol and 500µg norethisterone in white tablets marked C over 535. *Used for*: oral contraception. *Dosage*: 1 per day for 21 days commencing on the fifth day of menstruation, then 7 days without tablets. *Special care*: hypertension, Raynaud's disease (reduced blood supply to an organ of the body's extremities), asthma, severe depression, diabetes, varicose veins, multiple sclerosis, chronic kidney disease, kidney dialysis. Blood pressure, breasts and pelvic organs to be checked regularly; smoking not advised. *Avoid use*: history of heart disease, infectious hepatitis, sickle cell anaemia, porphyria, liver tumour, undiagnosed vaginal bleeding, pregnancy, hormone-dependent cancer, haemolytic uraemic syndrome (rare kidney disorder), chorea, otosclerosis. *Possible interaction*: barbiturates, tetracyclines, griseofulvin, rifampicin, primidone, phenytoin, chloral hydrate, ethosuximide, carbamazepine, glutethimide, dichloralphenazone. *Side effects*: fluid retention and bloating, leg cramps/pains, breast enlargement, depression, headaches, nausea, loss of libido, weight gain, vaginal discharge, cervical erosion (alteration of epithelial cells), chloasma (pigmentation of nose, cheeks or forehead), breakthrough bleeding (bleeding between periods). *Manufacturer*: Ortho.

NEOGEST

Description: a progestogen-only contraceptive, norgestrel (75µg) available in brown tablets. *Used for*: oral contraception. *Dosage*: starting on the first day of the cycle, 1 tablet each day at the same time, without a break. *Special care*: hypertension, thromboembolic disorders, liver disease, hormone-dependent cancer, ovarian cysts, migraine. Regular checks on blood pressure, breasts and pelvic organs. *Avoid use*: previous severe arterial or heart disease, benign liver tumours, undiagnosed vaginal bleeding, pregnancy, past ectopic pregnancy. Discontinue immediately for pregnancy, jaundice, thrombophlebitis or thromboembolism. *Possible interaction*: griseofulvin, rifampicin, meprobamate, chloral hydrate, carbamazepine, primidone, barbiturates, phenytoin, dichloralphenazone, ethosuximide, glutethimide. *Side effects*: acne, breast discomfort, headache, ovarian cysts, irregular menstrual bleeding. *Manufacturer*: Schering H.C.

NEOSPORIN

Description: a peptide and aminoglycoside, polymyxin B sulphate (5000 units) and neomycin sulphate (1700 units) with gramicidin (25 units/ml), as drops. *Used for*: bacterial infections, prevention of infections in the eye before and after surgery, removal of foreign bodies from the eye. *Dosage*: 1 or 2 drops 4 or more times per day. *Special care*: existing eye defect. *Manufacturer*: Dominion.

NEOTIGASON

Description: a vitamin A derivative, acitretin, used only in hospitals and available as brown/white (10mg) and brown/yellow capsules marked ROCHE. *Used for*: severe psoriasis, congenital ichthyosis, Darier's disease (skin disease with brown or black wart-like patches). *Dosage*: 25–30mg per day initially, for 2 to 4 weeks up to a maximum of 75mg per day. 25–50mg per day for maintenance. Maximum treatment period, 6 months. Not for children. *Special care*: teratogenic, effective contraception necessary during treatment and for 2 years after stopping. Diabetes, monitor liver, serum lipids and bone. Do not donate blood for 1 year afterwards. *Avoid use*: kidney or liver disease, pregnancy, lactation. *Possible interaction*: alcohol, tetracyclines, methotrexate, high doses or vitamin A. *Side effects*: hair loss, itching, erythema, dryness, erosion of mucous membranes, nausea, headache, sweating, drowsiness, myalgia, arthralgia, bone thickening, liver disorder. *Manufacturer*: Roche.

NEPHRIL

Description: a thiazide diuretic, polythiazide, available as white tablets (1mg) with NEP over 1 marked on one side and Pfizer on the reverse. *Used for*: oedema, hypertension. *Dosage*: 1–4mg per day for oedema, 500µg–4mg per day for hypertension. Not recommended for children. *Special care*: liver or kidney disease, liver cirrhosis, gout, SLE, diabetes, elderly, pregnancy, breast-feeding. Check glucose, electrolytes and fluid. *Avoid use*: liver or kidney failure, hypercalcaemia, Addison's disease, sensitivity to sulphonamides. *Possible interaction*: NSAIDs, cardiac glycosides, lithium corticosteroids, carbenoxolone, tubocurarine, alcohol, barbiturates, opioids, antidiabetic drugs. *Side effects*: rash, blood changes, dizziness, impotence, anorexia, pancreatitis, gastro-intestinal, electrolyte or metabolism upset, sensitivity to light. *Manufacturer*: Pfizer.

NERISONE

Description: a potent steroid, diflucortolone valerate (0.1%) available as a cream, oily cream or ointment. *Used for*: skin disorders that respond to steroids. *Dosage*: apply 2 or 3 times per day reducing to once per day for maintenance. On children under 4, do not use for more than 3 weeks. Also, **NERISONE FORTE**, a very potent form (0.3%) available as ointment and oily cream. *Used for*: initial treatment of resistant, severe skin disorders. *Dosage*: apply sparingly 2 or 3 times per day for a maximum of 2 weeks (maximum total use 60g/week). For maintenance use Nerisone. Not recommended for children under 4. *Special care*: thrombophlebitis, psychoses, recent intestinal anastomoses, chronic nephritis, certain cancers, osteoporosis, peptic ulcer, skin eruption/rash related to a disease, viral, fungal or active infections, tuberculosis. Hypertension, glaucoma, epilepsy, acute glomerulonephritis (inflammation of kidney glomerulus), diabetes, cirrhosis, hypothyroidism, pregnancy, stress. To be withdrawn gradually. *Possible interaction*: NSAIDs, oral anticoagulants, phenytoin, ephedrine, phenobarbitone, rifampicin, diuretics, cardiac glycosides, anticholinesterases, hypoglycaemics. *Side effects*: osteoporosis, depression, euphoria, hyperglycaemia, peptic ulcers, Cushingoid changes. *Manufacturer*: Schering H.C.

NETILLIN

Description: an aminoglycoside and anti-bacterial, netilmicin sulphate, available as ampoules containing 10, 50 or 100mg/ml. *Used for*: septicaemia, bacteraemia (bacteria in the blood), serious infections of the kidney, urinary tract, skin and soft tissues, respiratory tract. Gonorrhoea. *Dosage*: 4–6mg/kg once per day as 2 or 3 divided doses. For life-threatening infections, up to 7.5mg/kg per day in 3 divided doses, all by intramuscular or slow intravenous injection. Children (by the same means): over 2 years, 2–2.5mg/kg 8-hourly; 1 week to 2 years, 2.5–3mg/kg 8-hourly; under 1 week 3mg/kg 12-hourly. *Special care*: myasthenia gravis, Parkinsonism. Control total dosage in cases of kidney disease. *Avoid use*: pregnancy. *Possible interaction*: anaesthetics, etha crynic acid, frusemide, neuromuscular blockers. *Side effects*: nephrotoxicity and ototoxicity (affects hearing and balance). *Manufacturer*: Schering-Plough.

NEULACTIL

Description: a group II phenothiazine and antipsychotic, pericyazine, available as yellow tablets, marked with name (2.5mg) or marked with name and strength (10mg). Also **NEULACTIL FORTE SYRUP**, containing 10mg/5ml. *Used for*: schizophrenia, severe anxiety and tension, agitation, behavioural disorders, maintenance of sedation for psychotic states. *Dosage*: 15–75mg per day initially (elderly 5–30mg), to a maximum of 300mg daily. See literature for children. *Special care*: pregnancy, lactation, elderly during very hot or cold weather. *Avoid use*: heart failure, epilepsy, Parkinsonism, liver or kidney disorder, hypothyroidism, glaucoma, coma, bone marrow depression, enlarged prostate. *Possible interaction*: alcohol, CNS depressants, antihypertensives, analgesics, levodopa, antidepressants, anticonvulsants, antidiabetic drugs. *Side effects*: muscle spasms (eye, neck, back, face), restlessness, rigidity and tremor, tardive dyskinesia (repetitious muscular movements), dry mouth, blocked nose, difficulty in passing urine, tachycardia, blurred vision, hypotension, constipation, weight gain, impotence, galactorrhoea, gynaecomastia, amenorrhoea, blood and skin changes, lethargy, fatigue, ECG irregularities. *Manufacturer*: R.P.R.

NEUPOGEN

Description: a recombinant human granulocyte colony stimulating factor (G-CSF), filgrastim, available as 30 million units in a single dose vial, for specialist use. *Used for*: reduction of neutropenia during cytotoxic chemotherapy and after bone marrow transplantation. *Dosage*: chemotherapy, 500,000 units/kg per day by subcutaneous injection or intravenous infusion starting within 24 hours of chemotherapy and continuing until neutrophil count is normal (about 14 days). Bone marrow transplantation—1 million units/kg per day starting within 24 hours. *Special care*: risk of bone marrow tumour growth, pre-malignant bone marrow conditions. Monitor platelets, haemoglobin, osteoporosis, pregnancy, lactation. *Side effects*: temporary hypotension, urinary abnormalities, musculo-skeletal pain, disturbances in liver enzymes and serum uric acid. *Manufacturer*: Amgen-Roche.

NEURONTIN

Description: a GABA analogue, gabapentin, available as capsules: white (100mg), yellow (300mg); orange (400mg), all marked with name and strength. *Used for*: added treatment of seizures not controlled by other anticonvulsants. *Dosage*: 300mg once, twice and 3 times per day on days 1, 2 and 3 respectively, increasing to 400mg 3 times per day up to a maximum of 800mg. Not for children. *Special care*: haemodialysis, pregnancy, kidney disease, elderly, lactation, avoid sudden withdrawal (minimum 1 week). *Possible interaction*: antacids. *Side effects*: ataxia, dizziness, fatigue, headache, tremor, diplopia, nausea, vomiting, nystagmus (involuntary eye movements) rhinitis, amblyopia (reduced vision in an eye that appears normal structurally). *Manufacturer*: Parke-Davis.

NIFENSAR XL

Description: a class II calcium antagonist and antihypertensive, nifedipine, available as yellow, sustained-release tablets (20mg) marked N20. *Used for*: mild to moderate hypertension. *Dosage*: 2 once per day swallowed with food, adjusted according to response. 1 or 2 once per day for maintenance. Maximum 5 per day. Elderly, 1 per day initially. Not for children. *Special care*: diabetes, angina pectoris, kidney disease, weak heart. *Avoid use*: pregnancy, breast-feeding, liver disease. *Possible interaction*: other antihypertensives, digoxin, climetidine, quinidine, fentaryl. *Side effects*: nausea, oedema, headache, flushes, dizziness, ischaemic pain, jaundice, rash, lethargy, enlarged gums. *Manufacturer*: R.P.R.

NIMOTOP

Description: a class II calcium antagonist, nimodipine, available as 30mg off-white tablets marked Bayer and SK. *Used for*: prevention of ischaemic, neurological defects after a subarachnoid (intracranial) haemorrhage. *Dosage*: 2 tablets every 4 hours commencing within 4 days of the haemorrhage and continuing for 21 days. Also, **NIMOTOP INFUSION**, containing 0.2mg/ml in vial and bottle. *Used for*: neurological deficits after subarachnoid haemorrhage. *Dosage*: 1mg/hour by intravenous infusion for 2 hours, then 2mg/hour for 5 to 14 days. For bodyweights under 70kg, or for unstable blood pressure, start at 0.5mg/hour. Not for children. *Special care*: raised intracranial pressure, cerebral oedema, kidney disease, pregnancy. Check blood pressure. PVC apparatus should not be used—use polyethylene or polypropylene. *Possible interaction*: ß-blockers, other calcium antagonists. *Side effects*: flushes, headache, hypotension, heart rate changes. *Manufacturer*: Bayer.

NIPENT

Description: an adenosine deaminase inhibitor, and cytotoxic drug pentostatin, available as 10mg powder in vial for reconstitution, used in cancer chemotherapy. *Used for*: prolonged remission in the treatment of malignancies. *Dosage*: intravenously on alternate weeks. For specialist use only. *Side effects*: nausea and vomiting, bone marrow suppression, suppression of the immune system, hair loss, teratogenic. *Manufacturer*: Wyeth.

NIPRIDE

Description: a vasodilator, sodium nitroprusside available as powder (50mg) in ampoules. *Used for*: critical hypertension, heart failure, controlled hypotension in surgery. *Dosage*: for hypertension, 0.3µg/kg/minute by intravenous infusion to begin then adjust to response, usually 0.5–6µg/kg/minute (maximum 8 g/kg/minute). Lower doses for patients already taking antihypertensives. Lower doses also in surgery (up to 1.5µg/kg/minute). For heart failure, 10–15µg/minute by intravenous infusion increasing at 5 to 10 minute intervals to a maximum of 280µg/minute. Maximum treatment 72 hours, withdraw over 10 to 30 minutes. *Special care*: severe kidney disease, hypothyroidism, ischaemic heart disease, elderly, pregnancy, lactation, impaired circulation in the brain. Check blood pressure and concentration of cyanide in plasma. *Avoid use*: vitamin B_{12} deficiency, severe liver disease, optic atrophy (causing blindness). *Possible interaction*: ACE inhibitors, NSAIDs, alcohol, antipsychotics, antidepressants, ß-blockers, diuretics, anxiolytics and hypnotics, corticosteroids, sex hormones, baclofen, carbenoxolone, levodopa. *Side effects*: headache, nausea, dizziness, stomach pain, palpitations, sweating, reeduced platelet count. Also those due to high cyanide concentrations in plasma which *in addition* are tachycardia, metabolic acidosis. *Manufacturer*: Roche.

NITOMAN

Description: a dopamine reducing agent, tetrabenazine, available as yellow-buff tablets (25mg) marked ROCHE 120. *Used for*: Huntington's chorea, senile chorea, hemiballismus (violent involuntary movement). *Dosage*: 25mg 3 times per day initially, increasing by 25mg/day every 3 or 4 days to a daily maximum of 200mg. Not for children. *Special care*: pregnancy. *Avoid use*: breast-feeding. *Possible interaction*: levodopa, MAOIs, reserpine. *Side effects*: drowsiness, depression, hypotension on standing, rigidity, tremor. *Manufacturer*: Roche.

NITRAZEPAM

Description: a long-acting benzodiazepine, nitrazepam, available as tablets (5mg). Also, **NITRAZEPAM ORAL SUSPENSION** containing 2.5mg/5ml. *Used for*: insomnia over the short-term or when it is severe. *Dosage*: 5–10mg at bedtime; elderly, 2.5–5mg. Not for children. *Special care*: chronic liver or kidney disease, chronic lung disease, pregnancy, labour, lactation, elderly. May impair judgement. Withdraw gradually and avoid prolonged use. *Avoid use*: depression of respiration, acute lung disease; psychotic, phobic or obsessional states. *Possible interaction*: anticonvulsants, depressants of the CNS, alcohol. *Side effects*: ataxia, confusion, light-headedness, drowsiness, hypotension, gastrointestinal upsets, disturbances in vision and libido, skin rashes, retention of urine, vertigo. Sometimes jaundice or blood disorders. *Manufacturer*: non-proprietary—available from several suppliers.

NITROCINE

Description: a solution of glyceryl trinitrate (1mg/ml) in ampoules and bottles. *Used for*: prevention and treatment of angina, left ventricular failure. *Dosage*: 10–200μg/minute by intravenous infusion. *Special care*: hypotension, tolerance. *Avoid use*: anaemia, cerebral haemorrhage, head trauma, closed angle glaucoma. *Side effects*: flushes, headache, tachycardia, dizziness, hypotension on standing. *Manufacturer*: Schwarz.

NITRONAL

Description: a solution of glyceryl trinitrate (1mg/ml) in ampoules and vials. *Used for*: prevention and treatment of angina, left ventricular failure. *Dosage*: 10–200μg/minute by intravenous infusion. *Special care*: hypotension, tolerance. *Avoid use*: anaemia, cerebral haemorrhage, head trauma, closed angle glaucoma. *Side effects*: flushes, headache, tachycardia, dizziness, hypotension on standing. *Manufacturer*: Lipha.

NIVAQUINE

Description: a suppressive drug and 4-aminoquinoline, chloroquine sulphate, available as yellow tablet (150mg) marked NIVAQUINE 200. *Used for*: rheumatoid arthritis, malaria. *Dosage*: 1 tablet per day (arthritis); for malaria prevention, 2 tablets in 1 dose on the same week day for 2 weeks before being subjected to possible infection and for 4 weeks after. Children should use the syrup. Also, **NIVAQUINE SYRUP**, 50mg/5ml chloroquine sulphate. *Dosage*: 3mg/kg per day for arthritis; prevention of malaria, 5mg/kg at weekly intervals, for 2 weeks before and 4 weeks after being subjected to possible infection. For treatment see literature. Also, **NIVAQUINE INJECTION**, 40mg/ml in ampoules. *Used for*: emergency treatment. *Dosage*: see literature. *Special care*: porphyria, kidney or liver disorders, severe gastro-intestinal, blood or neurological disorders, psoriasis, pregnancy, lactation, history of epilepsy. Regular eye tests before and during treatment. *Side effects*: gastro-intestinal upset, headache, skin eruptions, loss of pigment, hair loss, blurred vision, damage to retina, blood disorders, allergic reactions, opacities in cornea. *Manufacturer*: R.P.R.

NIVEMYCIN

Description: an antibiotic and aminoglycoside, neomycin sulphate, available as 500mg tablets. Also, **NIVEMYCIN ELIXIR** containing 100mg/5ml. *Used for*: preparation before bowel surgery and an added treatment for hepatic coma. *Dosage*: 2 tablets per hour for 4 hours, then 2 every 4 hours for 2 to 3 days (pre-operation). Children: over 12 years, 2 tablets; 6 to 12 years, half to 1 tablet; 1 to 5 years, 10–20ml; under 1 year, 2.5–10ml. All taken 4 hourly for 2 to 3 days pre-operatively. *Special care*: Parkinsonism, hepatic coma, kidney disease. *Avoid use*: bowel obstruction. *Side effects*: gastro-intestinal upset. *Manufacturer*: Knoll.

NIZORAL

Description: an imidazole and antifungal, ketoconazole, available as white tablets (200mg) marked JANSSEN and K over 200. Also, **NIZORAL SUSPENSION** containing 100mg/5ml. *Used for*: systemic fungal infections, prevention of infections in patients with reduced immune response, chronic vaginal thrush and infections of the gastro-intestinal tract not responding to other teatment, skin and mucous membrane fungal infections. *Dosage*: 200–400mg daily with meals continuing 1 week after symptoms have ceased. For vaginal thrush 400mg once per day for 5 days. Children 3mg/kg daily. Also, **NIZORAL CREAM**, 2% ketoconazole. *Used for*: candidal vulvitis. *Dosage*: apply once or twice per day *Avoid use*: liver disease or liver abnormalities, pregnancy, hypersensitivity to other imidazoles. *Possible interaction*: antacids, anticoagulants, phenytoin, rifampicin, cyclosporin, astemizole, terfenadine, anticholinergics, H_2 antagonists. *Side effects*: hypersensitivity, rashes, headache, gastro-intestinal disturbances, hepatitis, thrombocytopenia (reduction in blood platelets), rarely breast enlargement. Nizoral Cream *also used for*: ringworm infections, skin infection, seborrhoeic dermatitis. Dosage: apply once or twice per day. *Side effects*: skin irritation. Also **NIZORAL SHAMPOO**, 20mg ketoconazole per ml of liquid. *Used for*: seborrhoeic dermatitis, dandruff, scaly skin rash (pityriasis). *Dosage*: dermatitis, use shampoo twice weekly for 2 to 4 weeks, and once every 1 or 2 weeks for prevention. Pityriasis, shampoo once per day for 5 days; prevention once daily for 3 days maximum. *Side effects*: skin irritation. *Manufacturer*: Janssen-Cilag.

NOBRIUM

Description: a long-acting benzodiazepine and anxiolytic medazepam, available as yellow/orange capsules (5mg) marked with strength and ROCHE. *Used for*: treatment of severe or disabling anxiety over the short-term whether it occcurs alone or with insomnia. *Dosage*: 15–40mg in divided doses; elderly 5–20mg. Not for children. *Special care*: chronic liver or kidney disease, chronic lung disease, pregnancy, labour, lactation, elderly. May impair judgement. Withdraw gradually and avoid prolonged use. *Avoid use*: depression of respiration, acute lung disease; psychotic, phobic or obsessional states. *Possible interaction*: anticonvulsants, depressants of the CNS, alcohol. *Side effects*: ataxia, confusion, light-headedness, drowsiness, hypotension, gastro-intestinal upsets, disturbances in vision and libido, skin rashes, retention of urine, vertigo. Sometimes jaundice or blood disorders. *Manufacturer*: Roche.

NOCTEC

Description: a sedative and hypnotic chloral hydrate, available as liquid-filled red capsules containing 500mg. *Used for*: insomnia. *Dosage*: 500mg–1g with water 15 to 30 minutes before bedtime. Daily maximum, 2g. Not for children. *Special care*: porphyria, lactation, impaired judgement and dexterity. *Avoid use*: gastritis, pregnancy, severe liver, heart or kidney disease. *Possible interaction*: anticoagulants, CNS depressants, alcohol. *Side effects*: headache, skin allergies, ketonuria, excitement, delirium. *Manufacturer*: Squibb.

NODS TROPICAMIDE

Description: an anticholinergic, tropicamide (125µg), available as sterile ophthalmic applicator strips. *Used for*: a short-acting dilator of the pupil and paralyser of the ciliary muscle of the eye. *Dosage*: 1 unit in lower conjunctival sac, repeating after 30–45 minutes if required. *Special care*: if driving or operating machinery. *Avoid use*: narrow angle glaucoma. *Manufacturer*: Chauvin.

NOLVADEX-D

Description: an antioestrogen and infertility drug, tamoxifen citrate, available as white octagonal tablets (20mg) marked NOVADEX-D and ICI. Also, **NOLVADEX FORTE**, as white elongated octagonal tablets (40mg) marked **NOLVADEX FORTE** and ICI. Also, **NOLVADEX**, 10mg white tablets marked NOLVADEX and ICI. *Used for*: infertility. *Dosage*: 20mg per day on 4 consecutive days starting on second day of menstruation, increasing to 40mg and 80mg for later courses, if necessary. *Avoid use*: pregnancy. *Possible interaction*:

warfarin. *Side effects*: vaginal bleeding, hot flushes, dizziness, gastro-intestinal upset. Stop if there are disturbances to vision. *Manufacturer*: Zeneca.

NOOTROPIL

Description: a GABA analogue, piracetam, available as white, oblong tablets (800 and 1200mg strengths) marked N. Also, NOOTROPIL SOLUTION, containing 333mg/ml. *Used for*: additional treatment for cortical myoclonus (sudden muscular spasms). *Dosage*: 7.2g per day initially, increasing by 4.8g daily at 3 or 4 day intervals to a maximum of 20g per day in 2 or 3 divided doses. Not for children under 16 years. *Special care*: kidney disease, elderly. Withdraw gradually. *Avoid use*: severe kidney dysfunction, liver disease, pregnancy, breast-feeding. *Possible interaction*: thyroid hormones. *Side effects*: insomnia, nervousness, weight gain, depression, diarrhoea, rash, hyperactivity. *Manufacturer*: UCB.

NORCURON

Description: a muscle relaxant, vercuronium bromide (10mg) as powder in vials with water for injections. *Used for*: short to medium duration muscle relaxant. *Dosage*: 80–100µg/kg by intravenous injection and 20–30µg/kg for maintenance. Infants over 5 months as for adult; up to 4 months 10–20µg/kg then increase gradually to obtain response. 50–80µg/kg/hour by intravenous infusion after initial injection of 40–100µg/kg. *Special care*: respiration should be assisted, reduce dose in kidney disease. *Possible interaction*: some cholinergics, nifedipine, verapamil. *Manufacturer*: Organon-Teknika.

NORDITROPIN

Description: a growth hormone, somatropin, available as a powder in a vial (12 units) plus diluent. *Used for*: failure of growth in children due to growth hormone deficiency, Turner's syndrome. *Dosage*: 0.07–0.1 units/kg body weight 6 to 7 times per week by subcutaneous injection (growth failure). For Turner's syndrome, 0.1 units/kg. Also, NORDITROPIN PENSET, 12 and 24 units somatropin as powder in vials with 2ml of solvent. *Dosage*: as above. *Special care*: diabetes, deficiency of ACTH (adrenocorticotrophic hormones), intrancranial lesion. Check thyroid function. *Avoid use*: pregnancy, lactation, tumour, closure of epiphyses. *Side effects*: oedema, hypothyroidism, pain at injection site. (Move site of injection to avoid lipoatrophy). *Manufacturer*: Novo Nordisk.

NORDOX

Description: a tetracycline, doxycycline, available in green capsules (100mg) marked NORDOX 100. *Used for*: infections of the respiratory tract including bronchitis and sinusitis. Acne. Infections of the genito-urinary tract. *Dosage*: 200mg on the first day, then 100mg per day with food or drink. Not for children. *Special care*: liver disease. *Avoid use*: pregnancy, breast-feeding. *Possible interaction*: mineral supplements, antacids. *Side effects*: allergic reactions, gastro-intestinal upset, superinfections. Stop if there is intracranial hypertension. *Manufacturer*: Panpharma.

NORFLEX

Description: an anticholinergic, orphenadrine citrate, available in ampoules (30mg/ml). *Used for*: musculoskeletal pain. *Dosage*: 60mg by intramuscular or slow intravenous injection, repeated every 12 hours if required. Not for children. *Special care*: pregnancy, tachycardia. *Avoid use*: glaucoma, lactation, myasthenia gravis, urine retention. *Side effects*: nausea, blurred vision, dizziness, dry mouth, confusion, tremor. *Manufacturer*: 3M Health Care.

NORGESTON

Description: a progestogen-only contraceptive, levonorgestrel, available in white tablets (30μg). *Used for*: oral contraception. *Dosage*: 1 at the same time each day without a break, starting on the first day of the cycle. *Special care*: hypertension, thromboembolic disorders, liver disease, hormone-dependent cancer, ovarian cysts, migraine. Regular checks on blood pressure, breasts and pelvic organs. *Avoid use*: previous severe arterial or heart disease, benign liver tumours, undiagnosed vaginal bleeding, pregnancy, past ectopic pregnancy. Discontinue immediately for pregnancy, jaundice, thrombophlebitis or thromboembolism. *Possible interaction*: griseofulvin, rifampicin, meprobamate, chloral hydrate, carbamazepine, primidone, barbiturates, phenytoin, dichloralphenazone, ethosuximide, glutethimide. *Side effects*: acne, breast discomfort, headache, ovarian cysts, irregular menstrual bleeding. *Manufacturer*: Schering H.C.

NORIDAY

Description: a progestogen-only contraceptive, norethisterone, as white tablets (350μg) marked NORIDAY and SYNTEX. *Used for*: oral contraception. *Dosage*: 1 at the same time each day without a break, starting on the first day of the cycle. *Special care*: hypertension, thromboembolic disorders, liver disease, hormone-dependent cancer, ovarian cysts, migraine. Regular checks on blood pressure, breasts and pelvic organs. *Avoid use*: previous severe arterial or heart disease, benign liver tumours, undiagnosed vaginal bleeding, pregnancy, past ectopic pregnancy. Discontinue immediately for pregnancy, jaundice, thrombophlebitis or thromboembolism. *Possible interaction*: griseofulvin, rifampicin, meprobamate, chloral hydrate, carbamazepine, primidone, barbiturates, phenytoin, dichloralphenazone, ethosuximide, glutethimide. *Side effects*: acne, breast discomfort, headache, ovarian cysts, irregular menstrual bleeding. *Manufacturer*: Schering H.C.

NORIMIN

Description: a combined oestrogen/progestogen contraceptive containing 35μg ethinyloestradiol and 1mg norethisterone in a peach tablet marked C over 135. *Used for*: oral contraception. *Dosage*: 1 per day for 21 days, starting on the fifth day of menstruation, then 7 days without tablets. *Special care*: hypertension, Raynaud's disease (reduced blood supply to an organ of the body's extremities), asthma, severe depression, diabetes, varicose veins, multiple sclerosis, chronic kidney disease, kidney dialysis. Blood pressure, breasts and pelvic organs to be checked regularly; smoking not advised. *Avoid use*: history of heart disease, infectious hepatitis, sickle cell anaemia, porphyria, liver tumour, undiagnosed vaginal bleeding, pregnancy, hormone-dependent cancer, haemolytic uraemic syndrome (rare kidney disorder), chorea, otosclerosis. *Possible interaction*: barbiturates, tetracyclines, griseofulvin, rifampicin, primidone, phenytoin, chloral hydrate, ethosuximide, carbamazepine, glutethimide, dichloralphenazone. *Side effects*: fluid retention and bloating, leg cramps/pains, breast enlargement, depression, headaches, nausea, loss of libido, weight gain, vaginal discharge, cervical erosion (alteration of epithelial cells), chloasma (pigmentation of nose, cheeks or forehead), breakthrough bleeding (bleeding between periods). *Manufacturer*: Searle.

NORINYL-1

Description: a combined oestrogen/progestogen contraceptive containing 50µg mestranol and 1mg norethisterone in a white tablet marked NORINYL and SYNTEX. *Used for*: oral contraception. *Special care*: hypertension, Raynaud's disease (reduced blood supply to an organ of the body's extremities), asthma, severe depression, diabetes, varicose veins, multiple sclerosis, chronic kidney disease, kidney dialysis. Blood pressure, breasts and pelvic organs to be checked regularly; smoking not advised. *Avoid use*: history of heart disease, infectious hepatitis, sickle cell anaemia, porphyria, liver tumour, undiagnosed vaginal bleeding, pregnancy, hormone-dependent cancer, haemolytic uraemic syndrome (rare kidney disorder), chorea, otosclerosis. *Possible interaction*: barbiturates, tetracyclines, griseofulvin, rifampicin, primidone, phenytoin, chloral hydrate, ethosuximide, carbamazepine, glutethimide, dichloralphenazone. *Side effects*: fluid retention and bloating, leg cramps/pains, breast enlargement, depression, headaches, nausea, loss of libido, weight gain, vaginal discharge, cervical erosion (alteration of epithelial cells), chloasma (pigmentation of nose, cheeks or forehead), breakthrough bleeding (bleeding between periods). *Manufacturer*: Searle.

NORISTERAT

Description: a depot progestogen contraceptive, norethisterone oenanthate, available as an oily solution in ampoules containing 200mg/ml. *Used for*: short-term highly effective contraception irrespective of errors by patient. *Dosage*: 200mg by deep intramuscular injection (in gluteal muscle) administered within the first 5 days of the cycle. May be repeated once after 8 weeks. *Special care*: liver disorder or diseases that are likely to worsen in pregnancy, severe depression. *Avoid use*: acute and severe chronic liver disease, pregnancy, history of thrombo-embolism, history during pregnancy of itching, idiopathic jaundice or pemphigoid gestationis (skin disorder with large blisters). *Side effects*: weight changes, breast discomfort, headache, dizziness, nausea, menstrual changes. *Manufacturer*: Schering H.C.

NORMAX

Description: a laxative and faecal softener containing danthron (50mg) and docusate sodium (60mg) in brown capsules marked NORMAX. *Used for*: constipation in the elderly, for those with heart failure, coronary thrombosis and constipation induced by analgesics. *Dosage*: 1 to 3 tablets at night. Children over 6 years, 1 at night. Not for children under 6 years. *Special care*: lactation. *Avoid use*: obstruction of the bowel. *Manufacturer*: Evans.

NORMEGON

Description: Human menopausal gonadotrophin. *Used for*: female or male infertility due to understimulation of the gonads by gonadotrophin. Superovulation for in-vitro fertilization. *Dosage*: by intramuscular injection, but see literature. *Special care*: exclude other possible causes including gonad abnormalities. Check oestrogen levels and size of ovaries regularly. *Avoid use*: ovarian, pituitary or testicular tumours. *Side effects*: risk of multiple pregnancy, miscarriage, rash. *Manufacturer*: Organon.

NORMISON^{CD}

Description: an intermediate-acting benzodiazepine, temazepam, available as yellow capsules marked N10 (10mg) and N20 (20mg). *Used for*: premedication, short-term treatment of insomnia when sedation during the day is not required. *Dosage*: 20–40mg half to 1 hour before surgery (premedication),. 10–30mg at bedtime (elderly 10mg), maximum 60mg for severe cases. Not for children. *Special care*: chronic liver or kidney disease, chronic lung disease, pregnancy, labour, lactation, elderly. May impair judgement. Withdraw gradually and avoid prolonged use. *Avoid use*: depression of respiration, acute lung disease; psychotic, phobic or obsessional states. *Possible interaction*: anticonvulsants, depressants of the CNS, alcohol. *Side effects*: ataxia, confusion, light-headedness, drowsiness, hypotension, gastro-intestinal upsets, disturbances in vision and libido, skin rashes, retention of urine, vertigo. Sometimes jaundice or blood disorders. *Manufacturer*: Wyeth.

NORPLANT

Description: a progestogen depot contraceptive, levonorgestrel, available as an implant (228mg) beneath the skin. *Used for*: long-term contraception that is reversible. *Dosage*: subdermal implant, for those aged 18–40, to be removed within 5 years. *Special care*: risk of arterial disease, hypertension, benign intracranial hypertension, migraine. Check blood pressure, breasts and pelvic organs before and during treatment. *Avoid use*: thromboembolic disorders, heart disease, liver disease, history of severe arterial disease, pregnancy, undiagnosed vaginal bleeding, hormone-dependent cancer, recent cancer of the uterus. *Possible interaction*: phenytoin, primidone, rifampicin, griseofulvin, barbiturates, carbamazepine, phenylbutazone, chronic use of tetracyclines. *Side effects*: amenorrhoea, ovarian cysts, irregular or extended menstrual bleeding, headache, nausea, weight gain, hirsutism, hair loss, enlargement of related organs. *Manufacturer*: Hoechst.

NORVAL

Description: a TCAD, mianserin hydrochloride, available as orange tablets in 10, 20 and 30mg strengths, marked with NORVAL and tablet strength. *Used for*: depression. *Dosage*: 30–40mg per day as 1 dose at night or in divided doses. Increase after a few days to maintenance levels of 30–90mg per day. Elderly, start no higher than 30mg per day, increase gradually. Not for children. *Special care*: elderly, pregnancy, heart block, myocardial infarction, epilepsy, glaucoma, enlarged prostate. *Avoid use*: lactation, severe liver disease, mania. *Possible interaction*: alcohol, anticoagulants, MAOIs. *Side effects*: drowsiness, blood changes. Blood tests advisable monthly for first 3 months. Withdraw if there develops infection, jaundice, convulsions or hypomania. *Manufacturer*: Bencard.

NOVA-T *Description*: an IUD comprising copper wire with a silver core on a plastic T-shaped carrier. *Used for*: contraception. *Special care*: diabetes, anaemia, history of endocarditis or pelvic inflammatory disease, epilepsy, hypermenorrhoea (or menorrhagia, long or heavy menstrual periods). Examine after 3 months, then annually. *Avoid use*: pregnancy, past ectopic pregnancy, uterus disorders, infection of vagina or cervix, acute pelvic inflammatory diseases, cervical cancer, abnormal vaginal bleeding, endometrial disease, immunosuppressive therapy, copper allergy, cancer of the genitalia. *Possible interaction*: anticoagulants. *Side effects*: pain, pelvic infection, perforation of the uterus, abnormal bleeding. On insertion there may be attack of asthma or epilepsy, bradycardia. Remove if persistent bleeding or cramps, perforation of cervix or uterus, pregnancy, persistent pelvic infection. *Manufacturer*: Schering H.C.

NOVAGARD

Description: an IUD comprising copper wire with a silver core on a plastic T-shaped carrier. *Used for*: contraception. *Special care*: diabetes, anaemia, history of endocarditis or pelvic inflammatory disease, epilepsy, hypermenorrhoea (or menorrhagia, long or heavy menstrual periods). Examine after 3 months, then annually. *Avoid use*: pregnancy, past ectopic pregnancy, uterus disorders, infection of vagina or cervix, acute pelvic inflammatory diseases, cervical cancer, abnormal vaginal bleeding, endometrial disease, immunosuppressive therapy, copper allergy, cancer of the genitalia. *Possible interaction*: anticoagulants. *Side effects*: pain, pelvic infection, perforation of the uterus, abnormal bleeding. *On insertion* there may be attack of asthma or epilepsy, bradycardia. Remove if persistent bleeding or cramps, perforation of cervix or uterus, pregnancy, persistent pelvic infection. *Manufacturer*: Pharmacia & Upjohn.

NOVANTRONE

Description: a cytotoxic antibiotic, mitozantrone hydrochloride, available as a solution in vials (2mg/ml). *Used for*: treatment of tumours (leukaemia, lymphoma, breast cancer, and solid tumours). *Dosage*: by intravenous infusion, see literature. *Special care*: check heart after total dose of 160mg/m^2 to avoid dose-related cardiotoxicity. *Side effects*: suppression of bone marrow, see literature. *Manufacturer*: Wyeth.

NOXYFLEX

Description: a combined antibacterial and antifungal compound, noxythiolin, available as powder (2.5g) in vials. *Used for*: solution to be instilled into bladder or other body cavities. *Dosage*: see literature. *Special care*: the solution must be freshly prepared and used within 7 days. *Manufacturer*: Geistlich.

NOZINAN

Description: a group I phenothiazine and antipsychotic, methotrimeprazine, available as white tablets (25mg) marked NOZINAN 25. *Used for*: schizophrenia, mental disorders where sedation is needed, control of terminal pain and accompanying vomiting or distress. *Dosage*: mental disorders, 25–50mg per day for patients who can walk about, 100–200mg for those who cannot. For pain, 12.5–50mg every 4 to 8 hours. Not for children. Also, **NOZINAN INJECTION**, 2.5% isotonic solution in ampoules. *Dosage*: for pain, 12.5–25mg by intramuscular injection or, after dilution, by intravenous injection, every 6 to 8 hours, up to 50mg for severe cases. Or 25–200mg per day diluted with saline, by continuous subcutaneous infusion. Not for children. *Special care*: liver disease, Parkinsonism, epilepsy, cardiovascular disease, pregnancy, lactation. *Avoid use*: bone marrow depression (unless terminal), coma. *Possible interaction*: alcohol, depressants of the CNS, antihypertensives, antidepressants, analgesics, antidiabetics, levodopa, anticonvulsants. *Side effects*: rigidity, tremor, dry mouth, muscle spasms in eye, neck, face and back, tardive dyskinesia (involuntary, repetitive muscle movements in the limbs, face and trunk), tachycardia, constipation, blocked nose, difficulty in urinating, hypotension, weight gain, impotence, galactorrhoea, gynaecomastia, blood changes, jaundice, dermatitis, ECG changes, fatigue, drowsiness, seizures. *Manufacturer*: Link.

NUBAIN

Description: an analgesic and opiate, nalbuphine hydrochloride, available as 10mg/ml in ampoules. *Used for*: moderate to severe pain. Pain associated with suspected myocardial infarction, pre and post-operative pain. *Dosage*: pain, 10–20mg by intravenous, intramuscular or subcutaneous injection. Myocardial infarction, 10–30mg by slow intravenous injection, followed within 30 minutes by 20mg if necessary. Children, starting with up to 0.3mg/kg by intravenous, intramuscular or subcutaneous injection, repeated up to twice if required. *Special care*: liver or kidney disease, head injury, pregnancy, labour, respiratory depression, history of opioid abuse. *Possible interaction*: depressants of the CNS. *Side effects*: sweating, dizziness, dry mouth, nausea, sedation. *Manufacturer*: DuPont.

NUELIN SA

Description: a xanthine and bronchodilator, theophylline, available as white sustained-release tablets (175mg) marked NLS175 and 3M. *Used for*: bronchitis, emphysema, narrowing of airways in asthma. *Dosage*: 1 to 2 tablets twice per day after food. Children over 6 years, 1 tablet twice per day. Not for children under 6. Also, **NUELIN SA-250**, containing 250mg and marked NLS 250 and 3M. *Dosage*: 1 to 2 tablets twice per day after food. Children over 6 years, half the adult dose. Not recommended for children under 6. Also, **NUELIN** containing 125mg, marked NL over 125 and 3M. *Dosage*: 1 to 2 tablets, 3 or 4 times per day, after food. Children aged 7 to 12, half the adult dose. Not for children under 7 years. Also, **NUELIN LIQUID**, containing 60mg theophylline hydrate (as sodium glycinate) per 5ml. *Dosage*: 10–20ml 3 or 4 times per day after food. Children aged 7 to 12, 10ml; aged 2 to 6, 5ml 3 or 4 times per day after food. Not for children under 2 years. *Special care*: pregnancy, breastfeeding, heart or liver disease, peptic ulcer. *Possible interaction*: B_2-agonists, steroids, interferon, erythromycin, diuretics, ciprafloxacin, cimetidine. *Side effects*: nausea, gastro-intestinal upset, headache, tachycardia, arrhythmias, insomnia. *Manufacturer*: 3M Health Care.

NUVELLE

Description: an oestrogen/progestogen compound available as 16 white tablets containing 2mg oestradiol valerate and 12 pink tablets containing in addition 75µg levonorgestrel. *Used for*: post-menopausal osteoporosis, hormone replacement therapy for climacteric syndrome (symptoms associated with the menopause). *Dosage*: 1 white tablet per day for 16 days then 12 days of taking 1 pink tablet. Start on fifth day of menses (discharge). *Special care*: those at risk of thrombosis or with liver disease. Women with any of the following disorders should be monitored: fibroids in the womb, multiple sclerosis, diabetes, tetany, porphyria, epilepsy, liver disease, hypertension, migraine, otosclerosis, gallstones. Breasts, pelvic organs and blood pressure should be checked at regular intervals during course of treatment. *Avoid use*: pregnant women, breast-feeding mothers, women with conditions which might lead to thrombosis, thrombophlebitis, serious heart, kidney or liver disease, breast cancer, oestrogen-dependent cancers including those of reproductive system, endometriosis, vaginal bleeding which is undiagnosed. *Possible interaction*: drugs which induce liver enzymes. *Side effects*: tenderness and enlargement of breasts, weight gain, breakthrough bleeding, giddiness, vomiting and nausea, gastro-intestinal upset. Treatment should be halted immediately if severe headaches occur, disturbance of vision, hypertension or any indications of thrombosis, jaundice. Also, in the event of pregnancy and 6 weeks before planned surgery. *Manufacturer*: Schering

H.C. NYCOPREN

Description: a propionic acid and NSAID, naproxen, available as white, oblong tablets (250 or 500mg strength). *Used for*: osteoarthrosis, rheumatoid arthritis, acute gout, ankylosing spondylitis, inflammatory musculoskeletal disorders, juvenile rheumatoid arthritis (JRA). *Dosage*: 250–500mg twice per day. Gout, start with 750mg followed by 250mg 8-hourly. Musculoskeletal, 500mg then 250mg 8-hourly. For JRA, over 50kg, 250–500mg twice per day, not recommended for under 50kg. *Special care*: elderly, kidney or liver disease, heart failure, history of gastro-intestinal lesions, pregnancy, asthma. Check kidney and liver for long-term treatment. *Avoid use*: lactation, allergy to aspirin or anti-inflammatory drugs, active peptic ulcer. *Possible interaction*: sulphonamides, sulphonylureas, anticoagulants, quinolones, ß-blockers, lithium, hydantoins, frusemide, methotrexate, probenecid. *Side effects*: headache, vertigo, blood changes, tinnitus, rash, gastro-intestinal intolerance. *Manufacturer*: Nycomed.

NYSTADERMAL

Description: an antibacterial and potent steroid, nystatin (100,000 units/g) and triamcinolone acetonide (0.1%) available as a cream. *Used for*: pruritus and eczema, skin infection and inflammation. *Dosage*: apply 2 to 4 times per day. *Special care*: thrombophlebitis, psychoses, recent intestinal anastomoses, chronic nephritis, certain cancers, osteoporosis, peptic ulcer, skin eruption/rash related to a disease, viral, fungal or active infections, tuberculosis. Hypertension, glaucoma, epilepsy, acute glomerulonephritis (inflammation of kidney glomerulus), diabetes, cirrhosis, hypothyroidism, pregnancy, stress. To be withdrawn gradually. *Possible interaction*: NSAIDs, oral anticoagulants, phenytoin, ephedrine, phenobarbitone, rifampicin, diuretics, cardiac glycosides, anticholinesterases, hypoglycaemics. *Side effects*: osteoporosis, depression, euphoria, hyperglycaemia, peptic ulcers, Cushingoid changes. *Manufacturer*: Squibb.

NYSTAFORM

Description: an antifungal and antibacterial cream containing 100,000 units of nystatin per gram and 1% chlorhexidine. *Used for*: skin infections. *Dosage*: apply liberally 2 to 3 times per day until 1 week after healing. *Manufacturer*: Bayer. NYSTAFORM-HC *Description*: an antifungal and mildly potent steroid containing 100,000 units of nystatin per gram, 1% chlorhexidine, and 0.5% hydrocortisone available as a cream. Also, **NYSTAFORM-HC OINTMENT** containing 100,000 units of nystatin, 1% chlorhexidine and 1% hydrocortisone. *Used for*: skin disorders where there is infection. *Dosage*: apply 2 or 3 times per day until 1 week after healing. *Special care*: thrombophlebitis, psychoses, recent intestinal anastomoses, chronic nephritis, certain cancers, osteoporosis, peptic ulcer, skin eruption/rash related to a disease, viral, fungal or active infections, tuberculosis. Hypertension, glaucoma, epilepsy, acute glomerulonephritis (inflammation of kidney glomerulus), diabetes, cirrhosis, hypothyroidism, pregnancy, stress. To be withdrawn gradually. *Possible interaction*: NSAIDs, oral anticoagulants, phenytoin, ephedrine, phenobarbitone, rifampicin, diuretics, anticholinesterases, cardiac glycosides, hypoglycaemics. *Side effects*: osteoporosis, depression, euphoria, hyperglycaemia, peptic ulcers, Cushingoid changes. *Manufacturer*: Bayer.

NYSTAN

Description: an antibiotic containing 500,000 units of nystatin, available as brown tablets. *Used for*: intestinal infection with *Candida*. *Dosage*: 1 to 2 tablets 4 times per day. Children should take the suspension. Also, **NYSTAN ORAL SUSPENSION** containing 100,000 units nystatin/ml in a ready-mixed suspension. Also, **NYSTAN FOR SUSPENSION** which in addition is free of lactose, sugar and corn starch. *Used for*: infections (candidiasis) of the mouth, oesophagus and intestines. *Dosage*: 1ml 4 times per day for oral infections, 5ml 4 times per day for infection of the intestines. Children, 1ml 4 times per day. Prevention in infants under 1 month, 1ml per day. For oral infections the suspension should be retained in the mouth. Continue for 2 days after cure. Also, **NYSTAN PASTILLES** containing 100,000 units nystatin per pastille. *Used for*: oral infections. *Dosage*: 1 pastille sucked slowly 4 times per day for 7 to 14 days. *Side effects*: nausea, vomiting and diarrhoea with high doses. Also, **NYSTAN** as 100,000 units of nystatin in yellow, diamond-shaped pessaries, marked SQUIBB 457; **NYSTAN VAGINAL CREAM** (100,000 units/4g); **NYSTAN GEL** (100,000 units/g); and **NYSTAN ORAL TABLETS** (500,000 units in brown tablets). *Used for*: candidal vaginitis (vaginal infection caused by *Candida*, thrush). *Dosage*: 1 to 2 pessaries or 1 to 2 applications of cream for 14 or more consecutive nights; irrespective of menstruation. Gel; applied topically to anogenital region 2 to 4 times per day for 14 days. Oral treatment, 1 tablet 4 times per day during vaginal treatment. Children use vaginal cream with oral treatment. *Side effects*: temporary burning and irritation. Also **NYSTAN** as cream, ointment and gel (100,000 units nystatin per gram). *Used for*: thrush of the skin and mucous membranes. *Dosage*: apply 2 to 4 times per day. *Manufacturer*: Squibb.

O

OCUFEN

Description: an NSAID which is a proprionic acid available in the form of eyedrops containing 0.03% flubiprofen sodium. *Used for*: to inhibit inflammation and constriction of the pupil (miosis) during operations of the eye. *Dosage*: as directed by physician. *Manufacturer*: Allergan.

OCUSERT PILO

Description: a cholinergic eye preparation containing pilocarpine 20 as elliptical-shaped sustained-release inserts delivering 40 micrograms/hour for a 1 week period. *Used for*: glaucoma. *Dosage*: place 1 insert under eyelid and replace each week. *Avoid use*: patients with severe inflammation or infection. *Side effects*: eye irritation, loss of sharpness of vision. *Manufacturer*: Dominion.

ODRIK

Description: an ACE inhibitor available as capsules of 3 strengths all containing trandolapril. Yellow/red capsules contain 0.5mg; orange/red contain 1mg; red/red contain 2mg. *Used for*: hypertension. *Dosage*: 0.5mg once each day at first increasing every 2 to 4 weeks to a maximum 4mg as a single daily dose. Maintenance dose is in the order of 1–2mg once each day. Any diuretics being taken should be discontinued 2 or 3 days before treatment starts. *Special care*: liver or kidney disease, receiving kidney dialysis, undergoing anaesthesia or surgery, congestive heart failure. Also, patients with low fluid and salt levels. *Avoid use*: pregnancy, breast-feeding, obstruction of blood outflow from heart or aortic stenosis (narrowing of aorta). Also, angioneurotic oedema due to previous treatment with an ACE inhibitor. *Possible interaction*: NSAIDs, potassium-sparing diuretics. *Side effects*: rash, cough, muscular weakness, headache, dizziness, palpitations, hypotension. Rarely, agranulocytosis (a blood disorder characterized by abnormal reduction in number of white blood cells (granulocytes), angioneurotic oedema, depression of bone marrow. *Manufacturer*: Hoechst.

OLBETAM

Description: a lipid-lowering nicotinic acid derivative available as pink/red-brown capsules containing 250mg acipimox marked with name. *Used for*: raised protein-bound lipid levels in blood (hyperlipoproteinaemia) of type IIa, IIb and IV. *Dosage*: adults, 2 or 3 tablets each day taken as divided doses with meals. Maximum dosage is 1200mg each day. *Avoid use*: pregnancy, breast-feeding, children, patients with peptic ulcer. *Side effects*: gastro-intestinal upset, flushing, headache, inflammation of skin and mucous membranes (erythema), malaise, skin rash. *Manufacturer*: Pharmacia & Upjohn.

OMNOPON[CD]

Description: an analgesic, opiate available as a solution in ampoules for injection containing 15.4mg papaveretum/ml. *Used for*: severe pain. *Dosage*: adults, 0.5–1ml given by subcutaneous, intravenous or intramuscular injection. Dose may be repeated after 4 hours. Children, under 1 year, 0.0075–0.01ml/kg body weight each day. Over 1 year, 0.01–0.015ml/kg. All given by subcutaneous, intravenous or intramuscular injection as a maximum single dose. Elderly, 0.5ml at first by same route. *Special care*: pregnancy, breast-feeding, elderly persons, newborn babies, patients with enlarged prostate gland, underactive thyroid gland, serious liver or kidney disease, having head injury. *Possible interaction*: alcohol, phenothiazines, MAOIs, CNS depressants. *Side effects*: drug dependence and tolerance, constipation, nausea, constipation. *Manufacturer*: Roche.

ONCOVIN

Description: a cytotoxic vinca alkaloid drug produced as a solution in vials for injection containing 1mg vincristine sulphate/ml. *Used for*: lymphomas, leukaemia, some solid tumours (e.g. lung and breast cancer). *Dosage*: by intravenous injection as directed by physician skilled in cancer chemotherapy. *Special care*: care in handling, contact with eyes must be avoided, tissue irritant. *Avoid use*: must not be given by intraethecal injection (i.e. into meninges (membrane linings) of the spinal cord). *Side effects*: damage to peripheral and autonomic nervous system characterized by muscle weakness and abdominal bloating. Hair loss, vomiting, nausea. *Manufacturer*: Lilly.

ONE-ALPHA

Description: a vitamin D analogue, alfacalcidol, available as capsules in 2 strengths; white capsules contain 0.25µg and brown capsules contain 1µg. **ALPHA SOLUTION** containing 0.2µg/ml and also **ONE-ALPHA INJECTION** in ampoules containing 2µg/ml. *Used for*: bone disorders due to kidney disease or loss of function, bone disease associated with under or overactivity of parathyroid glands, low calcium levels in newborn babies. Also, rickets and osteomalacia (bone softening). *Dosage*: 1µg at first adjusted according to response; children, under 20kg, 0.05µg/kg body weight each day at first; over 20kg, 1µg daily. Injection is given intravenously. *Special care*: pregnancy, breast-feeding, kidney failure. Levels of blood calcium must be checked at regular intervals during the course of treatment. *Possible interaction*: thiazide diuretics, colestipol, digitalis, barbiturates, antacids, cholestyramine, anticonvulsants, sucralfate, danazol, mineral oils, antacids. *Manufacturer*: Leo.

OPERIDINE^{CD}

Description: a narcotic analgesic which is a controlled drug available as a solution in ampoules for injection containing 1mg phenoperidine hydrochloride/ml. *Used for*: enhancement of anaesthetics and analgesia during surgery; as a depressant of respiration (especially doses above 1mg) in patients receiving longterm assisted ventilation. *Dosage*: up to 1mg by intravenous injection then 500µg every 40 to 60 minutes as needed. With assisted ventilation, 2–5mg then 1mg as needed. Children, 30–50µg/kg body weight. With assisted ventilation, 100–150µg/kg. Elderly persons receive lower doses. *Special care*: myasthenia gravis, serious respiratory or liver disease, underactive thyroid. If used in obstetrics, may cause depression of respiration in baby. *Avoid use*: obstructive airways disease or depression of respiration (unless being mechanically ventilated). *Possible interaction*: MAOIs, cimetidine. *Side effects*: convulsions with high doses, respiratory depression, nausea, vomiting, bradycardia, hypotension which is short-lived. *Manufacturer*: Janssen.

OPTHAINE

Description: local anaesthetic eyedrops containing 0.5% proxymetacaine hydrochloride. *Used for*: as local anaesthetic during ophthalmic procedures. *Dosage*: usual dose, 1 or 2 drops before procedure begins. Protect eye. *Side effects*: irritation of eye and, rarely, hypersensitive allergic reactions. *Manufacturer*: Squibb.

OPILON

Description: a selective alpha$_1$-blocker available as film-coated, pale yellow tablets containing 40mg thymoxamine as hydrochloride. *Used for*: short-term treatment of Raynaud's disease (a disease affecting the arteries of the fingers which makes them liable to spasm when the hands are cold). *Dosage*: 1 tablet 4 times each day increasing to 2 tablets 4 times each day if condition does not respond. If no significant improvement after 2 weeks, drug should be withdrawn. *Special care*: angina, recent heart attack, diabetes. *Avoid use*: pregnancy, breast-feeding, known hypersensitivity to thymoxamine. *Possible interaction*: diarrhoea, nausea, headache, vertigo. Drug should be withdrawn if liver function is affected. *Manufacturer*: Parke-Davis.

OPTICROM

Description: an NSAID preparation available in the form of eyedrops containing 2% sodium cromoglycate. Also, **OPTICROM EYE OINTMENT** containing 4% sodium cromoglycate. *Used for*: allergic conjunctivitis. *Dosage*: 1 or 2 drops in both eyes 4 times each day, or ointment 3 times daily. *Avoid use*: drops, patients wearing soft contact lenses; ointment, all types of contact lenses. *Side effects*: burning, stinging sensation in eye which is of short-lived duration. *Manufacturer*: R.P.R.

ORAMORPHCD

Description: an analgesic opiate preparation available in a variety of different forms, all containing morphine sulphate. **ORAMORPH SR** are sustained-release, film-coated tablets of different strengths: 10mg buff tablets; 30mg purple tablets; 60mg orange tablets; 100mg grey tablets. All are marked with strength. **ORAMORPH SOLUTION** contains 10mg morphine sulphate/5ml in a sugar-containing solution. **ORAMORPH UNIT DOSE** is a sugar-free solution in single dose vials containing 10mg, 30mg or 100mg morphine sulphate/5ml. **ORAMORPH CONCENTRATE** is a sugar-free solution containing 100mg morphine sulphate/5ml. *Used for*: severe pain. *Dosage*: Oramorph SR, 10–20mg every 12 hours at first, increasing as needed. Other preparations, 10–20mg at 4 hourly intervals. Children, all preparations except Oramorph SR, age 1 to 5 years, up to 5mg; 6 to 12 years, 5–10mg, both every 4 hours. *Special care*: elderly, breast-feeding, underactivity of thyroid gland, reduced function of adrenal glands, enlarged prostate gland, liver or kidney disease, shock, after surgery. *Avoid use*: pregnancy, children under 1 year, obstructive airways disease, disorders characterized by convulsions, depressed respiration, head injuries, coma, severe liver disease, severe alcoholism, raised intracranial pressure. *Possible interaction*: central nervous system depressants, MAOIs. *Side effects*: vomiting and nausea, constipation, sedation, drug dependence and tolerance. *Manufacturer*: Boehringer Ingelheim.

ORAP

Description: an antipsychotic drug, pimozide (a diphenylbutylpiperidine) available as tablets in 3 strengths: scored, white contain 2mg, marked on 1 side with O/2; scored green contain 4mg, marked on 1 side with O/4. Scored, white contain 10mg, marked 1 side with O/10. On the other side all are marked JANSSEN. *Used for*: schizophrenia. *Dosage*: adults, 10mg each day at first increasing by 2–4mg daily at weekly intervals. Maximum daily is 20mg. To prevent a relapse, 2mg each day. Usual daily dose is 2–20mg. *Special care*: pregnancy, imbalance in electrolyte (salts) levels, liver or kidney disorder, epilepsy, Parkinsonism, endogenous depression (resulting from factors within the body). Perform ECG before and during the course of treatment. Patients require careful monitoring. *Avoid use*: children, breast-feeding, those with a very long QT interval (part of the ECG) which can result in a potentially fatal type of tachycardia, history of heart arrhythmias. *Possible interaction*: analgesics, levodopa, CNS depressants, antidiabetics, alcohol, antidepressants, antihypertensives, anticonvulsants, some heart drugs and antipsychotics. *Side effects*: extrapyramidal effects (characterized by involuntary and reflex muscle movements, apathy, sleepiness, disturbance of sleep, depression. Blocked nose, dry mouth, constipation, blurring of vision, tachycardia, heart arrhythmias, hypotension. Changes in: EEG and ECG; breasts and menstrual cycle; blood and liver. Weight gain, impotence, rash, pigmentation of skin and eyes, sensitivity to light, haemolytic anaemia, difficulty in urination. *Manufacturer*: Janssen-Cilag.

ORBENIN

Description: an antibiotic penicillin which is penicillinase-resistant (i.e. resistant to the penicillinase enzymes produced by certain bacteria). Available as orange/black capsules containing 250mg or 500mg cloxacillin (as sodium salt) and marked with strength and name. Also **ORBENIN INJECTION**, available in vials containing 250mg and 500mg cloxacillin. *Used for*: infections caused by Gram-positive bacteria including resistant staphylococci. *Dosage*: tablets, 500mg every 6 hours taken half an hour to an hour before meals; injection, 250mg intramuscularly or 500mg intravenously every 4 to 6 hours. Children, over 2 years, half adult dose. *Avoid use*: children under 2 years. *Side effects*: gastro-intestinal upset, allergic responses, rash. *Manufacturer*: Forley.

ORELOX

Description: a cephalosporin antibiotic available as film-coated white tablets containing 100mg cefpodoxime (as proxetil) marked 208A. *Used for*: bronchitis, tonsilitis, pharyngitis, pneumonia, sinusitis. *Dosage*: adults, 1 or 2 tablets (depending upon infection) twice each day taken with a meal in the morning and evening. *Special care*: pregnancy, sensitivity to beta-lactam antibiotics, kidney disorders. *Avoid use*: children. *Possible interaction*: H_2 antagonists, antacids. *Side effects*: headache, gastro-intestinal upset, allergic responses, raised liver enzymes, colitis. *Manufacturer*: Hoechst.

ORGARAN

Description: an antithrombotic heparinoid preparation produced as a solution in ampoules for injection, containing 1250 units danaparoid sodium antifactor Xa activity/ml. *Used for*: prevention of deep vein thrombosis in patients undergoing surgery. *Dosage*: adults, 0.6ml by subcutaneous injection twice each day for 7 to 10 days before operation. The last dose should be given not less than 1 hour before surgery. *Special care*: patients with ulcer, liver or kidney disorder, asthma, history of heparin-induced thrombocytopenia who test positive to danaparoid. *Avoid use*: pregnancy, breast-feeding, children, bleeding disorders, stroke with haemorrhage, peptic ulcer, serious liver or kidney disease, bacterial endocarditis, serious hypertension, retinopathy (disorder of the blood vessels of the retina of the eye) associated with diabetes. *Side effects*: risk of haemorrhage, skin rash, haematoma, bruising. Also, changes in liver enzymes, thrombocytopenia. *Manufacturer*: Organon Teknika.

ORIMETEN

Description: an anti-cancer drug which inhibits steroid synthesis produced in the form of scored, off-white tablets containing 250mg aminoglutethimide marked GG and CG. *Used for*: advanced breast cancer in post-menopausal women or those whose ovaries have been removed. Also, advanced prostate cancer and Cushing's syndrome resulting from malignancy. *Dosage*: cancer, 1 tablet each day increasing by 1 tablet daily each week. Maximum daily dose is 4 tablets for breast cancer and 3 for prostate cancer. Cushing's syndrome, 1 each day slowly increasing if required to 4 daily in divided doses. Maximum dose is 8 tablets daily. *Special care*: regular monitoring of electrolytes and blood counts is required. Patients with breast or prostate cancer require glucocorticoids (adrenal gland hormones) and these may also be needed by those with Cushing's syndrome. Also, mineralocorticoids (adrenal gland hormones) may be needeed. *Avoid use*: pregnancy, breast-feeding. *Possible interaction*: synthetic glucocorticoids, anticoagulants, hypoglycaemics taken orally. *Side effects*: gastrointestinal upset, blood changes, effects on CNS, rash, thyroid disorders. If allergic alveolitis (inflammation of the air sacs, alveoli, of the lungs) occurs, the drug should be withdrawn. *Manufacturer*: Ciba.

ORTHO DIENOESTROL

Description: an hormonal oestrogen preparation available in the form of a vaginal cream with applicator containing 0.01% dienoestrol. *Used for*: inflammaion and irritation of the vagina and vulva, atrophic vaginitis. *Dosage*: 1 or 2 applicator doses into the vagina each day for 1 to 2 weeks, then reducing to half the initial dose for a further 1 or 2 weeks. Maintenance is 1 applicator dose 1, 2 or 3 times each week. *Special care*: patients considered at risk of thromboembolism, porphyria, multiple sclerosis, epilepsy, fibroids in the womb, migraine, tetany. Also, patients with otosclerosis, gallstones, liver disease. Pelvic organs, breasts and blood pressure should be checked regularly during treatment. *Avoid use*: pregnancy, breast-feeding, breast or other cancer of reproductive tract or one which is hormone-dependent. Also, thromboembolism-type disorders, undiagnosed vaginal bleeding or endometriosis, thrombophlebitis, heart, liver or kidney disease. Rotor or Dublin-Johnson syndrome. *Possible interaction*: drugs which induce liver enzymes. *Side effects*: enlargement and soreness of breasts, gastro-intestinal upset, dizziness, breakthrough bleeding, headache, vomiting and nausea, weight gain. *Manufacturer*: Janssen-Cilag.

ORTHO-GYNEST

Description: an hormonal oestrogen preparation available as vaginal pessaries containing 0.5mg oestriol. Also, **ORTHO-GYNEST CREAM** containing 0.01% oestriol, with applicator. *Used for*: vaginal, vulval and cervical inflammation and disorders in post-menopausal women; atrophic vaginitis. *Dosage*: 1 pessary or applicator dose inserted high up into the vagina at night. Maintenance is 1 pessary or applicator dose each week. *Special care*: patients considered at risk of thromboembolism, porphyria, multiple sclerosis, epilepsy, fibroids in the womb, migraine, tetany. Also, otosclerosis, gallstones, liver disease. Pelvic organs, breasts and blood pressure should be checked regularly during course of treatment. *Avoid use*: pregnancy, breast-feeding, breast or other cancer of reproductive tract or one which is hormone-dependent. Also, patients with thromboembolism-type disorders, undiagnosed vaginal bleeding or endometriosis, thrombophlebitis, heart, liver or kidney disease. Rotor or Dublin-Johnson syndrome. *Possible interaction*: drugs which induce liver enzymes. *Side effects*: enlargement and soreness of breasts, gastro-intestinal upset, dizziness, breakthrough bleeding, headache, vomiting and nausea, weight gain. *Manufacturer*: Janssen-Cilag.

ORTHO-NAVIN 1/50

Description: an hormonal combined oestrogen/progestogen preparation available as white tablets containing 50µg mestranol and 1mg norethisterone marked C over 50. *Used for*: oral contraception. *Dosage*: 1 tablet each day for 21 days starting on the fifth day of period followed by 7 tablet-free days. *Special care*: patients with multiple sclerosis, serious kidney disease or kidney dialysis, asthma, Raynaud's disease, abnormally high levels of prolactin in the blood (hyperprolactinaemia), varicose veins, hypertension. Also, patients suffering from severe depression. Thrombosis risk increases with smoking, age and obesity. During the course of treatment, regular checks on blood pressure, pelvic organs and breasts should be carried out. *Avoid use*: pregnancy, patients considered to be at risk of thrombosis, suffering from heart disease, pulmonary hypertension, angina, sickle cell anaemia. Also, undiagnosed vaginal bleeding, history of cholestatic jaundice during pregnancy, cancers which are hormone-dependent, infectious hepatitis, liver disorders. Also, porphyria, Dublin-Johnson and Rotor syndrome, otosclerosis, chorea, haemolytic uraemic syndrome, recent trophoblastic disease. *Possible interaction*: barbiturates, ethosuximide, glutethimide, rifampicin, phenytoin, tetracyclines, carbamazepine, chloral hydrate, griseofulvin, dichloralphenazone, primidone. *Side effects*: weight gain, breast enlargement, pains in legs and cramps, headaches, loss of sexual desire, depression, nausea, breakthrough bleeding, cervical erosion, brownish patches on skin (chloasma), vaginal discharge, oedema and bloatedness. *Manufacturer*: Janssen-Cilag.

ORUDIS

Description: an NSAID which is a propionic acid available as capsules in 2 strengths both containing ketoprofen. Purple/green capsules and pink capsules contain 50mg and 100mg respectively, both marked with strength and name. Also, **ORUDIS SUPPOSITORIES** containing 100mg. *Used for*: musculo-skeletal disorders, including osteoarthritis, rheumatoid arthritis, joint disorders, ankylosing spondylitis, gout, pain following orthopaedic surgery, dysmenorrhoea (period pain). *Dosage*: adults, capsules, 50–100mg twice daily with meals; suppositories, 1 at night with capsules taken during the day, if needed. *Special care*: pregnancy, elderly, heart failure, liver or kidney disorders. Patients taking the drug long-term should receive careful monitoring. *Avoid use*: children, patients with known allergy to aspirin or NSAID, history of or active stomach ulcer, asthma, serious kidney disease, recent proctitis (inflammation of rectum and anus). *Possible interaction*: hydantoins, anticoagulants, sulphonamides, high doses of methotrexate, quinolones. *Side effects*: rash, gastro-intestinal upset. *Manufacturer*: R.P.R.

ORUVAIL

Description: an NSAID which is a propionic acid available as capsules in 3 strengths all containing ketoprofen. Purple/pink, pink/pink and pink/white capsules contain 100mg, 150mg and 200mg respectively. All are continuous-release and marked with strength and name. Also, **ORUVAIL INJECTION** available as a solution in ampoules containing 50mg/ml. *Used for*: musculo-skeletal disorders including osteoarthritis, rheumatoid arthritis, joint disorders, ankylosing spondylitis, gout, pain following orthopaedic surgery, dysmenorrhoea (period pain). *Dosage*: capsules, 100–200mg once each day with meal; injection, 50–100mg every 4 hours by deep intramuscular injection. Maximum dose is 200mg each day for 3 days. *Special care*: pregnancy, elderly, liver or kidney disease, heart failure. *Avoid use*: children, known allergy to NSAID or aspirin, history of or active stomach ulcer, asthma, serious kidney disease. *Possible interaction*: hydantoins, anticoagulants, quinolones, high doses methotrexate, sulphonamides. *Side effects*: rash, gastro-intestinal upset. *Manufacturer*: R.P.R.

ORUVAIL GEL

Description: an NSAID which is a propionic acid available in the form of a gel containing 2.5% ketoprofen. *Used for*: sports injuries, strains, sprains, bruises, etc. *Dosage*: adults, 15g each day in 2 to 4 divided doses for up to 1 week; massage affected area after applying gel. *Special care*: pregnancy, avoid mucous membranes, eyes and broken skin. *Avoid use*: breast-feeding, patients with known allergy to NSAID or aspirin, history of asthma. *Side effects*: slight local irritation of skin. *Manufacturer*: R.P.R.

OTOMIZE

Description: a combined antibiotic and corticosteroid preparation available in the form of a suspension for use with a pump action spray. The solution contains 0.1% dexamethasone, 2% acetic acid and 3250 units neomycin/ml. *Used for*: inflammation of external ear. *Dosage*: 1 metered dose 3 times each day continuing for 2 days after condition has cleared. *Special care*: pregnant women, patients with perforated ear drum. *Side effects*: stinging or burning which is short-lived. *Manufacturer*: Stafford-Miller.

OTOSPORIN

Description: a combined antibiotic and corticosteroid preparation available in the form of ear drops containing 10,000 units polymixin B sulphate, 3400 units neomycin sulphate and 1% hydrocortisone. *Used for*: inflammation and bacterial infections of outer ear. *Dosage*: 3 drops 3 or 4 times each day or insert wick soaked in solution which is kept wet. *Special care*: avoid long-term use in infants. *Avoid use*: perforated eardrum. *Side effects*: superinfection. *Manufacturer*: Glaxo Wellcome.

OVESTIN

Description: an hormonal oestrogen preparation available as white tablets containing 1.0mg oestriol coded DG7, ORGANON and with *. Also, **OVESTIN CREAM** with applicator containing 0.1% oestriol. *Used for*: tablets, disorders of genital and urinary tract arising from infections when oestrogen is deficient. Cream, atrophic vaginitis, itching, dryness and atrophy of vulva in elderly women. Treatment of this area before vaginal operations. *Dosage*: tablets, 0.5–3mg each day for 4 weeks then 0.5–1mg daily. Cream, 1 applicator dose into vagina each day for 3 weeks with a maintenance dose of 1 applicatorful twice weekly. *Special care*: patients considered at risk of thromboembolism, porphyria, multiple sclerosis, epilepsy, fibroids in the womb, migraine, tetany. Also, patients with otosclerosis, gallstones, liver disease. Pelvic organs, breasts and blood pressure should be checked regularly during the course of treatment. *Avoid use*: pregnancy, breast-feeding, patients with breast or other cancer of reproductive tract or one which is hormone-dependent. Also, patients with thromboembolism-type disorders, undiagnosed vaginal bleeding or endometriosis, thrombophlebitis, heart, liver or kidney disease. Rotor or Dublin-Johnson syndrome. *Possible interaction*: drugs which induce liver enzymes. *Side effects*: enlargement and soreness of breasts, gastro-intestinal upset, dizziness, breakthrough bleeding, headache, vomiting and nausea, weight gain. *Manufacturer*: Organon.

OVRAN

Description: an hormonal combined oestrogen/progestogen preparation available as white tablets containing 50μg ethinyloestradiol and 250μg levonorgestrel. Also, **OVRAN 30**, white tablets containing 30μg ethinyloestradiol and 250μg levonorgestrel. Both are marked WYETH. *Used for*: oral contraception. *Dosage*: 1 tablet each day for 21 days starting on first day of period followed by 7 tablet-free days. *Special care*: patients with multiple sclerosis, serious kidney disease or kidney dialysis, asthma, Raynaud's disease, abnormally high levels of prolactin in the blood (hyperprolactinaemia), varicose veins, hypertension. Also, patients suffering from severe depression. Thrombosis risk increases with smoking, age and obesity. During the course of treatment, regular checks on blood pressure, pelvic organs and breasts should be carried out. *Avoid use*: pregnancy, patients considered to be at risk of thrombosis, suffering from heart disease, pulmonary hypertension, angina, sickle cell anaemia. Also, undiagnosed vaginal bleeding, history of cholestatic jaundice during pregnancy, cancers which are hormone-dependent, infectious hepatitis, liver disorders. Also, porphyria, Dublin-Johnson and Rotor syndrome, otosclerosis, chorea, haemolytic uraemic syndrome, recent trophoblastic disease. *Possible interaction*: barbiturates, ethosuximide, glutethimide, rifampicin, phenytoin, tetracyclines, carbamazepine, chloral hydrate, griseofulvin, dichloralphenazone, primidone. *Side effects*: weight gain, breast enlargement, pains in legs and cramps, headaches, loss of sexual desire, depression, nausea, breakthrough bleeding, cervical erosion, brownish patches on skin (chloasma), vaginal discharge, oedema and bloatedness. *Manufacturer*: Wyeth.

OVRANETTE

Description: an hormonal combined oestrogen/progestogen preparation, available as white tablets containing 30μg ethinyloestradiol and 150μg levonorgestrel, marked WYETH and 30. *Used for*: oral contraception. *Dosage*: 1 tablet each day for 21 days starting on first day of period followed by 7 tablet-free days. *Special care*: patients with multiple sclerosis, serious kidney disease or kidney dialysis, asthma, Raynaud's disease, abnormally high levels of prolactin in the blood (hyperprolactinaemia), varicose veins, hypertension. Also, patients suffering from severe depression. Thrombosis risk increases with smoking, age and obesity. During the course of treatment, regular checks on blood pressure, pelvic organs and breasts should be carried out. *Avoid use*: pregnancy, patients considered to be at risk of thrombosis, suffering from heart disease, pulmonary hypertension, angina, sickle cell anaemia. Also, undiagnosed vaginal bleeding, history of cholestatic jaundice during pregnancy, cancers which are hormone-dependent, infectious hepatitis, liver disorders. Also, porphyria, Dublin-Johnson and Rotor syndrome, otosclerosis, chorea, haemolytic uraemic syndrome, recent trophoblastic disease. *Possible interaction*: barbiturates, ethosuximide, glutethimide, rifampicin, phenytoin, tetracyclines, carbamazepine, chloral hydrate, griseofulvin, dichloralphenazone, primidone. *Side effects*: weight gain, breast enlargement, pains in legs and cramps, headaches, loss of sexual desire, depression, nausea, breakthrough bleeding, cervical erosion, brownish patches on skin (chloasma), vaginal discharge, oedema and bloatedness. *Manufacturer*: Wyeth.

OVYSMEN

Description: an hormonal combined oestrogen/progestogen preparation available as white tablets containing 35µg ethinyloestradiol and 500µg norethisterone marked C over 535. *Used for*: oral contraception. *Dosage*: 1 tablet each day for 21 days starting on fifth day of period followed by 7 tablet-free days. *Special care*: patients with multiple sclerosis, serious kidney disease or kidney dialysis, asthma, Raynaud's disease, abnormally high levels of prolactin in the blood (hyperprolactinaemia), varicose veins, hypertension. Also, patients suffering from severe depression. Thrombosis risk increases with smoking, age and obesity. During treatment, regular checks on blood pressure, pelvic organs and breasts should be carried out. *Avoid use*: pregnancy, patients considered to be at risk of thrombosis, suffering from heart disease, pulmonary hypertension, angina, sickle cell anaemia. Also, undiagnosed vaginal bleeding, history of cholestatic jaundice during pregnancy, cancers which are hormone-dependent, infectious hepatitis, liver disorders. Also, porphyria, Dublin-Johnson and Rotor syndrome, otosclerosis, chorea, haemolytic uraemic syndrome, recent trophoblastic disease. *Possible interaction*: barbiturates, ethosuximide, glutethimide, rifampicin, phenytoin, tetracyclines, carbamazepine, chloral hydrate, griseofulvin, dichloralphenazone, primidone. *Side effects*: weight gain, breast enlargement, pains in legs and cramps, headaches, loss of sexual desire, depression, nausea, breakthrough bleeding, cervical erosion, brownish patches on skin (chloasma), vaginal discharge, oedema and bloatedness. *Manufacturer*: Janssen-Cilag.

OXAZEPAM

Description: an anxiolytic drug and intermediate-acting benzodiazepine available as tablets in 3 strengths containing 10mg, 15mg and 30mg oxazepam. *Used for*: anxiety. *Dosage*: 15–30mg 3 or 4 times each day increasing to 60mg 3 times daily if exceptionally severe. Elderly persons take reduced dose of 10–20mg 3 to 4 times each day. *Special care*: chronic liver or kidney disease, chronic lung disease, pregnancy, labour, lactation, elderly. May impair judgement. Withdraw gradually and avoid prolonged use. *Avoid use*: depression of respiration, acute lung disease; psychotic, phobic or obsessional states. *Possible interaction*: anticonvulsants, depressants of the CNS, alcohol. *Side effects*: ataxia, confusion, light-headedness, drowsiness, hypotension, gastro-intestinal upsets, disturbances in vision and libido, skin rashes, retention of urine, vertigo. Sometimes jaundice or blood disorders. *Manufacturer*: non-proprietary but available from APS, Berk, Cox, Kerfoot, Norton, Wyeth.

OXIVENT

Description: an anticholinergic bronchodilator delivering 100µg oxitropium bromide per dose by metered dose inhaler. Also, **OXIVENT AUTOHALER** delivering 100µg oxitropium bromide per dose by breath-actuated metered dose aerosol. *Used for*: obstructive lung disease, asthma. *Dosage*: adults, 2 puffs 2 or 3 times each day. *Special care*: avoid eyes, patients with enlarged prostate gland, glaucoma. *Avoid use*: pregnancy, breast-feeding, children, allergy to ipratropium bromide or atropine. *Side effects*: dry mouth, nausea, irritation of throat, anticholinergic effects. If cough or wheezing develops, drug should be withdrawn. *Manufacturer*: Boehringer Ingelheim.

P

PABRINEX

Description: a combined preparation of vitamins B and C in paired ampoules for both intravenous and intramuscular injection. Pairs of intravenous ampoules contain 250mg thiamine hydrochloride, 4mg riboflavine, 50mg pyridoxine hydrochloride, 160mg nicotinamide, 500mg ascorbic acid and 1g anhydrous dextrose. Pairs of intramuscular ampoules contain the same but without anhydrous dextrose. *Used for*: severe deficiencies in vitamin B and C when oral doses cannot be taken or are not adequate. *Dosage*: by intravenous injection (over 10 minutes) or infusion, 2 to 4 pairs of ampoules every 4 to 8 hours for up to 2 days. Then 1 pair of intramuscular ampoules by intramuscular injection or 1 pair of intravenous ampoules by intravenous injection or infusion once each day for 5 to 7 days. *Special care*: anaphylaxis may occur hence treatment should only be given when it is essential and facilities for resuscitation must be available. *Possible interaction*: levodopa. *Side effects*: anaphylaxis. *Manufacturer*: Link.

PALFIUM^{CD}

Description: an analgesic opiate preparation which is a controlled drug available as scored, white tablets containing 5mg dextromoramide and scored peach tablets containing 10mg dextromoramide. Also, **PALFIUM SUPPOSITORIES** containinng 10mg dextromoramide astartrate. *Used for*: severe, intractable pain. *Dosage*: tablets, up to 5mg at first then adjusted according to response. Suppositories, 1 as required. Children, 80µg/kg body weight. *Special care*: pregnancy, elderly, underactive thyroid gland, liver disorders. *Avoid use*: women in labour, patients with obstructed airways and depression of respiration. *Possible interaction*: CNS depressants, MAOIs. *Side effects*: sweating, nausea dependence and tolerance. *Manufacturer*: B.M. UK.

PAMERGAN P100^{CD}

Description: a narcotic analgesic and sedative available in ampoules for injection containing 100mg pethidine hydrochloride and 50mg promethazine hydrochloride/2ml. *Used for*: relief of pain in labour, pain during and after operations, pre-medication enhancement of anaesthesia. *Dosage*: labour and severe pain, 1–2ml every 4 hours by intramuscular injection if necessary; pre-medication, 25–200mg by intramuscular injection 1 hour before surgery; enhancement of anaesthesia (with nitrous oxide), 10–25mg by slow intravenous injection. Children, pre-medication, age 8 to 12 years, 0.75ml; 13 to 16 years, 1ml all by intramuscular injection. *Special care*: pregnancy, breast-feeding. Elderly and debilitated persons should receive reduced doses. Also, liver disorders, asthma, respiratory depression, hypotension, underactivity of thyroid gland. If patient is terminally ill, the benefits may be considered to outweigh any risk. *Avoid use*: patients with serious kidney disorders, head injury or raised intracranial pressure. *Possible interaction*: MAOIs, cimetidine, anxiolytics and hypnotics. *Side effects*: convulsions with high doses, vomiting, nausea, constipation, drowsiness, difficulty passing urine, depression of respiration, hypotension, sweating, dry mouth, flushing palpitations, bradycardia, urticaria, rash, itching, miosis (constriction of pupil of the eye), vertigo. Hallucinations and mood swings. *Manufacturer*: Martindale.

PARAMAX

Description: an NSAID combining an analgesic and anti-emetic preparation available as scored, white tablets containing 500mg paracetamol and 5mg metaclopramide hydrochloride, marked PARAMAX. Also **PARAMAX SACHETS**, effervescent powder. *Used for*: migraine. *Dosage*: adults over 20 years, 2 tablets when attack starts followed by 2 every 4 hours up to maximum dose of 6 in 24 hours. Age 16 to 19 years and over 60kg body weight, 2 tablets at start of attack and maximum dose of 5 in 24 hours. 30–50kg body weight, 1 tablet at start of attack with a maximum of 3 in 24 hours. Age 12 to 14 years, over 30kg body weight, 1 tablet at start of attack with maximum of 3 in 24 hours. *Special care*: pregnancy, breast-feeding, liver or kidney disorder. *Avoid use*: children under 12 years, patients with phaeochromocytoma, breast cancer which is prolactin-dependent, recent surgery on gastro-intestinal tract. *Possible interaction*: phenothiazines, anticholinergics, butyrophenones. *Side effects*: drowsiness, raised blood levels of prolactin, diarrhoea, extrapyramidal reactions (characterized by reflex-type muscle movements and spasms). *Manufacturer*: Lorex.

PARAPLATIN

Description: an alkylating cytotoxic drug produced as a solution in vials for injection containing 10mg carboplatin/ml. *Used for*: ovarian cancer, small cell lung cancer. *Dosage*: as directed by physician skilled in cancer chemotherapy. *Special care*: patients with kidney disorders. *Possible interaction*: aminoglycosides, capreomycin, anticoagulants taken orally. *Side effects*: bone marrow suppression, nausea, vomiting, toxic effects on nerves, kidneys, hearing, hair loss. *Manufacturer*: Bristol-Myers.

PARLODEL

Description: a dopamine agonist available as scored white tablets in 2 strengths containing 1mg and 2.5mg bromocriptine (as mesylate) respectively, all marked with strength and name. Also, **PARLODEL CAPSULES** in 2 strengths, white/blue containing 5mg bromocriptine, coded PARLODEL 5 and white containing 10mg, coded PARLODEL 10. *Used for*: Parkinsonism, additional therapy in acromegaly (enlarged face, feet and hands due to a pituitary gland tumour producing an excess of growth hormone), tumours which are prolactin-dependent, abnormally high prolactin levels in blood, prevention and suppression of milk production after childbirth. Also, benign breast disorders connected with monthly cycle, breast pain, hormone-based infertility. *Dosage*: adults, for Parkinsonism, initial dose, 1–1.25mg taken at night for 1 week increasing gradually to 2.5mg 3 times each day in fourth week. Dose is then gradually increased to 10–40mg 3 times each day in divided doses. Drug should be taken with meals. Acromegaly and tumours dependent upon prolactin, initial dose, 1–1.25mg taken at night gradually increasing to 5mg every 6 hours (with daily meals). Prevention and suppression of lactation; 2.5mg on day of birth then 2.5mg twice each day with meals for 2 weeks. Excess prolactin levels in blood, 1–1.25mg taken at night increasing to 7.5mg each day in divided doses with meals with a maximum of 30mg daily. Benign breast disease and pain, 1–1.25mg taken at night increasing gradually to 2.5mg twice each day with meals. Infertility, 1–1.25mg taken at bedtime at first gradually increasing to 7.5mg each day in divided doses with meals, the maximum being 30mg daily. *Special care*: history of heart and circulatory disorders or psychoses. Regular gynaecological monitoring necessary for women and non-hormonal methods of contraception should be used for those not wishing to conceive as may cause ovulation. *Avoid use*: high blood pressure at time of childbirth, hypersensitivity to ergot alkaloids, toxaemia of pregnancy. Withdraw if conception occurs. *Possible interaction*: drugs affecting blood pressure, alcohol, metoclopramide, erythromycin. *Side effects*: vomiting, nausea, leg pains, slight constipation, dry mouth, vasospasm. Rarely, heart attack, stroke, headache, hypertension, convulsions, dizziness, confusion. Drug should be withdrawn if peritoneal fibrosis occurs. *Manufacturer*: Sandoz.

PARNATE

Description: an MAOI available as sugar-coated red tablets containing 100mg tranylcypromine (as sulphate), marked SKF. *Used for*: depression. *Dosage*: 1 tablet twice daily increasing to 1 tablet 3 times daily after 1 week. Maintenance dose is 1 tablet daily. *Special care*: elderly, epilepsy. *Avoid use*: children, patients with phaeochromocytoma, congestive heart failure, heart and circulatory diseases, blood changes, alcohol, hyperthyroidism, liver disease, disease of cerebral arteries. *Possible interaction*: ephedrine, TCADs, narcotic analgesics and pethidine, amphetamine, levodopa, methylphenidate, phenylpropanolamine, fenfluramine. Alcohol, barbiturates, hypnotics, hypoglycaemics, insulin, reserpine, anticholinergics, methyldopa, guanethidine. Many foods should be avoided including yeast extracts, Marmite, meat extracts, Oxo and Bovril, alcoholic drinks, broad bean pods, banana skins, flavoured textured soya protein, pickled herrings. Also any foods that are not completely fresh. *Side effects*: severe hypertensive responses with certain foods, constipation, blurred vision, difficulty passing urine, gastro-intestinal upset. Low blood pressure on rising, skin rash, swelling of ankles, fatigue, weariness, dizziness, jaundice, blood disorders, weight gain, changes in libido. Occasionally, confusion and mania. *Manufacturer*: SmithKline Beecham.

PARSTELIN

Description: an MAOI available as sugar-coated green tablets containing 10mg tranylcypromine as sulphate and 1mg trifluoperazine as hydrochloride, marked SKF. *Used for*: depression. *Dosage*: 1 tablet twice each day at first increasing to 1 tablet 3 times each day after 1 week. Maintenance dose is normally 1 daily tablet. *Special care*: elderly, epilepsy. *Avoid use*: children, phaeochromocytoma, congestive heart failure, heart and circulatory diseases, blood changes, hyperthyroidism, liver disease, disease of cerebral arteries. *Possible interaction*: ephedrine, TCADs, narcotic analgesics and pethidine, amphetamine, levodopa, methylphenidate, phenylpropanolamine, fenfluramine. Alcohol, barbiturates, hypnotics, hypoglycaemics, insulin, reserpine, anticholinergics, methyldopa, guanethidine. Many foods should be avoided including yeast extracts, Marmite, meat extracts, Oxo and Bovril, alcoholic drinks, broad bean pods, banana skins, flavoured textured soya protein, pickled herrings. Also any foods that are not completely fresh. *Side effects*: severe hypertensive responses with certain foods, constipation, blurred vision, difficulty passing urine, gastro-intestinal upset. Low blood pressure on rising, skin rash, swelling of ankles, fatigue, weariness, dizziness, jaundice, blood disorders, weight gain, changes in libido. Occasionally, confusion and mania. *Manufacturer*: SmithKline Beecham.

PARTOBULIN

Description: a preparation of human anti-D immunoglobulin available as a solution in ampoules for injection containing 1250 units/ml. *Used for*: rhesus (D) incompatibility. *Dosage*: antenatal prevention, 1250 units by intramuscular injection in weeks 28 and 34 of pregnancy and a further dose within 72 hours of birth. Following abortion or miscarriage or possible sensitizing procedure, e.g. amniocentesis, 1250 units within 72 hours by intramuscular injection. Following transplacental bleeding where more than 25ml of foetal blood has been transferred (1% of foetal red blood cells), 5000 units or 50 units/ml of foetal blood, by intramuscular injection. *Special care*: patients who have IGA antibodies or with known history of unusual reactions to transfused blood or blood products. *Possible interaction*: live vaccines. *Manufacturer*: Immuno.

PARVOLEX

Description: an amino acid preparation used to treat drug overdose and available as a solution in ampoules for injection containing 200mg acetylcysteine/ml. Acetylcysteine acts to protect the liver from damage. *Used for:* paracetamol overdose. *Dosage:* by intravenous infusion in glucose intravenous infusion; 150mg/kg body weight in 200ml over 15 minutes at first. Then 50mg/kg body weight in 500ml over 4 hours followed by 100mg/kg body weight in 1000ml over 16 hours. *Special care:* history of asthma. Vomiting should be induced if patient is treated within 4 hours of overdose. Plasma concentrations of paracetamol require monitoring. Patients who have taken alcohol, phenobarbitone, rifampicin, carbamazepine or phenytoin may be at risk of live toxicity at lower plasma-paracetamol concentrations. *Possible interaction:* metals and rubber. *Side effects:* rash, anaphylaxis. *Manufacturer:* Evans.

PAVULON

Description: a non-depolarizing muscle relaxant available as a solution in ampoules for injection containing 4mg pancuronium bromide/2ml. *Used for:* muscle relaxation for intubation of patients undergoing anaesthesia and mechanical ventilation in intensive care. *Dosage:* adults, 50–100µg/kg body weight at first (for intubation) then 10–20µg/kg body weight as needed to maintain relaxation. Children, 60–100µg/kg body weight at first then 10–20µg/kg. Newborn baby, 30–40µg/kg body weight at first followed by 10–20µg/kg. Intensive care patients, 60µg/kg body weight every hour to hour and a half. *Special care:* patients with liver and kidney disorders (reduced dose). *Possible interaction:* procainamide, quinidine, aminoglycosides, clindamycin, azloallin, colistin, propanolol, verapamil, nifedipine, ecothiopate, demacarium, pyridostigmine, neostigmine, magnesium salts. *Manufacturer:* Organon Teknika.

PENBRITIN

Description: an antibiotic broad-spectrum penicillin preparation available as black/red capsules in 2 strengths containing 250mg and 500mg ampicillin, marked with strength and name. Also, **PENBRITIN SYRUP** available as powder for reconstitution with water, then containing 125mg/5ml. **PENBRITIN SYRUP FORTE** contains 250mg/5ml (available as powder for reconstitution). **PENBRITIN PAEDIATRIC SUSPENSION** contains 125mg/1.25ml when reconstituted (available as powder). **PENBRITIN INJECTION** available as powder in vials containing 250mg and 500mg ampicillin sodium. *Used for:* ear, nose, throat and respiratory infections, soft tissue infections. Infections of urinary tract and gonorrhoea. *Dosage:* adults, oral preparations, 250mg–1g every 6 hours; injection, 250–500mg by intravenous or intramuscular injection, 4, 5 or 6 times each day. Children, oral preparations, 125–250mg every 6 hours; injection, half adult dose. *Special care:* patients with glandular fever. *Side effects:* gastro-intestinal upset, hypersensitivity reactions. *Manufacturer:* Beecham.

PENDRAMINE

Description: a penicillin derivative available as film-coated, scored, oblong white tablets containing 125mg and 250mg penicillamine respectively; the 250mg tablets are marked HB. *Used for*: severe rheumatoid arthritis. *Dosage*: 125–250mg each day for first 4 to 8 weeks, then increase every 4 weeks by 125–250mg to a maximum dose of 2g each day, if needed. Children, usual dose, 15–20mg/kg body weight each day. Start with lower dose then gradually increase every 4 weeks over period of 3 to 6 months. *Special care*: patients sensitive to penicillin checks on blood, urine and kidney function are required regularly during the course of treatment. *Avoid use*: pregnancy, breast-feeding, patients with kidney disorders, thrombocytopenia, SLE, agranulocytosis (serious reduction in number of white blood cells [granulocytes]). *Possible interaction*: phenylbutazone, zinc or iron salts, cytotoxic drugs, antimalarial drugs, gold salts, antacids. *Side effects*: blood changes, myasthenia gravis, anorexia, rash, fever, nausea, protein in urine, blood in urine, SLE, nephrotic syndrome (a kidney abnormality resulting from a number of diseases and conditions). *Manufacturer*: Asta Medica.

PENTACARINAT

Description: an antiprotozal preparation available as a powder in vials for reconstitution and injection containing 300mg pentamidine isethionate. Also, **PENTACARINAT SOLUTION** containing 300mg pentamidine isethionate/ 5ml for nebulization. *Used for*: pneumocystis carinii pneumonia, kala-azar, cutaneous leishmaniasis. *Dosage*: adults and children, pneumocystis carinii pneumonia, 4mg/kg body weight each day for 14 days; nebulized solution, 600mg each day for 3 weeks; prevention of secondary infection, 300mg every 4 weeks or 150mg every 2 weeks. Kala-azar, 3–4mg/kg body weight each day on alternate days up to a maximum of 10 deep intramuscular injections. May be repeated, if needed. Cutaneous leishmaniasis, 3–4mg/kg body weight by deep intramuscular injection once or twice each week until condition improves. Trypanosomiasis, 4mg/kg body weight by deep intramuscular injection or intravenous infusion each day on alternate days to a maximum of 7 to 10 injections. *Special care*: must only be given by specialist physician under close medical supervision. Risk of serious hypotension once dose has been given; patient must be lying down and blood pressure monitored. Patients with liver or kidney disorder (reduced dose), hyper or hypotension, anaemia, leucopenia, thrombocytopenia, hypo or hyperglycaemia. *Side effects*: severe and occasionally fatal reactions due to hypotension, pancreatitis, hypoglycaemia, cardiac arrhythmias. Also, leucopenia, thrombocytopenia, hypocalcaemia, serious kidney failure. Vomiting, dizziness, nausea, fainting, rash, flushing, constriction of airways on inhalation, pain, disturbance of sense of taste. Tissue and muscle damage, abscess and pain at injection site. *Manufacturer*: R.P.R.

PENTASA

Description: a colorectal salicylate preparation available as an enema containing 1g mesalazine. Also, **PENTASA SUPPOSITORY**, suppositories containing 1g mesalazine; PENTASA SR sustained-release scored tablets which are light grey and contain 250mg and 500mg mesalazine respectively, marked with strength and PENTASA. *Used for*: ulcerative colitis (inflammation and ulceration of the colon and rectum). *Dosage*: adults, 1 enema or suppository at night; tablets, 2 500mg tablets 3 times each day increasing to 8 500mg tablets (maximum dose), if needed. Maintenance dose is 500mg 3 times each day. *Special care*: pregnancy, breast-feeding, elderly, protein in urine or raised levels of blood urea. *Avoid use*: children. *Side effects*: headache, abdominal pain, nausea. *Manufacturer*: Yamanouchi.

PEPCID

Description: an H$_2$ blocker available as square, beige tablets and square, brown tablets containing 20mg and 40mg famotidine respectively, both marked with strength and name. *Used for*: treatment of stomach and duodenal ulcers, prevention of relapse of duodenal ulcers. Prevention and treatment of reflux disease of stomach and oesophagus, treatment of Zollinger-Ellison syndrome. *Dosage*: treatment of ulcers, 40mg taken at night for 4 to 8 weeks; prevention of relapse of duodenal ucer, 20mg taken at night. Gastro-oesophageal reflux disease, 20mg twice each day for 6 weeks to 3 months (or 40mg, if damage or ulceration is present). Prevention, 20mg twice each day. Zollinger-Ellison syndrome, 20mg 6 hours at first adjusted according to response to a maximum dose of 800mg each day. *Special care*: pregnancy, breast-feeding, stomach cancer or kidney disease. *Avoid use*: children. *Side effects*: nausea, diarrhoea, constipation, rash, gastro-intestinal upset, dry mouth, headache, anorexia, dizziness, weariness. Rarely there may be enlargement of breasts in males (reversible). *Manufacturer*: Morson.

PERFAN

Description: a phosphodiesterase inhibitor available in ampoules for injection containing 5mg enoximone/ml. *Used for*: congestive heart failure where filling pressures are increased and cardiac output reduced. *Dosage*: adults, by slow intravenous injection, 0.5–1mg/kg body weight at first then 500µg/kg every half hour until condition improves or 3mg/kg may be given every 3 to 6 hours, as needed. By intravenous infusion, 90µg/kg body weight/ minute at first over 10 to 30 minutes. Then intermittent or continuous infusion of 20µg/kg body weight. Total maximum dose should not be greater than 24mg/kg body weight in 24 hours. Plastic apparatus must be used as crystals form in glass. *Side effects*: tachycardia, heart arrhythmias, unusual heartbeats, nausea, vomiting, headache, diarrhoea, hypotension, insomnia, fever, chills, urine retention, reduced ability to produce and pass urine, pains in limbs. *Manufacturer*: Hoechst.

PERGONAL

Description: an hormonal gonadotrophin preparation available as a powder in ampoules for reconstitution and injection containing menotrophin (equivalent to 75 units of both follicle-stimulating hormone and luteinizing hormone, with solvent). *Used for*: underactivity (infertility) of testes due to lack of gonadotrophin. Female infertility due to lack of ovulation. Superovulation for in vitro fertilization. *Dosage*: male adults, 1 ampoule 3 times each week along with

2000 units chorionic gonadotrophin twice each week for at least 4 months. Female infertility, by intramuscular injection according to levels of oestrogen. Superovulation, 2 or 3 ampoules each day. *Special care*: patients with hormonal disorders or intracranial lesions must have these corrected before therapy begins. *Avoid use*: pregnancy. *Side effects*: overstimulation of ovaries may lead to enlargement and rupture, allergic responses, multiple pregnancy. *Manufacturer*: Serono.

PERINAL

Description: a colorectal preparation combining a steroid and local anaesthetic available in the form of a metered dose spray containing 0.2% hydrocortisone and 1% lignocaine hydrochloride. *Used for*: pain in anal area. *Dosage*: 2 sprays up to 3 times each day. *Special care*: short-term use only, pregnancy. *Avoid use*: patients with infections of fungal, viral and bacterial origin. *Side effects*: systemic corticosteroid effects, e.g. changes as in Cushing's syndrome. *Manufacturer*: Dermal.

PERSANTIN

Description: an anti-platelet drug available as sugar-coated orange and white tablets containing 25mg and 100mg dipyridamole, marked with strength and name. *Used for*: additional therapy along with oral anticoagulants to prevent thrombosis of artificial heart valves. *Dosage*: 300–600mg each day in 3 or 4 doses taken before meals. Children, 5mg/kg body weight as divided dose each day. *Special care*: recent heart attack, worsening angina, narrowing of aorta below valves. *Possible interaction*: antacids. *Side effects*: gastro-intestinal upset, giddiness, headache. *Manufacturer*: Boehringer Ingelheim.

PERTOFRAN

Description: a TCAD available as sugar-coated pink tablets containing 25mg desipramine hydrochloride, marked EW and CG. *Used for*: depression. *Dosage*: 1 tablet 3 times each day at first increasing to 2, 3 or 4 times daily if needed. Elderly, start with 1 tablet daily. *Special care*: elderly, epilepsy. *Avoid use*: children, phaeochromocytoma, congestive heart failure, heart and circulatory diseases, blood changes, hyperthyroidism, liver disease, disease of cerebral arteries. *Possible interaction*: ephedrine, TCADs, narcotic analgesics and pethidine, amphetamine, levodopa, methylphenidate, phenylpropanolamine, fenfluramine. Alcohol, barbiturates, hypnotics, hypoglycaemics, insulin, reserpine, anticholinergics, methyldopa, guanethidine. Many foods should be avoided including yeast extracts, Marmite, meat extracts, Oxo and Bovril, alcoholic drinks, broad bean pods, banana skins, flavoured textured soya protein, pickled herrings. Also any foods that are not completely fresh. *Side effects*: severe hypertensive responses with certain foods, constipation, blurred vision, difficulty passing urine, gastro-intestinal upset. Low blood pressure on rising, skin rash, swelling of ankles, fatigue, weariness, dizziness, jaundice, blood disorders, weight gain, changes in libido. Occasionally, confusion and mania. *Manufacturer*: Geigy.

PEVARYL TC

Description: a preparation in the form of a cream which combines an antifungal and potent steroid, containing 1% econazole nitrate and 0.1% triamcinolone acetonide. *Used for*: inflammatory skin conditions where fungal infection is present.. *Dosage*: rub into affected area twice each day for 14 days. *Special care*: short-term use only. *Avoid use*: children, long-term or extensive use especially in pregnancy, patients with untreated bacterial or fungal infections or skin infections of tuberculous or viral origin or due to ringworm. Also, dermatitis in area of mouth, acne, leg ulcers or scabies. *Side effects*: suppression of adrenal glands, skin thinning, abnormal hair growth, changes as in Cushing's syndrome. *Manufacturer*: Janssen-Cilag.

PHARMORUBICIN

Description: a cytotoxic antibiotic preparation available as a powder in vials for reconstitution and injection containing 10mg, 20mg or 50mg epirubicin hydrochloride. Also, **PHARMORUBICIN SOLUTION** containing 2mg/ml. *Used for*: breast cancer, papillary tumours of bladder. *Dosage*: adults, breast cancer, by intravenous injection as directed by physician. Papillary tumours, solution of 50mg in 50ml sterile water is instilled each week for 8 weeks. Prevention, once each week for 4 weeks then once each month for 11 months. *Special care*: care in handling, irritant to tissues. Patients with liver disease (reduced doses). *Side effects*: bone marrow suppression, nausea, vomiting, hair loss, effects on fertility. *Manufacturer*: Pharmacia & Upjohn.

PHYSEPTONE^{CD}

Description: an opiate analgesic preparation which is a controlled drug available as scored, white tablets containing 5mg methadone hydrochloride marked WELLCOME L4A. Also, **PHYSEPTONE INJECTION**, containing 10mg/ml in ampoules for injection. *Used for*: severe pain. *Dosage*: tablets, 5–10mg every 6 to 8 hours or same dose by subcutaneous or intramuscular injection. *Special care*: pregnancy, underactive thyroid gland or serious liver disease. *Avoid use*: children, depression of respiration, obstructive airways disease, obstetric patients, those who are not confined to bed. *Possible interaction*: central nervous system depressants, MAOIs. *Side effects*: dizziness, nausea, sedation, euphoria, drug tolerance and dependence. *Manufacturer*: Glaxo Wellcome.

PIPORTIL DEPOT

Description: a phenothiazine group II available as a depot oily injection in ampoules containing 50mg pipothiazine palmitate/ml. *Used for*: ongoing treatment of certain psychiatric disorders particularly schizophrenia. *Dosage*: a test dose at first of 25mg by deep intramuscular injection into the gluteal muscle (buttock), then adjusted by 25mg or 50mg increments until best response is achieved. The usual maintenance dose is in the order of 50–100mg every 4 weeks with a maximum of 200mg. *Special care*: pregnancy, breast-feeding, history of convulsions, severe extrapyramidal responses to phenothiazines taken orally. *Avoid use*: children, severe heart disorder, liver or kidney failure, phaeo-chromocytoma, depression of bone marrow function, severe hardening of cerebral arteries. *Possible interaction*: alcohol, anaesthetics, antacids, anti-muscarines, anxiolytics, hypnotics, calcium channel blockers, lithium. *Side effects*: extrapyramidal symptoms, changes in ECG and EEG, tachycardia and heart arrhythmias, apathy, drowsiness, insomnia, depression. Dry mouth, blocked nose, difficulty passing urine, constipation, hypotension, blurred vision. Changes in breasts and menstrual cycle, weight gain, impotence, blood changes, effects on liver, jaundice, rash, pigmentation of skin and eyes (especially higher doses). *Manufacturer*: R.P.R.

PIPRIL

Description: an antibiotic broad-spectrum penicillin available as powder in vials in strengths of 1g, 2g and 4g piperacillin (as sodium salt), with diluent, for injection (1g and 2g) and infusion (4g). *Used for*: local and systemic infections; prevention of infection during operations. *Dosage*: adults, by intramuscular or slow intravenous injection or by intravenous infusion. 100–150mg/kg body weight in divided doses each day at first. Severe infections may require up to 200–300mg/kg with 16g or more daily if life is threatened. Single doses over 2g must be given by intravenous injection or infusion. Children may require lesser doses. *Special care*: pregnancy, kidney disorder. *Side effects*: gastro-intestinal upset, hypersensitive allergic reactions. *Manufacturer*: Wyeth.

PIPTALIN

Description: an anti-spasmodic used for digestive disorders, combining an anti-cholinergic and deflatulent drug, available as a sugar-free elixir containing 4mg pipenzolate bromide and 40mg activated dimethicone/5ml. *Used for*: flatulence, pain due to spasm and overactivity of gastro-intestinal tract, abdominal extension due to gas build-up. *Dosage*: 10ml 3 or 4 times each day taken 15 minutes before meal. Children, up to 10kg body weight, 2.5ml; 10–20kg, 2.5–5ml; 20–40kg, 5ml. All taken 15 minutes before meals 3 or 4 times each day. *Special care*: urine retention, enlarged prostate gland, glaucoma. *Avoid use*: pregnancy, breast-feeding, myasthenia gravis, various disorders of gastro-intestinal tract including obstruction, paralytic ileus, pyloric stenosis, ulcerative colitis. Also, liver or kidney disorders, tachycardia, unstable angina. *Possible interaction*: benzodiazepines, TCADs, antihistamines. *Side effects*: constipation, urine retention, vomiting and nausea, dry mouth, visual disorder, weakness, tachycardia, blushing, palpitations, insomnia. *Manufacturer*: B.M. Pharmaceuticals.

PITRESSIN

Description: A preparation of antidiuretic hormone available as a solution in ampoules for injection containing 20 units agipressin (synthetic vasopressin)/ml. *Used for*: pituitary diabetes insipidus. *Dosage*: by intramuscular or subcutaneous injection, 5–20 units every 4 hours. By intravenous infusion, 20 units over 15 minutes. *Special care*: pregnancy, conditions which might be made worse by water retention, asthma, heart failure, migraine, epilepsy, kidney disorders. Careful checks on amount of water retention required. *Avoid use*: disease of arteries especially coronary arteries, severe nephritis. *Side effects*: constriction of coronary arteries possibly leading to angina and reduction in blood flow to heart, hypersensitive allergic reactions, feeling of needing to defecate, belching, abdominal pains, nausea, pallor. *Manufacturer*: Goldshield.

PLAQUENIL

Description: an NSAID which is a 4-aminoquinolone available as sugar-coated orange tablets containing 200mg hydroxychloroquine sulphate. *Used for*: rheumatoid arthritis and juvenile rheumatoid arthritis, lupus erythematosus (a severe inflammatory disease affecting internal organs and skin). *Dosage*: 2 tablets each day with meals at first, with a maintenance dose of 1 or 2 tablets daily. The maximum dose is 6.5mg/kg body weight each day. If no improvement is seen after 6 months, drug should be withdrawn. Children, 6.5mg/kg body weight each day. *Special care*: breast-feeding, porphyria, liver or kidney disease, a history of blood, gastro-intestinal or neurological disorders. Patients on long-term therapy should receive regular eye tests. *Avoid use*: pregnancy, patients with maculopathy (a disorder of the eye spot of the retina). *Possible interaction*: antacids, drugs which may damage the eyes, aminoglycosides. *Side effects*: opacity of the cornea and changes in the retina of the eye, reduced eye accommodation (discontinue if this occurs). Also, gastro-intestinal intolerance, baldness, skin responses, bleaching of hair. *Manufacturer*: Sanofi Winthrop.

PLENDIL

Description: an antihypertensive class II calcium antagonist available as film-coated sustained-release tablets containing 5mg and 10mg felodipine. *Used for*: hypertension. *Dosage*: 5mg once each day increasing if necessary to a usual maintenance dose of 5–10mg. The maximum daily dose is 20mg. *Special care*: recent problems of poor blood circulation to the heart or serious liver disease. *Avoid use*: pregnancy, breast-feeding. *Possible interaction*: phenytoin, phenobarbitone, cimetidine, carbamazepine. *Side effects*: flushing, swelling of ankles, weariness, giddiness, headache, slight swelling of gums, palpitations. *Manufacturer*: Astra.

PNEUMOVAX II

Description: a preparation of pneumococcal vaccine, available as a solution for injection, containing 25µg of 23 types of pneumococcus/0.5ml as a purified mixture of capsular polysaccharides. *Used for*: immunization against pneumococcal disease. *Dosage*: adults and children age 2 years and over, 0.5ml by intramuscular or subcutaneous injection. *Special care*: patients with weak hearts or lungs, respiratory diseases or feverish illnesses, revaccination of high risk children. *Avoid use*: pregnancy, breast-feeding, children under 2 years, patients with Hodgkin's disease who have had chemotherapy or radiation treatment. Patients who have recently received immunosuppressive treatment, revaccination of adults. *Side effects*: fever, local skin reactions, relapse of patients with stabilized thrombocytopenic purpura (a bleeding disorder characterized by haemorrhage beneath the skin and mucous membranes). *Manufacturer*: Pasteur Merieux MSD.

POLYFAX

Description: a preparation of peptide antibiotics available as an ointment containing 10,000 units polymyxin B sulphate and 500 units bacitracin zinc per gram. *Used for*: eye infections including conjunctivitis, keratitis, styes, blepharitis. Prevent infection after removal of foreign objects from the eye or surgery. Also, impetigo, infected burns and skin infections. *Dosage*: apply thinly at least twice per day. *Special care*: patients with extensive, open wounds. *Side effects*: skin sensitization, toxic effects on kidneys. *Manufacturer*: Dominion.

POLYTRIM

Description: A combined antibacterial preparation available in the form of eyedrops containing 1mg trimethoprim and 10,000 units polymyxin B sulphate/ml. Also, **POLYTRIM OINTMENT** containing 5mg trimethoprim and 10,000 units polymyxin B sulphate/gram. *Used for*: bacterial eye infections. *Dosage*: apply 3 or 4 times each day continuing for 2 days after symptoms have cleared. *Manufacturer*: Dominion.

PONDERAX PACAPS

Description: an anti-obesity serotoninergic drug available as blue/clear sustained-release capsules, with white pellets containing 60mg fenfluramine hydrochloride marked P and PA60. *Used for*: severe obesity. *Dosage*: adults 1 tablet daily half an hour before a meal for a maximum period of 3 months. *Special care*: therapy should last for up to 3 months and drug gradually withdrawn over last 1 or 2 weeks. *Avoid use*: patients suffering from depression, epilepsy, psychiatric disorder or drug or alcohol abuse. *Possible interaction*: antidiabetics, MAOIs, alcohol, antihypertensives, sedatives, anti-anoretics. *Side effects*: dry mouth, nervousness, sedation, hallucinations, frequency of urination, depression (especially if drug abruptly stopped), diarrhoea. *Manufacturer*: Pacaps Servier.

PONDOCILLIN

Description: an antibiotic preparation which is a broad-spectrum penicillin available as film-coated, oval, white tablets containing 500mg pivampicillin coded with symbol and 128. Also, **PONDOCILLIN SUSPENSION** containing 175mg pivampicillin/5ml available as granules for reconstitution. *Used for*: skin, soft tissue infections, bronchitis, pneumonia, gonorrhoea and urinary tract infections. *Dosage*: adults, 1 tablet or 15ml suspension twice each day with drink or food. Children, under 1 year, 40–60mg/kg; 1 to 5 years, 10–15ml; 6 to 10 years, 15–20ml. All as daily divided doses with food or drink. *Special care*: kidney disease. *Avoid use*: patients with glandular fever. *Side effects*: gastro-intestinal upset, hypersensitive allergic reactions. *Manufacturer*: Leo.

PONSTAN FORTE

Description: an NSAID available as blue/ivory capsules containing 250mg mefenamic acid marked PONSTAN 250. Also, **PONSTAN FORTE** film-coated, yellow tablets containing 500mg marked with name. **PONSTAN PAEDIATRIC SUSPENSION** containing 50mg/5ml. *Used for*: pain, period pain, headache, rheumatoid pain (Stills disease), osteoarthritis, heavy menstrual bleeding. *Dosage*: adults, 500mg 3 times each day (on first day of period in patients with heavy menstrual bleeding). Children, use paediatric suspension, aged 6 months to 1 year, 5ml; 2 to 4 years, 10ml; 5 to 8 years, 15ml; 9 to 12 years, 20ml. All doses at 8 hour intervals for no more than 1 week. *Special care*: pregnancy, breast-feeding, elderly, allergies, asthma, heart failure, epilepsy. *Avoid use*: known allergy to NSAID or aspirin, ulcer, liver or kidney disorder, inflammatory bowel disease. *Possible interaction*: sulphonylureas, anticoagulants, hydantoins, quinolones. *Side effects*: kidney disorder, gastro-intestinal intolerance, raised level of liver enzymes. Rarely, blood changes. Withdraw drug if skin rash occurs. *Manufacturer*: Elan.

POTABA

Description: an antifibrotic preparation which dissolves fibrous tissue, available as powder in sachets containing 3g potassium p-aminobenzoate. Also, **POTABA TABLETS** white, containing 500mg. **POTABA CAPSULES**, red/white, containing 500mg. *Used for*: scleroderma (thickened skin), Peyronie's disease (fibrous hardening of the penis). *Dosage*: adults, 12g each day in 4 divided doses with meals. *Special care*: kidney disease. *Possible interaction*: sulphonamides. *Side effects*: anorexia, nausea (discontinue if these occur). *Manufacturer*: Glenwood.

PRAXILENE

Description: a preparation that is a peripheral and cerebral activator which improves the use of glucose and oxygen by the tissues, increasing the level of ATP (the energy molecules of cells) and decreasing lactic acid levels. It is available as pink capsules containing 100mg naftidrofuryl oxalate. Also, **PRAXILENE FORTE** available in ampoules for injection containing 20mg naftidrofuryl oxalate/ml. *Used for*: disorders of cerebral and peripheral arteries. *Dosage*: 1 or 2 tablets 3 times each day. *Special care*: use of Praxilene Forte in patients with very weak heart or conduction disorders. *Avoid use*: children. Use of Forte in patients with heart block. *Side effects*: nausea, stomach ache. *Manufacturer*: Lipha.

PRECORTISYL

Description: a glucocorticoid corticosteroid preparation available as white tablets containing 1mg prednisolone and scored, white tablets containing 5mg prednisolone. Also, **PRECORTISYL FORTE** scored, white tablets containing 25mg prednisolone. *Used for*: Precortisyl, allergic and rheumatic disorders; Forte, rheumatic fever, systemic lupus erythematosus (severe inflammatory disorder affecting many parts of the body), blood disorders. *Dosage*: Precortisyl, 20–40mg each day in divided doses at first, then reducing by 2.5–5mg every third or fourth day until a maintenance dose, in the order of 5–20mg daily, is achieved. Forte, 75mg in 3 divided doses. Children, Precortisyl, age 1 to 7 years, quarter to half adult dose; 7 to 12 years, half to three-quarters adult dose. *Special care*: pregnancy, diabetes, kidney inflammation, hypertension, thrombophlebitis, epilepsy, secondary cancer, underactive thyroid, peptic ulcer, glaucoma, recent surgical anastomoses of intestine. Also, patients suffering from stress, psychoses, liver cirrhosis, infections of fungal or viral origin, tuberculosis, other infections. Also avoid contact with chicken pox or *Herpes zoster* and seek medical advice if this occurs or if infected. *Avoid use*: children under 1 year. *Possible interaction*: diuretics, hypoglycaemics, phenytoin, NSAIDs, rifampicin, anticholinesterases, ephedrine, anticoagulants taken orally, phenobarbitone, cardiac glycosides, diuretics. *Side effects*: mood changes, depression and euphoria, changes as in Cushing's syndrome, osteoporosis, peptic ulcer, hyperglycaemia. *Manufacturer*: Roussel.

PRED FORTE

Description: a corticosteroid preparation available as eyedrops, containing 1% prednisolone acetate. *Used for*: inflammation of eyes where no infection is present. *Dosage*: 1 or 2 drops 2, 3 or 4 times each day. 2 drops every hour may be needed during the first 48 hours. *Special care*: pregnancy, babies. *Avoid use*: fungal, viral or tuberculous eye infections or those producing pus. Also, glaucoma, dendritic ulcer, those wearing soft contact lenses. *Side effects*: formation of cataracts, thinning of cornea, rise in pressure within eye, secondary fungal or viral infections. *Manufacturer*: Allergan.

PREDENEMA

Description: a steroid colorectal agent available as an enema containing 20mg prednisolone (as metasulphobenzoate sodium). *Used for*: ulcerative colitis. *Dosage*: adults, 1 enema at night for 2, 3 or 4 weeks. *Special care*: pregnancy, avoid long-term use. *Avoid use*: children. Patients with perforated bowel, infections, fistulae, obstruction of the bowel, peritonitis. *Manufacturer*: Pharmax.

PREDFOAM

Description: a steroid colorectal agent available as a white aerosol foam containing 20mg prednisolone (as meta-sulphobenzoate sodium) per metered dose. *Used for*: ulcerative colitis, proctitis (inflammation of the rectum). *Dosage*: adults, 1 metered dose into rectum twice each day for 2 weeks continuing for another 2 weeks if condition improves. *Special care*: pregnancy, short-term use only. *Avoid use*: children, patients with perforated bowel, infections, fistulae, obstruction of the bowel, peritonitis. *Manufacturer*: Pharmax.

PREDNESOL

Description: a glucocorticoid corticosteroid preparation available as scored, pink tablets containing 5mg prednisolone (as disodium phosphate) marked with name and GLAXO. *Used for*: rheumatic, allergic and inflammatory disorders responsive to steroids. *Dosage*: adults, 10–100mg in water each day at first, in divided doses, then reducing to lowest dose which is effective. Children, age 1 to 7, quarter to half adult dose; 7 to 12, half to three-quarters adult dose. *Special care*: thrombophlebitis, psychoses, recent intestinal anastomoses, chronic nephritis, certain cancers, osteoporosis, peptic ulcer, skin eruption/rash related to a disease, viral, fungal or active infections, tuberculosis. Hypertension, glaucoma, epilepsy, acute glomerulonephritis (inflammation of kidney glomerulus), diabetes, cirrhosis, hypothyroidism, pregnancy, stress. To be withdrawn gradually. *Possible interaction*: NSAIDs, oral anticoagulants, phenytoin, ephedrine, phenobarbitone, rifampicin, diuretics, cardiac glycosides, anticholinesterases, hypoglycaemics. *Side effects*: osteoporosis, depression, euphoria, hyperglycaemia, peptic ulcers, Cushingoid changes. *Manufacturer*: Glaxo Wellcome.

PREDSOL

Description: a steroid colorectal agent available as an enema containing 20mg prednisolone as disodium phosphate. Also, **PREDSOL SUPPOSITORIES** containing 5mg prednisolone (as disodium phosphate). *Used for*: enema, ulcerative colitis; suppositories, proctitis (inflammation of rectum) and anal disorders resulting from Crohn's disease (a disorder of the intestine or part of digestive tract in which there is inflammation and ulceration). *Dosage*: adults, enema, 1 at night for 2, 3 or 4 weeks; suppositories, 1 every night and morning after passing stool. *Special care*: pregnancy, short-term use only. *Avoid use*: children, bacterial, fungal, tuberculous or viral infections. *Side effects*: systemic glucocorticoid effects, e.g. mood swings, euphoria and depression, changes as in Cushing's syndrome, peptic ulcer, hyperglycaemia, osteoporosis. *Manufacturer*: Evans.

PREFERID

Description: a potent topical steroid preparation available as cream and ointment containing 0.025% budesonide. *Used for*: psoriasis, all types of dermatitis, eczema. *Dosage*: apply thinly 2 or 3 times each day. *Special care*: thrombophlebitis, psychoses, recent intestinal anastomoses, chronic nephritis, certain cancers, osteoporosis, peptic ulcer, skin eruption/rash related to a disease, viral, fungal or active infections, tuberculosis. Hypertension, glaucoma, epilepsy, acute glomerulonephritis (inflammation of kidney glomerulus), diabetes, cirrhosis, hypothyroidism, pregnancy, stress. To be withdrawn gradually. *Possible interaction*: NSAIDs, oral anticoagulants, phenytoin, ephedrine, phenobarbitone, rifampicin, diuretics, cardiac glycosides, anticholinesterases, hypoglycaemics. *Side effects*: osteoporosis, depression, euphoria, hyperglycaemia, peptic ulcers, Cushingoid changes. *Manufacturer*: Yamanouchi.

PREGNYL

Description: a preparation of human chorionic gonadotrophin available as powder in ampoules, with solvent for reconstitution and injection, at strengths of 500, 1500 and 5000 units. *Used for*: underdevelopment of male sexual organs, deficient production of sperm, delayed puberty in males; infertility due to lack of maturing of follicles and ovulation in females. Along with human menopausal gonadotrophin to produce superovulation for in vitro fertilization treatment. *Dosage*: male adults, hypogonadism, 500–1000 units 2 or 3 times each week by intramuscular injection. Delayed puberty, 1500 units twice each week by intramuscular injection for at least 6 months. Females, infertility, following treatment with human menopausal gonadotrophin, 5000–10000 units by intramuscular injection. Then 3 further injections of 5000 units during the next 9 days. Superovulation, 30 to 40 hours after injection with human menopausal gonadotrophin, 5000–10000 units by intramuscular injection. *Special care*: patients with heart or kidney disorders, epilepsy, hypertension, migraine, hormone levels should be monitored in female patients. *Avoid use*: children, patients with androgen-dependent cancers. *Side effects*: skin rashes, salt and water retention. *Manufacturer*: Organon.

PREMARIN

Description: an oestrogen preparation available as sugar-coated, oval, maroon tablets and sugar-coated, oval, yellow tablets containing 0.625mg and 1.25mg conjugated oestrogens. Also, **PREMARIN VAGINAL CREAM** containing 0.625mg/g conjugated oestrogens. *Used for*: tablets, hormone replacement therapy for menopausal women who have had a hysterectomy. Prevention of osteoporosis following menopause. Relief of symptoms of some breast cancers in post-menopausal women. Cream, atrophic vaginitis and urethritis (inflammation due to atrophy of the tissues of the vagina and urethra), Kraurosis vulvae (a disease of the external genital area, characterized by degeneration of tissues and itching, affecting elderly women). *Dosage*: tablets, for hormone replacement therapy, 0.625mg–1.25mg each day for 12 to 18 months. Prevention of osteoporosis, same dose for 5 to 10 years. Breast cancer, up to 10mg 3 times each day for at least 9 months. Cream, 1–2g applied daily to affected area or intra-vaginally (using applicator) for 3 weeks followed by 1 week without treatment. *Special care*: those at risk of thromboembolism or with history of disorders relating to this, those with porphyria, gallstones, diabetes, otosclerosis, fibroids in the uterus, tetany, epilepsy, mild liver disease. Blood pressure, breasts and pelvic organs should be checked regularly during the course of treatment. *Avoid use*: thromboembolism, thrombophlebitis, vaginal bleeding which is not diagnosed, or endometriosis, genital tract cancer or other oestrogen-dependent cancers. Serious kidney, liver, heart disease, Dublin-Johnson or Rotor syndrome. *Possible interaction*: drugs which induce liver enzymes. *Manufacturer*: Wyeth.

PREMPAK-C

Description: an oestrogen and progestogen preparation available in the form of sugar-coated oval tablets in 2 strengths, 28 maroon or 28 yellow containing 0.625mg or 1.25mg conjugated oestrogens respectively. Also, 12 sugar-coated brown tablets containing 0.15mg norgestrel in same pack. *Used for*: hormone replacement therapy in women who have not had a hysterectomy, for meno-pausal symptoms, prevention of osteoporosis following menopause. *Dosage*: 1 maroon or yellow tablet for 16 days then 1 maroon or yellow tablet and 1 brown tablet for 12 days, starting on first day of period if present. *Special care*: pa-tients with history of, or considered to be at risk of thrombosis. Women with any of the following should receive careful monitoring: epilepsy, gallstones, porphyria, multiple sclerosis, otosclerosis, diabetes, migraine, hypertension, tetany, fibroids in the uterus. Blood pressure, breasts and pelvic organs should be examined regularly during the treatment especially in women who may be at risk of breast cancer. *Avoid use*: pregnancy, breast-feeding, with breast cancer, cancer of reproductive system or other hormonally dependent cancer, inflam-mation of veins or other thromboembolic conditions, endometriosis, undiag-nosed vaginal bleeding, serious liver, kidney or heart disease, Dublin-Johnson or Rotor syndrome. *Possible interaction*: drugs which induce liver enzymes. *Side effects*: soreness and enlargement of breasts, breakthrough bleeding, weight gain, gastro-intestinal upset, dizziness, nausea, headache, vomiting. If frequent, severe, migraine-like headaches, disturbance of vision, rise in blood pressure, jaundice or indications of thrombosis occur, drug should immediately be with-drawn, and also in the event of pregnancy. Drug should be stopped 6 weeks before planned major surgery. *Manufacturer*: Wyeth.

PREPIDIL

Description: a prostaglandin preparation available as a sterile cervical gel in single use syringes containing 500µg dinoprostone/3g gel. *Used for*: induction of labour, softening and dilation of cervix. *Dosage*: 1 dose into cervical canal, repeated as directed by physician. *Special care*: glaucoma, asthma, raised pres-sure within eye; high doses may cause rupture of uterus. Should not be given continuously for more than 2 days. *Avoid use*: patients at risk of rupture of uterus, those in whom delivery is complicated, e.g. placenta praevia, those with serious toxaemia, untreated pelvic infection, multiple pregnancy, previous his-tory of difficult delivery, inflammation of vagina or cervix. *Side effects*: chills, shivering, flushing, headache, nausea, vomiting, diarrhoea, raised level of white blood cells, short-lived fever, abnormal increase in muscle tone of uterus, se-vere contractions. *Manufacturer*: Pharmacia & Upjohn.

PREPULSID

Description: a prokinetic drug acting on the gastro-intestinal tract, which pro-motes the movement of food through the oesophagus and stomach. It is avail-able as scored, white tablets containing 10mg cisapride (as monohydrate). Also,

PREPULSID SUSPENSION, cherry-flavoured solution containing 5mg cisapride/5ml. *Used for*: gastro-oesophageal reflux, maintenance treatment of reflux oesophagitis, dyspepsia, relief of symptoms when gastric emptying is delayed as in systemic sclerosis, diabetes, autonomic neuropathy. *Dosage*: gastro-oesophageal reflux, 20mg before breakfast and at night time or 10mg 3 times each day for 12 weeks. Then a maintenance dose of 20mg once each day at bedtime or 10mg twice each day before breakfast and at night. Dyspepsia, 10mg 3 times each day for 4 weeks. Delayed gastric emptying, 10mg 3 or 4 times each day, for 6 weeks. *Special care*: breast-feeding, elderly, kidney or liver disorders. *Avoid use*: pregnancy, children, patients with gastro-intestinal obstruction, haemorrhage or perforation. *Possible interaction*: anticholinergics, anticoagulants taken orally, central nervous system depressants. *Side effects*: abdominal rumbling and pain, diarrhoea; rarely, extrapyramidal effects, headache, convulsions. *Manufacturer*: Janssen-Cilag.

PRESCAL

Description: an antihypertensive preparation which is a class II calcium antagonist, available as scored yellow tablets containing 2.5mg isradipine marked NM and CIBA. *Used for*: hypertension. *Dosage*: 1 tablet in the morning and at night, increasing after 3 or 4 weeks to 2 twice each day if needed. Maximum dose is 4 twice daily. Elderly, half a tablet twice each day at first. *Special care*: pregnancy, breast-feeding, narrowing of aorta (aortic stenosis), sick sinus syndrome. *Avoid use*: children. *Possible interaction*: anticonvulsants. *Side effects*: tachycardia, palpitations, headache, giddiness, flushing, fluid retention in hands and feet, pain in abdomen, gain in weight, tiredness, skin rashes. Rise in level of transaminase enzymes in blood. *Manufacturer*: Ciba.

PRESTIM

Description: an antihypertensive preparation which combines a non-cardioselective ß-blocker and thiazide diuretic available as white, scored tablets containing 10mg timolol maleate and 2.5mg bendrofluazide, marked with a lion and 132. Also, **PRESTIM FORTE** scored, white tablets containing 20mg timolol maleate and 5mg bendrofluazide, marked with a lion and 146. *Used for*: hypertension. *Dosage*: Prestim, 1 to 4 tablets each day. Prestim Forte, half dose. *Special care*: pregnancy, breast-feeding, patients with weak hearts may require diuretics and digitalis, those with diabetes, undergoing general anaesthesia, kidney or liver disorders, gout. Electrolyte (salts) levels may need to be monitored. *Avoid use*: history of bronchospasm or obstructive airways disease, heart block, heart shock, uncompensated heart failure, disease of peripheral arteries, bradycardia. Serious or worsening kidney failure or anuria. *Possible interaction*: sympathomimetics, class I antiarrhythmics, central nervous system depressants, clonidine withdrawal, ergot alkaloids, cardiac depressant anaesthetics, verapamil, reserpine, indomethacin, hypoglycaemics, cimetidine, other antihypertensives. Digitalis, potassium supplements, potassium-sparing diuretics, lithium. *Side effects*: cold hands and feet, disturbance of sleep, fatigue on exercise, bronchospasm, bradycardia, gastro-intestinal disturbances, heart failure, blood changes, gout, sensitivity to light, muscle weakness. If skin rash or dry eyes occur, withdraw drug gradually. *Manufacturer*: Leo.

PRIADEL

Description: an antidepressant preparation which is a lithium salt available as scored, white, continuous-release tablets in 2 strengths. Capsule-shaped tablets contain 200mg lithium carbonate marked P200. Tablets, marked PRIADEL, contain 400mg lithium carbonate. Also, **PRIADEL LIQUID**, a sugar-free solution containing 520mg lithium citrate/5ml. *Used for*: tablets, manic depression, mania, aggressive and self-harming behaviour, recurrent bouts of depression. *Dosage*: tablets, 400–1200mg as a single dose each day at first; liquid 400–1200mg in 2 divided daily doses at first. Dosage then adjusted to maintain a certain blood level. *Special care*: levels in blood must be monitored along with heart, kidney and thyroid function. *Avoid use*: children, pregnancy, breastfeeding, hypothyroidism, Addison's disease, heart or kidney disorders, disturbance of salt balance. *Possible interaction*: diazepam, metoclopramide, diuretics, flupenthixol, methyldopa, tetracyclines, phenytopin, haloperidol, NSAIDs, carbamazepine. *Side effects*: trembling hands, diarrhoea, nausea, disturbance of ECG and central nervous system, gain in weight, hypo and hyperthyroidism, skin rashes, oedema, passing of large quantities of urine, thirstiness, oedema. *Manufacturer*: Delandale.

PRIMACOR

Description: a heart drug and phosphodiesterase inhibitors, which have a mode of action resembling stimulation by the sympathetic nervous system. Primacor is available in ampoules for injection containing 10mg milrinone/ml. *Used for*: acute, post-operative heart failure after cardiac surgery; short-term treatment of congestive heart failure which has not responded to other drugs. *Dose*: 50µg/kg body weight by slow intravenous injection over 10 minutes. Then by intravenous infusion at a rate of 375–750 nanograms/kg/minute. This is for up to 12 hours in post-operative patients and for 48–72 hours in those with congestive heart failure. The maximum daily dose is 1.13mg/kg. *Special care*: certain types of heart failure associated with disease of heart valves and outflow obstruction. Patients with kidney disorder should receive reduced dose. Monitoring of fluid, electrolyte levels, blood pressure, central venous blood pressure, heart rate, ECG, liver enzymes, platelet counts must be carried out. *Side effects*: unusual heart beats, hypotension, arrhythmias, vomiting, nausea, insomnia, headache, diarrhoea. Less commonly, chills, pains in limbs, reduced production of urine, urine retention, fever. *Manufacturer*: Sanofi Winthrop.

PRIMALAN

Description: an anti-allergic antihistamine preparation which is a phenothiazine type drug, available as white tablets containing 5mg mequitazine marked

PRIMALAN. *Used for*: hay fever, itching, urticaria, inflammation of the nose. *Dosage*: 1 tablet twice each day. *Avoid use*: pregnancy, liver disease, enlarged prostate gland, epilepsy. *Possible interaction*: central nervous system depressants, some sympathomimetics (indirect acting), alcohol, MAOIs. *Side effects*: sleepiness, impaired reactions, extrapyramidal responses, anticholinergic side effects. *Manufacturer*: R.P.R.

PRIMAXIN IV

Description: an antibiotic compound preparation, combining a carbapenem and enzyme inhibitor. It is available as 250mg or 500mg of powder in vials for reconstitution and injection, containing equal parts of imipenem (as monohydrate) and cilastin (as sodium salt). Also, **PRIMAXIN IM**, a preparation containing 500mg cilastin and 500mg imipenem as powder in vials for reconstitution and intramuscular injection. *Used for*: septicaemia, bone, skin, joint, soft tissue infections, infections of urinary, genital and lower respiratory tracts, abdominal and gynaecological infections. Also, prevention of infection after surgery. *Dosage*: adults, Primaxin IV, 250 mg–1g by intravenous infusion every 6 to 8 hours, depending upon nature and severity of infection. Prevention of infection, 1g when patient is anaesthetized followed by a further 1g dose 3 hours later. Primaxin, depending upon nature and severity of infection, in the order of 500–750mg by deep intramuscular injection. Maximum dose is 1.5g each day. Patients with gonococcal inflammation and infection of urethra or cervix receive 500mg as a single dose. Children, Primaxin IV only, age over 3 months, 15mg/kg body weight every 6 hours, the maximum daily dose being 2g. *Special care*: pregnancy, breast-feeding, patients with kidney disorders, gastro-intestinal diseases (especially inflammation of bowel), those with known allergy to penicillin. *Avoid use*: children under 3 months. *Possible interaction*: ganciclovir, probenecid. *Side effects*: diarrhoea, colitis (inflammation of the large intestine or bowel), nausea, vomiting, blood changes. Disturbance of central nervous system, convulsions, rise in level of liver enzymes, creatinine and urea in blood. *Manufacturer*: M.S.D.

PRIMOLUT N

Description: an hormonal progestogen preparation available as white tablets containing 5mg norethisterone marked AN inside a hexagon shape. *Used for*: abnormal menstrual bleeding, other menstrual disorders, postponement of menstruation, endometriosis. *Dosage*: adults, heavy menstrual bleeding, 1 tablet twice or 3 times each day from day 19 to day 26 of cycle. Postponement of menstruation, 1 tablet 3 times each day, beginning 3 days before expected start of period. Endometriosis, 2 tablets each day beginning on fifth day of cycle, increasing to 4 or 5 daily if spotting takes place. 2 tablets each day should be taken for at least 4 to 6 months. *Special care*: migraine or epilepsy. *Avoid use*: pregnancy, history of itching or idiopathic jaundice during pregnancy, serious liver disorders, Dublin-Johnson and Rotor syndromes.. *Side effects*: disturbance of liver function, masculinization. *Manufacturer*: Schering H.C.

PRIMOTESTON DEPOT

Description: an hormonal preparation of a depot androgen available as a solution in ampoules for injection containing 250mg testosterone oenanthate/ml. *Used for*: underactivity of testes, breast cancer. *Dosage*: underactivity of testes, 250mg by intramuscular injection every 2 or 3 weeks. Same for maintenance once every 2 or 3 weeks. Female breast cancer, 200mg by intramuscular injection every 2 weeks. *Special care*: epilepsy, migraine, hypertension heart, kidney or liver disease. *Avoid use*: liver or prostate cancer, untreated heart failure, heart disease due to insufficient blood supply. *Possible interaction*: drugs that induce liver enzynmes. *Side effects*: weight gain, oedema, liver tumours. Males, decrease in fertility, premature closure of epiphyses, priapism (abnormal, prolonged and painful erection of penis, not associated with sexual arousal but with underlying disorder or caused by a drug). Females, masculinization, withdraw drug if hypercalcaemia occurs. *Manufacturer*: Schering H.C.

PRO-BANTHINE

Description: an anticholinergic preparation available as sugar-coated, peach-coloured tablets containing 15mg propantheline bromide. *Used for*: peptic ulcer, irritable bowel syndrome, enuresis (incontinence of urine). *Dosage*: ulcer, 1 tablet 3 times each day taken before meals, and 2 at bedtime; irritable bowel syndrome, up to 8 tablets each day in divided doses. Enuresis, 1 to 2 tablets 3 times each day, with a daily maximum of 8 in divided doses. *Special care*: elderly, liver or kidney disease, ulcerative colitis, serious heart disease, degenerative disease of autonomic nervous system. *Avoid use*: children, patients with glaucoma, obstruction of gastro-intestinal or urinary tracts. *Possible interaction*: digoxin. *Side effects*: anticholinergic side effects. *Manufacturer*: Baker Norton.

PRO-VIRON

Description: an hormonal androgen preparation available as white, scored tablets containing 25mg mesterolone. *Used for*: androgen deficiency, male infertility. *Dosage*: 25mg 3 or 4 times each day redcued to 50–70mg in divided doses as a daily maintenance dose. *Special care*: elderly patients with kidney or liver disorders, epilepsy, secondary bone cancers (risk of hypercalcaemia, hypertension, ischaemic heart diesease). Boys before age of puberty. *Avoid use*: kidney disorder, hypercalcaemia, breast cancer in men, prostate cancer. *Possible interaction*: liver-inducing enzymes. *Side effects*: premature closure of epiphyses in boys before puberty, precocious sexual development in boys, suppression of sperm production in men, hypercalcaemia. Increase in bone growth, priapism (prolonged, painful erection of penis not associated with sexual arousal but symptom of underlying disorder or drug), oedema with salt retention. *Manufacturer*: Schering Health.

PROCAINAMIDE DURULES

Description: a class I antiarrhythmic drug available as pale yellow, sustained-release tablets containing 500mg procainamide hydrochloride. *Used for*: heart arrhythmias, some disorders of muscles. *Dosage*: usually 2 to thee tablets 3 times each day. *Special care*: heart, liver or kidney failure. Regular blood tests required. *Avoid use*: patients with myasthenia gravis, SLE, heart block, asthma. *Side effects*: effects on CNS, blood changes, SLE, gastro-intestinal upset. *Manufacturer*: Astra.

PROCTOFOAM H.C.

Description: a colorectal preparation combining a steroid and local anaesthetic available as an aerosol foam containing 1% hydrocortisone acetate and 1% pramoxine hydrochloride with applicator. *Used for*: haemorrhoids, anal fissures, proctitis (inflammation of rectum and anus), cryptitis (inflammation of a crypt—a blind pit or small sac in the anal region). *Dosage*: 1 applicator dose into the rectum 2 or 3 times each day and after passing stool. Apply to external anal area as needed. *Special care*: pregnancy, short-term use only. *Avoid use*: children, patients with fungal, viral or tuberculous infections. *Side effects*: systemic corticosteroid side effects. *Manufacturer*: Stafford-Miller.

PROCTOSEDYL

Description: a colorectal preparation combining a steroid and local anaesthetic available as suppositories containing hydrochloride. Also, **PROCTOSEDYL OINTMENT** containing 0.5% hydrocortisone and 0.5% cinchocaine hydrochloride. *Used for*: haemorrhoids, anal itching, inflammation. *Dosage*: 1 suppository and/or 1 application of ointment in the morning and at night, and after passing motion. *Special care*: pregnancy, short-term use only. *Avoid use*: patients with fungal, viral or tuberculous infections. *Side effects*: systemic corticosteroid side effects. *Manufacturer*: Hoechst.

PROFASI

Description: a gonadotrophin preparation available as powder in ampoules along with solvent for reconstitution and injection in different strengths containing 500 units, 1000 units, 2000 units, 5000 units and 10,000 units chorionic gonadotrophin. *Used for*: underactivity of testes (infertility), undescended testicles, female infertility due to lack of ovulation, superovulation for in vitro fertilization treatment. *Dosage*: underactive testes, 2000 units twice each week; undescended testicles, 500–1000 units every other day. Females, lack of ovulation, up to 10,000 units in middle of monthly cycle; superovulation, up to 10,000 units. All doses in males given intramuscularly, in females by intramuscular or subcutaneous injection. *Special care*: any other hormonal disorders should be corrected before treatment starts. Hormone levels in females require monitoring. *Side effects*: oedema, allergic reactions, over-stimulation of ovaries. *Manufacturer*: Serono.

PROGESIC

Description: an NSAID available as yellow tablets containing 200mg fenprofen (as calcium salt) marked LILLY 4015. *Used for*: pain, rheumatic and arthritic disorders including osteoarthritis, rheumatoid arthritis, ankylosing spondylitis. *Dosage*: 200–600mg 3 or 4 times each day with a maximum of 3g daily. *Special care*: pregnancy, breast-feeding, elderly, history of gastro-intestinal bleeding or peptic ulcer, liver or kidney disease, heart failure, asthma. *Avoid use*: children, allergy to aspirin or antiinflammatory drug, severe kidney disease. *Possible interaction*: aspirin, loop diuretics, anticoagulants, sulphonylureas, hydantoins, phenobarbitone, quinolones. *Side effects*: liver and kidney disorders, allergic reactions, gastro-intestinal bleeding and intolerance. *Manufacturer*: Lilly.

PROGYNOVA

Description: an hormonal oestrogen preparation available in the form of beige, sugar-coated tablets, containing 1mg and blue, containing 2mg oestradiol valerate respectively. *Used for*: short-term treatment of menopausal symptoms. *Dosage*: 1mg each day for 21 days then 7 tablet-free days. 2mg tablets should only be used when needed. *Special care*:those at risk of thromboembolism, porphyria, multiple sclerosis, epilepsy, fibroids in the womb, migraine, tetany. Also, otosclerosis, gallstones, liver disease. Pelvic organs, breasts and blood pressure should be checked regularly during course of treatment. *Avoid use*: pregnancy, breast-feeding, breast or other cancer of reproductive tract or 1 which is hormone-dependent. Also, thromboembolism-type disorders, undiagnosed vaginal bleeding or endometriosis, thrombophlebitis, heart, liver or kidney disease, Rotor or Dublin-Johnson syndrome. *Possible interaction*: drugs which induce liver enzymes. *Side effects*: enlargement and soreness of breasts, gastro-intestinal upset, dizziness, breakthrough bleeding, headache, vomiting and nausea, weight gain. *Manufacturer*: Schering H.C.

PROLEUKIN

Description: a highly toxic drug which is a recombinant interleukin-2 available as a powder in vials for reconstitution and injection containing 18 million units aldesleukin. *Used for*: secondary cancer of kidney cells in some patients. *Dosage*: as individually directed by physician; by intravenous infusion. *Special care*: for use in specialist cancer units only. *Possible interaction*: antihypertensives. *Side effects*: pulmonary oedema, hypotension, serious toxic effects on liver, kidneys, bone marrow, thyroid and central nervous system. *Manufacturer*: Chiron.

PROLUTON DEPOT

Description: a depot hormonal preparation of a progestogen containing 250mg hydroxyprogesterone hexanoate/ml in ampoules for oily injection. *Used for*: habitual abortion. *Dosage*: 250–500mg by intramuscular injection each week during the first 5 months of pregnancy. *Special care*: hypertension, kidney or heart disease. *Avoid use*: pregnancy, liver disease, cancer of breast or reproductive tract, undiagnosed vaginal bleeding, porphyria, serious disease of the arteries. *Side effects*: weight changes, oedema, disturbance of menstrual cycle and pre-menstrual symptoms, depression, discomfort in breasts, change in libido, urticaria, acne, baldness, unusual hair growth, anaphylactoid-type reactions. Sleepiness, insomnia; rarely, jaundice. *Manufacturer*: Schering H.C.

PROMINAL^{CD}

Description: an anticonvulsant preparation and barbiturate available as white tablets containing 30mg, 60mg and 200mg methylphenobarbitone, marked P30, P60 and P200 respectively. *Used for*: focal and grand mal epilepsy. *Dosage*: 100–600mg each day, children 5–15mg/kg body weight each day. *Special care*: kidney and liver disorders, serious lung insufficiency. *Avoid use*: pregnancy, breast-feeding, elderly, patients who are debilitated, suffering from porphyria, pain which is not controlled, history of drug or alcohol abuse. *Possible interaction*: CNS depressants, griseofulvin, alcohol, phenytoin, systemic steroids, chloramphenicol, rifampicin, metronidazole, anticoagulants of the coumarin type. *Side effects*: headache, respiratory depression, dizziness, unsteadiness, sleepiness, confusion, agitation, allergic responses. Drug tolerance and dependence may occur. Drug is metabolized to phenobarbitone. *Manufacturer*: Sanofi Winthrop.

PRONDOL

Description: a TCAD available as yellow tablets containing 15mg iprindole (as hydrochloride) marked WYETH. *Used for*: depression. *Dosage*: 15–30mg 3 times daily at first with a maximum of 60mg 3 times daily. Elderly start with 15mg 3 times daily. *Special care*: liver disorders, hyperthyroidism, glaucoma, lactation, epilepsy, diabetes, adrenal tumour, heart disease, urine retention. Psychotic or suicidal patients. *Avoid use*: children, heart block, heart attacks, severe liver disease, pregnancy. *Possible interaction*: MAOIs (or within 14 days of their use), alcohol, anti-depressants, barbiturates, anticholinergics, local anaesthetics that contain adrenaline or noradrenaline, oestrogens, cimetidine, antihypertensives. *Side effects*: constipation, urine retention, dry mouth, blurred vision, palpitations, tachycardia, nervousness, drowsiness, insomnia. Changes in weight, blood and blood sugar, jaundice, skin reactions, weakness, ataxia, hypotension, sweating, altered libido, gynaecomastia, galactorrhoea. *Manufacturer*: Wyeth.

PRONESTYL

Description: a class I antiarrhythmic preparation available as scored, white tablets containing 250mg procainamide hydrochloride marked SQUIBB 754. Also, **PRONESTYL INJECTION**, a solution in vials containing 100mg procainamide hydrochloride/ml. *Used for*: heart arrhythmias. *Dosage*: tablets, up to 50mg/kg body weight each day as divided doses every 3 to 6 hours. Injection, for acute condition, rate not greater than 50mg/minute by slow intravenous injection (or 100mg with monitoring of ECG). This is repeated every 5 minutes until arrhythmia is controlled. Maximum dose 1g. By intravenous infusion, 500–600mg over 25 to 30 minutes while ECG is monitored. Then a maintenance dose of 2–6mg/minute followed by tablets, if needed, 3 to 4 hours after infusion has been given. *Special care*: elderly persons, pregnant women, patients with heart or liver failure, myasthenia gravis, regular blood tests should be carried out during the course of treatment. *Avoid use*: children, SLE or heart block. *Possible interaction*: other antiarrhythmics, terfenadine, astemizole, phenothiazines, cimetidine, neostigmine, pyridostigmine. *Side effects*: SLE, blood changes (leucopenia and agranulocytosis—severe reduction in some white blood cells due to chemicals or drugs), gastro-intestinal upset. *Manufacturer*: Squibb.

PROPADERM

Description: a potent topical steroid prepartion available as cream or ointment containing 0.025% beclomethasone dipropionate. *Used for*: inflammatory skin conditions responsive to steroids. *Dosage*: apply thinly to affected area twice each day. *Special care*: thrombophlebitis, psychoses, recent intestinal anastomoses, chronic nephritis, certain cancers, osteoporosis, peptic ulcer, skin eruption/rash related to a disease, viral, fungal or active infections, tuberculosis. Hypertension, glaucoma, epilepsy, acute glomerulonephritis (inflammation of kidney glomerulus), diabetes, cirrhosis, hypothyroidism, pregnancy, stress. To be withdrawn gradually. *Possible interaction*: NSAIDs, oral anticoagulants, phenytoin, ephedrine, phenobarbitone, rifampicin, diuretics, cardiac glycosides, anticholinesterases, hypoglycaemics. *Side effects*: osteoporosis, depression, euphoria, hyperglycaemia, peptic ulcers, Cushingoid changes. *Manufacturer*: Glaxo Wellcome.

PROPINE

Description: a sympathomimetic preparation available as eyedrops containing 0.1% dipivefrin hydrochloride. *Used for*: hypotension in eye, open angle glaucoma. *Dosage*: adults, 1 drop into eye every 12 hours. *Special care*: patients without whole or part of lens (aphakia) e.g. as in surgical removal of cataracts, narrow angle between iris and cornea of eye. *Avoid use*: children, patients with closed angle glaucoma, wearing soft contact lenses. *Side effects*: short-lived stinging, allergic responses, increased blood flow; rarely, raised blood pressure. *Manufacturer*: Allergan.

PROSCAR

Description: a preparation which is a selective 5-alpha reductase inhibitor available as film-coated, apple-shaped blue tablets containing 5mg finasteride marked with name and MSD. *Used for*: benign enlargement of the prostate gland. *Dosage*: 1 tablet each day for at least 6 months, then continuing long-term if condition is responding. *Special care*: obstruction or disease of genital tract. Women may absorb drug via semen through sexual intercourse or by handling tablets—risk in pregnancy. *Avoid use*: patients with prostate cancer. *Side effects*: decreased libido, impotence, reduced volume of ejaculation possibly affecting fertility. *Manufacturer*: M.S.D.

PROSTAP SR

Description: a gonadotrophin-releasing hormone analogue available as powder in microcapsule in vial with diluent for depot injection containing 3.75mg leuprorelin acetate. *Used for*: advanced cancer of the prostate gland. *Dosage*:

3.75mg as a single dose by subcutaneous or intramuscular injection each month. *Special care*: patients may require additional treatment with an anti-androgen starting 2 or 3 days before Prostap is given and continuing for 2 to 3 weeks. *Special care*: in patients at risk of compression of spinal cord or obstruction of ureter. *Side effects*: short-lived bone pain and obstruction of urine, decreased libido, impotence; rarely, swelling of hand and feet due to oedema, decreased libido, nausea, fatigue. *Manufacturer*: Wyeth.

PROSTIGMIN

Description: an anticholinesterase preparation available as scored, white tablets containing 15mg neostigmine bromide marked PROSTIGMIN. Also, **PROST-IGMIN INJECTION** available in ampoules containing 2.5mg neostigmin methylsulphate. *Used for*: myasthenia gravis, urine retention following surgery, paralytic ileus (decrease or absence of movement—peristalsis—along the intestine due to injury or surgery). *Dosage*: urine retention, paralytic ileus, 1 to 2 tablets as needed; myasthenia gravis, 5 to 20 tablets in divided doses each day. Injection, urine retention, paralytic ileus 0.5–2.5mg by subcutaneous or intramuscular injection; myasthenia gravis, 1.0–2.5mg by subcutaneous or intramuscular injection. Children, urine retention, paralytic ileus, 2.5–15mg as required; myasthenia gravis, newborn babies, 1–5mg every 4 hours, other ages 15–90mg in divided doses each day. Injection, urine retention, paralytic ileus, 0.125–1mg by intramuscular or subcutaneous injection; myasthenia gravis, newborn babies, 50–250 g every 4 hours, 30 minutes before feeds. Other ages, 200–500 g as needed. *Special care*: Parkinsonism, asthma, heart disease, epilepsy, vagotonia (increased activity of and effects resulting from stimulation of vagus nerve). *Avoid use*: patients with obstruction of intestine or urinary tract. *Possible interaction*: cyclopropane, halothane, depolarizing muscle relaxants. *Side effects*: vomiting, nausea, diarrhoea, pains in abdomen, over-production of saliva. *Manufacturer*: Roche.

PROSTIN E₂ ORAL

Description: a prostaglandin preparation available as rectangular, white tablets containing 500µg dinoprostone marked 76 on one side and U on the other. Also, **PROSTIN E₂ VAGINAL TABLETS**, white tablets containing 3mg, marked 715 and UPJOHN. **PROSTIN E₂ SOLUTIONS**, alcoholic solution in ampoules in 2 strengths containing 1mg and 10mg/ml. PROSTIN E₂ VAGINAL GEL, in 2 strengths containing 1mg and 2mg/3g gel. *Used for*: induction of labour. *Dosage*: tablets, 500µg then 0.5–1mg hourly, the maximum dose being 1.5mg. Vaginal tablets, 3mg inserted high into vagina followed by further 3mg 6 to 8 hours later if labour has not begun. Maximum dose is 6mg. Vaginal gel,1mg intravaginally at first followed by further 1–2mg after 6 hours if labour has not begun. Maximum dose is 3mg; (exceptionally, 4mg maximum dose may be needed). *Special care*: higher doses may cause rupture of uterus, should not be given for more than 2 days. Glaucoma, raised pressure within eye, asthma.

Avoid use: previous history of difficult or traumatic birth, multiple pregnancy, risk of uterine rupture, obstruction or failure of uterine contractions, untreated pelvic infections, foetal distress, serious toxaemia. *Side effects*: vomiting, diarrhoea, nausea, dizziness, headache, shivering, flushing, temporary fever, raised white blood cell count, exceptionally high muscle tone of uterus, very severe contractions. *Manufacturer*: Pharmacia & Upjohn.

PROSTIN F₂

Description: a prostaglandin available as a solution in ampoules for injection into amniotic fluid containing 5mg dinoprost (as tromethamine salt)/ml. *Used for*: induction of labour—rarely used. *Special care*: higher doses may cause rupture of uterus, should not be given for more than 2 days. Patients with vaginitis or cervicitis (inflammation of vagina or cervix), glaucoma, raised pressure within eye, asthma. *Avoid use*: previous history of difficult or traumatic birth, multiple pregnancy, risk of uterine rupture, obstruction or failure of uterine contractions, untreated pelvic infections, foetal distress, serious toxaemia. *Side effects*: vomiting, diarrhoea, nausea, dizziness, headache, shivering, flushing, temporary fever, raised white blood cell count, exceptionally high muscle tone of uterus, very severe contractions. *Manufacturer*: Upjohn.

PROSTIN VR

Description: a prostaglandin preparation available as an alcoholic solution in ampoules for infusion containing 0.5mg alprostadil/ml. *Used for*: newborn babies with congenital heart defects, before corrective surgery. *Dosage*: 50–100 nanograms/kg body weight/minute at first then lowest effective dose. *Special care*: risk of haemorrhage, arterial blood pressure must be monitored. *Avoid use*: newborn babies with hyaline membrane disease (respiratory distress syndrome) in which lungs are not properly expanded, (usually premature infants between 32 and 37 weeks of gestation). *Side effects*: apnoea (especially babies less than 2kg body weight), hypotension, oedema, fever, diarrhoea, tachycardia and bradycardia, flushing, convulsions, cardiac arrest. Effects on blood, weakening of walls of pulmonary artery and ductus arteriosus. *Manufacturer*: Pharmacia & Upjohn.

PROTHIADEN

Description: a TCAD preparation available as brown/red capsules containing 25mg dothiepin hydrochloride marked P25. Also, PROTHIADEN TABLETS, sugar-coated red tablets containing 75mg dothiepin hydrochloride marked P75. *Used for*: depression and anxiety. *Dosage*: adults, 75–150mg each day either as divided doses or taken as single dose at night. *Special care*: liver disorders, hyperthyroidism, glaucoma, lactation, epilepsy, diabetes, adrenal tumour, heart disease, urine retention. Psychotic or suicidal patients. *Avoid use*: children, heart block, heart attacks, severe liver disease, pregnancy. *Possible interaction*: MAOIs (or within 14 days of their use), alcohol, antidepressants, barbiturates, anticholinergics, local anaesthetics that contain adrenaline or noradrenaline, oestrogens, cimetidine, antihypertensives. *Side effects*: constipation, urine retention, dry mouth, blurred vision, palpitations, tachycardia, nervousness, drowsiness, insomnia. Changes in weight, blood and blood sugar, jaundice, skin reactions, weakness, ataxia, hypotension, sweating, altered libido, gynaecomastia, galactorrhoea. *Manufacturer*: Knoll.

PROVERA

Description: an hormonal progestogen preparation available as scored tablets in 3 strengths all containing medroxyprogesterone acetate. Orange, 2.5mg, marked U64; blue, 5mg, marked 286; white, 10mg, marked Upjohn 50. *Used for*: abnormal uterine bleeding, endometriosis, secondary ammenorrhoea (situation where menstrual periods stop due to underlying physical, psychiatric or environmental factors). Breast cancer in women after menopause, renal cell and endometrial cancer. *Dosage*: abnormal uterine bleeding 2.5–10mg each day for 5 to 10 days, repeated for 2 or 3 monthly cycles. Endometriosis, 10mg 3 times each day starting on first day of cycle and and continuing for 90 days without a break. Ammenorrhoea, 2.5–10mg each day for 5 to 10 days beginning on what is thought to be 16th continuing to 21st day of cycle. Repeat for 3 monthly cycles without break. Breast cancer, 400–800mg each day, renal cell and endometrial cancer, 200–400 mg daily. *Special care*: diabetes, asthma, heart or kidney disorders, migraine, history of depression. *Avoid use*: pregnancy, cancer of genital tract, liver disease, history of or present thromboembolic conditions. *Side effects*: gain in weight, abnormal production of breast milk, slight oedema, breast pain. Gastro-intestinal upset, central nervous system effects, skin and mucous membrane reactions. *Manufacturer*: Pharmacia & Upjohn.

PROZAC

Description: an antidepressant preparation which is a 5HT reuptake inhibitor, promoting the availability of this neurotransmitter. It is available as white/green capsules containing 20mg fluoxetine hydrochloride marked DISTA 3105. Also, **PROZAC LIQUID**, a syrup containing 20mg/5ml. *Used for*: depression especially when sedation is not needed. Obsessive-compulsive disorders, bulimia nervosa (over-eating phase of anorexia nervosa). *Dosage*: depression, usual dose in the order of 20mg each day; obsessive compulsive disorder, 20–60mg each day; bulimia nervosa, 60mg each day. *Special care*: pregnancy, heart disease, epilepsy, diabetes, kidney disorder, liver failure, heart disease. *Avoid use*: children, breast-feeding, severe kidney failure, unstable epilepsy. *Possible interaction*: vinblastine, MAOIs, lithium, carbamazepine, TCADs, flecainide, encainide, tryptophan. *Side effects*: diarrhoea, vomiting, nausea, insomnia, headache, dizziness, drowsiness, anxiety, weakness, fever, hypomania, convulsions, mania. Withdraw drug if allergic reactions or rash occur. *Manufacturer*: Dista.

PULMADIL

Description: a bronchodilator which is a selective beta$_2$-agonist available as a metered dose aerosol delivering 0.2mg rimiterol hydrobromide per dose. *Used for*: bronchospasm resulting from chronic bronchitis and bronchial asthma. *Dosage*: 1 to 3 doses which can be repeated after half an hour, if needed. Maximum of 24 doses in 24 hours. *Special care*: pregnancy, weak heart, arrhythmias, angina, hyperthyroidism, hypertension. *Possible interaction*: sympathomimetics. *Side effects*: dilation of peripheral blood vessels, headache. *Manufacturer*: 3M Health Care.

PULMICORT

Description: a bronchodilator corticosteroid preparation delivering 200µg budesonide per metered dose aerosol, suitable for use with a standard inhaler, nebuhaler or collapsible space delivery unit. Also, **PULMICORT LS** delivering 50µg per dose. **PULMICORT TURBOHALER** for use with a powder inhaler delivering 100, 200 or 400µg budesonide per metered dose. **PULMICORT RESPULES** available at strengths of 0.25mg and 0.5mg per ml available in ampoules for nebulization. *Used for*: bronchial asthma. *Dosage*: Pulmicort, 1 puff twice daily up to 8 puffs daily in severe attack. Pulmicort turbohaler 200–1600µg in divided doses daily. Pulmicort respules, in the order of 1–2mg twice each day with a maintenance dose of 0.5–1mg twice daily. Children, Pulmicort, 1 to 2 puffs twice each day. Pulmicort LS (children only), 1 to 8 puffs each day. Pulmicort turbohaler, 200–800µg in divided doses daily. Pulmicort respules, age 3 months to 12 years, 0.5–1mg twice each day with a maintenance dose of 0.25–0.5mg twice daily. *Special care*: pregnancy, pulmonary tuberculosis either active or statis, those transferring from other (systemic) steroids. *Side effects*: candidiasis of throat and mouth, dryness and hoarseness. *Manufacturer*: Astra.

PUMP-HEP

Description: an anticoagulant preparation of sodium heparin available in single dose ampoules for continuous infusion, at a strength of 1000 units/ml. *Used for*: pulmonary embolism and deep vein thrombosis. *Dosage*: 15,000 units; children 250 units/kg body weight, both 12 hourly. Both following on from first doses given by intravenous infusion or injection. *Special care*: pregnancy, kidney or liver disease. Drug should be withdrawn gradually if taken for more than 5 days. Platelet counts are required if taken for more than 5 days. *Avoid use*: patients with bleeding disorders, haemophilia, serious hypertension, recent operation on eye or nervous system, cerebral aneurysm, serious liver disease, peptic ulcer, allergy to heparin, thrombocytopenia. *Possible interaction*: aspirin, dipyridamole, glyceryl trinitrate infusion. *Side effects*: allergic reactions, skin necrosis, osteoporosis (if taken long-term). Stop drug immediately if thrombocytopenia occurs. *Manufacturer*: Leo.

PURI-NETHOL

Description: a cytotoxic drug available as scored, fawn-coloured tablets containing 50mg mercaptopurine coded WELLCOME 04A. *Used for*: leukaemia, especially in children. *Dosage*: adults and children, 2.5mg/kg bod yweight each day at first, used for maintenance treatment. *Special care*: pregnancy, kidney disorder. Dosage should be reduced if allopurinol is also being received. *Possible interaction*: allopurinol, warfarin. *Side effects*: vomiting, nausea, bone marrow suppression, anorexia, toxic effects on liver. *Manufacturer*: GlaxoWellcome.

PYOPEN

Description: an antibiotic preparation of penicillin available as powder in vials for reconstitution and injection containing 1g and 5g carbenicillin sodium. *Used for*: endocarditis, meningitis, septicaemia, infected burns and wounds, urinary and respiratory tract infections, sepsis within abdomen, infections following operations. *Dosage*: by rapid infusion, 5g every 4 to 6 hours; children, 250–400mg/kg body weight in divided doses each day. *Special care*: kidney disorders. *Side effects*: gastro-intestinal upset, allergic hypersensitivity reactions, hypokalaemia, change in function of blood platelets. *Manufacturer*: Link.

PYROGASTRONE

Description: a compound preparation combining an antacid and cytoprotectant available as off-white tablets containing 20mg carbenoxolone sodium, 60mg magnesium trisilicate, 600mg alginic acid, 240mg dried aluminium hydroxide, 210mg sodium bicarbonate marked PG and with symbol. Also, **PYROGASTRONE LIQUID** containing 10mg carbenoxolone sodium, 150mg dried aluminium hydroxide/5ml. *Used for*: gastro-oesophageal reflux, oesophagitis. *Dosage*: 1 tablet or 10ml suspension 3 times each day after meals plus 2 tablets or 20ml suspension at bedtime. *Special care*: patients with fluid and salt retention. *Avoid use*: pregnancy, children, elderly, hypokalaemia, liver or kidney failure. *Possible interaction*: diuretics, digoxin. *Side effects*: hypertension, heart failure, hypokalaemia, retention of water and salt. *Manufacturer*: Sanofi Winthrop.

Q

QUESTRAN A

Description: a bile acid sequestrant available as a low sugar powder in sachets containing 4g cholestyramine. Also, **QUESTRAN**, powder in sachets containing 4g cholestyramine. *Used for*: diarrhoea resulting from surgery, radiation, Crohn's disease, damage or disease of vagus nerve, itching resulting from liver disease. Also, prevention of coronary heart disease in men with very high lipid/cholesterol levels in the blood who are aged between 35 and 59. Treatment of type II hyperlipoproteinaemias (high levels of lipid-bound proteins). *Dosage*: diarrhoea and elevated lipid and lipid/protein levels, 1 sachet each day at first gradually increasing to 3 to 6 each day after 3 or 4 weeks, taken as single or divided doses; daily maximum is 9 sachets. Itching, 1 or 2 sachets daily; children over 6 years of age, dose in proportion to that of adult weighing 70kg.

Special care: pregnancy, breast-feeding, dietary supplements of vitamins A, D amd K may be needed with high doses taken long term, patients with phenylketonuria (abnormal presence of phenylketones in urine) taking Questran A. Any other drugs should be taken 1 hour before Questran A or 4 hours afterwards. *Avoid use*: children under 6 years of age, total obstruction of bile duct. *Possible interaction*: antibiotics, digitalis, diuretics. *Side effects*: increased tendency for bleeding in patients taking drug long-term due to deficiency in vitamin K, constipation. *Manufacturer*: Bristol-Myers.

QUINOCORT

Description: a topical preparation combining a mildly potent steroid and antifungal, antibacterial agent available as a cream containing 0.5% potassium hydroxyquinolone sulphate and 1% hydrocortisone. *Used for*: inflammatory, infected skin conditions responsive to steroids. *Dosage*: apply thinly 2 or 3 times each day. *Special care*: thrombophlebitis, psychoses, recent intestinal anastomoses, chronic nephritis, certain cancers, osteoporosis, peptic ulcer, skin eruption/rash related to a disease, viral, fungal or active infections, tuberculosis. Hypertension, glaucoma, epilepsy, acute glomerulonephritis (inflammation of kidney glomerulus), diabetes, cirrhosis, hypothyroidism, pregnancy, stress. To be withdrawn gradually. *Possible interaction*: NSAIDs, oral anticoagulants, phenytoin, ephedrine, phenobarbitone, rifampicin, diuretics, cardiac glycosides, anticholinesterases, hypoglycaemics. *Side effects*: osteoporosis, depression, euphoria, hyperglycaemia, peptic ulcers, Cushingoid changes. *Manufacturer*: Quinoderm.

R

RAPIFEN^{CD}

Description: a narcotic analgesic and controlled drug, alfentanil hydrochloride, available in ampoules containing 500μg/ml. Also **RAPIFEN INTENSIVE CARE** (5mg/ml). *Used for*: analgesia during short operations, enhancement of anaesthesia, suppression of respiration for patients in intensive care receiving assistance with ventilation. *Dosage*: 500μg over 30 seconds to start then 250μg; with assisted ventilation (for adult and child) 30–50μg/kg then 15μg/kg, all by intravenous injection. 50–100μg/kg over 10 minutes by intravenous infusion for adult or child with assisted ventilation. For analgesia and respiratory suppression, 2mg/hour adjusted according to response. *Special care*: myasthenia gravis, elderly, liver disease, pregnancy, respiratory disease. *Avoid use*: respiratory depression, diseases causing obstruction of the airways. *Possible interaction*: erythromycin, anxiolytics and hypnotics, cimetidine, cisapride, antidepressants. *Side* *effects*: respiratory depression, temporary hypotension, nausea, vomiting, brady-cardia. *Manufacturer*: Janssen-Cilag.

RASTINON

Description: a sulphonylurea, tolbutamide, available as white tablets (500mg) marked with symbol and RASTINON 0.5. *Used for*: maturity-onset diabetes. *Dosage*: 2 per day at the start, adjusted depending upon response. Maintenance dose of 1 to 3 per day as a single or divided dose. Not for children. *Special care*: the elderly or patients with kidney failure. *Avoid use*: during pregnancy or lactation; juvenile, growth-onset or unstable brittle diabetes (insulin-dependent diabetes mellitus); ketoacidosis; severe kidney or liver disorders; stress, infections or surgery; endocrine disorders. *Possible interaction*: MAOIs, corticosteroids, ß-blockers, diuretics, corticotrophin (ACTH), oral contraceptives, alcohol. Also aspirin, oral anticoagulants, and the generic drugs bezafibrate, clofibrate, phenylbutazone, cyclophosphamide, rifampicin, sulphonamides and chloramphenicol. Also glucagon. *Side effects*: skin rash and other sensitivity reactions. Other conditions tend to be rare, e.g. hyponatraemia (low blood sodium concentration) or aplastic anaemia. *Manufacturer*: Hoechst.

RAZOXIN

Description: a cytotoxic and antineoplastic drug, razoxone, available as white tablets (125mg), marked ICI. *Used for*: leukaemias. *Dosage*: 150–500mg/m² per day for 3 to 5 days. *Side effects*: nausea, vomiting, bone marrow suppression, hair loss, suppression of the immune system, teratogenic. *Manufacturer*: Zeneca.

RECORMON

Description: recombinant human erythropoietin (hormone-regulating red blood cell production) available as powder in vials (1000, 2000, 5000 units epoetin beta). *Used for*: anaemia in patients with chronic kidney failure and on dialysis. *Dosage*: 20 units/kg 3 times per week for 4 weeks, by subcutaneous injection, or 40 units/kg by intravenous injection with the same frequency. Dose may be doubled depending upon haemoglobin response. May be increased by 20 units/kg at monthly intervals to a maximum of 720 units/kg per week. For maintenance, reduce the dosage to half and adjust weekly. Children over 2 as per adults; not recommended for children under 2. *Special care*: history of epilepsy, thrombocytosis (increase in blood platelet count giving an increased tendency to blood clots), hypertension, chronic liver failure, pregnancy, lactation. May need iron supplements, check haemoglobin, blood pressure, platelet count and serum electrolytes. *Side effects*: symptoms resembling flu, hypertension, clotting in atrio-ventricular fistula. *Manufacturer*: B.M. UKm.

REDEPTIN

Description: an antipsychotic and diphe-nylbutylpiperidine, fluspirilene, available as 2mg/ml in ampoules and 6ml vials. *Used for*: schizophrenia. *Dosage*: starting with 2mg per week by intramuscular injection increasing as necessary by 2mg per week to a maximum of 20mg. Dose for maintenance, 2–8mg per week. Elderly, start with 0.5mg per week and adjust depending upon response. Not for children. *Special care*: lactation, epilepsy, liver or kidney disease, Parkinsonism. *Avoid use*: pregnancy. *Possible interaction*: alcohol, depressants of the CNS, antihypertensives, antidepressants, analgesics, antidiabetics, levodopa, anticonvulsants. *Side effects*: rigidity, tremor, dry mouth, muscle spasms in eye, neck, face and back, tardive dyskinesia (involuntary, repetitive muscle movements in the limbs, face and trunk), tachycardia, constipation, blocked nose, difficulty in urinating, hypotension, weight gain, impotence, galactorrhoea, gynaecomastia, blood changes, jaundice, dermatitis, ECG changes, fatigue, drowsiness, seizures. *Manufacturer*: S.H. & F.

REFOLINON

Description: Folinic acid (as a calcium salt) available as pale yellow tablets (15mg) marked F and CF. *Used for*: megaloblastic anaemia, antidote or rescue after treatment with methotrexate. *Dosage*: 1 tablet daily for anaemia, see literature for antidote use. Also, **REFOLINON INJECTION**, containing 3mg/ml. *Avoid use*: vitamin B_{12} deficiency anaemia. *Manufacturer*: Pharmacia & Upjohn.

REGAINE

Description: a hair restorer, minoxidil, available as a liquid containing 20mg/ml. *Used for*: alopecia. *Dosage*: 1ml applied to the scalp 2 times per day for at least 4 months. Hair loss will recur if treatment ceases. *Special care*: hypotension, broken skin, check blood pressure in susceptible patients. *Side effects*: dermatitis. *Manufacturer*: Upjohn.

RELIFEX

Description: an NSAID and naphthylalkanone, nabumetone, available as red tablets (500mg) marked RELIFEX 500. Also, **RELIFEX SUSPENSION** (500mg/5ml). *Used for*: rheumatoid arthritis and osteoarthritis. *Dosage*: 2 tablets or 10ml as 1 dose at bedtime. An extra 1 to 2 tablets or 5–10ml may be taken in the morning for severe cases. Elderly, 1 to 2 tablets or 5–10ml per day. Not for children. *Special care*: elderly, allergy-induced by aspirin or anti-inflammatory drugs, liver or kidney disease, history of peptic ulcer. *Avoid use*: active peptic ulcer, pregnancy, breast-feeding, severe liver disease. *Possible interaction*: sulphonylurea, hypoglycaemics, hydantoin, oral anticoagulants, anticonvulsants. *Side effects*: nausea, diarrhoea, abdominal pain, dyspepsia, constipation, headache, dizziness, rashes, sedation. *Manufacturer*: Bencard.

REMEDEINE

Description: an analgesic containing 500mg paracetamol, 20mg dihydrocodeine tartrate in white tablets marked PD/20. Also, **REMEDEINE FORTE** containing 500mg paracetamol and 30mg dihydrocodeine tartrate in white tablets marked PD/30. *Used for*: severe pain. *Dosage*: 1 to 2 tablets 4 to 6 hourly up to a daily maximum of 8 tablets. Not for children. *Special care*: chronic liver disease, hypothyroidism, allergies, kidney disease. *Avoid use*: raised intracranial pressure, depression of respiration, diseases causing obstruction of the respiratory tract. *Possible interaction*: alcohol, MAOIs. *Side effects*: nausea, vomiting, drowsiness, headache, vertigo, constipation, retention of urine. *Manufacturer*: Napp.

RESPACAL

Description: a ß$_2$-agonist and bronchodilator, tulobuterol hydrochloride, available as white tablets (2mg) marked ucb. *Used for*: prevention and control of bronchospasm in asthma. *Dosage*: 1 tablet twice per day increasing to 3 times per day if required. Children over 10 years, ^{1}/2 to 1 tablet twice per day. Not for children under 10. Also, **RESPACAL SYRUP**, 1mg per 5ml. *Dosage*: 10ml 2 or 3 times perday. Children over 10 years, 5–10ml; 6 to 10 years, 2.5–5ml both twice per day. Not for children under 6. *Special care*: epilepsy, hypertension, hyperthyroidism, diabetes, disease of the heart and blood vessels. *Avoid use*: acute liver failure or chronic liver disease, kidney failure. *Side effects*: tremor, palpitations, tachycardia, possible serious hypokalaemia. *Manufacturer*: UCB.

RESTANDOL

Description: an androgen, testosterone undecanoate, available as brown, oval gelatin capsules (40mg strength), marked ORG and DV3. *Used for*: osteoporosis caused by androgen deficiency, deficiency in the male of the secretory activity of the testis whether due to castration or other disorder. *Dosage*: starting with 3 to 4 capsules per day for 2 to 3 weeks, adjusting to 1 to 3 depending upon response. *Special care*: epilepsy, hypertension, heart, liver or kidney disease, migraine. *Avoid use*: untreated heart failure, cancer of the liver or prostate, abnormal condition of the kidney (nephrosis/nephrotic syndrome), ischaemic heart disease. *Possible interaction*: drugs that induce liver enzymes. *Side effects*: oedema, weight increase, tumours of the liver, lower fertility, premature epiphyseal closure, extended erection of the penis not associated with sexual arousal. *Manufacturer*: Organon.

RETIN-A

Description: a vitamin A derivative, tretinoin, available as a 0.025% lotion. Also, **RETIN-A GEL** (0.01% and 0.025%), **RETIN-A CREAM** (0.025% and 0.05%). *Used for*: acne vulgaris (common in adolescents) where there are pustules, papules (solid, raised lesion less than 1cm across) and comedones (blackheads). *Dosage*: apply once or twice per day for at least 8 weeks. Not for children. *Special care*: pregnancy, avoid UV light. *Avoid use*: eczema, abrasions, cuts. Do not get on eyes or mucous membranes. *Possible interaction*: keratolytics. *Side effects*: irritation, erythema, alteration to skin pigmentation. *Manufacturer*: Janssen-Cilag.

RETROVIR

Description: an antiviral compound, zidovudine, available as white capsules (100mg) marked 100 and Y9C and white/blue capsules (250mg) marked 250 and H2F. Both bear the company logo and a blue securiband. Also, **RETROVIR SYRUP**, 50mg/5ml, a pale-yellow strawberry-flavoured solution. *Used for*: HIV disease. *Dosage*: adults (asymptomatic) 500–1500mg per day in 4 or 5 divided doses; 6 200mg per day if tolerable for symptomatic HIV. Children over 3 months, 180mg/m² 4 times per day. Not for children under 3 months. *Special care*: blood tests every 2 weeks for the first 3 months, then monthly. Alter dose should there be anaemia or bone marrow suppression. Kidney or liver disease, elderly, pregnancy. *Avoid use*: low neutrophil (white blood cell) counts or low levels of haemoglobin, lactation. *Possible interaction*: analgesics (paracetamol particularly), potentially nephrotoxics or bone marrow suppressives, probenecid, methadone, drugs affecting liver activity. Warn patients about accompanying use of self-administered drugs. *Side effects*: neutropenia, leucopenia, nausea, anaemia, abdominal pain, fever, rash, headache, muscle pain, insomnia, numbness or tingling sensations. *Manufacturer*: Glaxo-Wellcome.

REVANIL

Description: a dopamine agonist, lysuride maleate, available as white tablets (200μg) marked CM in a hexagon. *Used for*: Parkinsonism. *Dosage*: start with 1 tablet at bedtime with food increasing weekly by 1 tablet daily to a maximum of 25 daily. Not for children. *Special care*: pregnancy, tumour of the pituitary. *Avoid use*: weak heart, disturbance of peripheral circulation. *Possible interaction*: dopamine antagonists, psychotropics (affecting behaviour and psychic functions). *Side effects*: nausea, vomiting, hypotension, headache, dizziness, lethargy, drowsiness, abdominal pain, constipation, psychiatric reactions. *Manufacturer*: Roche.

RHEUMOX

Description: a benzotriazine and NSAID, azapropazone dihydrate, available as orange capsules (300mg) marked RHEUMOX and AHR. Also, **RHEUMOX TABLETS** containing 600mg in orange, oblong tablets marked RHEUMOX 600. *Used for*: gout, hyperuricaemia (high blood uric acid), rheumatoid arthritis, osteoarthritis, ankylosing spondylitis. *Dosage*: acute gout, 2.4g in divided doses over 24 hours then 1.8g per day and 1.2g per day; 600mg morning and night for chronic gout. For other conditions, 1.2g per day in 2 or 4 divided doses. Elderly, 300mg morning and night up to a maximum of 900mg per day if kidneys function normally. Not for children. *Special care*: pregnancy, heart failure, elderly, liver or kidney disease (monitor if on long-term treatment), past peptic ulcer. *Avoid use*: kidney disorder, past blood changes, peptic ulcer. *Possible interaction*: sulphonamides, hypoglycaemics, anticoagulants, methotrexate, phenytoin. *Side effects*: oedema, gastro-intestinal bleeding, sensitivity to light, alveolitis (allergic lung reaction to substances inhaled). Discontinue upon a positive Coomb's test (antiglobulin test—an antibody against globulin). *Manufacturer*: Wyeth.

RHINOCORT

Description: a corticosteroid, budesonide, available as a metered dose (50μg) nasal aerosol. *Used for*: rhinitis. *Dosage*: apply twice to each nostril twice per day, reducing to 1 application twice daily. Not recommended for long-term continuous treatment for children. Also, **RHINOCORT AQUA**, a 100μg metered pump nasal spray. *Dosage*: start with 2 applications in each nostril every morning; 1 application for maintenance. Not for children. *Special care*: pregnancy, infections of a fungal, viral or tuberculous nature. *Side effects*: sneezing. *Manufacturer*: Astra.

RHINOLAST

Description: an antihistamine, azelastine hydrochloride, available as a 0.1% metered dose nasal spray. *Used for*: rhinitis. *Dosage*: 1 application per nostril twice per day. Not for children. *Special care*: pregnancy, breast-feeding. *Side effects*: nasal irritation, effect on taste. *Manufacturer*: Asta Medica.

RIDAURA

Description: a gold salt, auranofin, available as pale yellow square tablets (3mg). *Used for*: progressive rheumatoid arthritis not controlled by NSAIDs. *Dosage*: start with 6mg per day and continue for 3 to 6 months minimum. Dosage can be increased to 3mg 3 times per day if response is inadequate. Cease after a further 3 months if response still inadequate. Not for children. *Special care*: kidney and liver disorders, rash, past bone marrow depression, bowel inflammation. Blood and urinary protein should be monitored before and during treatment. Women should use effective contraception during and 6 months after treatment. *Avoid use*: past necrotizing enterocolitis (an acute inflammatory bowel disorder affecting large and small intestines), exfoliative dermatitis, severe blood disorders, kidney disease, severe liver disease, SLE, pregnancy, breast-feeding, pulmonary fibrosis. *Side effects*: nausea, abdominal pain, diarrhoea, rashes, itching, hair loss, ulcerative enterocolitis, inflammation of the mouth (stomatitis), conjunctivitis, nephrotic syndrome (oedema, low protein in the urine and low blood albumin levels), upset to taste. *Manufacturer*: Yamanouchi.

RIFADIN

Description: an antibiotic and antimalarial, rifampicin, available as blue/red capsules (150mg) and red capsules (300mg), marked LEPETIT. Also, **RIFADIN SYRUP** (100mg/5ml) and **RIFADIN INFUSION** as 600mg powder in a vial with 10ml solvent in an ampoule. *Used for*: prevention of meningococcal meningitis, treatment of carriers of *Haemophilus influenzae*, additional therapy for brucellosis, Legionnaire's disease and serious staphylococcal infections, tuberculosis and mycobacterial infections, leprosy. *Dosage*: meningitis—600g twice per day for 2 days; influenza—20mg/kg per day for 4 days; brucellosis—600-1200mg per day as 2 to 4 doses; tuberculosis—8-12mg/kg per day thirty minutes before or 2 hours after a meal; leprosy—600mg once per month or 10mg/kg per day. Children: meningitis—1 to 12 years, 10mg/kg twice per day for 2 days; 3 months to 1 year, 5mg/kg, not for children under 3 months; influenza—20mg/kg daily for 4 days, infants up to 1 month 10mg/kg daily for 4 days; tuberculosis—10-30mg/kg per day to a daily maximum of 600mg; leprosy—as adult dose. *Special care*: pregnancy, breast-feeding, liver disease, elderly, poorly nourished or the very young. *Avoid use*: jaundice. *Possible interaction*: digitalis, hypoglycaemics, cyclosporin, corticosteroids, anticoagulants, oral contraceptives, dapsone, quinidine, phenytoin, narcotics. *Side effects*: rashes, gastro-intestinal upset, flu-like symptoms, upset liver function, orange discolouration of urine and secretions. *Manufacturer*: Hoechst.

RIFATER

Description: a compound drug containing 50mg isoniazid, 300mg pyrazinamide and 120mg rifampicin in pink-beige tablets. *Used for*: pulmonary tuberculosis in the initial intensive phase. *Dosage*: a single dose thirty minutes before or 2 hours after a meal—over 65kg, 6 tablets per day; 50–64kg, 5 tablets; 40–49kg, 4 tablets; under 40 kg, 3 tablets per day, to continue for 2 months followed by rifampicin/isoniazid compound. For the initial period, the additional use of ethambutol or streptomycin is advised. For children contact the manufacturer. *Special care*: history of epilepsy, gout, liver disease, haemoptysis (coughing up blood). *Avoid use*: jaundice. *Possible interaction*: digitalis, hypoglycaemics, cyclosporin, corticosteroids, anticoagulants, oral contraceptives, dapsone, quinidine, phenytoin, narcotics. *Side effects*: rashes, gastro-intestinal upset, flu-like symptoms, upset liver function, orange discolouration of urine and secretions. *Manufacturer*: Hoechst.

RIFINAH

Description: a combination of rifampicin (150mg) and isoniazid (100mg) in pink tablets marked RH150 and also orange tablets, coded RH300 containing 300mg rifampicin and 150mg isoniazid. *Used for*: tuberculosis. *Dosage*: 2 Rifinah 300 daily if over 50kg; 3 Rifinah 150 daily if under 50kg, as a single dose thirty minutes before or 2 hours after a meal. Not for children. *Special care*: pregnancy, lactation, undernourished, elderly, liver disease (monitor). *Avoid use*: jaundice. *Possible interaction*: digitalis, hypoglycaemics, cyclosporin, corticosteroids, anticoagulants, oral contraceptives, dapsone, quinidine, phenytoin, narcotics. *Side effects*: rashes, gastro-intestinal upset, flu-like symptoms, upset liver function, orange discolouration of urine and secretions. *Manufacturer*: Hoechst.

RIMACTANE

Description: a rifamycin, rifampicin, available in red capsules coded JZ 150 (150mg) and red/brown capsules coded CS 300 (300mg), both also marked CG. Also, **RIMACTANE SYRUP** (100mg/5ml). *Used for*: prevention of meningococcal meningitis, additional treatment in tuberculosis and certain mycobacterial infections. *Dosage*: (meningitis) 600mg twice per day for 2 days; children 1 to 12 years 10mg/kg; up to 1 year, 5mg/kg both twice per day for 2 days. For tuberculosis etc., 450–600mg thirty minutes before breakfast; children up to 20mg/kg per day to a maximum single dose of 600mg. Also, **RIMACTANE INFUSION** as 300mg rifampicin powder in a vial. *Special care*: porphyria, pregnancy, breast-feeding, liver disease (monitor), elderly, poorly nourished or the very young. *Avoid use*: jaundice. *Possible interaction*: corticosteroids, digitalis, anticoagulants, hypoglycaemics, cyclosporin, oral contraceptives, phenytoin, quinidine, antacids, dapsone, anticholinergics, opiates. *Side effects*: rashes, gastro-intestinal upset, flu-like symptoms, upset liver function, discolouration of urine and secretions. *Manufacturer*: Ciba.

RIMACTAZID

Description: a combination of rifampicin and isoniazid in pink tablets '150' marked EI and CG (150mg/100mg respectively) and orange oblong tablets '300' marked DH and CG (300mg/150mg respectively). *Used for*: tuberculosis. *Dosage*: 2 300 tablets per day before breakfast (for over 50kg) or 3 150 tablets per day (for under 50kg). Not for children. *Special care*: porphyria, elderly, epilepsy, pregnancy, lactation, liver disease (monitor). *Avoid use*: acute liver disease, neuritis (peripheral), past drug-induced hepatitis. *Possible interaction*: anticoagulants, anticholinergics, corticosteroids, antacids, digitalis, hypoglycaemics, cyclosporin, oral contraceptives, phenytoin, dapsone, narcotics, quinidine, disulfiram. *Side effects*: rashes, gastro-intestinal upset, flu-like symptoms, upset liver function, discoloration of urine and secretions. *Manufacturer*: Ciba.

RIMSO-50

Description: a bladder irrigator, dimethyl sulphoxide (50%, sterile solution). *Used for*: relief of interstitial cystitis. *Dosage*: see literature. *Special care*: malignancy of the urinary tract. Check liver and kidney function and eyes regularly. *Side effects*: hypersensitivity reactions because of histamine release. *Manufacturer*: Britannia.

RINATEC

Description: an anticholinergic nasal spray, ipratropium bromide, in 20µg metered dose spray. *Used for*: rhinorrhoea (runny nose) associated with perennial rhinitis. *Dosage*: 1 or 2 sprays in the nostrils up to 4 times per day. Not for children. *Special care*: enlarged prostate, glaucoma. *Side effects*: irritation, nasal dryness. *Manufacturer*: Boehringer Ingelheim.

RISPERDAL

Description: an antipsychotic and benzisoxazole derivative, risperidone available as 1mg white (Ris/1), 2mg orange (Ris/2), 3mg yellow (Ris/3) and 4mg green oblong tablets (Ris/4), all marked Janssen. *Used for*: schizophrenia and other psychoses. *Dosage*: (over 15 years) 1mg on first day, 2mg on second day, 3mg on third day, all twice per day. Maximum 8mg twice per day. Elderly, start with 0.5mg, increasing by 0.5mg to 1–2mg twice daily. Not for children. *Special care*: epilepsy, elderly, disease of kidney, liver or heart and blood vessels, Parkinsonism, pregnancy, breast-feeding. If driving or operating machine. Cease if signs of tardive dyskinesia. *Possible interaction*: levodopa, dopamine agonists, drugs acting centrally. *Side effects*: hypotension when standing, tachycardia, galactorrhoea, sexual disorders, extrapyramidal symptoms, anxiety, insomnia, headache, fatigue, dizziness, weight gain, gastro-intestinal upset, rash, rhinitis, blurred vision, poor concentration. *Manufacturer*: Janssen/Organon.

RIVOTRIL

Description: an anticonvulsant and benzodiazepine, clonazepam, available as beige tablets (0.5mg) and white tablets (2mg) marked RIV and with tablet strength. *Used for*: epilepsy. *Dosage*: start with maximum daily dose of 1mg increasing to maintenance of 4–8mg per day. Elderly, 0.5mg daily maximum initially. Children: 5 to 12 years, 0.5mg maximum per day initially rising to maintenance of 3–6mg per day; 1 to 5 years, 0.25mg, and 1–3mg (same criteria); up to 1 year, 0.25mg and 0.5–1mg (same criteria). Gradually increase all to maintenance dose. Also, **RIVOTRIL INJECTION**, 1mg in solvent in ampoules (with diluent). *Used for*: status epilepticus (continual seizures producing brain damage unless halted). *Dosage*: 1mg by slow intravenous injection. Children, 0.5mg by same means, but see literature. *Special care*: chronic lung insufficiency, chronic liver or kidney disease, the elderly, pregnant, during labour or lactation. Judgement and dexterity may be affected, long-term use is to be avoided. To be withdrawn gradually. *Avoid use*: acute lung insufficiency, depression of respiration (except in cases of acute muscle spasms). Also when treating anxiety, obsessional states or chronic psychosis. *Possible interaction*: alcohol and other depressants of the central nervous system, anticonvulsants. *Side effects*: vertigo, gastro-intestinal upsets, confusion, ataxia, drowsiness, light-headedness, hypotension, disturbance of vision, skin rashes. Also urine retention, changes in libido. Dependence a potential problem. *Manufacturer*: Roche.

RO-A-VIT

Description: Vitamin A as 50,000 units per ml in an aqueous solution (in ampoules). *Used for*: vitamin A deficiency. *Dosage*: ½ to 1 ampoule by deep intramuscular injection, weekly or monthly. *Special care*: do not mix with other vitamin injections, liver disease. Monitor. *Side effects*: possible hypervitaminosis (toxic effects of excessive doses) in children and infants. *Manufacturer*: Cambridge.

ROACCUTANE

Description: a vitamin A derivative, isotretinoin, available in red/white gelatin capsules (5 and 20mg) marked with R and strength. *Used for*: acne, especially severe forms unresponsive to antibiotics. *Dosage*: start with 0.5mg/kg with food for 4 weeks adjusting depending upon response within the range 0.1–1.0mg/kg for an additional 8 to 12 weeks. Not normally repeated. Not for children. *Special care*: (hospital use only) exclude pregnancy, effective contraception necessary 1 month before and up to 4 weeks after treatment. Check liver function and blood lipids regularly. *Avoid use*: pregnancy, breast-feeding, liver or kidney disease. *Possible interaction*: high doses of vitamin A. *Side effects*: hair loss, dryness, mucosal erosion, nausea, headache, drowsiness, sweating, seizures, menstrual disorders, mood changes, rise in liver enzymes; sometimes hearing loss, thrombo-cytopenia. *Manufacturer*: Roche.

ROBAXIN

Description: a carbamate and muscle relaxant, methocarbamol, available as white, oblong tablets marked AHR (750mg strength). *Used for*: skeletal muscle spasm. *Dosage*: 2 tablets 4 times per day. Elderly—1 tablet 4 times per day. Not for children. Also, **ROBAXIN INJECTABLE** (100mg/ml in ampoules). *Special care*: liver or kidney disease, pregnancy, breast-feeding. *Avoid use*: coma, brain damage, myasthenia gravis, epilepsy. *Possible interaction*: depressants and stimulants of the CNS, alcohol, anticholinergics. *Side effects*: allergies, drowsiness. *Manufacturer*: Shire.

ROBAXISAL FORTE

Description: a carbamate and salicylate and muscle relaxant comprising 400mg methocarbamol and 325g aspirin in pink/white, two-layered tablets marked AHR. *Used for*: skeletal muscle spasms. *Dosage*: 2 tablets (elderly 1) 4 times daily. Not for children. *Special care*: pregnancy, breast-feeding, liver or kidney disease, past bronchospasm, allergy to anti-inflammatory drugs. *Avoid use*: brain damage, coma, myasthenia gravis, peptic ulcer, epilepsy, haemophilia. *Possible interaction*: anticholinergics, alcohol, stimulants and depressants of the CNS, hypoglycaemics, hydantoins, anticoagulants. *Side effects*: gastro-intestinal bleeding, allergies, drowsiness. *Manufacturer*: Shire.

ROBINUL

Description: an anticholinergic, glyco-pyrronium bromide, available as ampoules containing 0.2mg/ml. Also, **ROBINUL NEOSTIGMINE** which contains 0.5mg glycopyrronium bromide and 2.5mg/ml neostigmine methysulphate in ampoules. *Used for*: reduction of secretions during anaesthesia. *Dosage*: for premedication 200–400µg Robinul by intramuscular or intravenous injection (child: 4–8µg/kg to a maximum of 200µg). Robinul neostigmine: 1–2ml (child 0.02ml) by intravenous injection over 10 to thirty seconds. *Special care*: cardiovascular disease, atropine should be given, asthma, epilepsy, peptic ulcer, pregnancy, breast-feeding, hypotension, Parkinsonism, bradycardia, recent myocardial infarction. *Possible interaction*: cisapride, antihistamines, nefopam, disopyramide, TCADs, MAOIs, phenothiazines, amantadine. *Side effects*: nausea, vomiting, diarrhoea, abdominal cramps, tachycardia. *Manufacturer*: Anpharm.

ROCALTROL

Description: a vitamin D analogue, calcitriol, available as capsules containing 0.25µg (red/white) and 0.5µg (red). *Used for*: in cases of renal osteodystrophy (bone development defect due to kidney disorder affecting calcium and phosphorus metabolism). *Dosage*: 1–2µg per day increasing if required to 2–3µg by 0.25–0.5µg increments. Not for children. *Special care*: pregnancy, do not use other vitamin D preparations. Check serum calcium levels. *Avoid use*: hypercalcaemia metastatic calcification (due to spread of malignancy). *Side effects*: hypercalciuria (calcium in urine), hypercalcaemia. *Manufacturer*: Roche.

ROCEPHIN

Description: a cephalosporin, ceftriaxone, available as a powder in vials (250mg, 1g and 2g). *Used for*: meningitis, pneumonia, septicaemia. Infections of bone, skin and soft tissue. Gonorrhoea, preventitive for operations, infections in patients with neutropenia. *Dosage*: 1g per day by deep intramuscular injection, slow intravenous injection or infusion. 2–4g as 1 dose, per day, for severe infections. Gonorrhoea—250mg intramuscularly; preventitive—1g intra-muscularly or slow intravenous injection; also colorectal surgery—2g intramuscularly or by slow intravenous injection or infusion. Children (over 6 weeks only): 20–50mg/kg daily by the same means, up to 80mg/kg for severe infections. *Special care*: severe liver or kidney disease, hypersensitivity to ß-lactam. *Avoid use*: pregnancy. *Side effects*: primarily skin infections, blood changes, gastro-intestinal upset. *Manufacturer*: Roche.

ROFERON-A

Description: an interferon, interferon alfa-2a, available in vials of 3, 4.5 and 18 million units, with syringe, needles and water for injection. *Used for*: AIDS-related Kaposi's sarcoma, some leukaemias, T-cell lymphoma, hepatitis B, renal cell carcinoma. *Dosage*: by subcutaneous and intramuscular injection. See literature. *Avoid use*: pregnancy. *Possible interaction*: theophylline. *Side effects*: (dose-related) depression, flu-like symptoms, bone marrow suppression, hypo- and hypertension, arrhythmia, rash, seizures; rarely, coma. *Manufacturer*: Roche.

ROGITINE

Description: an alpha-blocker and antihypertensive, phentolamine mesylate, in ampoules of 10mg/ml. *Used for*: hypertension associated with phaeochromocytoma. *Dosage*: 2–5mg by intravenous injection, repeated if required. Children: 1mg. *Special care*: asthma, gastritis, kidney disorder, peptic ulcer. Elderly, pregnancy, lactation. Monitor blood. *Avoid use*: hypotension, weak heart, myocardial infarction, hypersensitivity to sulphites, disease of coronary arteries. *Possible interaction*: antihypertensives, antipsychotics. *Side effects*: weakness, dizziness, tachycardia, hypotension, flushes, blocked nose, gastro-intestinal upset. *Manufacturer*: Ciba.

ROHYPNOL

Description: an hypnotic and intermediate-acting benzodiazepine, flunitrazepam, in diamond-shaped purple tablets (1mg) marked ROHYPNOL. *Used for*: short-term treatment of severe or disabling insomnia, to induce sleep at unusual times. *Dosage*: ½ to 1 tablet at bedtime (elderly, ½ tablet). Not for children. *Special care*: chronic liver or kidney disease, chronic lung disease, pregnancy, labour, lactation, elderly. May impair judgement. Withdraw gradually and avoid prolonged use. *Avoid use*: depression of respiration, acute lung disease; psychotic, phobic or obsessional states. *Possible interaction*: anticonvulsants, depressants of the CNS, alcohol. *Side effects*: ataxia, confusion, light-headedness, drowsiness, hypotension, gastro-intestinal upsets, disturbances in vision and libido, skin rashes, retention of urine, vertigo. Sometimes jaundice or blood disorders. *Manufacturer*: Roche.

ROWACHOL

Description: Essential oils comprising 32mg menthol, 17mg a and ß-pinenes, 6mg menthone, 5mg camphene, 5mg borneol and 2mg cineole in green, spherical, soft, gelatin capsules. *Used for*: additional treatment for disposal of stones in the common bile duct (with chenodeoxycholic acid). *Dosage*: start with 1 capsule 3 times per day, increasing to 1 to 2 capsules 3 times per day, before meals. Not for children. *Possible interaction*: oral contraceptives, oral anticoagulants. *Manufacturer*: Rowa.

ROWATINEX

Description: Essential oils comprising 31mg a and ß pinenes, 15mg camphene, 10mg borneol, 4mg anethol, 4mg fenchone, 3mg cineole in yellow, spherical, soft, gelatin capsules. *Used for*: stones in the urinary tract or kidney, mild urinary tract infections. *Dosage*: 1 capsule 3 or 4 times per day before meals. Not for children. *Possible interaction*: oral contraceptives, oral anticoagulants. *Manufacturer*: Rowa.

RUBAVAX

Description: a live attenuated virus, Rubella vaccine, with 25µg neomycin per dose, as powder in vial with syringe of diluent (0.5ml). *Used for*: immunization of girls aged 10 to 14 and women (not pregnant) who are seronegative. *Dosage*: 0.5ml by deep subcutaneous or intramuscular injection. Not for children under 10. *Avoid use*: pregnancy, or pregnancy within 3 months of injection, acute infections. *Possible interaction*: live vaccines, immunoglobulin, transfusions of blood or plasma. *Side effects*: rash, joint pain, sore throat, fever, malaise, disorder of the lymph system. *Manufacturer*: Pasteur Merieux MSD.

RYTHMODAN

Description: a class I antiarrhythmic, disopyramide, available as green/beige capsules (100mg) marked RY RL. *Used for*: disturbance in heart beat. *Dosage*: 300–800mg per day in divided doses. Not for children. Also, **RYTHMODAN RETARD**, 250mg disopyramide phosphate in white, sustained-release tablets marked RY and R with symbol. *Dosage*: 1–1½ tablets twice per day. Not for children. Also, **RYTHMODAN INJECTION**, 10mg/ml in ampoules. *Special care*: 1st degree atrioventricular block (slowed conduction or stopped heart impulse), heart, liver or kidney failure, enlarged prostate, urine retention, hyperkalaemia, glaucoma. *Avoid use*: 2nd or 3rd degree atrioventricular block, severe heart failure. *Possible interaction*: ß-blockers, anticholinergics, diuretics, other class I antiarrhythmics, erythromycin. *Side effects*: anticholinergic effects, sometimes jaundice, hypoglycaemia, psychosis. *Manufacturer*: Roussel.

S

SABRIL

Description: an anticonvulsant preparation which is an analogue of a gamma-aminobutyric acid available as oval, white, scored tablets containing 500mg vigabatrin. Also, **SABRIL SACHET** containing 500mg vigabatrin as powder. *Used for*: control of epilepsy which has not responded to other drugs. *Dosage*: 2g each day as single or divided doses, at first along with any other drug being taken. Then dose altered according to response with a maximum of 4g daily. Children, 40mg/kg body weight each day at first increasing, if needed, to a maximum of 80–100mg/kg. *Special care*: elderly, kidney disorders, history of psychiatric illness or behavioural problems. Neurological function should be monitored during the course of treatment. Withdraw drug gradually. *Avoid use*: pregnancy, breast-feeding. *Possible interaction*: other anti-epileptic drugs. *Side effects*: behavioural disturbances, irritability, aggression, dizziness, sleepiness, fatigue, disturbance of vision and memory, nervousness. Children may show agitated behaviour. Patients with a certain type of convulsion (myoclonic) may experience an increase in frequency. *Manufacturer*: Hoechst.

SAIZEN

Description: a preparation of growth hormone as powder in vials containing 4 units and 10 units somatropin for reconstitution and injection. *Used for*: failure of growth in children due to deficiency in growth hormone. Turner syndrome. *Dosage*: children, deficiency of growth hormone, 0.07–0.08 units/kg body weight each day by intramuscular or subcutaneous injection. Or, 0.2 units/kg 3 times each week. Turner syndrome, 0.09–0.1 units/kg each day at first then 0.11–0.14 units/kg if needed. *Special care*: diabetes, lesion on the brain, deficiency in ACTH (adrenocorticotrophic hormone). Thyroid function should be monitored. *Avoid use*: Girls who are pregnant or breast-feeding, children with fusion of epiphyses or tumour. *Side effects*: pain at site of injection, breakdown of fat beneath skin at injection site, oedema, hypothyroidism. *Manufacturer*: Serono.

SALAMOL

Description: a preparation which is a bronchodilator and selective β_2-agonist available as a metered dose aerosol delivering 100μg salbutamol per dose. Also, **SALAMOL STERI-NEB** available as a preservative-free solution for nebulization containing 2.5mg and 5mg salbutamol as sulphate/2.5ml, as single dose units. *Used for*: Salamol, bronchospasm as in bronchitis, emphysema and asthma. Salamol Steri-Neb, severe bronchospasm and acute severe asthma which has failed to respond to other drugs. *Dosage*: Salamol, adults, for attack,

1 or 2 puffs; prevention, 2 puffs 3 to 4 times each day. Salamol Steri-Neb, 2.5mg nebulized 3 or 4 times each day increasing to 5mg if needed. Children, Salamol, half adult dose. *Special care*: pregnancy, weak heart, heart arrhythmias, angina, hypertension, hyperthyroidism. *Possible interaction*: ß-blockers, sympathomimetics. *Side effects*: headache, dilation of peripheral blood vessels, tremor, hypokalaemia. *Manufacturer*: Baker Norton.

SALAZOPYRIN

Description: a colorectal NSAID which is a salicylate and sulphonamide, available as scored, yellow tablets containing 500mg sulphasalazine marked with logo. Also, **SALAZOPYRIN EN-TABS**, enteric-coated yellow tablets (500mg) marked with logo. **SALAZOPYRIN SUSPENSION**, fruit-flavoured containing 250mg/5ml. **SALAZOPYRIN ENEMA** containing 3g; **SALAZOPYRIN SUPPOSITORIES** containing 500mg. *Used for*: ulcerative colitis (inflammation of colon), Crohn's disease. Salazopyrin En-Tabs, rheumatoid arthritis which has not responded to other NSAIDs. *Dosage*: oral preparations, for ulcerative colitis and Crohn's disease, 2 to 4 tablets or 20–40ml 4 times each day with a maintenance dose of 4 tablets or 40ml in divided doses daily. Enema, 1 at night; suppositories, 2 in the morning and after passing stool in addition to oral dose. Rheumatoid arthritis, 1 En-Tab daily for 1 week increasing over 6 weeks to 6 each day in divided doses. Children, over 2 years of age, oral preparations, 40–60mg/kg body weight each day with a maintenance dose of 20–30mg/kg daily. Suppositories, a reduced dose in proportion to that for 70kg adult. *Special care*: patients with allergies, liver or kidney disorders. Any ill effects should be reported and patients should receive regular checks of liver function and blood. *Avoid use*: children under 2 years. *Possible interaction*: rash, nausea, fever, headache, appetite loss, gastro-intestinal disturbance. Effects on CNS and kidneys, blood changes, allergic hypersensitivity reactions. Reduced production of, and presence of abnormal spermatozoa in males. *Manufacturer*: Pharmacia & Upjohn.

SALBULIN

Description: a bronchodilator which is a selective β_2-agonist available as a metered dose aerosol delivering 100µg salbutamol/dose. *Used for*: bronchospasm in bronchitis, emphysema, asthma. *Dosage*: adults, attack, 1 or 2 puffs; prevention, 2 puffs 3 or 4 times each day. Children, half adult dose. *Special care*: pregnancy, hyperthyroidism. *Possible interaction*: ß-blockers, sympathomimetics. *Side effects*: headache, dilation of peripheral blood vessels, nervousness, tremor. *Manufacturer*: 3M Health Care.

SALOFALK

Description: a colorectal preparation and salicylate available as oval, yellow, enteric-coated tablets containing 250mg mesalazine. *Used for*: ulcerative colitis, maintenance treatment. Dosage: adults, for active condition, 6 tablets each day in 3 divided doses. Maintenance treatment, 3 to 6 tablets each day in divided doses. *Special care*: pregnancy, kidney disorder. *Avoid use*: children, blood clotting disorders, serious liver or kidney disease, allergy to salicylates, peptic ulcer. *Possible interaction*: preparations that make the stools more acid, lactulose. *Side effects*: allergic hypersensitivity responses, increased haemoglobin levels. *Manufacturer*: Thames.

SALURIC

Description: a thiazide diuretic available as scored, white tablets containing 500mg chlorothiazide marked MSD 432. *Used for*: hypertension, oedema. *Dosage*: hypertension, half to 1 tablet in single or divided doses each day with a maximum of 2 tablets. Oedema, ½ to 2 tablets once or twice each day or on days when required, with a maximum of 4 daily. Children, age under 6 months, 35mg/kg body weight each day; 6 months to 2 years, 125–375mg each day. 2 to 12 years, 375mg–1g each day. All in 2 divided doses. *Special care*: elderly, pregnancy, breast-feeding, gout, liver or kidney disorders, SLE, liver cirrhosis, diabetes. Glucose, electrolyte and fluid levels should be monitored during the course of treatment. *Avoid use*: hypercalcaemia, allergy to sulphonamides, serious liver or kidney failure. Addison's disease. *Possible interaction*: NSAIDs, lithium opioids, corticosteroids, alcohol cardiac glycosides, barbiturates, tubocurarine, carbenoxolone, antidiabetic drugs. *Side effects*: gastro-intestinal upset, dizziness, disturbance of metabolism and electrolyte balance, blood changes, pancreatitis, impotence, anorexia. *Manufacturer*: M.S.D.

SANDIMMUN

Description: a fungal metabolite immunosuppressant available as a yellow, sugar-free, oily solution containing 100mg cyclosporin/ml. Also, **SANDIMMUN CAPSULES** available in 3 strengths, oval, light pink 25mg; oblong, yellow, 50mg; and oblong, deep pink, 100mg all containing cyclosporin. **SANDIMMUN INTRAVENOUS INFUSION** available in ampoules containing 50mg/ml. *Used for*: serious rheumatoid arthritis which has not responded to other drugs, suppression of immune system in patients undergoing bone marrow or organ transplants, prevention and treatment of graft-versus-host disease. Serious atopic dermatitis and psoriasis which has not responded to other drugs or where these are not considered to be suitable. *Dosage*: 1.25–5mg/kg body weight per day depending upon condition. See literature. *Special care*: pregnancy, breast-feeding, hyperkalaemia, herpes, hyperuricaemia (raised levels of uric acid in blood). Treatment must be given in specialist unit and close monitoring of blood potassium levels, blood pressure, liver and kidney function is required before and during treatment. Avoid sunbathing. *Avoid use*: malignant diseases (except of skin), kidney disorders, uncontrolled infections or hypertension. *Possible interaction*: barbiturates, systemic antibiotics, rifampicin, live vaccines, ketoconazole, erythromycin, phenytoin, carbamazepine, itraconazole, fluconazole, ACE inhibitors, oral contraceptives, calcium antagonists, certain enzyme inhibitors, colchicine, drugs with toxic effects on kidneys. Potassium supplements and potassium-sparing diuretics, prednisolone, lipid solutions, methyl prednisolone, NSAIDs, propafenone. *Side effects*: weakness, tiredness, muscle cramps, burning sensation in feet and hands, tremor, gastro-intestinal upset. Rarely, other blood changes, headache, weight gain, oedema, rash, fits, colitis, pancreatitis. Also, hyperkalaemia, rise in uric acid levels in blood, damage to nerves, effects on menstruation, enlargement of breasts. If uncontrolled hypertension or liver and kidney disorders occur, drug should be withdrawn. *Manufacturer*: Sandoz.

SANDOGLOBULIN

Description: a freeze-dried preparation of human normal immunoglobulin available with diluent for intravenous infusion. *Used for*: globulin deficiencies in newborn babies, thrombocytopenic purpura (a bleeding disorder). *Dosage*: deficiency, 0.1–0.3g/kg body weight every 2 to 4 weeks. Thrombocytopenic purpura, 0.4g/kg each day for 5 days. Then maintenance dose of same order when needed. *Special care*: during infusion, patients must be monitored for signs of anaphylaxis. *Avoid use*: patients with selective immunoglobulin A deficiency who have antibodies to Ig A and who are sensitized. *Possible interaction*: live viral vaccines. *Side effects*: allergic anaphylactoid-type reactions, inflammatory responses which may be delayed. *Manufacturer*: Sandoz.

SANDOSTATIN

Description: a sandostatin analogue available as a solution in ampoules for injection at strengths of 0.05mg, 0.1mg and 0.5mg/ml and 1mg/5ml multi-dose vial, all containing octreotide (as acetate). *Used for*: short-term treatment of acromegaly (abnormal enlargement of face, hands and feet due to excess secretion of growth hormone by a pituitary gland tumour), before surgery or X-ray therapy. Relief of symptoms of certain tumours of the gastro-intestinal tract and pancreas, and carcinoid tumours which release hormones. *Dosage*: acromegaly, 0.1–0.2mg 3 times each day. Tumours, 0.05mg once or twice each day increasing to 0.2mg 3 times daily if needed. Carcinoid tumours, stop drug if no improvement after 1 week. *Special care*: diabetes. Those taking drug long-term require monitoring of thyroid function and for development of gallstones. *Avoid use*: pregnancy, breast-feeding. *Possible interaction*: cimetidine, cyclosporin. *Side effects*: pain, swelling and soreness at injection site, pain in abdomen, vomiting, diarrhoea, steatorrhoea (increased amount of fat in faeces which are pale, frothy and foul-smelling), anorexia, gallstones. *Manufacturer*: Sandoz.

SANOMIGRAN

Description: a serotonin antagonist available as sugar-coated, ivory-coloured tablets containing 0.5mg and 1.5mg pizotifen (as hydrogen maleate), marked SMG and SMG 1.5 respectively. Also, **SANOMIGRAN ELIXIR** containing 0.25mg/5ml as a sugar-free solution. *Used for*: prevention of migraine. *Dosage*: 1.5mg each day in 3 divided doses or 1 dose at night. Dosage may be increased to a maximum of 4.5mg each day if needed with up to 3mg as a maximum single dose. Children, up to 1.5mg each day in divided doses or 1mg as a single night time dose. *Special care*: urine retention, glaucoma. *Side effects*: gain in weight, sleepiness. *Manufacturer*: Sandoz.

SAVENTRINE

Description: a heart stimulant and ß-agonist available as mottled white tablets containing 30mg isoprenaline hydrochloride marked with a P inside a hexagon shape. Also, **SAVENTRINE I.V.** available as a solution in ampoules for injection containing 1mg/ml. *Used for*: heart block, severe bradycardia, Stokes Adams attacks. *Dosage*: tablets (rarely used) 30mg every 6 hours with usual dose in the order of 90–840mg each day. Infusion, 0.5–10μg/minute. *Special care*: diabetes or hypertension. *Avoid use*: hyperthyroidism, serious heart disease, tachycardia, ventricular fibrillation, cardiac asthma. *Side effects*: headache, tremor, sweating, diarrhoea, palpitations. *Manufacturer*: Pharmax.

SCHERING PC4

Description: an oestrogen/progestogen preparation available as sugar-coated white tablets containing 50μg ethinyloestradiol and 0.5mg norgestrel. *Used for*: emergency and contraception (the "morning-after" pill) to be taken within 72 hours of unprotected sexual intercourse. *Dosage*: 2 tablets taken as soon as possible after intercourse followed, 12 hours later, by another 2 tablets. *Special care*: porphyria, gallstones, liver disorders, heart, kidney, circulatory diseases, diabetes, epilepsy, hypertension, history of severe depression. If patient still becomes pregnant, monitoring required to ensure pregnancy is not ectopic. Intercourse should be avoided for the remainder of the cycle. *Avoid use*: patients with overdue menstrual period, those not within 72 hours of unprotected intercourse. *Possible interaction*: barbiturates, chlorpromazine, rifampicin, chloral hydrate, glutethimide, tetracyclines, dichloralphenazone, griseofulvin, ethosuximide, phenytoin, carbamazepine, primidone. *Side effects*: vomiting (reduces drug's effect) and nausea. Period normally starts later than expected, following treatment. *Manufacturer*: Schering H.C.

SCHERIPROCT

Description: a combined steroid and local anaesthetic preparation available as an ointment containing 0.19% prednisolone hexanoate and 0.5% cinchocaine hydrochloride. Also, **SCHERIPROCT SUPPOSITORIES** containing 1.3mg prednisolone hexanoate and 1mg cinchocaine hydrochloride. *Used for*: anal fissure, haemorrhoids, proctitis (inflammation of rectum), anal itching. *Dosage*: apply ointment 2, 3 or 4 times each day; insert 1 suppository 1, 2 or 3 times each day after passing stool. *Special care*: pregnant women, short-term use only. *Avoid use*: patients with tuberculous, viral or fungal infections. *Side effects*: systemic corticosteroid side effects. *Manufacturer*: Schering H.C.

SCOLINE

Description: a depolarizing muscle relaxant of short-lived duration available as a solution in ampoules for injection containing 50mg suxamethonium chloride/ml. *Used for*: paralysis following induction of anaesthesia usually to allow tracheal tube to be inserted. Has duration of action lasting 5 minutes and repeated doses may be given to allow longer-lasting procedures to be carried out. *Special care*: with unusual or low concentration of pseudocholinesterase enzymes in whom more prolonged paralysis may occur. Dual block involving longer-lasting paralysis may develop after repeated doses of suxamethonium. *Avoid use*: liver disease or burns. *Possible interaction*: digoxin, ecothiopate, demacarium, eyedrops, neostigmine, pyndostigmine, thiotepa, cyclophoshamide, bambuterol. *Side effects*: short-lived rise in creatine, phosphokinase (enzyme) and potassium levels in blood plasma, post-operative muscle pains. *Manufacturer*: Evans.

SCOPODERM

Description: an anti-emetic, anticholinergic preparation available as a self-adhesive pink patch containing 1.5mg hyoscine. *Used for*: motion sickness. *Dosage*: adults and children over 10 years, apply patch to clean, dry skin behind ear 5 to 6 hours before travelling. Replace after 72 hours if needed and remove when travelling is finished. *Special care*: pregnancy, breast-feeding, liver or kidney disorders, obstruction of intestine, bladder or pyloric stenosis. *Avoid use*: children under 10 years, glaucoma. Consumption of alcohol. *Possible interaction*: drugs affecting CNS, anticholinergics, alcohol. *Side effects*: skin rashes and irritation, urine retention, dry mouth, disturbance of vision, sleepiness, dizziness. Rarely, withdrawal symptoms. *Manufacturer*: Ciba.

SECADREX

Description: an antihypertensive preparation combining a cardioselective ß-blocker and thiazide diuretic available as film-coated white tablets containing 200mg acebutolol (as hydrochloride) and 12.5mg hydrochlorothiazide, marked SECADREX. *Used for*: hypertension. *Dosage*: 1 to 2 tablets as a single dose each day. *Special care*: pregnancy, breast-feeding, patients with weak hearts may require diuretics and digitalis, diabetes, undergoing general anaesthesia, kidney or liver disorders, gout. Electrolyte (salts) levels may need to be monitored. *Avoid use*: history of bronchospasm or obstructive airways disease, heart block, heart shock, uncompensated heart failure, disease of peripheral arteries, bradycardia. Serious or worsening kidney failure or anuria. *Possible interaction*: sympathomimetics, class I antiarrhythmics, CNS depressants, clonidine withdrawal, ergot alkaloids, cardiac depressant anaesthetics, verapamil, reserpine, indomethacin, hypoglycaemics, cimetidine, other antihypertensives. Digitalis, potassium supplements, potassium-sparing diuretics, lithium. *Side effects*: cold hands and feet, disturbance of sleep, fatigue on exercise, bronchospasm, bradycardia, gastro-intestinal disturbances, heart failure, blood changes, gout, sensitivity to light, muscle weakness. If skin rash or dry eyes occur, withdraw drug gradually. *Manufacturer*: R.P.R.

SECONAL SODIUM^{CD}

Description: a barbiturate preparation available as 50mg and 100mg orange capsules, coded F42 and F40 respectively, both containing quinalbarbitone sodium. *Used for*: short-term treatment of serious insomnia. *Dosage*: 50–100mg taken at night. *Special care*: extremely dangerous, addictive drug with narrow margin of safety. Liable to abuse by overdose leading to coma and death or if combined with alcohol. Easily produces dependence and severe withdrawal symptoms. Drowsiness may persist next day affecting driving and performance of skilled tasks. *Avoid use*: should be avoided if possible in all patients. Not to be used for children, young adults, pregnant and nursing mothers, elderly, those with drug or alcohol related problems, patients with liver, kidney or heart disease or porphyria. Insomnia where the cause is pain. *Possible interaction*: alcohol, CNS depressant drugs, Griseofulvin, metronidazone, rifampicin, phenytoin, chloramphenicol. Anticoagulant drugs of the coumarin type, steroid drugs including contraceptive pill. *Side effects*: hangover with drowsiness, shakiness, dizziness, headache, anxiety, confusion, excitement, rash and allergic responses, gastro intestinal upsets, urine retention, loss of sexual desire. *Manufacturer*: Flynn.

SECTRAL

Description: an anti-arrhythmic, anti-anginal preparation which is a cardioselective ß-blocker available as capsules in 2 strengths, both containing acebutolol (as hydrochloride). White/buff, 100mg and pink/buff 200mg both marked with strength and SECTRAL. Also, **SECTRAL TABLETS**, white, film-coated, containing 400mg marked SECTRAL 400. *Used for*: heart arrhythmias, angina. *Dosage*: adults, arrhythmias, maintenance dose of 400–1200mg in 2 or 3 divided doses each day. Angina, 400mg once each day taken with breakfast or 200mg twice daily. The maximum is 1.2g each day. *Special care*: history of bronchospasm and certain ß-blockers, diabetes, liver or kidney disease, pregnancy, lactation, general anaesthesia. Withdraw gradually. Not for children. *Avoid use*: heart block or failure, bradycardia, sick sinus syndrome (associated with sinus node disorder); certain ß-blockers, severe peripheral arterial disease. *Possible interaction*: verapamil, hypoglycaemics, reserpine, clonidine withdrawal, some antiarrhythmics and anaesthetics, antihypertensives, depressants of the CNS, cimetidine, indomethacin, sympathomimetics. *Side effects*: bradycardia, cold hands and feet, disturbance to sleep, heart failure, gastro-intestinal upsets, tiredness on exertion, bronchospasm. *Manufacturer*: R.P.R.

SECURON SR

Description: a class I calcium antagonist available as film-coated, oblong, scored, green, sustained-release tablets containing 240mg verapamil hydrochloride and marked with logo. Also, **HALF SECURON SR**, white, film-coated, sustained-release tablets containing 120mg marked 120 SR and company name. Also, **SECURON TABLETS** white, film-coated and available in strengths of 40mg,

80mg and 120mg, all marked with strength, name and KNOLL. Also, **SECURON I.V.** available as a solution in pre-filled syringes containing 2.5mg/ml. *Used for*: supraventricular tachycardia, angina, hypertension. *Dosage*: tachycardias, Securon Tablets, 40–120mg 3 times each day. Angina, Securon SR, Half Securon SR or Securon Tablets, 120mg 3 times each day. Hypertension, Securon SR or Half Securon SR, 240mg once each day with a maximum of 480mg in divided doses daily. Patients who have not taken verapamil before start with lower dose of 120mg once daily. Securon Tablets, 120mg twice each day at first increasing to 160mg twice daily if needed. Maximum dose is 480mg in divided doses daily. Children, for tachycardias, Securon Tablets only, age under 2 years, 20mg; age over 2 years, 20–40mg, both 2 or 3 times each day. *Special care*: pregnancy, breast-feeding, patients with liver or kidney disorders, heart conduction disturbances, bradycardia, 1st degree heart block. Patients with weak hearts require digitalis and/or diuretics. *Avoid use*: some kinds of heart block, heart shock, sick sinus syndrome, serious bradycardia, heart attack, severe hypotension, uncompensated heart failure, certain types of heart flutter or fibrillation. Patients should not receive intravenous ß-blockers at same time. *Possible interaction*: digoxin, ß-blockers, cimetidine, muscle relaxant drugs, inhaled anaesthetics, cyclosporin, rifampicin, antihypertensives, lithium, carbamazepine, theophylline, phenobarbitone, phenytoin. *Side effects*: constipation; rarely, nausea, headache, dizziness, allergic reactions, hypotension, enlargement of breasts, increased growth of gum tissues, flushes. (Effects on heart rate, heart muscle and hypotension when given intravenously). *Manufacturer*: Knoll.

SECUROPEN

Description: an antibiotic preparation which is an antipseudomonal penicillin available as powder in vials for reconstitution and injection at strengths of 500mg, 1g, 2g and 5g all containing azlocillin (as monosodium). *Used for*: local and systemic infections especially those caused by pseudomonas bacteria. *Dosage*: adults, 2g every 8 hours by intravenous injection; serious infections, 5g every 8 hours by intravenous infusion. Children, premature baby, 50mg/kg body weight every 12 hours; newborn baby, 100mg/kg every 12 hours; aged 1 week to 1 year, 100mg/kg every 8 hours; 1 to 14 years, 75mg/kg every 8 hours. *Special care*: pregnancy, kidney disorders. *Possible interaction*: tubocurarine and other non-depolarizing muscle relaxants, methotrexate. *Side effects*: gastro-intestinal upset, allergic hypersensitive responses. *Manufacturer*: Bayer.

SEMPREX

Description: an antihistamine preparation of the arylalkylamine type available as white capsules containing 8mg acrivastine marked with symbol, 09C and company name. *Used for*: allergic rhinitis, urticaria. *Dosage*: adults, 1 tablet 3 times each day. *Special care*: pregnancy, breast-feeding. *Avoid use*: children, elderly, kidney failure. *Possible interaction*: CNS depressants, alcohol. *Side effects*: rarely, drowsiness. *Manufacturer*: Glaxo Wellcome.

SEPTRIN

Description: an antibiotic preparation combining a folic acid inhibitor and sulphonamide available as white tablets and orange dissolvable tablets, both containing 80mg trimethoprim and 400mg sulphamethoxazole. Tablets are both marked with maker's name, tablet name and coded Y2B. **SEPTRIN ADULT SUSPENSION** same components/5ml. **SEPTRIN PAEDIATRIC SUSPENSION**, sugar-free, containing 40mg trimethoprim and 200mg sulphamethoxazole/5ml. Also, **SEPTRIN FOR INFUSION** available in ampoules containing 80mg trimethoprim and 400mg sulphamethoxazole/5ml. *Used for*: infections of skin, gastro-intestinal, respiratory and urinary tracts. *Dosage*: tablets, 1 to 3 twice each day; suspension, 5–15ml twice daily; Septrin Forte, 1 to 1½ tablets twice each day. Infusion, 960mg every 12 hours increasing to 1.44g if infection is extremely severe, given intravenously. Children, Paediatric Suspension, 6 weeks to 6 months, 2.5ml; 6 months to 6 years, 5ml; over 6 years, 10ml, all twice each day. Tablets, children over 6 years, 1 tablet or 5ml adult suspension. Infusion, 36mg/kg body weight each day in 2 divided doses increasing to 54mg/kg in the case of severe infections. *Special care*: breast-feeding, elderly, patients with kidney disorders (require reduced or less frequent doses). Regular blood tests should be carried out in patients taking the drug long-term. *Avoid use*: pregnancy, newborn babies, severe liver or kidney disorders, blood changes. *Possible interaction*: anticonvulsants, folate inhibitors, hypoglycaemics, anticoagulants. *Side effects*: vomiting, nausea, inflammation of tongue, blood changes, skin rashes, folate deficiency; rarely erythema multiformae (allergic disorder affecting skin and mucous membranes), Lyell syndrome. *Manufacturer*: Glaxo Wellcome.

SERC

Description: an anti-emetic preparation which is a histamine analogue available as white tablets in 2 strengths containing 8mg and 16mg betahistine, dihydrochloride, marked Duphar 256 or 267 respectively. *Used for*: symptoms associated with Ménière's syndrome including hearing loss, tinnitus and vertigo. *Dosage*: 16mg 3 times each day at first with a maintenance dose of 24–48mg daily. *Special care*: patients with peptic ulcer, bronchial asthma. *Avoid use*: phaeochromocytoma. *Side effects*: gastro-intestinal upset. *Manufacturer*: Solvay.

SERENACE

Description: an anti-depressant preparation which is a butyrophenone available as green/light green capsules containing 0.5mg haloperidol marked Norton 500 and SERENACE. Also, **SERENACE TABLETS** in 4 strengths all containing haloperidol; white, 1.5mg; pink, 5mg; 10mg and 20mg all marked with strength on one side and SERENACE on other, and coded NORTON. **SERENACE LIQUID**, containing 2mg/ml; **SERENACE INJECTION** available as a solution in ampoules for injection in strengths of 5mg and 10mg/ml. *Used for*: capsules, additional treatment for anxiety; tablets and liquid, manic states, psychoses, schizophrenia, behaviour disorders in children. *Dosage*: capsules, 1 twice each day; tablets or liquid, 1.5–20mg each day at first increasing as needed to control disorder. Then decreasing to a maintenance dose in the order of 3–10mg each day. The maximum daily dose is 200mg. Injection, for emergency treatment, 5–30mg by intravenous or intramuscular injection every 6 hours, then preparations taken by mouth. Children, tablets or liquid only, 0.025–0.05mg/kg body weight each day at first. Usual daily maximum is 10mg. *Special care*: pregnancy, tardive dyskinesia (disorder characterized by repeated involuntary muscle movements), hyperthyroidism, kidney or liver failure, serious heart or circulatory disorders, epilepsy. *Avoid use*: breast-feeding, Parkinsonism, coma. *Possible interaction*: rifampicin, fluoxetine, carbamazepine, anxiolytics, hypnotics. *Side effects*: extrapyramidal side effects, drowsiness, hypothermia, insomnia, pallor, nightmares, depression, constipation, dry mouth, blocked nose, difficulty in urination. Changes in ECG and EEG, effects on heart, e.g. tachycardia, arrhythmias, blood changes, changes in endocrine system, e.g. effects on menstruation, breasts, impotence, weight gain. Effects on liver, jaundice, sensitivity to light, purple pigmentation of skin and eyes. *Manufacturer*: Baker Norton.

SEREVENT

Description: a bronchodilator and selective ß$_2$-agonist available as a metered dose aerosol delivering 25µg salmeterol (as xinafoate) per dose. Also, **SEREVENT DISKHALER**, using disks containing 4 x 50µg blisters salmeterol (as xinafoate) with breath-actuated delivery system. *Used for*: various types of asthma along with anti-inflammatory therapy. *Dosage*: adults, Serevent, 2 puffs twice each day, 4 puffs if exceptionally severe. Serevent Diskhaler, 1 blister twice each day or 2 if very severe. Children, Serevent, age over 4 years, 2 puffs twice each day. Serevent Diskhaler, 1 blister twice each day. *Special care*: pregnancy, breast-feeding, thyrotoxicosis, acute symptoms of asthma or if unstable and severe. Steroid therapy should be continued. *Avoid use*: children under 4 years. *Possible interaction*: ß-blockers. *Side effects*: paradoxical bronchospasm, hypokalaemia; rarely, skin eruptions, pain in chest, joints and muscles, headache, palpitations, tremor, irritation of throat. *Manufacturer*: A. & H.

SEROPHENE

Description: an antioestrogen preparation available as scored, white tablets containing 50mg clomiphene citrate. *Used for*: female infertility caused by disorder of hypothalamus-pituitary gland function. Also, with gonadotrophins in invitro fertilization treatment. *Dosage*: infertility, 1 tablet each day for 5 days, ideally starting within 5 days of menstruation. Superovulation, 2 tablets each day starting on day 2 continuing to day 6 of monthly cycle. *Special care*: ensure patient is not pregnant before and during course of treatment. *Avoid use*: patients with undiagnosed bleeding from uterus, large cyst on ovary, cancer of endometrium, liver disorder. *Side effects*: pain or discomfort in abdomen, enlargement of ovaries, flushes. Withdraw drug if blurring of vision occurs. *Manufacturer*: Serono.

SEROXAT

Description: an antidepressant available as film-coated, oval, scored tablets in 2 strengths; containing 20mg (white) and 30mg (blue) paroxetine (as hydrochloride). Both marked with strength and name. *Used for*: depression and depressive illness with anxiety. *Dosage*: 20mg once each day at first, taken in the morning with breakfast. Then increasing gradually every 2 or 3 weeks by 10mg to a maximum daily dose of 50mg. Elderly persons start with lower dose of 20mg once each day increasing gradually to 40mg daily, if needed. *Special care*: pregnancy, breast-feeding, serious liver or kidney disorders, heart disease or disease of arteries of heart, epilepsy, history of mania. *Avoid use*: children. *Possible interaction*: anticonvulsants, tryptophan, drugs affecting liver enzymes, phenytoin, MAOIs, anticonvulsants. *Side effects*: dry mouth, sweating, sleepiness, tremor, nausea, weakness, effects on sexual habits. *Manufacturer*: SmithKline Beecham.

SEVREDOL[CD]

Description: an analgesic opiate available as film-coated, capsule-shaped, scored tablets in 2 strengths, blue containing 10mg, and pink containing 20mg morphine sulphate. Both are marked with strength and IR. *Used for*: severe pain. *Dosage*: 10mg every 4 hours at first increasing dose if necessary. Children, age 3 to 5 years, 5mg every 4 hours; 6 to 12 years, 5–10mg every 4 hours. *Special care*: elderly, enlarged prostate gland, underactive thyroid, liver or kidney disease, paralytic ileus, respiratory problems, reduced function of adrenal glands, following surgery. *Avoid use*: pregnancy, breast-feeding, children under 3 years, obstructive airways disease, serious liver disease, head injuries, raised pressure within brain, coma, depression of respiration, alcoholism. *Possible interaction*: CNS depressants, MAOIs. *Side effects*: nausea, vomiting, constipation, sedation, drug tolerance and addiction. *Manufacturer*: Napp.

SIMPLENE

Description: a sympathomimetic preparation available in the form of eyedrops in 2 strengths containing 0.5% and 1% adrenaline. *Used for*: primary open angle and secondary glaucoma. *Dosage*: 1 drop twice each day. *Avoid use*: patients with narrow angle glaucoma or diabetes. *Possible interaction*: MAOIs, ß-blockers, tricyclics. *Side effects*: pain or discomfort in eye, headache, skin reactions, pigmentation with melanin. Rarely, systemic side effects. *Manufacturer*: Chauvin.

SINEMET

Description: an anti-Parkinsonism preparation combining a dopamine precursor and dopa decarboxylase inhibitor available in the form of tablets. "LS" scored, oval, yellow tablets contain 50mg levodopa and 12.5mg carbidopa (as monohydrate), marked with name. "Plus" scored, oval, yellow tablets contain 100mg and 25mg marked with name. "110" scored, oval, blue tablets contain 100mg and 10mg, marked MSD 647. "275" scored, oval, blue tablets contain 250mg and 25mg marked MSD 654. Also, **SINEMET CR**, oval, mottled, peach-coloured, continuous-release tablets containing 200mg and 50mg marked 521 and DPP. Also, **HALF SINEMET CR**, oval, pink, continuous-release tablets containing 100mg and 25mg marked 601 and DPP. *Used for*: Parkinsonism. *Dosage*: adults over 18 years, not receiving levodopa, 1 "LS" or 1 "Plus" tablet 3 times each day at first increasing by 1 tablet every other day to the equivalent of 8 "Plus" tablets each day. Patients who have been taking levodopa should stop this 8 hours before taking Sinemet. Sinemet CR, 1 tablet twice each day in first instance, if not receiving levodopa, then adjusted according to response. *Special care*: liver or kidney disease, disease of heart or heart blood vessels, endocrine disorders, peptic ulcer, wide angle glaucoma. Liver, kidney and heart function should be monitored and blood values checked regularly if patients are taking drug long-term. *Avoid use*: children, pregnancy, breast-feeding, narrow angle glaucoma, history of malignant melanoma, severe psychoses. *Possible interaction*: MAOIs, sympathomimetics, antihypertensives, drug acting on central amines. *Side effects*: CNS effects, low blood pressure on rising, discolouration of urine, vomiting, nausea, involuntary muscle movements, anorexia. *Manufacturer*: DuPont.

SINEQUAN

Description: a TCAD preparation available as tablets in different strengths, all containing doxepin (as hydrochloride). Red, 10mg capsules, coded SQN; red/blue 25mg capsules, coded SQN 25; blue, 50mg capsules, coded SQN 50; blue/yellow 75mg capsules coded SQN 75. All are marked PFIZER. *Used for*: depression. *Dosage*: 10–100mg 3 times each day or a maximum of 100mg as a single night-time dose. *Special care*: liver disorders, hyperthyroidism, glaucoma, lactation, epilepsy, diabetes, adrenal tumour, heart disease, urine retention. Psychotic or suicidal patients. *Avoid use*: heart block, heart attacks, severe liver disease, pregnancy. *Possible interaction*: MAOIs (or within 14 days of their use), alcohol, antidepressants, barbiturates, anticholinergics, local anaesthetics that contain adrenaline or noradrenaline, oestrogens, cimetidine, antihypertensives. *Side effects*: constipation, urine retention, dry mouth, blurred vision, palpitations, tachycardia, nervousness, drowsiness, insomnia. Changes in weight, blood and blood sugar, jaundice, skin reactions, weakness, ataxia, hypotension, sweating, altered libido, gynaecomastia, galactorrhoea. *Manufacturer*: Pfizer.

SINTHROME

Description: a coumarin anticoagulant preparation available as white tablets containing 1mg nicoumalone, marked CG and AA. *Used for*: thromboembolic disorders. *Dosage*: 8–12mg on first day, 4–8mg on following day, then according to response. *Special care*: breast-feeding, elderly, serious heart failure, liver disorders, hypertension, disorders of absorption from gastro-intestinal tract, reduced protein binding. Risk of haematoma (accumulation of leaked blood which forms a solid mass within tissues) with intramuscular injections. *Avoid use*: pregnancy, children, if surgery or undergone labour in last 24 hours, liver or kidney disorders, serious hypertension, blood changes, inflammation of or leakage of fluid from pericardium, bacterial endocarditis. Patients who are uncooperative. *Possible interaction*: quinidine, corticosteroids, NSAIDs, antibiotics, oral hypoglycaemics, cimetidine, sulphonamides, phenformin. Drugs affecting the halting of bleeding, liver enzymes, vitamin K, absorption. *Side effects*: allergic responses, damage to liver, reversible hair loss, haemorrhage. Rarely, headache, nausea, skin necrosis, anorexia. *Manufacturer*: Geigy.

SKINOREN

Description: an antibacterial preparation available as a cream containing 20% azelaic acid. *Used for*: acne. *Dosage*: apply in the morning and evening to affected skin and rub in, maximum dose is 10g daily. Treatment should be continued according to response but for no more than 6 months. *Special care*: pregnancy, breast-feeding, avoid eyes. *Side effects*: sensitivity to light, local skin irritation. *Manufacturer*: Schering H.C.

SLO-PHYLLIN

Description: a xanthine bronchodilator available as sustained-release capsules enclosing white pellets, in 3 strengths, all containing theophylline. White/clear 60mg, brown/clear 125mg and blue/clear 250mg capsules are all marked with strength, SLO-PHYLLIN and LIPHA. *Used for*: bronchospasm in asthma, emphysema, bronchitis. *Dosage*: 250–500mg twice each day; children, age 2 to 6 years, 60–120mg; 6 to 12 years, 125–250mg; all twice each day. *Special care*: pregnancy, breast-feeding, peptic ulcer, liver or heart disease. *Avoid use*: children under 2 years. *Possible interaction*: interferon, erythromycin, diuretics, ß₂-agonists, cimetidine, steroids, ciprofloxacin. *Side effects*: gastro-intestinal upset, nausea, heart arrhythmias, tachycardia, headache, insomnia. *Manufacturer*: Lipha.

SLOW-FE FOLIC

Description: a haematinic preparation available as film-coated, cream-coloured tablets containing 160mg dried ferrous sulphate and 400µg folic acid, marked TP and CIBA. *Used for*: prevention of iron and folic acid deficiencies in pregnant women. *Dosage*: 1 to 2 tablets each day. *Possible interaction*: anticonvulsants, penicillamine, tetracyclines, antacids, zinc salts. *Side effects*: constipation nausea. *Manufacturer*: Ciba.

SLOW-TRASICOR

Description: an antianginal, antihypertensive preparation available as film-coated, white, sustained-release tablets containing 160mg oxprenolol hydrochloride, marked with name and manufacturer's name. *Used for*: angina, hypertension. *Dosage*: angina, 1 each morning at first increasing to 2 or 3 if needed. If nocturnal angina is present, an evening dose may be taken. Hypertension, 1 tablet each morning. *Special care*: history of bronchospasm and certain ß-blockers, diabetes, liver or kidney disease, pregnancy, lactation, general anaesthesia. Withdraw gradually. Not for children. *Avoid use*: heart block or failure, bradycardia, sick sinus syndrome (associated with sinus node disorder), certain ß-blockers, severe peripheral arterial disease. *Possible interaction*: verapamil, hypoglycaemics, reserpine, clonidine withdrawal, some antiarrhythmics and anaesthetics, antihypertensives, depressants of the CNS, cimetidine, indomethacin, sympathomimetics. *Side effects*: bradycardia, cold hands and feet, disturbance to sleep, heart failure, gastro-intestinal upset, tiredness on exertion, bronchospasm. *Manufacturer*: Ciba.

SNO-PHENICOL

Description: a broad-spectrum antibiotic preparation available as eyedrops containing 0.5% chloramphenicol. *Used for*: bacterial infections of the eye. *Dosage*: 1 or more drops into eye, as needed. Children, 1 drop as needed. *Side effects*: local allergic hypersensitive responses (stop immediately). Rarely, aplastic anaemia. *Manufacturer*: Chauvin. SNO-PILO *Description*: a cholinergic eye preparation available in the form of drops in different strengths containing 1%, 2% and 4% pilocarpine. *Used for*: glaucoma. *Dosage*: 1 or 2 drops 4 times each day. *Avoid use*: severe inflammation of iris, wearing soft contact lenses. *Side effects*: short-lived loss of visual sharpness. *Manufacturer*: Chauvin.

SODIUM AMYTAL^{CD}

Description: an hypnotic barbiturate preparation, available as blue capsules in 2 strengths containing 60mg and 200mg amylobarbitone sodium, coded LILLY F23 or F33 respectively. *Used for*: insomnia, which has not responded to other drugs. *Dosage*: tablets, 60–200mg taken at night. *Special care*: extremely dangerous, addictive drug with narrow margin of safety. Liable to abuse by overdose leading to coma and death or if combined with alcohol. Easily produces dependence and severe withdrawal symptoms. Drowsiness may persist next day affecting driving and performance of skilled tasks. *Avoid use*: should be avoided if possible in all patients. Not to be used for children, young adults, pregnant and nursing mothers, elderly pesons, those with drug or alcohol related problems, patients with liver, kidney or heart disease, porphyria. Insomnia where the cause is pain. *Possible interaction*: alcohol, CNS depressant drugs, Griseofulvin, metronidazone, rifampicin, phenytoin, chloramphenicol. Anticoagulant drugs of the coumarin type, steroid drugs including contraceptive pill. *Side effects*: hangover with drowsiness, shakiness, dizziness, headache, anxiety, confusion, excitement, rash and allergic responses, gastro intestinal upsets, urine retention, loss of sexual desire. *Manufacturer*: Kite.

SODIUM AMYTAL INJECTION^{CD}

Description: a barbiturate preparation, available as a powder in vials for reconstitution and injection containing 500mg amylobarbitone sodium. *Used for*: status epilepticus (but not grand mal epilepsy). *Dosage*: 250 mg–1g by slow intravenous or intramuscular injection. Children, age over 6 years, 65–500mg by slow intravenous or intramuscular injection. *Special care*: kidney and liver disorders, serious lung insufficiency. *Avoid use*: pregnancy, breast-feeding, elderly, patients who are debilitated, porphyria, pain which is not controlled, history of drug or alcohol abuse. *Possible interaction*: CNS depressants, griseofulvin, alcohol, phenytoin, systemic steroids, chloramphenicol, rifampicin, metronidazole, anticoagulants of the coumarin type. *Side effects*: headache, respiratory depression, dizziness, unsteadiness, sleepiness, confusion, agitation, allergic responses. Drug tolerance and dependence may occur. *Manufacturer*: Flynn.

SOFRA-TULLE

Description: a gauze dressing for wounds impregnated with 1% framycetin sulphate available in individual foil sachets. *Used for*: burns, wounds, ulcers, infected areas. *Dosage*: apply to affected area. *Avoid use*: large open wounds—danger of ototoxicity (damage to organs of balance and hearing), especially in children, elderly and patients with kidney disorders. *Manufacturer*: Hoechst.

SOFRADEX

Description: a compound preparation combining a corticosteroid, aminoglycoside and antibiotic available in the form of drops containing 0.05% dexamethasone, 0.5% framycetin sulphate and 0.005% gramicidin. Also, **SOFRADEX OINTMENT** containing 0.05% dexamethasone, 0.5% framycetin sulphate and 0.005% gramicidin. *Used for*: inflammation and infection of outer ear. Inflammation of eye and prevention of infection, short term only, blepharitis (inflammation of hair follicles of eye lashes which may be caused by infection). *Dosage*: drops, ear, apply 2 to 3 drops 3 or 4 times each day; ointment, ear, apply once or twice daily. Drops, eye, 1 or 2 drops up to 6 times each day or more frequently if necessary. Ointment, eye, apply 2 or 3 times each day or at night if drops are being used. *Special care*: pregnant women. *Avoid use*: longterm use in babies or by pregnant women, perforated eardrum (if for ear infections), eye infections producing pus or those with tuberculous, fungal or viral origin. *Side effects*: superinfection, use in eyes may lead to thinning of cornea, fungal infection, cataract, rise in pressure within eye. *Manufacturer*: Hoechst.

SOFRAMYCIN

Description: an antibiotic aminoglycoside preparation available in the form of drops containing 0.5% framycetin sulphate. Also, **SOFRAMYCIN OINTMENT** containing 0.5% framycetin sulphate. *Used for*: eye infections, styes, blepharitis (inflammation and infection of hair follicles of eye lashes), conjunctivitis. Ointment also used for bacterial infections of skin. *Dosage*: eyes, apply 1 or 2 drops 3 or 4 times each day; apply ointment 2 or 3 times each day or at night if drops are being used. Skin, apply to affected area up to 3 times each day. *Special care*: use on more extensive areas of skin. *Side effects*: sensitization, ototoxicity (damage to organs of balance and hearing). *Manufacturer*: Hoechst.

SOLPADOL

Description: a compound analgesic preparation available as scored, white, effervescent tablets containing 500mg paracetamol and 30mg codeine phosphate. Also, **SOLPADOL CAPLETS**, capsule-shaped, white tablets containing the same. *Used for*: severe pain. *Dosage*: 2 tablets every 4 hours with a maximum of 8 in any 24 hour period. *Special care*: labour, pregnancy, breast-feeding, elderly, liver or kidney disorders, underactive thyroid gland, obstruction or inflammation of the bowel. *Avoid use*: children, depression of respiration, obstruction of airways, head injury, raised pressure within brain, alcoholism, surgery to the biliary tract (bile duct, gall bladder). *Possible interaction*: CNS depressants, MAOIs. *Side effects*: constipation, blurred vision, dizziness, dry mouth, nausea, sedation, drug dependence and tolerance. *Manufacturer*: Sanofi Winthrop.

SOLU-CORTEF

Description: a glucocorticoid-mineralocorticoid (corticosteroid) preparation available in vials with diluent for reconstitution and injection, containing 100mg hydrocortisone (as sodium succinate). *Used for*: medical emergencies requiring rapid corticosteroid dose, e.g. anaphylaxis, asthma. *Dosage*: 100–500mg by slow intravenous injection. Children, may require reduced doses but not less than 25mg each day. *Special care*: thrombophlebitis, psychoses, recent intestinal anastomoses, chronic nephritis, certain cancers, osteoporosis, peptic ulcer, skin eruption/rash related to a disease, viral, fungal or active infections, tuberculosis. Hypertension, glaucoma, epilepsy, acute glomerulonephritis (inflammation of kidney glomerulus), diabetes, cirrhosis, hypothyroidism, pregnancy, stress. To be withdrawn gradually. *Possible interaction*: NSAIDs, oral anticoagulants, phenytoin, ephedrine, phenobarbitone, rifampicin, diuretics, cardiac glycosides, anticholinesterases, hypoglycaemics. *Side effects*: osteoporosis, depression, euphoria, hyperglycaemia, peptic ulcers, Cushingoid changes. *Manufacturer*: Pharmacia & Upjohn.

SOLU-MEDRONE

Description: a glucocorticoid corticosteroid preparation as powder in vials for reconstitution and injection, in 4 strengths of 40mg, 125mg, 500mg and 1g all containing methylprednisolone. Also, **SOLU-MEDRONE 2G** available in vials with diluent, containing 2g methylprednisolone (all as sodium succinate). *Used for*: Solu-Medrone: allergic conditions, ulcerative colitis, Crohn's disease, Stevens-Johnson syndrome, removal of stomach contents by aspiration, cerebral oedema resulting from tumour, transplant operations. Solu-Medrone 2G: serious spinal cord injuries. *Dosage*: Solu-Medrone, transplants, up to 1g each day; other conditions, 10–500mg by slow intravenous or intramuscular injection over 30 minutes or more. Solu-Medrone 2G, 30mg/kg body weight by intravenous injection over 15 minutes starting within 8 hours of injury. Further dose after 45 minutes at 5.4mg/kg/hour for 23 hours, by intravenous infusion. Children, Solu-Medrone only, up to 30mg/kg each day depending upon condition; status asthmaticus (severe, prolonged asthma attack), 1–4mg/kg each day for 1 to 3 days. *Special care*: thrombophlebitis, psychoses, recent intestinal anastomoses, chronic nephritis, certain cancers, osteoporosis, peptic ulcer, skin eruption/rash related to a disease, viral, fungal or active infections, tuberculosis.

Hypertension, glaucoma, epilepsy, acute glomerulonephritis (inflammation of kidney glomerulus), diabetes, cirrhosis, hypothyroidism, pregnancy, stress. Withdraw gradually. *Possible interaction*: NSAIDs, oral anticoagulants, phenytoin, ephedrine, phenobarbitone, rifampicin, diuretics, cardiac glycosides, anticholinesterases, hypoglycaemics. *Side effects*: osteoporosis, depression, euphoria, hyperglycaemia, peptic ulcers, Cushingoid changes. *Manufacturer*: Pharmacia & Upjohn.

SONERYL^{CD}

Description: an hypnotic barbiturate available as pink, scored tablets containing 100mg butobarbitone marked SONERYL. *Used for*: insomnia which has not responded to other drugs. *Dosage*: 1–2 tablets taken at bedtime. *Special care*: extremely dangerous, addictive drug with narrow margin of safety. Liable to abuse by overdose leading to coma and death or if combined with alcohol. Easily produces dependence and severe withdrawal symptoms. Drowsiness may persist next day affecting driving and performance of skilled tasks. *Avoid use*: should be avoided if possible in all patients. Not to be used for children, young adults, pregnant and nursing mothers, elderly pesons, those with drug or alcohol related problems, patients with liver, kidney or heart disease, porphyria. Insomnia where the cause is pain. *Possible interaction*: alcohol, CNS depressants, griseofulvin, metronidazole, rifampicin, phenytoin, chloramphenicol. Anticoagulant drugs of the coumarin type, steroid drugs including contraceptive pill. *Side effects*: hangover with drowsiness, shakiness, dizziness, headache, anxiety, confusion, excitement, rash and allergic responses, gastro intestinal upsets, urine retention, loss of sexual desire. *Manufacturer*: Concord.

SOTACOR

Description: a non-cardioselective ß-blocker available as white tablets in 2 strengths of 80mg and 160mg containing solatol hydrochloride, both marked with strength and name. Also, **SOTACOR INJECTION** available as a solution in ampoules for injection containing 10mg/ml. *Used for*: prevention of second heart attack, arrhythmias, angina, hypertension. *Dosage*: prevention of heart attack, 320mg once each day starting 5 to 14 days after first attack. Arrhythmias, 160–240mg each day in divided or single doses. Angina, 160mg each day in single or divided doses; hypertension, 160mg each day at first increasing to 320mg daily if needed. *Special care*: history of bronchospasm and certain ß-blockers, diabetes, liver or kidney disease, pregnancy, lactation, general anaesthesia. Withdraw gradually. Not for children. *Avoid use*: heart block or failure, bradycardia, sick sinus syndrome (associated with sinus node disorder), certain ß-blockers, severe peripheral arterial disease. *Possible interaction*: verapamil, hypoglycaemics, reserpine, clonidine withdrawal, some antiarrhythmics and anaesthetics, antihypertensives, depressants of the CNS, cimetidine, indomethacin, sympathomimetics. *Side effects*: bradycardia, cold hands and feet, disturbance to sleep, heart failure, gastro-intestinal upset, tiredness on exertion, bronchospasm. *Manufacturer*: Bristol-Myers.

SOTAZIDE

Description: an antihypertensive compound with a non-cardioselective ß-blocker and thiazide diuretic, available as oblong, scored, blue tablets containing 160mg solatol hydrochloride and 25mg hydrochlorothiazide. *Used for*: hypertension. *Dosage*: 1 tablet each day increasing to 2 if needed. *Special care*: pregnancy, breast-feeding, patients with weak hearts may require diuretics and digitalis, those with diabetes, undergoing general anaesthesia, kidney or liver disorders, gout. Electrolyte (salts) levels may need to be monitored. *Avoid use*: history of bronchospasm or obstructive airways disease, heart block, heart shock, un-compensated heart failure, disease of peripheral arteries, bradycardia. Serious or worsening kidney failure or anuria. *Possible interaction*: sympathomimetics, class I antiarrhythmics, CNS depressants, clonidine withdrawal, ergot alkaloids, cardiac depressant anaesthetics, verapamil, reserpine, indomethacin, hypo-glycaemics, cimetidine, other antihypertensives. Digitalis, potassium supple-ments, potassium-sparing diuretics, lithium. *Side effects*: cold hands and feet, disturbance of sleep, fatigue on exercise, bronchospasm, bradycardia, gastro-intestinal disturbances, heart failure, blood changes, gout, sensitivity to light, muscle weakness. If skin rash or dry eyes occur, withdraw drug gradually. *Manu-facturer*: Bristol-Myers.

SPARINE

Description: an antipsychotic and group I phenothiazine available as a yellow suspension containing promazine embonate equivalent to 50mg promazine hydrochloride/5ml. Also, SPARINE INJECTION containing 50mg promazine hydrochloride/ml as a solution in ampoules. *Used for*: additional therapy in treatment of agi-tation, restlessness and agitation in elderly people, prolonged hiccough. Injec-tion additionally used for vomiting and nausea, EEG and cardiac investigative proceudres in children. *Dosage*: 100–200mg 4 times each day; elderly, half adult dose or 25–50mg for agitation and restlessness. Injection, 50mg every 6 to 8 hours by intramuscular injection; elderly, half adult dose. Children, injection only, 0.7mg/kg body weight given intramuscularly. *Special care*: pregnancy, breast-feeding, Parkinsonism, liver disorders, disease of heart or arteries of heart. *Avoid use*: depresssed bone marrow function or in coma. *Possible inter-action*: alcohol, anaesthetics, anticonvulsants, levodopa, analgesics, antidiabetic drugs, antihypertensives, antidepressants, tranquillizers. *Side effects*: extrapy-ramidal side effects, drowsiness, hypothermia, insomnia, pallor, nightmares, depression, constipation, dry mouth, blocked nose, difficulty in urination. Changes in ECG and EEG, effects on heart, e.g. tachycardia, arrhythmias, blood changes, changes in endocrine system, e.g. effects on menstruation, breasts, impotence, weight change. Effects on liver, jaundice, sensitivity to light, purple pigmentation of skin and eyes. *Manufacturer*: Wyeth.

SPIROCTAN

Description: a potassium-sparing diuretic, available in the form of blue tablets containing 25mg and green tablets containing 50mg spironolacetone, coded BM B2 and BM A8 respectively. Also, **SPIROCTAN CAPSULES**, green, containing 100mg, coded BM A7. Also, **SPIROCTAN-M**, available as a solution in ampoules containing 20mg cannrenoate potassium/ml. *Used for*: congestive heart failure, cirrhosis of the liver, nephrotic syndrome (a kidney abnormality), primary aldosteronism (a disease of the adrenal glands in which an excess of aldosterone, the hormone which regulates blood levels of sodium and potassium, is produced). Also, ascites (a collection of fluid in the peritoneal cavity of the abdomen, resulting from various diseases or disorders). *Dosage*: tablets and capsules, 50–200mg each day which may be increased, if needed, to a maximum of 400mg. The maximum single dose is 100mg. Spiroctan-M, 200–400mg, maximum 800mg, each day. Children, tablets or capsules, 1.5–3mg/kg body weight each day. *Special care*: liver or kidney disorders, long-term use in young people. Fluid, electrolyte and levels of blood urea nitrogen should be monitored. *Avoid use*: pregnancy, breast-feeding, Addison's disease, serious kidney disorders, hyperkalaemia. *Possible interaction*: potassium-sparing diuretics, potassium supplements, carbenoxolone, ACE inhibitors, NSAIDs, cardiac glycosides. *Side effects*: disturbance of metabolism and electrolyte levels, menstrual changes, gastro-intestinal upset, enlargement of breasts, deepening of voice, rash, loss of coordination, confusion. *Manufacturer*: B.M. UK.

SPORANOX

Description: a triazole antifungal drug available as pink/blue capsules enclosing coated pellets containing 100mg itraconazole. *Used for*: candidiasis (fungal infections) of vagina, oropharynx (the part of the pharynx containing the tonsils), skin disorders. *Dosage*: vulvo-vaginal infections, 2 tablets twice for 1 day; infections of oropharynx, 1 tablet each day for 15 days (2 tablets daily in patients with AIDS or who are neutropenic). Skin disorders, 1 tablet each day for 15 days or 30 days or 2 for 7 days, depending upon condition. *Special care*: liver disease or those who have suffered toxic effects to the liver from taking other drugs. *Avoid use*: elderly, children, pregnancy, breast-feeding. Contraception must be used during treatment and for 1 month following taking Sporanox. *Possible interaction*: antacids, astemizole, rifampicin, terfenadine, cyclosporin, H_2 antagonists. *Side effects*: pain in abdomen, indigestion, nausea, headache. *Manufacturer*: Janssen-Cilag.

STAFOXIL

Description: a penicillinase-resistant penicillin (i.e. resistant to the enzymes produced by some bacteria), available as brown/cream capsules in 2 strengths, containing 250mg and 500mg flucloxacillin (as sodium salt). *Used for*: soft tissue, skin, ear, nose and throat infections caused by Gram-positive bacteria. *Dosage*: 250mg 4 times each day taken 1 hour before meals. Children, over 2 years, half adult dose. *Avoid use*: children under 2 years. *Side effects*: gastro-intestinal upset, allergic hypersensitive reactions; rarely, cholestatic jaundice. *Manufacturer*: Yamanouchi.

STARIL

Description: an antihypertensive and ACE inhibitor available as diamond-shaped, white tablets containing 10mg fosinopril sodium marked with star, 158 and SQUIBB. Also, white 20mg tablets, marked with star, 609 and SQUIBB. *Used for*: hypertension which has not responded to other drugs or where these are not appropriate. *Dosage*: 10mg once each day at first with a maintenance dose in the order of 10–20mg daily. The maximum daily dose is 40mg. Any diuretic being taken should be stopped a few days before treatment starts but can be resumed after 4 weeks, if needed. *Special care*: congestive heart failure, kidney or liver disorders, receiving dialysis, depletion of fluid or salts. *Avoid use*: pregnancy, breast-feeding, children. *Possible interaction*: antacids, potassium-sparing diuretics, potassium supplements, lithium, NSAIDs, antihypertensives. *Side effects*: chest and muscle pains, rash, gastro-intestinal upset, fatigue, dizziness, palpitations, cough, disturbance of sense of taste; rarely, pancreatitis. If angioneurotic oedema occurs, withdraw drug. *Manufacturer*: Squibb.

STD INJECTION

Description: a sclerosant drug available as a solution in ampoules for injection at strengths of 0.5%, 1% and 3% all containing sodium tetradecyl sulphate. *Used for*: varicose veins in the leg by compression sclerotherapy. *Dosage*: for large veins, 0.25–1ml of 3% solution into section of vein by intravenous injection followed immediately by compression applied continuously. Maximum treatment of 4 sites in any 1 session of treatment. Small veins, 0.25–1ml of 1% solution in same way as for large veins. Maximum treatment of 10 sites in any 1 session. Very small veins or venules, 0.1–1ml of 0.5% solution as above. Maximum treatment of 10 sites in any 1 session. *Special care*: pregnancy, breast-feeding, disease of the arteries, history of allergy. Treatment must be carried out by specialist with emergency equipment available in the event of anaphylaxis. *Avoid use*: thrombophlebitis, infections, varicose veins caused by tumours, diabetes which is not controlled. Patients who are obese or immobile, taking oral contraceptives. *Manufacturer*: STD.

STELAZINE

Description: an anxiolytic, antidepressant and anticonvulsant preparation which is a phenothiazine group II drug. It is available as sugar-coated, blue tablets in 2 strengths containing 1mg and 5mg trifluoperazine (as hydrochloride), and marked SKF. Also, **STELAZINE SYRUP** containing 1mg/5ml; **STELAZINE SPANSULES**, yellow/clear, sustained-release capsules containing 2mg, 10mg and 15mg as white and blue pellets, marked 2. **STELAZINE CONCENTRATE**, containing 10mg/ml; **STELAZINE INJECTION** available as a solution in ampoules containing 1mg/ml. *Used for*: anxiety and agitation which may be accompanied by depression, psychosis, schizophrenia, disturbed behaviour; vomiting and nausea. *Dosage*: anxiety, Stelazine tablets, syrup, spansules, 2–

4mg each day with a maximum of 6mg. Schizophrenia, psychosis, disturbed behaviour, tablets or syrup, 5mg twice each day at first increasing to 15mg after 7 days. If needed, dosage may be further increased every 3 days by 5mg until condition is controlled and then reduced again for maintenance. Spansules, 1 10mg strength each day at first, increasing to 1 15mg spansule daily after 7 days. Injection, 1–3mg each day in divided doses, by intramuscular injection. Nausea and vomiting, tablets, syrup, spansules, 2–6mg each day. Elderly persons, tablets or syrup, all disorders, 1mg each day at first which may require gradual increase according to response. Children, usually use syrup, all disorders, age 3 to 5 years, up to 1mg; 6 to 12 years, up to 4mg, all as daily divided doses. *Special care*: pregnancy, breast-feeding, elderly, heart disease or disease of heart blood vessels, epilepsy, Parkinsonism, vomiting which is undiagnosed. *Avoid use*: children under 3 years, depressed bone marrow function, liver damage, coma. *Possible interaction*: analgesics, alcohol, CNS depressants, antihypertensives. *Side effects*: dry mouth, blurring of vision, disturbance of CNS, changes to ECG, hormonal changes. Rarely, extrapyramidal side effects and allergic responses with low doses. Judgement and performance of skilled tasks may be impaired. *Manufacturer*: S.K. & F.

STEMETIL

Description: an antipsychotic and anticonvulsant and phenothiazine group III drug, available as cream tablets 5mg and 25mg (scored) both containing prochlorperazine maleate and marked with strength and name. Also, **STEMETIL SYRUP** containing 5mg prochlorperazine mesylate/5ml. **STEMETIL EFF**, effervescent granules in sachets for reconstitution in water containing 5mg prochlorperazine mesylate. Also, **STEMETIL SUPPOSITORIES**, available in strengths of 5mg and 25mg containing prochlorperazine. **STEMETIL INJECTION** available as a solution in ampoules for injection containing 1.25% prochlorperazine mesylate. *Used for*: psychoses, schizophrenia, minor psychiatric and emotional disorders, severe vomiting and nausea, migraine, vertigo resulting from Ménière's disease (an inner ear disorder accompanied by ringing in the ears and progressive deafness). *Dosage*: psychiatric disorders, oral preparations, 15–25mg each day, maximum 40mg for minor illnesses; 75–100mg daily for schizophrenia, all in divided doses. Suppositories, 25mg 2 or 3 times each day, then oral preparations. Injection, 12.5–25mg 2 or 3 times each day by deep intramuscular injection then oral preparations. Vertigo, oral preparations, 5mg 3 times each day with a maximum of 30mg. Nausea, vomiting, 20mg as single dose then 10mg after 2 hours if needed. Prevention, 5–10mg 2 or 3 times each day. Suppositories, for vertigo, nausea and vomiting, 25mg as single dose then oral preparations after 6 hours, if needed. Injection, 12.5mg by deep intramuscular injection, then oral preparations if needed. Children, use syrup for nausea, vomiting only, over 10kg in weight, 0.25mg/kg body weight 2 or 3 times each day. *Special care*: breast-feeding, heart disease or disease of heart blood vessels, Parkinsonism, prolonged vomiting which is not diagnosed. *Avoid use*:

pregnancy, children under 10kg body weight, epilepsy, depressed bone marrow function, liver or kidney disorders, coma. *Possible interaction*: alcohol, antidiabetics, CNS depressants, antihypertensives, anti-cholinergics, analgesics, anticonvulsants. *Side effects*: anticholinergic side effects and disturbance of CNS, hypotension on rising (following injection), blood disorders, jaundice. At low doses there may rarely be endocrine changes, extrapyramidal side effects and allergic responses. Judgement and performance of skilled tasks may be impaired. *Manufacturer*: R.P.R.

STER-ZAC DC

Description: a disinfectant preparation available as a cream containing 3% hexachlophane. *Used for*: disinfection of hands prior to surgery. *Dosage*: wash hands with 3–5ml used as soap. *Special care*: children under 2 years. *Manufacturer*: Seton.

STESOLID

Description: a preparation for use rectally, with applicator, which is a long-acting benzodiazepine, available as a solution in single doses containing 5mg or 10mg diazepam. *Used for*: agitation, acute anxiety, convulsions, status epilepticus in which rapid treatment is necessary but injection intravenously is not desirable. Also, muscle spasm and pre-medication. *Dosage*: for all conditions, 10mg via rectum, elderly persons, 5mg. Children, age 1 to 3 years, 5mg; over 3 years, 10mg. *Special care*: chronic liver or kidney disease, chronic lung disease, pregnancy, labour, lactation, elderly. May impair judgement. Withdraw gradually and avoid prolonged use. *Avoid use*: children under 1 year, depression of respiration, acute lung disease; psychotic, phobic or obsessional states. *Possible interaction*: anticonvulsants, depressants of the CNS, alcohol. *Side effects*: ataxia, confusion, light-headedness, drowsiness, hypotension, gastro-intestinal upsets, disturbances in vision and libido, skin rashes, retention of urine, vertigo. Sometimes jaundice or blood disorders. *Manufacturer*: Dumex.

STIEDEX

Description: a topical potent steroid preparation available as an oily cream containing 0.25% desoxymethasone. **STIEDEX LP**, a moderately potent steroid preparation available as an oily cream containing 0.05%. Also, **STIEDEX LOTION**, combining a potent steroid and keratolytic agent in a lotion containing 0.25% desoxymethasone and 1% salicylic acid. *Used for*: Stiedex cream and LP cream, skin inflammations responsive to steroids. Lotion, psoriasis, especially of scalp and various other skin conditions. *Dosage*: creams, apply thinly 2 or 3 times each day and rub in. Lotion, apply once or twice each day in morning and/or evening and rub in. When condition improves, use once each day. *Special care*: thrombophlebitis, psychoses, recent intestinal anastomoses, chronic nephritis, certain cancers, osteoporosis, peptic ulcer, skin eruption/rash related to a disease, viral, fungal or active infections, tuberculosis. Hypertension, glaucoma, epilepsy, acute glomerulonephritis (inflammation of kidney glomerulus), diabetes, cirrhosis, hypothyroidism, pregnancy, stress. To be withdrawn gradually. *Avoid use*: children (Stiedex). *Possible interaction*: NSAIDs, oral anticoagulants, phenytoin, ephedrine, phenobarbitone, rifampicin, diuretics, cardiac glycosides, anticholinesterases, hypoglycaemics. *Side effects*: osteoporosis, depression, euphoria, hyperglycaemia, peptic ulcers, Cushingoid changes. *Manufacturer*: Stiefel.

STIEMYCIN

Description: an antibiotic solution containing 2% erythromycin. *Used for*: acne. *Dosage*: adults, apply twice each day in the morning and evening after washing. *Side effects*: possible slight irritation and dryness of skin at site of application. *Manufacturer*: Stiefel.

STREPTASE

Description: a fibrinolytic preparation available as powder in vials for reconstitution and injection containing 250,000 units or 750,000 units streptokinase. Also, **STREPTASE 1.5 MEGA UNITS**, as powder in vials for reconstitution and injection containing 1,500,000 units streptokinase. *Used for*: Streptase, pulmonary embolism, deep vein thrombosis, blockage of peripheral arteries, thrombosis of retinal blood vessels. Streptase 1.5 Mega Units, acute heart attack. *Dosage*: Streptase, initial dose of 250,000 units by intravenous infusion, then 100,000 units by infusion/hour for 24–72 hours depending upon response. Streptase 1.5 Mega Units, single dose over 1 hour by intravenous infusion of 1.5 million units, accompanied by oral doses of 150mg aspirin each day for at least 4 weeks. Children, Streptase only, initial dose adjusted according to condition, body weight then 20 units/ml of blood volume. *Special care*: heart disorders; blood tests and anticoagulant therapy are also required. *Avoid use*: pregnancy, patients who have received streptokinase treatment in last 5 days to 12 months, those with known allergy to streptokinase. Patients with recent bleeding disorders, clotting disorders, liver or kidney damage, brain growth, lung disease, inflammation and bacterial infection of endocardium, serious bronchitis, pancreatitis, diabetes. Having recently had surgery or with history of bleeding. *Possible interaction*: drugs affecting blood platelets, anticoagulants. *Side effects*: feverish reactions, heart arrhythmias, hypotension, pulmonary oedema, haemorrhage, embolism caused by cholesterol. Rarely, anaphylaxis. *Manufacturer*: Hoechst.

STROMBA

Description: an anabolic steroid available as white, scored tablets containing 5mg stanozolol marked STROMBA. *Used for*: Behcet's disease, (a rare disease affecting the blood vessels of the eye), prevention of angio-oedema which is hereditary. *Dosage*: Behcet's disease, 10mg each day; angio-oedema, 2.5–10mg each day at first then reduce dose as condition responds. Children, angio-oedema, aged 1 to 6 years, 2.5mg each day at first; 6 to 12 years, 2.5–5mg daily in first instance. Dose is then adjusted according to response. *Special care*: use for long periods in children, women past menopause, patients with kidney or heart disorders. Monitoring of liver function is required if patient has history of jaundice. *Avoid use*: pregnancy, porphyria, cancer of prostate gland, liver disease, type 1 diabetes. *Possible interaction*: oral anticoagulants. *Side effects*: indigestion, headache, skin rash, pains and cramps; toxic effects on liver, masculinizing effects on women and children before puberty. *Manufacturer*: Sanofi Winthrop.

SUBLIMAZE^{CD}

Description: a narcotic analgesic available as a solution in ampoules containing 50µg fentanyl/ml. *Used for*: analgesia during operations, enhancement of analgesic, respiratory depression in patients receiving artificial ventilation. *Dosage*: adults breathing unaided, 50–200µg at first then 50µg as needed. Adults being ventilated, 0.3–3.5mg at first then 100–200µg as needed. Children, 3 to 5 µg/kg body weight then 1µg/kg as needed. Child being ventilated, 15µg/kg then 1–3 µg/kg as needed. *Special care*: liver disease, underactive thyroid, respiratory disorders, myasthenia gravis. If used in obstetric patients, may cause depression of respiration in baby. *Avoid use*: obstructive airways disease or depression of respiration unless being artificially ventilated. *Possible interaction*: MAOIs, anxiolytics, hypnotics, cimetidine. *Side effects*: depression of respiration, bradycardia, vomiting, nausea, short-lived hypotension. *Manufacturer*: Janssen-Cilag.

SULPITIL

Description: an antipsychotic preparation and substituted benzamide available as scored, white tablets containing 200mg sulpiride marked L113. *Used for*: schizophrenia. *Dosage*: adults and young persons over 14 years, 200–400mg twice each day with a maximum of 1800mg daily. Elderly, 50–100mg twice each day at first increasing slowly to normal adult dose. *Special care*: pregnancy, epilepsy, kidney disorders, hypertension, hypomania. *Avoid use*: breast-feeding, phaeochromocytoma, porphyria. *Possible interaction*: alcohol, anxiolytics, hypnotics, tetrabenazine, calcium channel blockers, cimetidine. *Side effects*: extrapyramidal side effects, ECG and EEG changes. Effects on heart rhythm, blocked nose, dry mouth, constipation, blurring of vision, difficulty passing urine, drowsiness, apathy, depression, insomnia. Blood changes involving white blood cells, hormonal changes, e.g. enlargement of breasts, change in libido, impotence, sensitivity to light, effects on liver, changes in weight. *Manufacturer*: Pharmacia & Upjohn.

SULTRIN

Description: a compound sulphonamide antibacterial preparation available as lozenge-shaped, white, vaginal tablets (with applicator) containing 172.5mg sulphathiazole, 143.75mg sulphacetamide and 184mg sulphabenzamide marked with C and symbol. Also, **SULTRIN CREAM** containing 3.42% sulphathiazole, 2.86% sulphacetamide, 3.7% sulphabenzamide, with applicator. *Used for*: inflammation and infection of vagina and cervix caused by bacteria, post-cervical cautery, post-operative treatment. *Dosage*: tablets, 1 intravaginally twice each day for 10 days. Cream, 1 applicator dose intravaginally twice each day for 10 days which may need to be reduced to 1 dose daily, depending upon response. *Avoid use*: children, kidney disorders. *Side effects*: allergic reactions. *Manufacturer*: Janssen-Cilag.

SUPRAX

Description: an antibiotic cephalosporin available as film-coated, scored white tablets containing 200mg cefixime marked LL200 and SUPRAX. Also, **SUPRAX PAEDIATRIC SUSPENSION** containing 100mg/5ml solution. *Used for*: infections of urinary and respiratory tract. *Dosage*: 200–400mg as single or 2 divided doses for 7 to 14 days. Children, age 6 to 12 months, 3.75ml; 1 to 4 years, 5ml; 5 to 10 years, 10ml; 11 to 12 years, 15ml. All as daily doses of paediatric suspension. *Special care*: pregnancy, breast-feeding, allergy to ß-lactams, serious kidney disorders. *Avoid use*: children under 6 months. *Side effects*: rashes, gastro-intestinal upset, headache, dizziness. Rarely, pseudomembranous colitis. *Manufacturer*: R.P.R.

SUPRECUR

Description: a preparation which is a GnRH (gonadotrophin-releasing hormone) analogue that acts on the pituitary gland inhibiting the release of gonadotrophin, resulting in a lowering of the levels of oestrogen produced by the ovaries. It is available in the form of a nasal spray, with pump, delivering a metered dose of 150µg buserelin (as acetate) per application. *Used for*: endometriosis, pituitary desensitization prior to controlled stimulation of the ovaries (with gonadotrophins) as a part of infertility treatment. *Dosage*: for endometriosis, 1 spray into each nostril in the morning, middle of the day and evening for a maximum period of 6 months. Treatment should begin on first or second day of monthly cycle. Infertility, 1 spray in 1 nostril 4 times each day, as directed by specialist, usually for 2 to 3 weeks. *Special care*: patients subject to depression or at risk of osteoporosis. Barrier methods of contraception must be used. *Avoid use*: pregnancy, breast-feeding, hormone-dependent tumours, undiagnosed vaginal bleeding. *Possible interaction*: nasal decongestants. *Side effects*: local irritation of nose, menopausal symptoms, e.g. hot flushes, change in libido, vaginal dryness, sweating, nausea, headache, changes in breasts and tenderness, cysts on ovaries, backache, dry skin, acne, rash, palpitations, changes in density of bones. *Manufacturer*: Shine.

SUPREFACT

Description: a gonadotrophin-releasing hormone analogue, acting on pituitary gland receptors resulting in the inhibition of the release of luteinizing hormone and lower levels of testosterone in the blood. Suprefact is available in vials for injection containing 1mg buserelin (as acetate)/ml. Also, **SUPREFACT NASAL SPRAY** containing 100 µg per dose. *Used for*: Stage C or D cancer of the prostate gland in which it is desirable for levels of testosterone to be reduced. *Dosage*: 0.5ml every 8 hours by subcutaneous injection for 1 week. Then 1 spray in each nostril 6 times each day as maintenance dose. *Special care*: anti-androgens may be needed. *Avoid use*: patients with tumours that are not responsive to hormones; those who have had 1 or both testes surgically removed (orchidectomy). *Side effects*: short-lived irritation of nostrils, loss of libido, hot flushes. *Manufacturer*: Shine.

SURGAM SA

Description: an NSAID which is a propionic acid available as sustained-release maroon/pink capsules enclosing white pellets containing 300mg tiaprofenic acid, marked SURGAM SA. Also, **SURGAM TABLETS**, white, in strengths of 200mg and 300mg, marked with symbol on one side and name and strength on the reverse. *Used for*: disorders of joints, skeleton and muscles including osteoarthritis, rheumatoid arthritis, lumbago, ankylosing spondylitis, injuries. *Dosage*: capsules, 2 as a single daily dose; tablets, 600mg as divided doses each day. *Special care*: pregnancy, breast-feeding, elderly, heart failure, liver or kidney disorders, known allergy to aspirin or NSAID. *Avoid use*: children, history of or active peptic ulcer. *Possible interaction*: sulphonamides, hypoglycaemics, diuretics, anticoagulants, hydantoins. *Side effects*: headache, gastro-intestinal upset, sleepiness, rash. Withdraw if cystitis and haematuria (blood in urine) occur (rare). *Manufacturer*: Hoechst.

SURMONTIL

Description: a TCAD preparation available as white tablets in strengths of 10mg and 25mg containing trimipramine (as maleate), both marked with strength and SURMONTIL. Also, **SURMONTIL CAPSULES**, white/green containing 50mg marked SU50. *Used for*: depression and/or anxiety, agitation, disturbance of sleep. *Dosage*: mild or moderate symptoms, 50–75mg as single dose, 2 hours before going to bed. Continue for a minimum of 3 weeks. Moderate to severe symptoms, 75mg each day under specialist supervision gradually increasing according to condition. Usual dose is in the order of 150–300mg each day then reducing for maintenance once condition improves. Elderly, 10–25mg 3 times each day. *Special care*: liver disorders, hyperthyroidism, glaucoma, lactation, epilepsy, diabetes, adrenal tumour, heart disease, urine retention. Psychotic or suicidal patients. *Avoid use*: heart block, heart attacks, severe liver disease, pregnancy. *Possible interaction*: MAOIs (or within 14 days of their use), alcohol, antidepressants, barbiturates, anticholinergics, local anaesthetics that contain adrenaline or noradrenaline, oestrogens, cimetidine, antihypertensives. *Side effects*: constipation, urine retention, dry mouth, blurred vision, palpitations, tachycardia, nervousness, drowsiness, insomnia. Changes in weight, blood and blood sugar, jaundice, skin reactions, weakness, ataxia, hypotension, sweating, altered libido, gynaecomastia, galactorrhoea. *Manufacturer*: R.P.R.

SURVANTA

Description: a lung surfactant available as a solution in single dose vials containing 25mg beractant (a natural lung extract)/ml. *Used for*: newborn babies with respiratory distress undergoing mechanical ventilation whose birthweight exceeds 700g and who are receiving continuous monitoring. *Dosage*: 100mg/kg body weight in volume not greater than 4ml/kg by endotracheal tube. Best given within 8 hours of birth and a maximum of 4 further doses at a minimum of 6 hourly intervals, may be given within 48 hours. *Special care*: continuous monitoring of oxygen level in arterial blood required. *Side effects*: endotracheal tube may become blocked by mucous, possible haemorrhage in lung. *Manufacturer*: Abbott.

SUSTAMYCIN

Description: a tetracycline antibiotic preparation available as sustained-release capsules in light and darker blue containing 250mg tetracycline hydrochloride. *Used for*: infections responsive to tetracyclines, severe acne. *Dosage*: infections, 2 capsules twice each day at first reducing to 1 as condition improves. Acne, 4 tablets each day for first 2 to 3 weeks then 1 for 3 to 4 months. *Special care*: liver or kidney disorders. *Avoid use*: pregnancy, breast-feeding, children. *Possible interaction*: mineral supplements, milk, antacids, oral contraceptives. *Side effects*: allergic responses, superinfections, gastro-intestinal upset. *Manufacturer*: B.M. Pharmaceuticals.

SUSTANON 100

Description: an hormonal depot androgen preparation available in ampoules for injection containing 20mg testosterone propionate, 40mg testosterone phenylpropionate, 40mg testosterone isocaproate/ml. Also, **SUSTANON 250** available in ampoules for injection containing 30mg testosterone propionate, 60mg testosterone phenylpropionate, 60mg testosterone isocaproate and 100mg testosterone decanoate/ml. *Used for*: androgen deficiency in males, osteoporosis resulting from androgen deficiency. *Dosage*: 1ml by deep intramuscular injection every 2 weeks; Sustanon 250, 1ml by deep intramuscular injection every 3 weeks. *Special care*: heart, liver or kidney disorders, migraine, hypertension, epilepsy. *Avoid use*: heart disease, heart failure which is untreated, cancer of prostate gland or liver, nephrotic syndrome (a kidney abnormality resulting from various diseases and disorders). *Possible interaction*: drugs which induce liver enzymes. *Side effects*: weight gain, liver tumours, oedema, reduced fertility, premature closure of epiphyses, priapism (painful and prolonged erection of penis not connected with sexual arousal but caused by drug treatment or sickle-cell trait. Causes tissue damage if not relieved by decompression). *Manufacturer*: Organon.

SYMMETRAL

Description: a dopaminergic, tricyclic amine preparation available as reddish-brown capsules containing 100mg amantadine hydrochloride marked GEIGY. Also, **SYMMETRAL SYRUP** containing 50mg amantadine hydrochloride/ml. *Used for*: Parkinsonism, prevention and treatment of patients with certain strains of influenza (A$_2$, A/New Jersey) who are at risk from complications. *Herpes zoster* infections. *Dosage*: Parkinsonism, 100mg capsules of syrup each day for 7 days at first then same dose twice daily. Influenza, treatment, 1 capsule twice each day for 5 to 7 days; prevention, 1 capsule twice each day for 7 to 10 days. *Herpes zoster*, 1 capsule or 10ml syrup twice each day for 14 to 28 days. Children, for influenza age over 10 years, treatment and prevention, 1 capsule in morning for 7 to 10 days. *Special care*: pregnancy, congestive heart failure, liver or kidney disorders, suffering from confusion. *Avoid use*: children under 10 years, serious kidney disease, history of or active stomach ulcer, history of convulsions. *Possible interaction*: anticholinergics, levodopa, CNS stimulants. *Side effects*: livedo reticularis (a disorder of the veins resulting in a mottled "fish-net" appearance of legs and occasionally arms), oedema in hands and feet, skin rash, gastro-intestinal upset, disturbance of vision, effects on central nervous system. *Manufacturer*: Geigy.

SYNACTHEN DEPOT

Description: a depot preparation of adrenal stimulating hormone available in ampoules for injection containing 1mg tetracosactrin acetate and zinc complex/ml. *Used for*: collagen and rheumatic disorders, Crohn's disease, ulcerative colitis. *Dosage*: acute treatment, 1–2g by intramuscular injection each day with reduced doses for maintenance. Children, age 1 month to 2 years, 0.25mg by intramuscular injection each day at first; 2 to 5 years, 0.25–0.5mg by intramuscular injection each day at first; 5 to 12 years, 0.25–1mg by intramuscular injection each day at first. For maintenance, these doses are repeated every 2 to 8 days. *Special care*: thrombophlebitis, psychoses, recent intestinal anastomoses, chronic nephritis, certain cancers, osteoporosis, peptic ulcer, skin eruption/rash related to a disease, viral, fungal or active infections, tuberculosis. Hypertension, glaucoma, epilepsy, acute glomerulonephritis (inflammation of kidney glomerulus), diabetes, cirrhosis, hypothyroidism, pregnancy, stress. To be withdrawn gradually. *Avoid use*: allergic conditions, asthma. *Possible interaction*: NSAIDs, oral anticoagulants, phenytoin, ephedrine, phenobarbitone, rifampicin, diuretics, cardiac glycosides, anticholinesterases, hypoglycaemics. *Side effects*: osteoporosis, depression, euphoria, hyperglycaemia, peptic ulcers, Cushingoid changes. *Manufacturer*: Ciba.

SYNALAR

Description: a potent topical steroid preparation available as cream and ointment containing 0.025% fluocinolone acetonide. **SYNALAR 1:4**, a moderately potent steroid cream and ointment containing 0.00625%. **SYNALAR CREAM 1:10**, a mildly potent steroid cream containing 0.0025%. **SYNALAR C** a combined potent steroid, antibacterial, antifungal cream and ointment containing 0.025% fluocinolone acetonide and 3% clioquinol. **SYNALAR N**, a potent steroid and antibacterial cream and ointment containing 0.025% fluocinolone acetonide and 0.5% neomycin sulphate. Also, **SYNALAR GEL** containing 0.025%

fluocinolone acetate. *Used for*: Synalar steroid preparations, skin conditions responsive to steroid treatment; Synalar combined preparations, infected skin conditions responsive to steroid treatment. Synalar Gel, skin conditions of the scalp responsive to steroid treatment. *Dosage*: apply thinly 2 or 3 times each day and rub in. Synalar Gel, rub into scalp in the morning and at night at first and then once or twice each week for maintenance. *Special care*: thrombophlebitis, psychoses, recent intestinal anastomoses, chronic nephritis, certain cancers, osteoporosis, peptic ulcer, skin eruption/rash related to a disease, viral, fungal or active infections, tuberculosis. Hypertension, glaucoma, epilepsy, acute glomerulonephritis (inflammation of kidney glomerulus), diabetes, cirrhosis, hypothyroidism, pregnancy, stress. To be withdrawn gradually. *Avoid use*: use only mild steroid preparations in children. *Possible interaction*: NSAIDs, oral anticoagulants, phenytoin, ephedrine, phenobarbitone, rifampicin, diuretics, cardiac glycosides, anticholinesterases, hypoglycaemics. *Side effects*: osteoporosis, depression, euphoria, hyperglycaemia, peptic ulcers, Cushingoid changes. *Manufacturer*: Zeneca.

SYNARD

Description: a gonadotrophin-releasing hormone analogue available as a nasal spray delivering 200µg nafarelin (as acetate) per metered dose. It acts on the pituitary gland to lower the levels of oestrogen produced by the ovaries and endometrial growth. *Used for*: endometriosis. *Dosage*: 1 spray into 1 nostril in the morning and then a second spray into the other nostril in the evening. Treatment should continue for a maximum period of 6 months and start between day 2 and 4 of monthly cycle. *Special care*: patients at risk of osteoporosis. Barrier methods of contraception should be used. *Avoid use*: pregnancy, breast-feeding, undiagnosed vaginal bleeding. Treatment should not be repeated. *Possible interaction*: nasal decongestants. *Side effects*: changes in libido and bone density, changes in breast size and tenderness. Menopausal symptoms, e.g. hot flushes, sweating, vaginal dryness, mood changes, depression, aches and cramps. Migraine, palpitations, cysts on ovaries, allergic hypersensitive responses, hair loss, blurring of vision. *Manufacturer*: Syntex.

SYNFLEX

Description: an NSAID available as film-coated orange tablets containing 275mg napoxen sodium marked SYNTEX. *Used for*: period pain, pain following operations, migraine, muscle and bone pains, strains and sprains. *Dosage*: age over 16 years, usual dose, 2 tablets as 1 dose then 1 tablet 6 to 8-hourly as required. Maximum dose is 4 tablets daily. Migraine, 3 tablets as first dose then 1 or 2 tablets 6 to 8-hourly with a daily maximum of 5. *Special care*: pregnancy, breast-feeding, elderly, liver or kidney disorders, history of lesions in gastrointestinal tract, heart failure, asthma. Patients taking drug long-term require careful monitoring. *Avoid use*: children under 16 years, known allergy to NSAID or aspirin, peptic ulcer. *Possible interaction*: sulphonylureas, anticoagulants, frusemide, ß-blockers, quinolones, ACE inhibitors, hydantoins, lithium probenecid, methotrexate. *Side effects*: blood changes, gastro-intestinal intolerance, vertigo, rash, tinnitus. *Manufacturer*: Roche.

SYNPHASE

Description: a combined oestrogen/progestogen oral contraceptive preparation available as: 7 white tablets containing 35µg ethinyloestradiol, 0.5mg norethisterone; 9 yellow tablets containing 35µg and 1mg norethisterone; 5 white tablets containing 35µg and 0.5mg respectively. All are marked SYNTEX and the white tablets also with a B. *Used for*: oral contraception. *Dosage*: 1 tablet each day starting on fifth day of period then 7 tablet-free days. *Special care*: multiple sclerosis, serious kidney disease or kidney dialysis, asthma, Raynaud's disease, abnormally high levels of prolactin in the blood (hyperprolactinaemia), varicose veins, hypertension, severe depression. Thrombosis risk increases with smoking, age and obesity. During the course of treatment, regular checks on blood pressure, pelvic organs and breasts should be carried out. *Avoid use*: pregnancy, patients at risk of thrombosis, suffering from heart disease, pulmonary hypertension, angina, sickle cell anaemia. Also, undiagnosed vaginal bleeding, history of cholestatic jaundice during pregnancy, cancers which are hormone-dependent, infectious hepatitis, liver disorders. Also, porphyria, Dublin-Johnson and Rotor syndrome, otosclerosis, chorea, haemolytic uraemic syndrome, recent trophoblastic disease. *Possible interaction*: barbiturates, ethosuximide, glutethimide, rifampicin, phenytoin, tetracyclines, carbamazepine, chloral hydrate, griseofulvin, dichloralphenazone, primidone. *Side effects*: weight gain, breast enlargement, pains in legs and cramps, headaches, loss of sexual desire, depression, nausea, breakthrough bleeding, cervical erosion, brownish patches on skin (chloasma), vaginal discharge, oedema and bloatedness. *Manufacturer*: Searle.

SYNTARIS

Description: a corticosteroid preparation available as a nasal spray delivering 25µg flunisolide per metered dose. *Used for*: allergic and inflammatory conditions affecting the nose, e.g. hay fever. *Dosage*: 2 sprays into each nostril 2, or maximum of 3, times each day reducing to a minimum effective dose for control. Treatment should continue long-term. Children, age 5 to 12 years, 1 spray in each nostril 3 times each day. *Special care*: pregnancy, patients who have had recent trauma or surgery, ulcers of the nose. Also, special care in patients changing from other steroid drugs. *Avoid use*: children under 5, untreated infections of nose or eyes. *Side effects*: short-lived irritation of nose. *Manufacturer*: Roche.

SYNTOCINON

Description: a uterotropic hormonal preparation containing synthetic oxytocin used in obstetrics, available as a solution in ampoules for injection at strengths of 2 units/2ml, 5 units/ml, 10 units/ml, 50 units/5ml. *Used for*: to induce and augment labour, missed abortion. *Dosage*: by slow intravenous infusion as a solution with 1 unit per litre, adjusted as needed. *Special care*: disorders of heart and heart circulation, hypertension, previous Caesarian section, abnormal presentation of baby, multiple birth. *Avoid use*: placental praevia, serious toxaemia, obstruction of delivery, distress in baby, hypertonic (very active) activity of uterus, tendency to amniotic fluid embolism. *Side effects*: danger of severe uterine contractions leading to rupture (with higher doses), hypertension and subarachnoid haemorrhage in mother, heart arrhythmias, water intoxication and lung oedema (infusion volume must be low). *Manufacturer*: Sandoz.

SYNTOMETRINE

Description: a uterotropic hormonal preparation used in obstetrics available as a solution in ampoules for injection containing 0.5mg ergometrine maleate and 5 units synthetic oxytocin/ml. *Used for*: bleeding due to incomplete abortion (before surgery to remove contents of uterus), during delivery (third stage of labour) after or when baby's shoulders have emerged. *Dosage*: 1ml by intramuscular injection. *Special care*: porphyria, multiple birth, hypertension, heart disease, liver or kidney disease. *Avoid use*: serious heart, liver, kidney or lung disease, severe hypertension, sepsis, circulatory disease, toxaemia, in first or second stage of labour. *Side effects*: vomiting and nausea, short-lived hypertension, constriction of blood vessels, heart attack, stroke, lung oedema. *Manufacturer*: Sandoz.

SYNTOPRESSIN

Description: a vasopressin analogue available as a solution for use with a nasal spray delivering 50 units lypressin/ml. *Used for*: diabetes insipidus. *Dosage*: 1 or 2 sprays into one or both nostrils 3 to 7 times a day. *Special care*: pregnancy, patients with epilepsy, hypertension, disease of peripheral blood vessels, hypertension, advanced arteriosclerosis, heart failure. *Avoid use*: coronary heart disease, undergoing anaesthesia with cyclopropane or halothane. *Possible interaction*: chlorpropamide, lithium, carbamazepine, clofibrate. *Side effects*: blocked nose and ulceration of lining of nose, nausea, pain in abdomen, feeling of needing to defecate. *Manufacturer*: Sandoz.

T

TAGAMET

Description: an H_2 blocker cimetidine for treatment of ulcers, available in green tablets (200mg) and green oblong tablets (400mg) marked TAGAMET, SK & F and strength, and green oval tablets (800mg) marked SK & F and T 800. Also, **TAGAMET EFFERVESCENT**, 400mg white effervescent tablet and **TAGAMET SYRUP** (200mg/5ml). *Used for*: ulcers—duodenal, benign gastric, recurrent and stomach. Dyspepsia, oesophageal reflux and where gastric acid has to be reduced. *Dosage*: for duodenal ulcer, 800mg at bedtime or 400mg twice daily for 4 weeks, then half dose for maintenance. See literature for other conditions. Children over 1 year, 25–30mg/kg per day in divided doses. Also, **TAGAMET INJECTION** (200mg/2ml) and **TAGAMET INFUSION** (400mg in 100ml). *Special care*: eliminate malignancy first; kidney disorder, pregnancy, breast-feeding. *Possible interaction*: theophylline, oral anticoagulants, phenytoin. *Side effects*: rash, dizziness, tiredness, diarrhoea, confusion, gynaecomastia; rarely pancreatitis, thrombocytopenia, muscle and joint pain. *Manufacturer*: SmithKline Beecham.

TAMBOCOR

Description: a class I antiarrhythmic, flecainide acetate, available as white tablets marked 3M TR 50 (50mg) or 3M TR 100 (100mg). *Used for*: tachycardia, arrhythmias. *Dosage*: 50–100mg twice per day to a maximum of 400mg daily, depending upon condition, reduced after 3 to 5 days to the lowest possible maintenance dose. Not for children. Also, **TAMBOCOR INJECTION**, 10mg/ml in ampoules. *Dosage*: see literature. Not for children. *Special care*: start therapy in hospital. Pacemakers, weak liver or kidneys, heart disease, pregnancy. Monitor plasma levels. *Avoid use*: heart failure, past myocardial infarction, 2nd or 3rd degree atrioventricular block, sinus node disease, atrial fibrillation. *Possible interaction*: digoxin, other class I antiarrhythmics, cardiac depressants. *Side effects*: nausea, dizziness, vomiting, sight disturbances, sensitivity to light, jaundice, upset to liver enzymes, ataxia, tingling sensations. *Manufacturer*: 3m Health Care.

TAMOFEN

Description: an antioestrogen, tamoxifen citrate, available as white tablets with 10mg (marked T10), 20mg (T20) and 40mg (T40). *Used for*: infertility, breast cancer. *Dosage*: 20mg per day for 4 days starting on second day on menstruation increasing to 40g and then 80mg for later treatments if required. For breast cancer 20mg per day increasing to 40mg if required. *Avoid use*: pregnancy. *Possible interaction*: warfarin. *Side effects*: gastro-intestinal upset, hot flushes, vaginal bleeding, dizziness, disturbance to sight. *Manufacturer*: Pharmacia & Upjohn.

TAMPOVAGAN

Description: an oestrogen, stilboestrol, available as a pessary with 5% lactic acid. *Used for*: vaginitis after the menopause. *Dosage*: 2, high in the vagina at night for 2 to 3 weeks. Not for children. *Special care*: patients considered to be at risk of thrombosis or with liver disease. Women with any of the following disorders should be carefully monitored: fibroids in the womb, multiple sclerosis, diabetes, tetany, porphyria, epilepsy, liver disease, hypertension, migraine, otosclerosis, gallstones. Breasts, pelvic organs and blood pressure should be checked at regular intervals during the course of treatment. *Avoid use*: pregnancy, breast-feeding, conditions which might lead to thrombosis, thrombophlebitis, serious heart, kidney or liver disease, breast cancer, oestrogen-dependent cancers including those of reproductive system, endometriosis, vaginal bleeding which is undiagnosed. *Possible interaction*: drugs which induce liver enzymes. *Side effects*: tenderness and enlargement of breasts, weight gain, breakthrough bleeding, giddiness, vomiting and nausea, gastro-intestinal upset. Treatment should be halted immediately if severe headaches occur, disturbance of vision, hypertension or any indications of thrombosis, jaundice. Also, in the event of pregnancy and 6 weeks before planned surgery. *Manufacturer*: Co-Pharma.

TARCORTIN

Description: a mild steroid and anti-psoriatic, comprising 0.5% hydrocortisone and 5% coal tar extract in a cream. *Used for*: eczema, psoriasis and other skin disorders. *Dosage*: apply twice or more per day. *Special care*: thrombophlebitis, psychoses, recent intestinal anastomoses, chronic nephritis, certain cancers, osteoporosis, peptic ulcer, skin eruption/rash related to a disease, viral, fungal or active infections, tuberculosis. Hypertension, glaucoma, epilepsy, acute glomerulonephritis (inflammation of kidney glomerulus), diabetes, cirrhosis, hypothyroidism, pregnancy, stress. To be withdrawn gradually. *Possible interaction*: NSAIDs, oral anticoagulants, phenytoin, ephedrine, phenobarbitone, rifampicin, diuretics, cardiac glycosides, anticholinesterases, hypoglycaemics. *Side effects*: osteoporosis, depression, euphoria, hyperglycaemia, peptic ulcers, Cushingoid changes. *Manufacturer*: Stafford-Miller.

TARGOCID

Description: a glycopeptide and antibiotic, teicoplanin, available as powder in vials (200 and 400mg). *Used for*: serious Gram-positive infections or staphylococcal infections where there is no response or a sensitivity to penicillins or cephalosporins. *Dosage*: 400mg intravenously on first day, then 200mg per day. For severe infections, 400mg intravenously every 12 hours for 3 doses then 400mg daily. Over 85kg, 3–6mg/kg but see literature. If kidney disease, reduce dose from day 4. Children, up to 2 months, 16mg/kg on first day, tnen 8mg/kg per day; over 2 months, 10mg/kg every 12 hours for 3 doses then 6mg/kg per day. For severe infections 10mg/kg every 12 hours for 3 doses then same dose daily. *Special care*: check blood, liver and kidneys regularly. *Avoid use*: pregnancy, lactation. *Side effects*: thrombophlebitis, rash, fever, reaction at site of injection, bronchospasm, nausea, vomiting, dizziness, diarrhoea, blood changes. *Manufacturer*: Hoechst.

TARIVID

Description: a 4-quinolone antibiotic, ofloxacin, available as white, oblong tablets (200mg) and yellow, oblong tablets (400mg). *Used for*: infections of the urinary tract, respiratory tract. Sexually transmitted diseases. *Dosage*: 200–400mg per day depending upon the infection and its severity. Doses over 400mg to be given as 2 divided doses. Not for children. Also, **TARIVID INFUSION**,

2mg/ml ofloxacin hydrochloride. *Used for*: infections of the respiratory tract, upper and lower urinary tract, septicaemia. *Dosage*: 200–800mg per day for 7 to 10 days, varying according to infection and its severity. Not for children. *Special care*: kidney damage, psychiatric disorders, exposure to UV light or strong sunlight, when driving or operating machinery. *Avoid use*: pregnancy, breast-feeding, history of epilepsy, growing adolescents. *Possible interaction*: NSAIDs, anticoagulants, iron, antacids with aluminium or magnesium. Hypotensives, barbiturate anaesthetics (for injection). *Side effects*: skin reactions, convulsions, disturbances to CNS, gastro-intestinal upset, hypersensitivity reactions, colitis. For injection—thrombophlebitis, pain at the site of injection, hypotension. *Manufacturer*: Hoechst.

TAXOL

Description: a taxane, paclitaxel, available as a solution (6mg/ml) in vials. *Used for*: ovarian cancer (metastatic) resistant to treatment with platinum. *Dosage*: 175mg/m² by intravenous infusion over 3 hours, repeated 3-weekly. Additional, preliminary treatment necessary with antihistamines, H_2-antagonists and corticosteroids. *Special care*: abnormalities in heart conduction, disease of peripheral nerves, liver or kidney failure. Check blood. Have resuscitation equipment available. *Avoid use*: if neutrophils are low, pregnancy, lactation, severe liver damage. *Side effects*: peripheral nerve disease, suppression of bone marrow, joint and muscle pain, hair loss, hypotension, gastro-intestinal upset, bradycardia, oedema. *Manufacturer*: BMS.

TAZOCIN

Description: a ß-lactamase inhibitor (active against ß-lactamase-producing bacteria) and broad spectrum penicillin comprising piperacillin (2g) with tazobactam (250mg) both as sodium salts also as 4g/500mg both as powder in vials. *Used for*: infections of the lower respiratory tract, urinary tract, of the skin, abdominal. Septicaemia and infections caused by more than 1 organism. *Dosage*: 4.5g every 8 hours by slow intravenous infusion or injection. Not for children. *Special care*: pregnancy, breast-feeding, kidney failure, low potassium levels. *Possible interaction*: drugs that affect blood coagulation or platelet function, probenecid. *Side effects*: allergic reactions, superinfection, gastro-intestinal upset, skin reactions. *Manufacturer*: Wyeth.

TEGRETOL

Description: an iminostilbene and diben-zazepine, carbamazepine, available as white tablets (100 and 200mg) marked with name and strength, and white oblong tablets (400mg) marked with name and strength. Also, **TEGRETOL CHEWTABS**, 100 and 200mg as square, pale orange chewable tablets marked T, tablet strength and name. **TEGRETOL RETARD**, 200mg in continuous-release, orange, oblong tablets marked CG and 400mg tablets coloured brown and marked CG and ENE. Also, **TEGRETOL LIQUID**, a sugar-free liquid containing 100mg/5ml. *Used for*: prevention of manic depressive psychosis which does not respond to therapy with lithium, epilepsy, trigeminal neuralgia. *Dosage*: manic depression—start with 400mg per day in divided doses and increase until the symptoms are controlled (to a maximum of 1.6g per day), usually 400–600mg. Epilepsy, start with 100–200mg once or twice per day increasing to 800mg–1.2g and a maximum of 1.6g. Children, 10 to 15 years, 600mg–1g; 5 to 10 years, 400–600mg; 1 to 5 years, 200–400mg; up to 1 year, 100–200mg. All per day, in divided doses. Neuralgia, start with 100mg once or twice per day increasing to gain control, usually 600–800mg per day in divided doses (daily maximum 1.6g). *Special care*: pregnancy, breast-feeding, liver and kidney disease, elderly, severe cardiovascular disease. Check blood and liver function. *Avoid use*: abnormalities in atrioventricular conduction (heart conduction block). *Possible interaction*: MAOIs, combined oral contraceptives, oral anticoagulants, steroids, lithium, phenytoin, cimetidine, dextropropoxyphene, doxycycline, isoniazid, erythromycin, diltiazem, verapamil, viloxazine. *Side effects*: double vision, dry mouth, dizziness, drowsiness, gastric upset, oedema, rashes, blood changes, hair loss, toxic epidermal necrolysis (a rare skin disease producing exfoliation), kidney failure, hepatitis, enlargement of lymph nodes, changes in heart conduction, jaundice. *Manufacturer*: Geigy.

TEMAZEPAM CD

Description: an intermediate benzodiazepine and hypnotic, temazepam, available as a solution (10mg/5ml). Also, **TEMAZEPAM TABLETS** (10 and 20mg) and **TEMAZEPAM GEL FILLED**, 10, 15, 20 and 30mg gel-filled capsules. *Used for*: insomnia. *Dosage*: 10–30mg at bedtime (elderly, 5–15mg). For severe cases, up to 60mg maximum. Not for children. *Special care*: chronic liver or kidney disease, chronic lung disease, pregnancy, labour, lactation, elderly. May impair judgement. Withdraw gradually and avoid prolonged use. *Avoid use*: depression of respiration, acute lung disease; psychotic, phobic or obsessional states. *Possible interaction*: anticonvulsants, depressants of the CNS, alcohol. *Side effects*: ataxia, confusion, light-headedness, drowsiness, hypotension, gastrointestinal upsets, disturbances in vision and libido, skin rashes, retention of urine, vertigo. Sometimes jaundice or blood disorders. *Manufacturer*: non-proprietary.

TEMGESIC CD

Description: an opiate and analgesic, buprenorphine hydrochloride, available as white, sublingual tablets (200 and 400μg) marked with 2 or 4 and symbol. *Used for*: moderate to severe pain. *Dosage*: 200–400μg sublingually every 6 to 8 hours or as required. Children, not for under 16kg; 16–25kg, 100μg; 25–37.5kg, 100–200μg; 37.5–50kg, 200–300μg, taken sublingually every 6 to 8 hours. Also, **TEMGESIC INJECTION** (300μg/ml in ampoules). *Dosage*: 300–600μg every 6 to 8 hours, by intramuscular or slow, intravenous injection. Children, not for under 6 months; over 6 months, 3–6μg/kg every 6 to 8 hours to a maximum of 9μg/kg. *Special care*: pregnancy, labour, reduced breathing or liver functions, dependence on narcotics or large doses previously. *Possible interaction*: depressants of the CNS, MAOIs. *Side effects*: nausea, dizziness, drowsiness, sweating. *Manufacturer*: Reckitt & Colman.

TEMOPEN

Description: a penicillin, temocillin (as sodium) that is resistant to penicillinase, available as powder (1g) in vials. *Used for*: septicaemia, infections of the urinary and lower respiratory tracts caused by Gram-negative bacilli which are susceptible to temocillin. *Dosage*: 1–2g every 12 hours intramuscularly or intravenously. For urinary tract infection, 1g per day. Contact manufacturer re dosage for children. *Special care*: pregnancy, breast-feeding, kidney disease. *Side effects*: pain at the point of injection, diarrhoea. Discontinue if rash occurs. *Manufacturer*: Bencard.

TENIF

Description: a cardioselective ß-blocker and class II calcium antagonist, atenolol (50mg) with nifedipine (20mg) available in red-brown capsules marked with TENIF and logo. *Used for*: angina, hypotension. *Dosage*: 1 capsule twice per day (angina); 1 per day increasing to 2 per day if necesssary (elderly, 1) for hypertension. Not for children. *Special care*: anaesthesia, diabetes, liver or kidney disease, weak heart or heart conduction defect. *Avoid use*: heart failure, heart block, cardiagenic shock, pregnancy, breast-feeding. *Possible interaction*: heart depressants, quinidine, cimetidine. *Side effects*: oedema, headache, dizziness, flushes, rash, dry eyes, jaundice, hyperplasia of the gums. *Manufacturer*: Zeneca.

TENORET 50

Description: a cardioselective ß-blocker and thiazide diuretic comprising 50mg atenolol and 12.5mg chlorthalidone in brown tablets marked TENORET 50 and logo. *Used for*: hypertension, especially in the elderly. *Dosage*: 1 tablet per day. Not for children. *Special care*: history of bronchospasm and certain ß-blockers, diabetes, liver or kidney disease, pregnancy, lactation, general anaesthesia, gout, check electrolyte levels, K^+ supplements may be required depending on the case. Withdraw gradually. Not for children. *Avoid use*: heart block or failure, slow heart rate (bradycardia), sick sinus syndrome (associated with sinus node disorder), certain ß-blockers, severe peripheral arterial disease, pregnancy, lactation, severe kidney failure, anuria, hepatic cornea. Possible interaction: verapamil, hypoglycaemics, reserpine, clonidine withdrawal, some antiarrhythmics and anaesthetics, antihypertensives, depressants of the CNS, cimetidine, indomethacin, sympathomimetics, lithium, potassium supplements with potassium-sparing diuretics, digitalis. *Side effects*: bradycardia, cold hands and feet, disturbance to sleep, heart failure, gastro-intestinal upset, tiredness on exertion, bronchospasm, gout, weakness, blood disorders, sensitivity to light. *Manufacturer*: Zenecon.

TENORETIC

Description: a cardioselective ß-blocker and thiazide diuretic containing 100mg atenolol, 25mg chlorthalidone in brown tablets marked with logo and TENORETIC. *Used for*: hypertension. *Dosage*: 1 tablet per day. Not for children. *Special care*: history of bronchospasm and certain ß-blockers, diabetes, liver or kidney disease, pregnancy, lactation, general anaesthesia, gout, check electrolyte levels, K^+ supplements may be required depending on the case. Withdraw gradually. Not for children. *Avoid use*: heart block or failure, slow heart rate (bradycardia), sick sinus syndrome (associated with sinus node disorder), certain ß-blockers, severe peripheral arterial disease, pregnancy, lactation, severe kidney failure, anuria, hepatic cornea. *Possible interaction*: verapamil, hypoglycaemics, reserpine, clonidine withdrawal, some antiarrhythmics and anaesthetics, antihypertensives, depressants of the CNS, cimetidine, indomethacin, sympathomimetics, lithium, potassium supplements with potassium-sparing diuretics, digitalis. *Side effects*: bradycardia, cold hands and feet, disturbance to sleep, heart failure, gastro-intestinal upset, tiredness on exertion, bronchospasm, gout, weakness, blood disorders, sensitivity to light. *Manufacturer*: Zeneca.

TENORMIN

Description: a cardioselective ß-blocker, atenolol, available in white tablets (25mg, marked with TENORMIN, 25 and logo) and orange tablets (100mg, marked with TENORMIN and logo). Also, **TENORMIN LS**, 50mg orange tablets marked 9 with name and **TENORMIN SYRUP**, a lemon-lime sugar-free syrup containing 25mg/ml. Also available as **TENORMIN INJECTION** (0.5mg/ml in 10ml ampoule). *Used for*: cardiac arrhythmias, early treatment of acute myocardial infarction, angina, hypertension. *Dosage*: 50–100mg per day, reduced for the elderly or where there is kidney disorder. Not for children. *Special care*: history of bronchospasm and certain ß-blockers, diabetes, liver or kidney disease, pregnancy, lactation, general anaesthesia. Withdraw gradually. Not for children. *Avoid use*: heart block or failure, slow heart rate (bradycardia), sick sinus syndrome (associated with sinus node disorder), certain ß-blockers, severe peripheral arterial disease. *Possible interaction*: verapamil, hypoglycaemics, reserpine, clonidine withdrawal, some antiarrhythmics and anaesthetics, antihypertensives, depressants of the CNS, cimetidine, indomethacin, sympathomimetics. *Side effects*: bradycardia, cold hands and feet, disturbance to sleep, heart failure, gastro-intestinal upset, tiredness on exertion, bronchospasm. *Manufacturer*: Zeneca.

TENUATE DOSPAN^{CD}

Description: a CNS stimulant, diethylpropion hydrochloride, available as sustained-release, white, oblong tablets marked MERRELL. *Used for*: obesity. *Dosage*: 1 tablet mid-morning. Not for children. *Special care*: angina, peptic ulcer, hypertension, arrhythmias. *Avoid use*: severe hypertension, arteriosclerosis, hyperthyroidism, glaucoma, pregnancy, breast-feeding, past drug or alcohol abuse or psychiatric illness. *Possible interaction*: other anoretics, antihypertensives, antidiabetics, guanethidine, methyldopas, MAOIs, sympathomimetics, psychotropics. *Side effects*: dependence, tolerance, psychoses, agitation, sleeplessness. Do not use over long period. *Manufacturer*: Merrell Dow.

TEOPTIC

Description: a ß-blocker, carteolol hydrochloride, available as 1% and 2% drops. *Used for*: hypertension in the eye, certain glaucomas. *Dosage*: start with 1 drop of 1% solution in affected eye twice per day. Use 2% solution if 1% is ineffective. Not for children. *Special care*: heart block, cardiogenic shock, diabetes. *Avoid use*: heart failure, asthma, serious lung disease, pregnancy, soft or gaspermeable contact lenses. *Possible interaction*: other ß-blockers. *Side effects*: blurred vision, burning sensation, pain, irritation of the eye, hyperaemia (greater than normal amount of blood in the vessels). *Manufacturer*: Ciba Vision.

TERRA-CORTRIL

Description: an antibiotic 0.5% oxytetracycline hydrochloride, with a mild steroid, 0.17% hydrocortisone, in a spray. *Used for*: infected eczema, infected intertrigo (dermatitis of skin surfaces in contact), insect bites. *Dosage*: spray 2 to 4 times per day. Not for children. Also **TERRA-CORTRIL OINTMENT**, 3% oxytetracycline hydrochloride with 1% hydrocortisone. *Dosage*: use 2 to 4 times per day. Not for children. Also, **TERRA-CORTRIL NYSTATIN**, as for the ointment but with 100,000 units nystatin (an antifungal). *Used for*: infected skin conditions. *Dosage*: apply 2 to 4 times per day. Not for children. *Special care*: thrombophlebitis, psychoses, recent intestinal anastomoses, chronic nephritis, certain cancers, osteoporosis, peptic ulcer, skin eruption/rash related to a disease, viral, fungal or active infections, tuberculosis. Hypertension, glaucoma, epilepsy, acute glomerulonephritis (inflammation of kidney glomerulus), diabetes, cirrhosis, hypothyroidism, pregnancy, stress. To be withdrawn gradually. *Possible interaction*: NSAIDs, oral anticoagulants, phenytoin, ephedrine, phenobarbitone, rifampicin, diuretics, cardiac glycosides, anticholinesterases, hypoglycaemics. *Side effects*: osteoporosis, depression, euphoria, hyperglycaemia, peptic ulcers, Cushingoid changes. *Also*, an antibiotic/corticosteroid combination with 5mg oxytetracycline hydrochloride, 15mg hydrocortisone acetate and 10,000 units/ml polymyxin in B sulphate, in drop form. *Used for*: external ear infections. *Dosage*: 2 to 4 drops 3 times per day for up to 7 days. Not for children. *Avoid use*: pregnancy, perforated ear drum, infections of a viral, fungal or tuberculous nature or those containing pus. *Side effects*: superinfection, allergy. *Manufacturer*: Pfizer.

TERRAMYCIN

Description: a tetracycline, oxytetracycline, available as yellow tablets (250mg) marked Pfizer. Also, **TERRAMYCIN CAPSULES**, 250mg in yellow capsules marked TER 250 and Pfizer. *Used for*: infections sensitive to Terramycin; severe acne. *Dosage*: 250–500mg 4 times per day. Not for children. *Special care*: liver or kidney disease. *Avoid use*: pregnancy, breast-feeding. *Possible interaction*: antacids, mineral supplements, milk, oral contraceptives. *Side effects*: superinfections, allergic reactions, gastro-intestinal upsets. *Manufacturer*: Pfizer.

TERTROXIN

Description: a thyroid hormone, liothyronine sodium (20µg), in white tablets marked with EVANS and name. *Used for*: severe thyroid deficiency, myxoedema coma. *Dosage*: start with 10–20µg 8-hourly increasing after 7 days if required to 60µg per day in divided doses. For elderly and children, start with 5µg per day in divided doses. *Special care*: diabetes, breast-feeding. *Avoid use*: angina caused by effort, cardiovascular problems. *Possible interaction*: phenytoin, anticoagulants, tricyclics, cholestyramine. *Side effects*: tachycardia, arrhythmias, muscle cramps or weakness, anginal pain, flushes, headache, sweating, diarrhoea, weight loss, excitability. *Manufacturer*: Link.

TETAVAX

Description: a purified tetanus toxoid vaccine containing 40 units/0.5ml on aluminium hydroxide in syringes, ampoules and vials. *Used for*: immunization and booster doses. *Dosage*: first immunization: 0.5ml, then 0.5ml after 1 month and 0.5ml after 1 more month. Reinforcing (booster) doses: 0.5ml 10 years after first immunization. When required after injuries, 0.5ml single dose unless a booster has been administered in previous 12 months. All given by deep subcutaneous or intramuscular injection. *Special care*: hypersensitivity may occur if a dose is given within 12 months of a booster. *Avoid use*: acute infectious disease unless in a wound susceptible to tetanus. *Side effects*: malaise, fever. *Manufacturer*: Pasteur Merieux MSD.

TETRABID

Description: 250mg tetracycline hydrochloride in purple/yellow sustained-release capsules. *Used for*: acne, infections sensitive to this drug such as bronchitis. *Dosage*: 1 capsule per day for at least 3 months (acne). For infections, start with 2 capsules then 1 every 12 hours. Not for children. *Special care*: liver or kidney disorder. *Avoid use*: pregnancy, breast-feeding. *Possible interaction*: antacids, mineral supplements, milk, digoxin, oral anticoagulants, oral contraceptives. *Side effects*: superinfections, allergic reactions, gastro-intestinal upset. Cease use if there is intracranial hypertension. *Manufacturer*: Organon.

TETRALYSAL

Description: a tetracycline, lymecycline (408mg), in white capsules marked Farmitalia. *Used for*: acne; infections of the skin and soft tissue; ear, nose and throat or the respiratory tract. *Dosage*: 1 twice per day (for at least 8 weeks in the case of acne). Not for children. *Special care*: liver and kidney disorders. *Avoid use*: pregnancy, breast-feeding. *Possible interaction*: mineral supplements, antacids, oral contraceptives. *Side effects*: superinfections, allergic reactions, gastro-intestinal upset. *Manufacturer*: Galderma.

TICAR

Description: a penicillin, ticarcillin sodium, available as a 5g infusion bottle and powder in vials. *Used for*: septicaemia, peritonitis, infections of the urinary or respiratory tract, infected wounds, endocarditis and post-operative infections especially those caused by *Pseudomonas aeruginosa*. *Dosage*: up to 20g by slow intravenous injection or rapid infusion (children 300mg/kg) or up to 4g per day intramuscularly and in divided doses (children 100mg/kg). *Special care*: kidney disease. *Side effects*: gastro-intestinal upset, hypersensitivity reactions. *Manufacturer*: Link.

TILADE SYNCRONER

Description: an anti-inflammatory and non-steroid, nedocromil sodium, available as a mint-flavoured suspension delivered by aerosol with spacer device (2mg). Also, **TILADE**, utilizing a metered dose aerosol *Used for*: bronchial asthma where anti-inflammatory control is required. *Dosage*: start with 2 puffs 4 times per day (2 puffs twice per day for maintenance). Not for children. *Special care*: pregnancy. *Side effects*: cough, passing headache, gastro-intestinal upset. *Manufacturer*: R.P.R.

TILDIEM

Description: a class III calcium antagonist, diltiazem hydrochloride, available as off-white tablets (60mg) marked TILDIEM 60. *Used for*: angina. *Dosage*: 60mg 3 times per day to a maximum of 480mg per day in divided doses. Not for children. Also, **TILDIEM RETARD**, white, sustained-release tablets (90 and 120mg). *Dosage*: start with 90mg or 120mg twice per day increasing if required to a maximum of 2 120mg tablets twice per day. Elderly; 60mg twice per day, increasing to 90 or 120mg. Not for children. Also, **TILDIEM LA**, white/yellow, sustained-release capsules containing 300mg. *Used for*: hypertension. *Dosage*: 1 at the same time every day. For the elderly, start with Retard 120mg each day. Using Retard–120mg twice per day increasing if required to 180mg twice daily. Elderly, 120mg daily to a maximum of 120mg twice per day. Not for children. *Special care*: check heart rate in elderly or cases of liver and kidney disorder. Monitor patients with mild bradycardia. *Avoid use*: pregnancy, bradycadia, heart block, sick sinus syndrome. *Possible interaction*: other antihypertensives, ß-blockers, heart depressants, digoxin, dantrolene infusion, cyclosporin, diazepam, lithium cimetidine, theophylline, carbamazepine. *Manufacturer*: Lorex.

TIMECEF

Description: a cephalosporin antibiotic, cefodizime (as sodium salt) available in vials (1g). *Used for*: infections of the urinary and lower respiratory tracts. *Dosage*: 1g twice per day (respiratory tract), 2g per day as 1 or divided doses (urinary tract) by intravenous injection, infusion or intramuscular injection.

Not for children. *Special care*: sensitivity to penicillin, severe kidney disorder, pregnancy, breast-feeding, colitis. *Possible interaction*: aminoglycosides, loop diuretics. *Side effects*: gastro-intestinal upset, passing rise in liver enzymes, hypersensitivity reactions, eosinophilia (increase of eosinophils, a type of white blood cell, in the blood). *Manufacturer*: Hoechst.

TIMENTIN

Description: a ß-lactamase inhibitor with penicillin, comprising clavulanic acid (as potassium salt) with ticarcillin (as sodium salt) available as powder in vials (1.6 or 3.2g containing 100mg/1.5g and 200mg/3g). *Used for*: severe infections in patients in hospital with poor host defence to infection. *Dosage*: 3.2g every 6 to 8 hours by intermittent intravenous infusion to a maximum frequency of 4-hourly. Children up to 1 month, 80mg/kg every 12 hours, increasing to 8-hourly; others 80mg/kg every 6 to 8 hours. *Special care*: kidney disorder, severe liver disorder. *Side effects*: gastro-intestinal upset, hypersensitivity reactions, hepatitis. *Manufacturer*: Beecham.

TIMODINE

Description: a combined antifungal, mild steroid and disinfectant comprising 100,000 units/g nystatin, 0.5% hydrocortisone, 0.2% benzalkonium chloride solution with 10% dimethicone. *Used for*: skin disorders, severe nappy rash infected with *Candida*. *Dosage*: apply sparingly 3 times per day or at nappy change. *Special care*: thrombophlebitis, psychoses, recent intestinal anastomoses, chronic nephritis, certain cancers, osteoporosis, peptic ulcer, skin eruption/rash related to a disease, viral, fungal or active infections, tuberculosis. Hypertension, glaucoma, epilepsy, acute glomerulonephritis (inflammation of kidney glomerulus), diabetes, cirrhosis, hypothyroidism, pregnancy, stress. To be withdrawn gradually. *Possible interaction*: NSAIDs, oral anticoagulants, phenytoin, ephedrine, phenobarbitone, rifampicin, diuretics, cardiac glycosides, anticholinesterases, hypoglycaemics. *Side effects*: osteoporosis, depression, euphoria, hyperglycaemia, peptic ulcers, Cushingoid changes. *Manufacturer*: Reckitt & Colman.

TIMOPTIL

Description: a ß-blocker, timolol maleate, available as metered dose drops (0.25% and 0.5%). *Used for*: ocular hypertension, certain glaucomas. *Dosage*: 1 drop of 0.25% solution twice per day increasing to 0.5% solution if required. Not for children. *Special care*: pregnancy, breast-feeding, withdraw gradually. *Avoid use*: heart failure, heart block, asthma, sinus bradycardia, past obstructive lung disease, soft lenses. *Possible interaction*: adrenaline, antihypertensives, verapamil. *Side effects*: irritation, systemic ß-blocker effects (e.g. cold hands and feet, tiredness, stomach upset, rash). *Manufacturer*: M.S.D.

TINSET

Description: an antihistamine and mast cell stabilizer, oxatomide, available as white tablets (30mg) marked JANSSEN and Ox over 30. *Used for*: allergic rhinitis, urticaria, other allergic conditions. *Dosage*: 1 to 2 tablets twice per day; children over 5 up to 1 tablet twice per day. Not for children under 5. *Possible interaction*: depressants of the CNS, alcohol. *Side effects*: drowsiness, slowed reactions. *Manufacturer*: Janssen.

TOBRALEX

Description: an aminoglycoside, tobramycin, available as 0.3% drops. *Used for*: bacterial infections of the eye. *Dosage*: 1 or 2 drops every 4 hours, up to 2 drops every hour for severe cases. Reduce dose before ceasing treatment. *Side effects*: passing irritation. *Manufacturer*: Alcon.

TOFRANIL

Description: a TCAD, imipramine hydrochloride, available as red-brown triangular (10mg) and round (25mg) tablets, both marked GEIGY. Also, **TOFRANIL SYRUP** (25mg/5ml). *Used for*: depression; bedwetting in children. *Dosage*: 25mg 3 times per day, up to 150–200mg per day after 7 days. Maintenance dose, 50–100mg per day. Elderly, 10mg per day increasing to 30–50mg. Children: over 11 years, 10–15ml; 8 to 11 years, 5–10ml; 6 to 7 years, 5ml; at bedtime for 3 months maximum (withdraw gradually). Not for children under 6 years. *Special care*: liver disorders, hyperthyroidism, glaucoma, lactation, epilepsy, diabetes, adrenal tumour, heart disease, urine retention. Psychotic or suicidal patients. *Avoid use*: heart block, heart attacks, severe liver disease, pregnancy. *Possible interaction*: MAOIs (or within 14 days of their use), alcohol, antidepressants, barbiturates, anticholinergics, local anaesthetics that contain adrenaline or noradrenaline, oestrogens, cimetidine, antihypertensives. *Side effects*: constipation, urine retention, dry mouth, blurred vision, palpitations, tachycardia, nervousness, drowsiness, insomnia. Changes in weight, blood and blood sugar, jaundice, skin reactions, weakness, ataxia, hypotension, sweating, altered libido, gynaecomastia, galactorrhoea. *Manufacturer*: Geigy.

TOLANASE

Description: a sulphonylurea, tolazamide, available as white tablets marked UPJOHN 70 (100mg) or UPJOHN 114 (250mg). *Used for*: maturity-onset diabetes. *Dosage*: 100–250mg per day to a maximum of 1g if necessary (in divided doses). Not for children. *Special care*: elderly, kidney failure. *Avoid use*: during pregnancy or lactation; juvenile, growth-onset or unstable brittle diabetes (insulin-dependent diabetes mellitus); ketoacidosis; severe kidney or liver disorders; stress, infections or surgery; endocrine disorders. *Possible interaction*: MAOIs, corticosteroids, ß-blockers, diuretics, corticotrophin (ACTH), oral contraceptives, alcohol. Also aspirin, oral anticoagulants, and the generic drugs bezafibrate, clofibrate, phenylbutazone, cyclophosphamide, rifampicin, sulphonamides and chloramphenicol. Also glucagon. *Side effects*: skin rash and other sensitivity reactions. Other conditions tend to be rare, e.g. hyponatraemia (low blood sodium concentration) or aplastic anaemia. *Manufacturer*: Pharmacia & Upjohn.

TOLECTIN

Description: a derivative of acetic acid, tolmetin (as sodium salt), available as orange/ivory capsules marked T200 (200mg) or orange capsules marked T400 (400mg). *Used for*: osteoarthritis, rheumatoid arthritis, ankylosing spondylitis, juvenile rheumatoid arthritis, joint disorders. *Dosage*: 600–1800mg per day in 2 to 4 divided doses. Children, 20–25mg/kg per day in 3 or 4 divided doses. *Special care*: liver or kidney disease (check on long-term treatment), heart failure, past gastro-intestinal disease, pregnancy, breast-feeding, elderly. *Avoid use*: allergy to aspirin or anti-inflammatory drugs, active peptic ulcer. *Side effects*: oedema, rash, epigastric pain. *Manufacturer*: Cilag.

TOLERZIDE

Description: a non-cardioselective ß-blocker and thiazide diuretic comprising 80mg sotalol hydrochloride and 12.5mg hydrochlorothiazide in a lilac tablet marked TOLERZIDE. *Used for*: hypertension. *Dosage*: 1 tablet per day. Not for children. *Special care*: history of bronchospasm and certain ß-blockers, diabetes, liver or kidney disease, pregnancy, lactation, general anaesthesia, gout, check electrolyte levels, K^+ supplements may be required depending on the case. Withdraw gradually. *Avoid use*: heart block or failure, slow heart rate (bradycardia), sick sinus syndrome (associated with sinus node disorder), certain ß-blockers, severe peripheral arterial disease, pregnancy, lactation, severe kidney failure, anuria, hepatic cornea. *Possible interaction*: verapamil, hypoglycaemics, reserpine, clonidine withdrawal, some antiarrhythmics and anaesthetics, antihypertensives, depressants of the CNS, cimetidine, indomethacin, sympathomimetics, lithium, potassium supplements with potassium-sparing diuretics, digitalis. *Side effects*: bradycardia, cold hands and feet, disturbance to sleep, heart failure, gastro-intestinal upset, tiredness on exertion, bronchospasm, gout, weakness, blood disorders, sensitivity to light. *Manufacturer*: Bristol-Myers.

TONOCARD

Description: a class I antiarrhythmic, tocainide hydrochloride, available as yellow tablets marked A/TT (400mg). *Used for*: life-threatening ventricular arrhythmias. *Dosage*: 1.2g per day in 2 or 3 divided doses, to a maximum of 1.8–2.4g. Not for children. *Special care*: severe liver or kidney disease, elderly, heart failure, pregnancy. *Avoid use*: heart block in the absence of a pacemaker. *Possible interaction*: other anti-arrhythmics. *Side effects*: leucopenia, agranulocytosis, tremor, SLE, dizziness, gastro-intestinal upset. *Manufacturer*: Astra.

TOPICYCLINE

Description: an antibiotic, tetracycline hydrochloride, available as a 0.22% solution. *Used for*: acne. *Dosage*: apply liberally twice per day until the skin is wet. Not for children. *Special care*: kidney disease, pregnancy, breast-feeding. Avoid mouth, eyes and mucous membranes. *Side effects*: stinging. *Manufacturer*: Monmouth.

TOPILAR

Description: a potent steroid, fluclorolone acetonide, available as a cream (0.025%). Also **TOPILAR OINTMENT** (0.025%). *Used for*: skin disorders that respond to steroids, plaque psoriasis of soles and palms. *Dosage*: apply 2 times per day. *Special care*: thrombophlebitis, psychoses, recent intestinal anastomoses, chronic nephritis, certain cancers, osteoporosis, peptic ulcer, skin eruption/rash related to a disease, viral, fungal or active infections, tuberculosis. Hypertension, glaucoma, epilepsy, acute glomerulonephritis (inflammation of kidney glomerulus), diabetes, cirrhosis, hypothyroidism, pregnancy, stress. To be withdrawn gradually. *Possible interaction*: NSAIDs, oral anticoagulants, phenytoin, ephedrine, phenobarbitone, rifampicin, diuretics, cardiac glycosides, anticholinesterases, hypoglycaemics. *Side effects*: osteoporosis, depression, euphoria, hyperglycaemia, peptic ulcers, Cushingoid changes. *Manufacturer*: Bioglan.

TORADOL

Description: an NSAID, ketorolac trometamol, available as solutions (10mg/ml and 30mg/ml) in ampoules. *Used for*: short-term control of moderate or severe post-operative pain. *Dosage*: start with 10mg intravenously or intramuscularly then 10–30mg 4 to 6 hourly. Maximum 90mg daily for 2 days. Elderly, maximum 60mg daily for 2 days. Not for children under 16. Also, **TORADOL TABLETS**, 10mg in white tablets marked TORADOL 10 and SYNTEX. *Dosage*: 1 tablet 4 to 6 hourly, maximum 4 per day, for up to 7 days. If following injections, 90mg maximum dose on day 1 and 40mg thereafter. Elderly, 1 tablet 6 to 8-hourly for up to 7 days. Maximum dose after injections 60mg on day 1 and then 40mg. Not for children under 16. *Special care*: elderly; heart, liver kidney or allergic disease, gastro-intestinal disease. *Avoid use*: allergy to aspirin or anti-inflammatory drugs, pregnancy, breast-feeding, peptic ulcer, angioneurotic oedema, asthma, blood coagulation disorders, kidney disease, gastro-intestinal or cerebrovascular bleeding, low volume of circulating blood, dehydration, high risk of haemorrhage induced by surgery. *Possible interaction*: NSAIDs, anticoagulants, lithium, methotrexate, probenecid, frusemide, oxypentifylline. *Side effects*: ulcers, wound haemorrhage, gastro-intestinal upsets, drowsiness, oedema, kidney failure, bronchospasm, anaphylaxis, pain at site of injection, abnormal liver functions. *Manufacturer*: Roche.

TOTAMOL

Description: a cardioselective ß-blocker, atenolol, available as orange tablets (25, 50 and 100mg) each marked ATL, CP and with tablet strength. *Used for*: cardiac arrhythmias, early treatment of acute myocardial infarction; angina; hypertension. *Dosage*: 50–100mg per day, less for the elderly or where there is impaired kidney function. Not for children. *Special care*: history of bronchospasm and certain ß-blockers, diabetes, liver or kidney disease, pregnancy, lactation, general anaesthesia. Withdraw gradually. Not for children. *Avoid use*: heart block or failure, bradycardia, sick sinus syndrome (associated with sinus node disorder), certain ß-blockers, severe peripheral arterial disease. *Possible interaction*: verapamil, hypoglycaemics, reserpine, clonidine withdrawal, some antiarrhythmics and anaesthetics, antihypertensives, depressants of the CNS, cimetidine, indomethacin, sympathomimetics. *Side effects*: bradycardia, cold hands and feet, disturbance to sleep, heart failure, gastro-intestinal upset, tiredness on exertion, bronchospasm. *Manufacturer*: C.P. Pharm.

TRACRIUM

Description: a muscle relaxant, atracurium besylate, available in ampoules (10mg/ml). *Used for*: surgery, long-term ventilation. *Dosage*: start with 300–600µg/kg, then 100–200µg/kg as required, by intravenous injection; 5–10µg/kg/minute by intravenous infusion. *Special care*: respiration should be assisted until drug is inactivated or antagonized. *Avoid use*: myasthenia gravis. *Possible interaction*: lithium, nifedipine, verapamil. *Manufacturer*: Glaxo Wellcome.

TRANCOPAL

Description: a muscle relaxant and tranquillizer, chlormezanone, available in yellow tablets (200mg) marked TR. *Used for*: short-term treatment of insomnia, and anxiety where there is muscle tension; painful muscle spasms. *Dosage*: 200mg up to 4 times per day or 1 400mg dose at night. Half doses for the elderly. Not for children. *Special care*: liver or kidney disease, pregnancy. Judgement and dexterity may be impaired. *Avoid use*: porphyria. *Possible interaction*: alcohol, MAOIs, CNS depressants. *Side effects*: headache, dry mouth, nausea, lethargy, dizziness, rashes, jaundice. *Manufacturer*: Sanofi Winthrop.

TRANDATE

Description: an a/ß-blocker, labetolol hydrochloride, available as orange tablets (50, 100, 200 and 400mg) marked with name and strength. *Used for*: angina, hypertension. *Dosage*: start with 100mg twice per day with food, increasing at intervals of 14 days to a maximum of 2.4g per day in divided doses. Elderly start with 50mg twice per day. Not for children. Also, **TRANDATE INJECTION**, ampoules containing 5mg/ml. *Special care*: history of bronchospasm and certain ß-blockers, diabetes, liver or kidney disease, pregnancy, lactation, general anaesthesia. Withdraw gradually. Not for children. *Avoid use*: heart block or failure, slow heart rate, sick sinus syndrome (associated with sinus node disorder), certain ß-blockers, severe peripheral arterial disease. *Possible interaction*: verapamil, hypoglycaemics, reserpine, clonidine withdrawal, some antiarrhythmics and anaesthetics, antihypertensives, depressants of the CNS, cimetidine, indomethacin, sympathomimetics. *Side effects*: bradycardia, cold hands and feet, disturbance to sleep, heart failure, gastro-intestinal upset, tiredness on exertion, bronchospasm. Withdraw if liver reaction (rare). *Manufacturer*: Evans.

TRANXENE

Description: a long-acting benzodiazepine, clorazepate potassium available in capsules containing 15mg (pink/grey) and 7.5mg (maroon/grey), marked with TRANXENE, capsule strength and symbol. *Used for*: anxiety whether or not depression is present. *Dosage*: 7.5–22.5mg per day, elderly 7.5mg. Not for children under 16. *Special care*: chronic liver or kidney disease, chronic lung disease, pregnancy, labour, lactation, elderly. May impair judgement. Withdraw gradually and avoid prolonged use. *Avoid use*: depression of respiration, acute lung disease; psychotic, phobic or obsessional states. *Possible interaction*: anticonvulsants, depressants of the CNS, alcohol. *Side effects*: ataxia, confusion, light-headedness, drowsiness, hypotension, gastro-intestinal upsets, disturbances in vision and libido, skin rashes, retention of urine, vertigo. Sometimes jaundice or blood disorders. *Manufacturer*: Boehringer Ingelheim.

TRASICOR

Description: a non-cardioselective ß-blocker, oxprenolol hydrochloride, available as tablets containing 20 or 40mg (white), 80mg (beige) and 160mg (orange) all marked with strength, CIBA and TRASICOR. *Used for*: cardiac arrhythmias, angina, hypertension, anxiety. *Dosage*: from 20–160mg 2 or 3 times per day, depending upon condition being treated. Maximum daily dose 480mg. Not for children. *Special care*: history of bronchospasm and certain ß-blockers, diabetes, liver or kidney disease, pregnancy, lactation, general anaesthesia. Withdraw gradually. Not for children. *Avoid use*: heart block or failure, bradycardia, sick sinus syndrome (associated with sinus node disorder), certain ß-blockers, severe peripheral arterial disease. *Possible interaction*: verapamil, hypoglycaemics, reserpine, clonidine withdrawal, some antiarrhythmics and anaesthetics, antihypertensives, depressants of the CNS, cimetidine, indomethacin, sympathomimetics. *Side effects*: bradycardia, cold hands and feet, disturbance to sleep, heart failure, gastro-intestinal upset, tiredness on exertion, bronchospasm. *Manufacturer*: Ciba.

TRASIDREX

Description: a non-cardioselective ß-blocker and thiazide, comprising 160mg oxprenolol hydrochloride in a sustained-release core and 0.25mg cyclopenthiazide in a red outer coat. The tablet is marked with Ciba and TRASIDREX. *Used for*: hypertension. *Dosage*: start with 1 tablet each morning increasing to 3 per day if required. Not for children. *Special care*: history of bronchospasm and certain ß-blockers, diabetes, liver or kidney disease, pregnancy, lactation, general anaesthesia, gout, check electrolyte levels, K^+ supplements may be required depending on the case. Withdraw gradually. Not for children. *Avoid use*: heart block or failure, bradycardia, sick sinus syndrome (associated with sinus node disorder), certain ß-blockers, severe peripheral arterial disease; pregnancy, lactation, severe kidney failure, anuria, hepatic cornea. *Possible interaction*: verapamil, hypoglycaemics, reserpine, clonidine withdrawal, some antiarrhythmics and anaesthetics, antihypertensives, depressants of the CNS, cimetidine, indomethacin, sympathomimetics, lithium, potassium supplements with potassium-sparing diuretics, digitalis. *Side effects*: bradycardia, cold hands and feet, disturbance to sleep, heart failure, gastro-intestinal upset, tiredness on exertion, bronchospasm, gout, weakness, blood disorders, sensitivity to light. *Manufacturer*: Ciba.

TRASYLOL

Description: a haemostatic and antifibrinolytic, aprotinin, available as vials containing 500,000 units per 50ml. *Used for*: where there is risk of major blood loss during open heart surgery, or where blood conservation is vital, haemorrhage. *Dosage*: by slow intravenous injection or infusion, up to 2 or 3 million units. *Side effects*: localized thrombophlebitis, sometimes hypersensitivity reactions. *Manufacturer*: Bayer.

TRAVOGYN

Description: an antifungal drug, isoconazole nitrate, available as white, almond-shaped vaginal tablets (300mg) marked with CT in a hexagon. *Used for*: vaginal infections from *Candida* or mixed fungal and Gram-positive bacteria. *Dosage*: 2 tablets inserted in 1 dose. Not for children. *Side effects*: passing irritation and burning sensation. *Manufacturer*: Schering H.C.

TRAXAM

Description: an NSAID, felbinac, available as a 3% gel. Also, **TRAXAM FOAM** (3.17%). *Used for*: strains, sprains and injury to soft tissue. *Dosage*: 1g rubbed into the area 2 to 4 times per day initially for 14 days. Maximum daily usage 25g. Not for children. *Special care*: pregnancy, breast-feeding. *Avoid use*: allergy to aspirin or anti-inflammatory drugs. *Side effects*: dermatitis, itching, erythema. *Manufacturer*: Wyeth.

TRENTAL

Description: a peripheral vasodilator and xanthine, oxpentifylline, available in pink, oblong, sustained-release tablets (400mg). *Used for*: disorders of the peripheral vascular system. *Dosage*: 400mg 2 or 3 times per day. Not for children. *Special care*: coronary artery disease, hypotension, kidney disease. *Avoid use*: porphyria. *Possible interaction*: antihypertensives. *Side effects*: flushes, vertigo, gastro-intestinal upsets. *Manufacturer*: Hoechst.

TRI-ADCORTYL

Description: a potent steroid with antifungal and antibacterial comprising 0.1% triamcinolone acetate, 100,000 units/g nystatin, 0.25% neomycin sulphate and 0.025% gramicidin, as cream and ointment. *Used for*: inflamed skin disorders with infection. *Dosage*: use 2 to 4 times per day. *Special care*: thrombophlebitis, psychoses, recent intestinal anastomoses, chronic nephritis, certain cancers, osteoporosis, peptic ulcer, skin eruption/rash related to a disease, viral, fungal or active infections, tuberculosis. Hypertension, glaucoma, epilepsy, acute glomerulonephritis (inflammation of kidney glomerulus), diabetes, cirrhosis, hypothyroidism, pregnancy, stress. To be withdrawn gradually. *Possible interaction*: NSAIDs, oral anticoagulants, phenytoin, ephedrine, phenobarbitone, rifampicin, diuretics, cardiac glycosides, anticholinesterases, hypoglycaemics. *Side effects*: osteoporosis, depression, euphoria, hyperglycaemia, peptic ulcers, Cushingoid changes. *Manufacturer*: Squibb.

TRI-ADCORTYL OTIC

Description: a combined preparation of corticosteroid, antibiotic and antifungal containing 0.1% triamcinolone acetonide, 0.25% neomycin sulphate, 0.025% gramicidin and 100,000 units/g nystatin. *Used for*: inflammation of the outer ear. *Dosage*: use 2 to 4 times per day. *Special care*: pregnancy, perforated ear drum, do not use long-term in infants. *Avoid use*: viral and tuberculous lesions. *Manufacturer*: Squibb.

TRI-CICATRIN

Description: a topical corticosteroid containing 1% hydrocortisone, 250 units/g bacitracin zinc, 3400 units/g neomycin sulphate and 100,000 units/g nystatin, as an ointment. *Used for*: mild inflammatory skin disorders. *Dosage*: use 2 to 3 times per day, less frequently upon improvement. *Special care*: thrombophlebitis, psychoses, recent intestinal anastomoses, chronic nephritis, certain cancers, osteoporosis, peptic ulcer, skin eruption/rash related to a disease, viral, fungal or active infections, tuberculosis. Hypertension, glaucoma, epilepsy, acute glomerulonephritis (inflammation of kidney glomerulus), diabetes, cirrhosis, hypothyroidism, pregnancy, stress. To be withdrawn gradually. *Possible interaction*: NSAIDs, oral anticoagulants, phenytoin, ephedrine, phenobarbitone, rifampicin, diuretics, cardiac glycosides, anticholinesterases, hypoglycaemics. *Side effects*: osteoporosis, depression, euphoria, hyperglycaemia, peptic ulcers, Cushingoid changes *Manufacturer*: Wellcome.

TRI-MINULET

Description: an oestrogen/progestogen compound containing ethinyloestradiol and gestodene in 6 beige tablets (30/50μg) 5 dark brown tablets (40/70μg) and 10 white tablets (30/100μg respectively). *Used for*: oral contraception. *Dosage*: 1 tablet daily for 21 days starting on first day of menstruation, then 7 days without tablets. *Special care*: hypertension, Raynaud's disease (reduced blood supply to an organ of the body's extremities), asthma, severe depression, diabetes, varicose veins, multiple sclerosis, chronic kidney disease, kidney dialysis. Blood pressure, breasts and pelvic organs to be checked regularly; smoking not advised. *Avoid use*: history of heart disease, infectious hepatitis, sickle cell anaemia, porphyria, liver tumour, undiagnosed vaginal bleeding, pregnancy, hormone-dependent cancer, haemolytic uraemic syndrome (rare kidney disorder), chorea, otosclerosis. *Possible interaction*: barbiturates, tetracyclines, griseofulvin, rifampicin, primidone, phenytoin, chloral hydrate, ethosuximide, carbamazepine, glutethimide, dichloralphenazone. *Side effects*: fluid retention and bloating, leg cramps/pains, breast enlargement, depression, headaches, nausea, loss of libido, weight gain, vaginal discharge, cervical erosion (alteration of epithelial cells), chloasma (pigmentation of nose, cheeks or forehead), breakthrough bleeding (bleeding between periods). *Manufacturer*: Wyeth.

TRIADENE

Description: an oestrogen/progestogen compound containing ethinyloestradiol and gestodene in 6 beige tablets (30/50μg) 5 dark brown tablets (40/70μg) and 10 white tablets (30/100μg respectively). *Used for*: oral contraception. *Dosage*: 1 tablet daily for 21 days starting on first day of menstruation, then 7 days without tablets. *Special care*: hypertension, Raynaud's disease (reduced blood supply to an organ of the body's extremities), asthma, severe depression, diabetes, varicose veins, multiple sclerosis, chronic kidney disease, kidney dialysis. Blood pressure, breasts and pelvic organs to be checked regularly; smoking not advised. *Avoid use*: history of heart disease, infectious hepatitis, sickle cell anaemia, porphyria, liver tumour, undiagnosed vaginal bleeding, pregnancy, hormone-dependent cancer, haemolytic uraemic syndrome (rare kidney disorder), chorea, otosclerosis. *Possible interaction*: barbiturates, tetracyclines, griseofulvin, rifampicin, primidone, phenytoin, chloral hydrate, ethosuximide, carbamazepine, glutethimide, dichloralphenazone. *Side effects*: fluid retention and bloating, leg cramps/pains, breast enlargement, depression, headaches, nausea, loss of libido, weight gain, vaginal discharge, cervical erosion (alteration of epithelial cells), chloasma (pigmentation of nose, cheeks or forehead), breakthrough bleeding (bleeding between periods). *Manufacturer*: Schering H.C.

TRIAM-CO

Description: a potassium-sparing diuretic and thiazide, triamterene (50mg) and hydrochlorothiazide (25mg) in peach tablets marked with logo and TTRIAM-CO. *Used for*: oedema, hypertension. *Dosage*: start with 1 per day for hypertension; 1 twice per day after meals for oedema, reducing to 1 daily or 2 on alternate days. Maximum 4 per day. Not for children. *Special care*: diabetes, gout, pancreatitis, acidosis, liver or kidney disease, pregnancy, breast-feeding. *Avoid use*: severe kidney failure, hyperkalaemia, hypercalcaemia, Addison's disease, diabetic ketoacidosis, liver disorder. *Possible interaction*: potassium supplements, potassium-sparing diuretics, digitalis, lithium, NSAIDs, ACE inhibitors, antihypertensives. *Side effects*: headache, cramps, weakness, diarrhoea, nausea, vomiting, dry mouth, rash, hypotension, hypercalcaemia, hyperglycaemia, SLE, reversible kidney failure. *Manufacturer*: Baker Norton.

TRIBIOTIC

Description: an aminoglycoside and antibiotic in aerosol form containing 500,000 units neomycin sulphate, 10,000 units bacitracin zinc and 150,000 units/110g polymyxin B sulphate. *Used for*: prevention and control of infection during surgery. *Dosage*: apply 1 aerosol sparingly for a maximum of 7 days; (children 1 second/kg/day). *Special care*: pregnancy, breast-feeding, loss of hearing, large areas of damaged skin. *Avoid use*: burns. *Possible interaction*: other aminoglycoside antibiotics. *Side effects*: sensitization, toxicity of the kidney or organs of hearing and balance. *Manufacturer*: 3M Health Care.

TRIDIL

Description: an antiarrhythmic and anti-anginal, glyceryl nitrate available in ampoules containing 0.5mg/ml. *Used for*: angina, arrhythmias. *Dosage*: see literature. *Special care*: hypotension, tolerance. *Avoid use*: anaemia, cerebral haemorrhage, certain glaucomas, head trauma. *Possible interaction*: anticoagulants. *Side effects*: flushes, headache, dizziness, tachycardia, hypotension on standing. *Manufacturer*: DuPont.

TRIMOPAN

Description: a folic acid inhibitor, trimethoprim, available in white tablets marked 2H7 (100mg) and 3H7 (200mg). *Used for*: infections sensitive to trimethoprim, urinary tract infections. *Dosage*: 200mg twice per day. Children should use the suspension. Also, **TRIMOPAN SUSPENSION** containing 50mg/5ml. *Dosage*: children, 6 to 12 years, 10ml; 2 to 6 years, 5ml; 4 months to 2 years, 2.5ml; all twice per day. Not for infants under 4 months. *Special care*: kidney disorder, folate deficiency, elderly, breast-feeding. Check blood during long-term treatment. *Avoid use*: pregnancy, infants up to 1 month, severe kidney disease where blood levels cannot be monitored. *Side effects*: folate deficiency, gastro-intestinal and skin reactions. *Manufacturer*: Berk.

TRIMOVATE

Description: a moderately potent steroid with antifungal and antibiotic comprising 0.05% clobetasone butyrate, 100,000 units/g nystatin, 3% oxytetracycline, as a cream. *Used for*: skin disorders that respond to steroids, especially in moist or covered areas where there may be infection. *Dosage*: use up to 4 times per day. *Special care*: thrombophlebitis, psychoses, recent intestinal anastomoses, chronic nephritis, certain cancers, osteoporosis, peptic ulcer, skin eruption/rash related to a disease, viral, fungal or active infections, tuberculosis. Hypertension, glaucoma, epilepsy, acute glomerulonephritis (inflammation of kidney glomerulus), diabetes, cirrhosis, hypothyroidism, pregnancy, stress. To be withdrawn gradually. *Possible interaction*: NSAIDs, oral anticoagulants, phenytoin, ephedrine, phenobarbitone, rifampicin, diuretics, cardiac glycosides, anticholinesterases, hypoglycaemics. *Side effects*: osteoporosis, depression, euphoria, hyperglycaemia, peptic ulcers, Cushingoid changes. *Manufacturer*: Glaxo Wellcome.

TRINORDIOL

Description: an oestrogen/progestogen combined contraceptive containing ethinyloestradiol and levonorgestrel as 6 brown tablets (30/50µg respectively), 5 white tablets (40/75µg) and 10 ochre tablets (30/125µg). *Used for*: oral contraception. *Dosage*: 1 tablet for 21 days starting on the first day of menstruation, then 7 days without tablets. *Special care*: hypertension, Raynaud's disease (reduced blood supply to an organ of the body's extremities), asthma, severe depression, diabetes, varicose veins, multiple sclerosis, chronic kidney disease, kidney dialysis. Blood pressure, breasts and pelvic organs to be checked regularly; smoking not advised. *Avoid use*: history of heart disease, infectious hepatitis, sickle cell anaemia, porphyria, liver tumour, undiagnosed vaginal bleeding, pregnancy, hormone-dependent cancer, haemolytic uraemic syndrome (rare kidney disorder), chorea, otosclerosis. *Possible interaction*: barbiturates, tetracyclines, griseofulvin, rifampicin, primidone, phenytoin, chloral hydrate, ethosuximide, carbamazepine, glutethimide, dichloralphenazone. *Side effects*: fluid retention and bloating, leg cramps/pains, breast enlargement, depression, headaches, nausea, loss of libido, weight gain, vaginal discharge, cervical erosion (alteration of epithelial cells), chloasma (pigmentation of nose, cheeks or forehead), breakthrough bleeding (bleeding between periods). *Manufacturer*: Wyeth.

TRINOVUM

Description: a combined oestrogen/progestogen contraceptive containing ethinyloestradiol and norethisterone as 7 white tablets marked C535 (35µg/0.5mg respectively), 7 light peach tablets marked C735 (35µg/0.75mg) and 7 peach tablets marked C135 (35µg/1mg). *Used for*: oral contraception. *Dosage*: 1 tablet per day for 21 days commencing on first day of menstruation then 7 days without tablets. Also, **TRINOVUM ED**, as for Trinovum but with 7 light-green inert lactose tablets marked CC. *Dosage*: starting on first day of menstruation, 1 tablet per day for 28 days with no break. *Special care*: hypertension, Raynaud's disease (reduced blood supply to an organ of the body's extremities), asthma, severe depression, diabetes, varicose veins, multiple sclerosis, chronic kidney disease, kidney dialysis. Blood pressure, breasts and pelvic organs to be checked regularly; smoking not advised. *Avoid use*: history of heart disease, infectious hepatitis, sickle cell anaemia, porphyria, liver tumour, undiagnosed vaginal bleeding, pregnancy, hormone-dependent cancer, haemolytic uraemic syndrome (rare kidney disorder), chorea, otosclerosis. *Possible interaction*: barbiturates, tetracyclines, griseofulvin, rifampicin, primidone, phenytoin, chloral hydrate, ethosuximide, carbamazepine, glutethimide, dichloralphenazone. *Side effects*: fluid retention and bloating, leg cramps/pains, breast enlargement, depression, headaches, nausea, loss of libido, weight gain, vaginal discharge, cervical erosion (alteration of epithelial cells), chloasma (pigmentation of nose, cheeks or forehead), breakthrough bleeding (bleeding between periods). *Manufacturer*: Janssen-Cilag.

TRIPTAFEN

Description: an anti-depressant combining a TCAD and group III phenothiazine, as 25mg amitryptiline hydrochloride with 2mg perphenazine in pink tablets marked 1D. Also, **TRIPTAFEN-M**, containing 10mg amitriptyline hydrochloride and 2mg perphenazine in pink tablets marked 2D. *Used for*: depression with anxiety. *Dosage*: 1 tablet 3 times per day plus 1 at bedtime if needed. Assess after 3 months. Not for children. *Special care*: pregnancy, breast-feeding, Parkinsonism, liver disorders, hyperthyroidism, epilepsy, diabetes, glaucoma, retention of urine, cardiovascular disease, psychotic patients. *Avoid use*: cardiovascular disease, bone marrow depression, heart block, acute myocardial infarction, severe liver disease. *Possible interaction*: antidepressants, anticonvulsants, alcohol, within 2 weeks of taking MAOIs, barbiturates, adrenaline, noradrenaline, antihypertensives, anticholinergics, oestrogens, cimetidine. *Side effects*: sleepiness, vertigo, light-headedness, unsteadiness, disturbance of vision, rash, hypotension, gastro-intestinal upset, changes in libido, retention of urine. Allergic reactions, dry mouth, constipation, sweating, tachycardia, nervousness, heart arrhythmias. Impotence, effects on breasts, weight loss or gain. *Manufacturer*: Forley.

TRISEQUENS

Description: an oestrogen/progestogen combination available as 12 blue tablets (marked 270) containing 2mg oestradiol and 1mg oestriol, 10 white tablets (marked 271) containing 2mg oestradiol, 1mg oestriol and 1mg norethisterone acetate and 6 red tablets (marked 272) containing 1mg oestradiol and 0.5mg oestriol. Also, **TRISEQUENS FORTE**, with the same components as 12 yellow tablets marked 273 (4mg/2mg), 10 white tablets marked 274 (4mg/2mg/1mg) and 6 red tablets marked 272 (1mg/0.5mg). *Used for*: symptoms of the menopause, prevention of post-menopausal osteoporosis. *Dosage*: 1 tablet per day without a break, starting on fifth day of discharge with a blue tablet (or yellow if Forte). *Special care*: patients considered to be at risk of thrombosis or with liver disease. Women with any of the following disorders should be carefully monitored: fibroids in the womb, multiple sclerosis, diabetes, tetany, porphyria, epilepsy, liver disease, hypertension, migraine, otosclerosis, gallstones. Breasts, pelvic organs and blood pressure should be checked at regular intervals during the course of treatment. *Avoid use*: pregnancy, breast-feeding, conditions which might lead to thrombosis, thrombophlebitis, serious heart, kidney or liver disease, breast cancer, oestrogen-dependent cancers including those of reproductive system, endometriosis, vaginal bleeding which is undiagnosed. *Possible interaction*: drugs which induce liver enzymes. *Side effects*: tenderness and enlargement of breasts, weight gain, breakthrough bleeding, giddiness, vomiting and nausea, gastro-intestinal upset. Treatment should be halted immediately if severe headaches occur, disturbance of vision, hypertension or any indications of thrombosis, jaundice. Also, in the event of pregnancy and 6 weeks before planned surgery. *Manufacturer*: Novo Nordisk.

TRITACE

Description: an ACE inhibitor, ramipril, available as yellow/white (1.25mg), orange/white (2.5mg) and crimson/white (5mg) capsules. *Used for*: hypertension. *Dosage*: start with 1.25mg per day moving to maintenance dose of 2.5–5mg per day; maximum of 10mg per day. Any diuretic should be stopped 2 to 3 days before taking Tritace. Not for children. *Special care*: start treatment in hospital for congestive heart failure or liver disease; haemodialysis, kidney disease (reduce dose and monitor during treatment). *Avoid use*: pregnancy, breast-feeding, narrowing of the aorta, past angioneurotic oedema, outflow obstruction. *Possible interaction*: lithium, potassium supplements, potassium-sparing diuretics, antihypertensives. *Side effects*: headache, fatigue, nausea, vomiting, dizziness, abdominal pain, cough, diarrhoea, hypersensitivity reactions. *Manufacturer*: Hoechst.

TRIVAX

Description: a vaccine containing the triple antigen for diphtheria, tetanus and whooping cough, available in ampoules. Also **TRIVAX-AD** which is adsorbed on aluminium hydroxide. *Used for*: active immunization against these diseases. *Dosage*: for children under 5, 3 doses of 0.5ml at 4 weekly intervals. Not for children over 5 or adults. *Avoid use*: acute fever, past convulsions, cerebral irritation, neurological diseases. Reaction to a preceding dose. Epilepsy in the family or history of severe allergies. *Side effects*: fever, loss of appetite, irritability, crying. *Manufacturer*: Evans.

TROBICIN

Description: an antibacterial compound similar to an aminoglycoside, spectinomycin, as powder (as dihydrochloride pentahydrate) in a vial (400mg/ml) with diluent. *Used for*: gonorrhoea. *Dosage*: 2g by deep intramuscular injection or 4g for severe cases. Children over 2, 40mg/kg. *Special care*: pregnancy, liver or kidney disease. *Possible interaction*: lithium. *Side effects*: fever, urticaria, nausea, dizziness, lower urine output. *Manufacturer*: Pharmacia & Upjohn.

TROSYL

Description: an imidazole antifungal, tioconazole, available as a solution containing 280mg/ml. *Used for*: nail infections caused by *Candida* and fungi. *Dosage*: apply 12 hourly for 6 to 12 months. *Avoid use*: pregnancy. *Side effects*: nail irritation. *Manufacturer*: Pfizer.

TRYPTIZOL

Description: a TCAD, amitriptyline hydrochloride, available as blue tablets marked MSD 23 (10mg), yellow tablets marked MSD 45 (25mg) and brown tablets marked MSD 102 (50mg). Also, **TRYPTIZOL CAPSULES**, 75mg orange, sustained-release capsules (marked MSD 649) and **TRYPTIZOL SYRUP** 10mg amitriptiline embonate/5ml. *Used for*: depression (adults), bedwetting (children). *Dosage*: 75mg up to 150mg per day, in divided doses and 50–100mg for maintenance usually as 1 bedtime dose. Elderly, 50mg per day in divided doses or as 1 bedtime dose. Children; 11 to 16 years, 25–50mg per day; 6 to 10 years, 10–20mg per day. Not for children under 6. Also, **TRYPTIZOL INJECTION** as 10mg/ml. *Dosage*: 10–20mg 4 times per day, intravenously or intramuscularly. Not for children. *Special care*: liver disorders, hyperthyroidism, glaucoma, lactation, epilepsy, diabetes, adrenal tumour, heart disease, urine retention. Psychotic or suicidal patients. *Avoid use*: children, heart block, heart attacks, severe liver disease, pregnancy. *Possible interaction*: MAOIs (or within 14 days of their use), alcohol, antidepressants, barbiturates, anticholinergics, local anaesthetics that contain adrenaline or noradrenaline, oestrogens, cimetidine, antihypertensives. *Side effects*: constipation, urine retention, dry mouth, blurred vision, palpitations, tachycardia, nervousness, drowsiness, insomnia. Changes in weight, blood and blood sugar, jaundice, skin reactions, weakness, ataxia, hypotension, sweating, altered libido, gynaecomastia, galactorrhoea. *Manufacturer*: Morson.

TUINAL^{CD}

Description: a barbiturate, quinal barbitone sodium and amylobarbitone sodium in equal amounts, available as orange/blue capsules (100mg) marked LILLY F65. *Used for*: short-term treatment of severe insomnia for those tolerant to barbiturates. *Dosage*: 100–200mg at bedtime. Not for children. *Special care*: extremely dangerous, addictive drug with narrow margin of safety. Liable to abuse by overdose leading to coma and death or if combined with alcohol. Easily produces dependence and severe withdrawal symptoms. Drowsiness may persist next day, affecting driving and performance of skilled tasks. *Avoid use*: should be avoided if possible in all patients. Not to be used for children, young adults, pregnancy, nursing mothers, elderly, those with drug- or alcohol-related problems, patients with liver, kidney or heart disease, porphyria. Insomnia where the cause is pain. *Possible interaction*: alcohol, central nervous system depressant drugs, Griseofulvin, metronidazone, rifampicin, phenytoin, chloramphenicol. Anticoagulant drugs of the coumarin type, steroid drugs including contraceptive pill. *Side effects*: hangover with drowsiness, shakiness, dizziness, headache, anxiety, confusion, excitement, rash and allergic responses, gastro intestinal upsets, urine retention, loss of sexual desire. *Manufacturer*: Flynn.

TYLEX

Description: an analgesic comprising 500mg paracetamol and 30mg codeine phosphate in red and white capsules marked C30. *Used for*: severe pain. *Dosage*: 1 or 2 capsules 4-hourly to a maximum of 8 per day. Not for children. *Special care*: head injury, raised intracranial pressure, bowel disorders, Addison's disease, hypothyroidism, liver or kidney disease, elderly. *Avoid use*: pregnancy, breast-feeding, chronic alcoholism, depression of respiration, diseases causing obstruction of airways. *Possible interaction*: CNS depressants, MAOIs. *Side effects*: nausea, dry mouth, blurred vision, dizziness, sedation, constipation, tolerance, dependence. *Manufacturer*: Schwarz.

TYPHIM VI

Description: an inactivated surface antigen of *Salmonella typhi* as 25µg/0.5ml in pre-filled syringe. *Used for*: active immunization against typhoid. *Dosage*: 0.5ml by intramuscular or deep subcutaneous injection. Children over 18 months, as adult dosage; under 18 months, assess risk of exposure. *Special *care*: pregnancy, breast-feeding. *Avoid use*: acute infections. *Side effects*: headache, fever, malaise, localized reactions. *Manufacturer*: Pasteur Merieux MSD.

U

UBRETID

Description: an anticholinesterase, distigmine bromide, available as white tablets (5mg) marked UBRETID, and **UBRETID INJECTION** as 1ml ampoules (0.5mg/ml). *Used for*: intestinal and ileal weakness after operations, myasthenia gravis, post-operative urine retention, neurogenic bladder (bladder disorder caused by a lesion of the nervous system). *Dosage*: 1 tablet daily, 30 minutes before breakfast up to 4 for myasthenia gravis (2 for children). Post-operative conditions, 0.5mg 12 hours intramuscularly after surgery then 24-hourly until normal function restored. Not for children. *Special care*: asthma, heart disease, epilepsy, Parkinsonism, peptic ulcer. *Avoid use*: pregnancy, post-operative shock, obstruction in intestines or urinary tract, weak circulation. *Possible interaction*: depolarizing muscle relaxants. *Side effects*: nausea, vomiting, colic, diarrhoea, increased salivation. *Manufacturer*: R.P.R.

UCERAX

Description: an antihistamine, hydroxyzine hydrochloride, available as white, oblong tablets (25mg). Also, **UCERAX SYRUP** (10mg/5ml). *Used for*: anxiety, skin disorders, pruritus (itching) due to urticaria. *Dosage*: 50–100mg 4 times per day for anxiety; otherwise 25mg at night up to 25mg 3 or 4 times per day if required. Children; over 6 years start with 15–25mg at night increasing to 50–100mg per day in divided doses; 6 months to 6 years, 5–15mg increasing to 50mg daily maximum in divided doses. *Special care*: kidney disease. Judgement and dexterity may be affected. *Avoid use*: pregnancy, breast-feeding. *Possible interaction*: depressants of the CNS, alcohol. *Side effects*: anticholinergic effects, drowsiness. *Manufacturer*: U.C.B.

UKIDAN

Description: a fibrinolytic, urokinase, available as powder in vials containing 5000, 25,000 and 100,000 units. *Used for*: pulmonary embolism, deep vein thrombosis, bleeding into the eye in front of the lens, clot in haemodialysis shunt, blockage in peripheral vessel. *Dosage*: see the literature. *Special care*: peptic ulcer. *Avoid use*: severe liver or kidney disease, pregnancy, severe hypertension, recent surgery. *Possible interaction*: glucose. *Side effects*: fever, haemorrhage. *Manufacturer*: Serono.

ULTRADIL

Description: a moderately potent steroid containing 0.1% fluocortolone pivalate and 0.1% fluocortolone hexanoate as cream and ointment. *Used for*: eczema, skin disorders and skin conditions that respond to steroids. *Dosage*: start by applying 3 times per day, reducing to once per day. *Special care*: thrombophlebitis, psychoses, recent intestinal anastomoses, chronic nephritis, certain cancers, osteoporosis, peptic ulcer, skin eruption/rash related to a disease, viral, fungal or active infections, tuberculosis. Hypertension, glaucoma, epilepsy, acute glomerulonephritis (inflammation of kidney glomerulus), diabetes, cirrhosis, hypothyroidism, pregnancy, stress. To be withdrawn gradually. *Possible interaction*: NSAIDs, oral anticoagulants, phenytoin, ephedrine, phenobarbitone, rifampicin, diuretics, cardiac glycosides, anticholinesterases, hypoglycaemics. *Side effects*: osteoporosis, depression, euphoria, hyperglycaemia, peptic ulcers, Cushingoid changes. *Manufacturer*: Schering H.C.

ULTRALANUM

Description: a moderately potent steroid containing 0.25% fluocortolone pivalate and 0.25% fluocortolone hexanoate as a cream. Also, **ULTRALANUM OINTMENT** containing 0.25% fluocortolone and 0.25% fluocortolone hexanoate. *Used for*: skin conditions responding to steroids. *Dosage*: apply 2 or 3 times per day and reduce to once per day. *Special care*: thrombophlebitis, psychoses, recent intestinal anastomoses, chronic nephritis, certain cancers, osteoporosis, peptic ulcer, skin eruption/rash related to a disease, viral, fungal or active infections, tuberculosis. Hypertension, glaucoma, epilepsy, acute glomerulonephritis (inflammation of kidney glomerulus), diabetes, cirrhosis, hypothyroidism, pregnancy, stress. To be withdrawn gradually. *Possible interaction*: NSAIDs, oral anticoagulants, phenytoin, ephedrine, phenobarbitone, rifampicin, diuretics, cardiac glycosides, anticholinesterases, hypoglycaemics. *Side effects*: osteoporosis, depression, euphoria, hyperglycaemia, peptic ulcers, Cushingoid changes. *Manufacturer*: Schering H.C.

ULTRAPROCT

Description: a steroid and local anaesthetic containing fluocortolone pivalate (0.61mg), fluocortolone hexanoate (0.63mg) and cinchocaine hydrochloride (1mg) as suppositories. *Used for*: haemorrhoids, anal fissure, itching, proctitis (inflammation of the rectum). *Dosage*: 1 to 3 per day, after defaecation. Not for children. Also, **ULTRAPROCT OINTMENT**, containing 0.092% fluocortolone pivalate, 0.095% fluocortolone hexanoate and 0.5% cinchocaine hydrochloride. *Dosage*: use 2 to 4 times per day. Not for children. *Special care*: pregnancy. Do not use for a long period. *Avoid use*: infections of a viral, fungal or tuberculous nature. *Side effects*: corticosteroid effects. *Manufacturer*: Schering H.C.

UNIHEP

Description: an anticoagulant, heparin sodium, available as 1000, 5000, 10,000 and 25,000 units in ampoules. *Used for*: treatment and prophylaxis of deep vein thrombosis and pulmonary embolism, angina, acute occlusion of peripheral arteries. *Dosage*: varies with condition, see literature. *Special care*: pregnancy, liver and kidney disease. Monitor platelet count if treatment exceeds 5 days and cease treatment should thrombocytopenia occur. *Avoid use*: thrombocytopenia, cerebral aneurysm, severe hypertension, haemophilia, haemorrhagic disorders, severe liver disease, recent eye or nervous system surgery, hypersensitivity to heparin. *Possible interaction*: aspirin, ketorolac, dipyridamole, glyceryl trinitrate. *Side effects*: thrombocytopenia, skin necrosis, haemorrhage, hypersensitivity reactions, osteoporosis with prolonged use. *Manufacturer*: Leo.

UNIPARIN

Description: an anticoagulant, heparin sodium, available as 5000 units/0.2ml in pre-filled syringe. Also, **UNIPARIN FORTE** (10,000 units/0.4ml) and **UNIPARIN Ca**, heparin calcium as 25,000 units per ml in pre-filled syringes. *Used for*: treatment and prophylaxis of deep vein thrombosis and pulmonary embolism, angina, acute occlusion of peripheral arteries. *Dosage*: by subcutaneous injection. See literature for dosage. *Special care*: pregnancy, liver and kidney disease. Monitor platelet count if treatment exceeds 5 days and cease treatment should thrombocytopenia occur. *Avoid use*: thrombocytopenia, cerebral aneurysm, severe hypertension, haemophilia, haemorrhagic disorders, severe liver disease, recent eye or nervous system surgery, hypersensitivity to heparin. *Possible interaction*: aspirin, ketorolac, dipyridamole, glyceryl trinitrate. *Side effects*: thrombocytopenia, skin necrosis, haemorrhage, hypersensitivity reactions, osteoporosis with prolonged use. *Manufacturer*: C.P. Pharm.

UNIROID-HC

Description: a steroid (5mg hydrocortisone) and local anaesthetic (5mg cinchocaine hydrochloride) available as suppositories. *Used for*: haemorrhoids, itching around the anus. *Dosage*: insert 1 dose 3 times per day, and after defaecation for up to 7 days. Not for children. Also, **UNIROID-HC OINTMENT** containing 5mg hydrocortisone and 5mg/g cinchocaine hydrochloride. *Dosage*: use 3 times per day and after defaecation, for up to 7 days. Not for children. *Special care*: pregnancy. Do not use over a prolonged period. *Avoid use*: infections of a viral, fungal or tuberculous nature. *Side effects*: corticosteroid effects. *Manufacturer*: Unigreg.

UNIVER

Description: a class I calcium antagonist, verapamil hydrochloride, available as sustained-release capsules coloured yellow/dark blue (120mg and 240mg, marked V120 and V240) and yellow (180mg, marked V180). *Used for*: angina, hypertension. *Dosage*: 360mg once per day to a maximum of 480mg (angina). For hypertension, 240mg once per day, unless new to verapamil in which case start with 120mg per day. *Special care*: 1st degree heart block, weak heart, liver or kidney disease, bradycardia, hypotension, disturbance in heart conduction, pregnancy. *Avoid use*: 2nd or 3rd degree heart block, heart failure, sick sinus syndrome. *Possible interaction*: quinidine, digoxin, ß-blockers. *Side effects*: flushes, constipation, occasionally nausea, vomiting, headache, allergy or liver disorder. *Manufacturer*: R.P.R.

URIBEN

Description: a quinolone, nalidixic acid, available as a suspension (300mg/5ml). *Used for*: infections of the gastro-intestinal tract caused by Gram-negative organisms, urinary tract infections. *Dosage*: gastro-intestinal tract infections: 10–15ml 4 times per day, children over 3 months 1ml/kg per day. Contact manufacturer regarding children under 3 months. For urinary tract infections: acute cases, 15ml 4 times per day for at least 7 days; chronic cases 10ml. Children's doses as above. *Special care*: severe kidney disease, liver disease, avoid excessive sunlight. *Avoid use*: past convulsions. *Possible interaction*: probenecid, anticoagulants. *Side effects*: rashes, blood disorders, seizures, disturbances in sight, gastro-intestinal upset. *Manufacturer*: Rosemont.

URISPAS

Description: an antispasmodic drug, flavoxate hydrochloride, available as white tablets containing 100mg and marked URISPAS, and 200mg (marked URISPAS 200). *Used for*: incontinence, frequent or urgent urination, painful urination, bedwetting. *Dosage*: 200mg 3 times per day. Not for children. *Special care*: pregnancy, glaucoma. *Avoid use*: conditions causing obstruction in the urinary or gastro-intestinal tracts. *Side effects*: diarrhoea, dry mouth, blurred vision, nausea, fatigue, headache. *Manufacturer*: Shine.

UROMITEXAN

Description: a protectant for the urinary tract, mesna, available as solution in ampoules (100mg/ml). *Used for*: prevention of toxicity in the urinary tract caused by the metabolite acrolein. *Dosage*: orally or intravenously. See literature for details. *Side effects*: fatigue, headache, gastro-intestinal upset, depression, irritability, rash, malaise, pain in the limbs. *Manufacturer*: ASTA Medica.

URSOFALK

Description: a bile acid, ursodeoxycholic acid, available as white capsules containing 250mg. *Used for*: dissolving cholesterol gallstones. *Dosage*: 8–12mg/kg/day in 2 divided doses after meals of which one must be the evening meal. Use for 3 to 4 months after the stones have been dissolved. Not for children. *Avoid use*: if gall bladder does not function. Women who are not using contraception. *Possible interaction*: drugs to lower cholesterol levels, oral contraceptives, oestrogens. *Manufacturer*: Thames.

UTINOR

Description: a 4-quinolone compound, norfloxacin, available as white, oval tablets (400mg) marked UTINOR. *Used for*: acute and chronic infections of the urinary tract. *Dosage*: 1 tablet twice per day. Duration depends upon the condition. Not for children. *Special care*: past epilepsy, kidney disorder. *Avoid use*: pregnancy, breast-feeding, growing adolescents and children before puberty. *Possible interaction*: NSAIDs, antacids, oral anticoagulants, cyclosporin, theophylline, nitrofurantoin, probenecid, sucralfate. *Side effects*: diarrhoea, nausea, headache, dizziness, heartburn, rash, abdominal cramp, irritability, convulsions, anorexia, disturbance to sleep. *Manufacturer*: M.S.D.

UTOVLAN

Description: a progestogen, norethisterone, available as white tablets (5mg) marked SYNTEX. *Used for*: dysmenorrhoea (painful menstruation), menorrhagia (long or heavy menstrual periods), uterine bleeding, metropathia haemorrhagica (endometrial hyperplasia—irregular bleeding due to excess activity of oestrogen). *Dosage*: 1 tablet 3 times per day for 10 days then twice per day for days 19–26 of the next 2 cycles. *Used for*: postponement of menses (discharge). *Dosage*: 1 tablet 3 times per day commencing 3 days before anticipated start. *Used for*: endometriosis. *Dosage*: 1 tablet 3 times per day for at least 6 months, increasing to 4 or 5 per day if necessary. *Used for*: pre-menstrual syndrome. *Dosage*: 1 per day from days 16–25 of the cycle. *Used for*: breast cancer. *Dosage*: start with 8 per day increasing to 12 if required. *Special care*: epilepsy, migraine, diabetes. *Avoid use*: not for children. Carcinoma of the breast dependent upon progestogen, past thromboembolic disorders, undiagnosed abnormal vaginal bleeding, liver disease, severe itching, pregnancy, jaundice, past herpes. *Side effects*: liver or gastro-intestinal upset. *Manufacturer*: Searle.

V

VAGIFEM

Description: an hormonal oestrogen preparation available as vaginal pessaries with applicator containing 25µg oestradiol. *Used for*: atrophic vaginitis. *Dosage*: adults, 1 pessary inserted into vagina each day for 2 weeks, then 1 twice each week for 3 months. *Special care*: those at risk of thrombosis or with liver disease. Women with any of the following disorders should be carefully monitored: fibroids in the womb, multiple sclerosis, diabetes, tetany, porphyria, epilepsy, liver disease, hypertension, migraine, otosclerosis, gallstones. Breasts, pelvic organs and blood pressure should be checked at regular intervals during the course of treatment. *Avoid use*: pregnancy, breast-feeding, women with conditions which might lead to thrombosis, thrombophlebitis, serious heart, kidney or liver disease, breast cancer, oestrogen-dependent cancers including those of reproductive system, endometriosis, vaginal bleeding which is undiagnosed. *Possible interaction*: drugs which induce liver enzymes. *Side effects*: tenderness and enlargement of breasts, weight gain, breakthrough bleeding, giddiness, vomiting and nausea, gastro-intestinal upset. Treatment should be halted immediately if severe headaches occur, disturbance of vision, hypertension or any indications of thrombosis, jaundice. Also, in the event of pregnancy and 6 weeks before planned surgery. *Manufacturer*: Novo Nordisk.

VALIUM

Description: a long-acting benzodiazepine drug available as white 2mg tablets, yellow 5mg tablets and blue 10mg tablets all containing diazepam. Tablets are scored and marked with ROCHE and strength. Also, **VALIUM SYRUP** containing 2mg diazepam/5ml; **VALIUM INJECTION** available as a solution in ampoules containing 5mg diazepam/ml. *Used for*: severe and disabling anxiety, insomnia, severe alcohol withdrawal symptoms, sleep disorders in children. Feverish convulsions, status epilepticus (injection only), spasm of muscles and cerebral spasticity, as a sedative during medical or surgical procedures. *Dosage*: oral preparations, 2–60mg in divided doses each day depending upon condition being treated. Injection, 10–20mg, or 0.2mg/kg body weight depending upon condition being treated, by intravenous or intramuscular injection every 4 hours. Status epilepticus, this dose may be repeated after half an hour to an hour with a maximum of 3mg/kg by intravenous infusion over 24 hours. Elderly, oral preparations, 1–30mg each day in divided doses; injection 5mg by intravenous or intramuscular injection every 4 hours. Children, oral preparations, 1–40mg each day in divided doses depending upon condition being treated; 1–5mg at bedtime for sleep disorders. Injection, status epilepticus and convulsions, 0.2–0.3mg/kg by intravenous or intramuscular injection. *Special care*: elderly, pregnancy, breast-feeding, liver or kidney disorders, lung disease. Drug should be gradually withdrawn. *Avoid use*: patients with serious lung disease, depression of respiration, obsessional and phobic disorders, severe psychosis. Avoid long-term use. *Possible interaction*: CNS depressants, anticonvulsants, alcohol. Drugs which induce or inhibit liver enzymes. *Side effects*: impaired judgement and performance of skilled tasks, confusion, shakiness, sleepiness, vertigo. Gastro-intestinal upset, retention of urine, disturbance of vision, changes in libido, skin rashes, hypotension. Thrombophlebitis at site of injection; rarely, jaundice and blood changes. The longer treatment lasts and the higher the dose the greater the risk of drug dependence. *Manufacturer*: Roche.

VALLERGAN

Description: an anti-allergic preparation, which is an antihistamine of the phenothiazine type, available as film-coated, blue tablets containing 10mg trimeprazine tartrate marked V10. Also, **VALLERGAN SYRUP** containing 7.5mg/5ml; **VALLERGAN FORTE SYRUP**, containing 30mg/5ml. *Used for*:

itching, urticaria, premedication before surgery in children. *Dosage*: 10mg 2 or 3 times each day with a maximum of 100mg daily. Elderly persons, 10mg once or twice daily. Children, for itching and allergic conditions age over 2 years, 2.5–5mg 3 or 4 times each day. Premedication, age 2 to 7 years, up to 2mg/kg body weight 1 or 2 hours before surgery. *Avoid use*: pregnancy, breast-feeding, liver or kidney disorders, Parkinson's disease, epilepsy, phaeochromocytoma, underactive thyroid gland, myasthenia gravis, glaucoma. *Possible interaction*: antihypertensives, hypoglycaemics, alcohol, sympathomimetics, anticholinergics, MAOIs, central nervous system depressants. *Side effects*: sleepiness, rash, drowsiness, impaired performance and reactions, heart disturbances, hypotension, depression of respiration. Anticholinergic and extrapyramidal effects, convulsions, raised levels of prolactin in blood, abnormally low level of white blood cells, jaundice, sensitivity to light (with high doses). *Manufacturer*: R.P.R.

VANCOCIN CP

Description: an antibiotic glycopeptide preparation available as powder in vials for reconstitution and injection containing 250mg, 500mg and 1g vancomycin (as hydrochloride). Also, **VANCOCIN MATRIGEL** available as peach/blue capsules containing 125mg (coded Lilly 3125); grey/blue capsules containing 250mg (coded Lilly 3126). *Used for*: potentially fatal infections caused by staphylococci which are resistant to other antibiotics. Vancocin Matrigel, staphylococcal enterocolitis and pseudo-membraneous colitis. *Dosage*: 500mg every 6 hours or 1g every 12 hours given by slow intravenous infusion over 1 hour. Children, 10mg/kg body weight by slow intravenous infusion over 1 hour at 6 hourly intervals. Vancocin Matrigel, 500mg each day for 7 to 10 days in divided doses with a daily maximum of 2g. Children, 40mg/kg for 7 to 10 days in 3 or 4 divided doses with a daily maximum of 2g. *Special care*: elderly, pregnancy, patients with existing loss of hearing, kidney disorders. Blood, kidney function and hearing shoudl be carefully monitored during the course of treatment. *Possible interaction*: drugs with toxic effects on central nervous system or kidneys, anaesthetics. *Side effects*: chills, fever, nausea, phlebitis, reduction in number of some white blood cells and rise in number of eosinophils, toxic effects on kidneys and organs of hearing and balance. Anaphylactoid allergic reactions. *Manufacturer*: Lilly.

VARIDASE

Description: a preparation of fibrinolytic and proteolytic enzymes available as powder in vials containing 100,000 units streptokinase and 25,000 units streptodomase. *Used for*: cleansing and removal of debris from wounds and ulcers. *Dosage*: apply as wet dressing once or twice each day. *Avoid use*: patients with active haemorrhage. *Manufacturer*: Wyeth.

VASCACE

Description: an antihypertensive which is an ACE inhibitor, available in the form of oval, film-coated, scored tablets in various strengths, all containing cilazapril and marked with strength and CIL. Pink, 0.25mg strength; white, 0.5mg strength; yellow, 1mg strength; red, 2.5mg strength and brown 5mg strength. *Used for*: hypertension and renovascular hypertension. *Dosage*: hypertension, 1mg once each day at first with a maintenance dose of 1–2.5mg daily. Any diuretic being taken should be withdrawn 2 or 3 days before treatment starts. Renovascular hypertension, 0.25–0.5mg once each day then adjusted according to response. Elderly, hypertension, 0.5mg each day at first; renovascular hypertension, 0.25mg once each day at first. *Special care*: liver or kidney disease, congestive heart failure, undergoing renal dialysis, anaesthesia or surgery, suffering from lack of fluid or salt. *Avoid use*: children, pregnancy, breast-feeding, patients wth outflow obstruction of the heart, aortic stenosis, ascites (abnormal collection of fluid in the peritoneal cavity – a complication of various diseases). *Possible interaction*: NSAIDs, potassium-sparing diuretics. *Side effects*: nausea, headache, fatigue, rash, indigestion, giddiness. Rarely, pancreatitis, changes in blood count, angioneurotic oedema. *Manufacturer*: Roche.

VASOCON-A

Description: an anti-inflammatory compound preparation combining an antihistamine and sympathomimetic, available as eyedrops containing 0.5% antazoline phosphate and 0.05% naphazoline hydrochloride. *Used for*: inflammatory eye conditions including allergic conjunctivitis. *Dosage*: adults, 1 or 2 drops up to 4 times each day. *Special care*: diabetes, hypertension, hyperthyroidism, disease of coronary arteries. *Avoid use*: narrow angle glaucoma, wearing soft contact lenses. *Possible interaction*: MAOIs. *Side effects*: sleepiness, tachycardia, headache, insomnia, short-lived stinging in eye. *Manufacturer*: Lolab.

VASOXINE

Description: an antiarrhythmic and α-agonist, available as a solution in ampoules for injection containing 20mg methoxamine hydrochloride. *Used for*: hypotension during anaesthesia. *Dosage*: adults, 5–10mg by slow intravenous injection or 5–20mg by intramuscular injection. *Special care*: pregnancy, patients with hyperthyroidism. *Avoid use*: serious disease of the coronary arteries or heart blood vessels. *Possible interaction*: anoretic drugs, cough and cold remedies. *Side effects*: hypertension, bradycardia, headache. *Manufacturer*: Glaxo Wellcome.

VELBE

Description: a drug which is a vinca alkaloid available as powder in vials with diluent containing 10mg vinblastine sulphate. *Used for*: leukaemias, lymphomas, some solid tumours, e.g. of lung and breast. *Dosage*: by intravenous injection as directed by specialist physician. *Special care*: caution in handling (trained personnel, protective clothing), irritant to tissues. *Avoid use*: intrathecal route. *Side effects*: bone marrow suppression, toxic effects on peripheral and autonomic nervous system, reversible hair loss, nausea, vomiting, effects on fertility. *Manufacturer*: Lilly.

VELOSEF

Description: an antibiotic preparation which is a cephalosporin available as capsules in 2 strengths both containing cephradine. Blue/orange 250mg capsules, coded SQUIBB 113 and blue 500mg capsules coded SQUIBB 114. Also, **VELOSEF SYRUP** containing 250mg/5ml. **VELOSEF INJECTION** as powder in vials for reconstitution and injection containing 500mg and 1g cephradine. *Used for*: infections of skin, soft tissues, respiratory, gastro-intestinal and urinary tracts, joints and bones. Also, endocarditis and septicaemia and for prevention of infection during surgery. *Dosage*: oral preparations, 1–2g each day in 2, 3 or 4 divided doses with a maximum daily dose of 4g. Injection, 2–4g by intramuscular or intravenous injection or intravenous infusion in divided daily doses. Children, oral preparations, 25–50mg/kg body weight in 2, 3 or 4 daily divided doses. For inflammation of middle ear, 75–100mg/kg each day in divided doses. Injection, 50–100mg/kg each day in divided doses. All treatment should continue for 48–72 hours after symptoms have disappeared. *Special care*: kidney disorders, known hypersensitivity to penicillins. *Possible interaction*: aminoglycosides. *Side effects*: gastro-intestinal upset, allergic hypersensitive responses. Rarely, blood changes involving white blood cells, rise in levels of urea and liver enzymes in blood, positive Coomb's test (a test to detect Rhesus antibodies), candidiasis. *Manufacturer*: Squibb.

VENTIDE

Description: a bronchodilator and anti-inflammatory which combines a selective ß-agonist and corticosteroid. Available as an aerosol delivering 100µg salbutamol and 50µg beclomethasone dipropionate per metered dose. Also, **VENTIDE ROTACAPS** available as clear/grey capsules containing 400µg salbutamol as sulphate and 200µg beclomethasone dipropionate, marked VENTIDE, for use with Rotahaler. Also, **VENTIDE PAEDIATRIC ROTACAPS**, clear/light grey capsules containing 200µg salbutamol as sulphate and 100µg beclomethasone dipropionate, for use with Rotahaler. *Used for*: long-term treatment of asthma which requires inhaled bronchodilator and corticosteroid therapy. *Dosage*: Ventide, 2 puffs 3 to 4 times each day; Ventide Rotacaps, 1 puff 3 to 4 times each day. Children, Ventide, 1 or 2 puffs 2, 3 or 4 times each day. Ventide Paediatric Rotacaps, 1 puff 2, 3 or 4 times each day. *Special care*: pregnancy, weak heart, angina, heart arrhythmias, hyperthyroidism, hypertension, tuberculosis. Special care in patients changing from systemic steroids. *Possible interaction*: sympathomimetics. *Side effects*: dilation of peripheral blood vessels, headache, nervous tension, tremor, fungal infections of throat and mouth and hoarseness. *Manufacturer*: A. & H.

VENTODISKS

Description: a bronchodilator, anti-inflammatory preparation, which is a selective ß₂-agonist, available as light blue disks of 200µg strength and dark blue disks of 400µg strength, containing salbutamol as sulphate. Both are marked with strength and name. *Used for*: bronchospasm occurring in bronchitis, emphysema and bronchial asthma. *Dosage*: acute attack, 200 or 400µg 3 to 4 times each day. Children, acute attack, 200µg as single dose; prevention, half the dose of adult. *Special care*: pregnancy, weak heart, angina, heart arrhythmias, hyperthyroidism, hypertension. *Possible interaction*: sympathomimetics. *Side effects*: headache, dilation of peripheral blood vessels, nervous tension, tremor. *Manufacturer*: A. & H.

VENTOLIN

Description: a bronchodilator/anti-inflammatory preparation which is a selective ß$_2$-agonist, available as pink tablets containing 2mg and 4mg salbutamol as sulphate, marked AH and IK and AH and 2K respectively. Also, **VENTOLIN SYRUP**, sugar and colour-free, containing 2mg/5ml. Also, **VENTOLIN INHALER**, a metered dose aerosol delivering 100µg salbutamol per puff. **VENTOLIN ROTACAPS** available as clear/light blue capsules containing 200µg and clear/dark blue capsules containing 400 µg, both marked with strength and name for use with Rotahaler. **VENTOLIN INJECTION** available as a solution in ampoules containing 50 and 500µg/ml. **VENTOLIN INFUSION**, available as a solution in ampoules containing 1mg/ml. **VENTOLIN RESPIRATOR SOLUTION**, for hospital use only containing 5mg/ml in bottles. **VENTOLIN NEBULES** for use with nebulizer available as single dose units containing 2.5mg and 5mg/2.5ml. *Used for*: bronchospasm occurring in bronchitis, emphysema and bronchial asthma. Injection, status asthmaticus and severe bronchospasm. *Dosage*: oral preparations, 2–8mg 3 or 4 times each day. Ventolin Inhaler, attack, 1 or 2 puffs; prevention, 2 puffs 3 or 4 times each day. Ventolin Rotacaps, acute attack, 200 or 400µg as 1 dose; prevention, 400µg 3 or 4 times each day. Injection, 8µg/kg body weight by intramuscular or subcutaneous injection. Or, 4 µg/kg by slow intravenous injection. Nebules, 2.5–5mg nebulized up to 4 times each day. Other preparations, see literature. Children, oral preparations, aged 2 to 6 years, 1–2mg; 6 to 12 years, 2mg, all 3 or 4 times each day. Ventolin Inhaler, half adult dose; Rotacaps, acute attack, 200µg as 1 dose; prevention, half adult dose. Nebules, same as adult dose. *Special care*: pregnancy, patients with hyperthyroidism, hypertension, weak heart, angina, heart arrhythmias. *Avoid use*: children under 2 years (oral preparations). *Possible interaction*: sympathomimetics. *Side effects*: headache, dilation of peripheral blood vessels, nervous tension, tremor. *Manufacturer*: A. & H.

VEPESID

Description: an anti-cancer drug which is a podophyllotoxin available as pink gelatin capsules containing 50mg and 100mg etoposide. Also, **VEPESID INJECTION** available as a solution in vials containing 20mg etoposide/ml. *Used for*: lymphomas, cancer of the bronchus, teratoma of the testes. *Dosage*: as directed by specialist but in divided doses over 3 to 5 days. Oral doses are double those of inection which is given intravenously. *Special care*: care in handling (trained staff, protective clothing), irritant to tissues. *Side effects*: hair loss, bone marrow suppression, vomiting, nausea, effects on fertility. *Manufacturer*: Bristol-Myers.

VERMOX

Description: an antihelmintic preparation available as a sugar-free suspension containing 100mg mebendazole/5ml. Also, **VERMOX TABLETS**, scored, pink, containing 100mg mebendazole marked Me/100 and JANSSEN. *Used for*: infestations of large roundworm, threadworm, common and American hookworm, whipworm. *Dosage*: adults and children aged over 2 years; threadworm, 100mg with dose repeated after 2 or 3 weeks if necessary. Other types of worm, 100mg morning and night for 3 days. *Avoid use*: pregnancy. *Side effects*: gastrointestinal upset. *Manufacturer*: Janssen-Cilag.

VIBRAMYCIN

Description: a tetracycline antibiotic preparation available as green capsules containing 100mg doxycycline (as hydrochloride), marked VBM 100 and Pfizer. Also, **VIBRAMYCIN-D**, off-white, dissolvable tablets containing 100mg vibramycin marked Pfizer and D-9. *Used for*: gastro-intestinal and respiratory tract infections, pneumonia, soft tissue, urinary tract infections, sexually transmitted diseases, eye infections, acne vulgaris. *Dosage*: all infections except sexually transmitted diseases, 200mg with food or drink on first day then 100–200mg daily. Acne, 50mg each day with food or drink for 6 to 12 weeks. (Sexually transmitted diseases, as advised in literature). *Special care*: patients with liver disease. *Avoid use*: pregnancy, breast-feeding, children. *Possible interaction*: carbamazepine, antacids, phenytoin, mineral supplements, barbiturates, methoxyflurane. *Side effects*: superinfections, gastro-intestinal upset, allergic responses. Withdraw if intracranial hypertension occurs. *Manufacturer*: Invicta.

VILLESCON

Description: a combined sympathomimetic and vitamin preparation available as a tonic containing 2.5mg prolintane hydrochloride, 1.67mg thiamine-hydrochloride, 1.36mg riboflavine sodium phosphate, 0.5mg pyridoxine hydrochloride, 5mg nicotinamide/5ml. *Used for*: a general tonic. *Dosage*: 10ml after breakfast with second dose in afternoon for 1 to 2 weeks. Children, age 5 to 12 years, 2.5–10ml twice each day. *Avoid use*: children under 5 years, patients with epilepsy or thyrotoxicosis. *Possible interaction*: levodopa, MAOIs. *Side effects*: nausea, insomnia, tachycardia, colic. *Manufacturer*: Boehringer Ingelheim.

VIRAZID

Description: an antiviral preparation available as a powder in vials for nebulization containing 20mg tribavirin/ml. *Used for*: serious respiratory syncitial virus bronchiolitis (inflammation and infection of bronchioles). *Dosage*: children only, delivery via an oxygen hood, tent or mask for 12 to 18 hours each day for at least 3 days and for a maximum of 7 days. *Special care*: patient and equipment require careful monitoring. *Avoid use*: pregnancy, females of child-bearing age. *Side effects*: worsening of respiratory condition, reticulocytosis (increase in number of reticulocytes—immature erythrocyte red blood cells), pneumothorax, bacterial pneumonia. *Manufacturer*: ICN.

VIRORMONE

Description: a sex hormone (androgen) preparation available as a solution in ampoules containing 50mg testosterone propionate/ml. *Used for*: cryptorchidism (undescended testicle), male hypogonadism (deficiency in secretion of hormones by testes), delayed puberty in males. Breast cancer after menopause in women. *Dosage*: for hypogonadism, 50mg 2 or 3 times each week; cryptorchidism or delayed puberty, 50mg each week. Breast cancer in women, 100mg 2 or 3 times each week, all by intramuscular injection. *Special care*: liver, kidney, or heart disorders, migraine, epilepsy, hypertension. *Avoid use*: cancer of liver or prostate gland, heart disease or heart failure which is untreated, kidney nephrosis (an abnormality resulting from various diseases or conditions). Hypercalcaemia, high levels of calcium in urine. *Possible interaction*: drugs that induce liver enzymes. *Side effects*: weight gain, reduced fertility, oedema, tumours of liver, priapism (painful and prolonged erection of penis not connected with sexual arousal but resulting from drug treatment or underlying disorder). Also, premature closure of epiphyses, increased bone growth, masculinization (women). *Manufacturer*: Ferring.

VIRUDOX

Description: an antiviral preparation available as a solution with applicator brush containing 5% idoxuridine, dimethyl sulphoxide to 100%. *Used for*: skin infections caused by *Herpes simplex* and *Herpes zoster*. *Dosage*: adults, apply to affected skin 4 times each day for 4 days. *Special care*: avoid mucous membranes and eyes. May damage clothing. *Avoid use*: pregnancy, breast-feeding, children. *Side effects*: stinging when applied, unusual, distinctive taste during treatment. Overuse may cause skin to soften and break down. *Manufacturer*: Bioglan.

VISKALDIX

Description: a non-cardioselective ß-blocker and thiazide, pindolol (10mg) with clopamide (5mg) in white tablets marked with name. *Used for*: hypertension. *Dosage*: start with 1 tablet in the morning increasing if required, after 2 or 3 weeks, to 2 or a maximum of 3 per day. Not for children. *Special care*: history of bronchospasm and certain ß-blockers, diabetes, liver or kidney disease, pregnancy, lactation, general anaesthesia, gout, check electrolyte levels, K$^+$ supplements may be required depending on the case. Withdraw gradually. Not for children. *Avoid use*: heart block or failure, bradycardia, sick sinus syndrome (associated with sinus node disorder), certain ß-blockers, severe peripheral arterial disease, pregnancy, lactation, severe kidney failure, anuria, hepatic cornea. *Possible interaction*: verapamil, hypoglycaemics, reserpine, clonidine withdrawal, some antiarrhythmics and anaesthetics, antihypertensives, depressants of the CNS, cimetidine, indomethacin, sympathomimetics, lithium, potassium supplements with potassium-sparing diuretics, digitalis. *Side effects*: bradycardia, cold hands and feet, disturbance to sleep, heart failure, gastro-intestinal upset, tiredness on exertion, bronchospasm, gout, weakness, blood disorders, sensitivity to light. *Manufacturer*: Sandoz.

VISKEN

Description: a non-cardioselective ß-blocker, pindolol, available as white tablets (5 and 15mg) marked with name and strength. *Used for*: angina, hypertension. *Dosage*: half to 1 tablet 3 times per day (angina); 10–15mg per day increasing weekly to a maximum of 45mg if necessary. Not for children. *Special care*: history of bronchospasm and certain ß-blockers, diabetes, liver or kidney disease, pregnancy, lactation, general anaesthesia. Withdraw gradually. Not for children. *Avoid use*: heart block or failure, bradycardia, sick sinus syndrome, certain ß-blockers, severe peripheral arterial disease. *Possible interaction*: verapamil, hypoglycaemics, reserpine, clonidine withdrawal, some antiarrhythmics and anaesthetics, antihypertensives, depressants of the CNS, cimetidine, indomethacin, sympathomimetics. *Side effects*: bradycardia, cold hands and feet, disturbance to sleep, heart failure, gastro-intestinal upset, tiredness on exertion, bronchospasm. *Manufacturer*: Sandoz.

VISTA-METHASONE

Description: a corticosteroid, betamethasone sodium phosphate, available as 0.1% drops. *Used for*: non-infected inflammatory conditions of the nose, ear and eye. Also, **VISTA-METHASONE N** (also includes 0.5% neomycin sulphate). *Used for*: infected inflammation of the nose, ear and eye. *Dosage*: 1 to 3 drops from 2 hourly to twice daily, depending upon condition. *Special care*: pregnancy; avoid prolonged use during pregnancy, or with infants. *Avoid use*: infections of a viral, fungal or tuberculous nature, perforated eardrum (for ear conditions), glaucoma or soft contact lenses (for eye conditions). *Side effects*: superinfection. For eyes—corneal thinning, cataract, fungal infection, rise in pressure within the eye. *Manufacturer*: Martindale.

VIVALAN

Description: an antidepressant and oxazine, viloxazine hydrochloride, in white tablets (50mg) marked V and ICI. *Used for*: depression, particularly where sedation is not required. *Dosage*: 300mg per day in divided doses (maximum 400mg/day). Elderly, start with 100mg per day. Not for children. *Special care*: heart block, heart failure, ischaemic heart disease, pregnancy, epilepsy, suicidal tendency. *Avoid use*: past peptic ulcer, liver disease, mania, recent myocardial infarction, breast-feeding. *Possible interaction*: phenytoin, levodopa, theophylline, CNS depressants, carbamazepine, clonidine, MAOIs. *Side effects*: anticholinergic effects, jaundice, convulsions, vomiting, headache, affected reactions. *Manufacturer*: Zeneca.

VIVOTIF

Description: a live attenuated vaccine, *Salmonella typhi*, Ty 21a strain in white/pink capsules. *Used for*: immunization against typhoid fever. *Dosage*: 1 capsule with cold drink 1 hour before a meal on days 1, 3 and 5. Annual boost of 3 capsules for those regularly at risk. Children over 6 years, adult dose. Not for children under 6. *Special care*: pregnancy, breast-feeding. *Avoid use*: acute fever or gastro-intestinal illness, immunosuppressed patients. *Possible interaction*: antibiotics, cytotoxics, immunosuppressants, sulphonamides, mefloquine. *Side effects*: mild gastro-intestinal upset. *Manufacturer*: Evans.

VOLITAL

Description: a stimulant of the CNS, pemoline, available as white tablets (20mg) marked P9. *Used for*: hyperkinesia (overactive restlessness) in children. *Dosage*: aged 6 to 12 years, start with 20mg in the morning increasing weekly by 20mg to 60mg/day, or possible 120mg if no improvement on lower doses. Not for children under 6. *Special care*: reduce dose if side effects occur (improvement usually happens within 6 weeks). *Possible interaction*: MAOIs. *Side effects*: weight loss, anorexia, headache, sweating, palpitations, dizziness, irritability. *Manufacturer*: L.A.B.

VOLMAX

Description: a selective β_2-agonist, salbutamol sulphate, in white hexagonal continuous-release tablets (4 and 9mg) marked with strength. *Used for*: chronic bronchitis, emphysema, bronchospasm. *Dosage*: 8mg twice per day. Children, aged 3 to 12 years, 4mg twice per day. Not for those under 3 years. *Special care*: angina, hypertension, cardiac arrhythmias, pregnancy, hyperthyroidism, weak heart. *Possible interaction*: sympathomimetics. *Side effects*: headache, dilatation of peripheral vessels, nervousness. *Manufacturer*: A. & H.

VOLRAMAN

Description: a phenylacetic acid, diclofenac sodium, in 25 and 50mg orange tablets. *Used for*: pain or inflammation associated with rheumatic disease, gout, musculo-skeletal disorders. *Dosage*: 75–150mg per day in divided doses after food. *Special care*: elderly, kidney, liver or heart disease. *Avoid use*: porphyria, hypersensitivity to aspirin or other NSAIDs, pregnancy, peptic ulcer. *Possible interaction*: ACE inhibitors, other NSAIDs, quinolones, anticoagulants, antidiabetics, antihypertensives, diuretics, lithium. *Side effects*: gastro-intestinal upset, nausea, diarrhoea, hypersensitivity reactions, dizziness, blood disorders, headache. *Manufacturer*: Eastern.

VOLTAROL

Description: a phenylacetic acid, diclofenac sodium, available as yellow (25mg) and brown (50mg) tablets marked with name, strength and GEIGY. *Used for*: rheumatoid arthritis, osteoarthrosis, ankylosing spondylitis, chronic juvenile arthritis, acute gout. *Dosage*: 75–150mg per day in divided doses. Children over

1 year, 1–3mg/kg/day. Also, **VOLTAROL DISPERSIBLE** as pink, triangular tablets (50mg) marked V and GEIGY. *Dosage*: 1 taken 3 times daily in water for a maximum of 3 months. Not for children. Also, **VOLTAROL SUSTAINED-RELEASE SR**, as pink, triangular tablets (75mg) marked V 75 SR and GEIGY, and RETARD as 100mg red tablets marked VOLTAROL R and GEIGY. *Dosage*: 1 SR once or twice per day, 1 Retard per day. Also, **VOLTAROL SUPPOSITORIES** (100mg). *Dosage*: 1 at night and **VOLTAROL PAEDIATRIC SUPPOSITORIES** (12.5mg). *Dosage*: children, 1–3mg/kg/day in divided doses. Also, **VOLTAROL INJECTION** (25mg/ml). *Used for*: back pain, post-operative pain, pain in trauma or from fractures. *Dosage*: 75mg intramuscularly once or twice per day for 2 days maximum. Continue with tablets or suppositories if required. *Special care*: monitor long-term treatment. Liver, kidney or heart disease, porphyria, past gastro-intestinal lesions, pregnancy, breast-feeding, elderly, blood disorders. *Avoid use*: allergy to aspirin or anti-inflammatory drugs, proctitis (inflammation of anus and rectum), peptic ulcer. *Possible interaction*: lithium, diuretics, digoxin, methotrexate, salicylates, cyclosporin, oral hypoglycaemics, NSAIDs, steroids, quinolones. *Side effects*: headache, oedema, gastro-intestinal upset. *Manufacturer*: Geigy.

VOLTAROL EMULGEL

Description: an NSAID, diclofenac diethy-lammonium salt as 1.16g in an aqueous gel (equivalent to 1g diclofenac sodium). *Used for*: soft tissue rheumatism, strains, sprains, bruises. *Dosage*: 2–4g rubbed into area 3 to 4 times per day. Not for children. *Special care*: pregnancy, breast-feeding, avoid eyes, mucous membrane, broken skin. *Avoid use*: allergy to aspirin or anti-inflammatory drugs. *Side effects*: itching, dermatitis, localized erythema, sensitivity to light. *Manufacturer*: Geigy.

VOLTAROL OPHTHA

Description: an NSAID, diclofenac sodium, available as 0.1% single dose eyedrops. *Used for*: reduction of miosis (excessive constriction of the sphincter muscle of the iris) in cataract surgery, post-operative inflammation. *Dosage*: see literature. *Possible interaction*: ACE inhibitors, other NSAIDs, quinolones, anticoagulants, antidiabetics, antihypertensives, diuretics, lithium. *Manufacturer*: Ciba Vision.

W

WARTICON

Description: a cytotoxic drug, 0.5% podophyllotoxin, available as a solution with applicator. Also, **WARTICON FEM** including mirror. *Used for*: external genital warts. *Dosage*: use twice per day over 3 days, repeated weekly for up to 4 weeks if necessary. Not for children. *Avoid use*: pregnancy, breast-feeding. *Side effects*: localized irritation. *Manufacturer*: Perstorp.

WELLDORM

Description: a sedative and hypnotic, chloral betaine, available in purple oval tablets (strength 707mg, equivalent to 414mg of chloral hydrate). *Used for*: insomnia over the short-term. *Dosage*: 1 or 2 tablets at bedtime to a maximum of 2g chloral hydrate equivalent per day. Also, **WELLDORM ELIXIR**, 143mg chloral hydrate/5ml. *Dosage*: 15–45ml at bedtime to a daily maximum of 2g. Children: 30–50mg/kg to a daily maximum of 1g. *Avoid use*: severe heart, kidney or liver disease, porphyria, gastritis, pregnancy, breast-feeding. *Possible interaction*: anticoagulants, anti-cholinergics, CNS depressants, alcohol. *Side effects*: headache, nausea, vomiting, flatulence, bloating, rashes, blood disorders, excitability. *Manufacturer*: S & N.

WELLFERON

Description: an interferon (affects immunity and cell function) interferon alfa-N1, available as vials containing 3 million units/ml. *Used for*: chronic hepatitis B, hairy-cell leukaemia. *Dosage*: by subcutaneous and intramuscular injection. See literature for dose. *Special care*: see literature. *Avoid use*: see literature. *Possible interaction*: theophylline. *Side effects*: lethargy, flu-like symptoms, depression, bone marrow depression, hypo- and hypertension, arrhythmias, rashes, seizures. *Manufacturer*: Glaxo Wellcome.

X

XANAX

Description: a long-acting benzodiazepine, alprazolam, available as white, oval tablets (250µg) marked UPJOHN 29 and pink, oval tablets (500µg) marked UPJOHN 55. *Used for*: short-term treatment of anxiety and anxiety with depression. *Dosage*: 250–500µg 2 or 3 times per day, elderly, 250µg, to a daily maximum of 3mg. Not for children. *Special care*: chronic liver or kidney disease, chronic lung disease, pregnancy, labour, lactation, elderly. May impair judgement. Withdraw gradually and avoid prolonged use. *Avoid use*: depression of respiration, acute lung disease; psychotic, phobic or obsessional states. *Possible interaction*: anticonvulsants, depressants of the CNS, alcohol. *Side effects*: ataxia, confusion, light-headedness, drowsiness, hypotension, gastro-intestinal upsets, disturbances in vision and libido, skin rashes, retention of urine, vertigo. Sometimes jaundice or blood disorders. *Manufacturer*: Pharmacia & Upjohn.

XATRAL

Description: a selective α₁-blocker, alfuzosin hydrochloride, available as white tablets (2.5mg) marked XATRAL 2.5. *Used for*: benign prostatic hypertrophy (enlargement of prostate gland). *Dosage*: 1 tablet 3 times per day to a maximum of 4. Elderly, 1 at morning and evening to start, to a maximum of 4. *Special care*: weak heart, hypertension. Monitor blood pressure especially when starting treatment. Stop 24 hours before anaesthesia, or if angina worsens. *Avoid use*: severe liver disease, past orthostatic hypotension (low blood pressure on standing). *Possible interaction*: antihypertensives, calcium antagonists, other α-blockers. *Side effects*: gastro-intestinal upset, headache, dizziness, vertigo, tachycardia, orthostatic hypotension, chest pain, fatigue, rash, flushing, oedema, itching, palpitations, fainting. *Manufacturer*: Lorex.

XURET

Description: a thiazide-like diuretic, metolazone, available as white tablets (0.5mg) marked X and GALEN. *Used for*: hypertension. *Dosage*: 1 per day each morning (maximum 2 per day). Not for children. *Special care*: diabetes, gout, SLE, elderly, cirrhosis of the liver, liver or kidney disease, pregnancy, breast-feeding. Check, fluid, glucose and electrolyte levels. *Avoid use*: Addison's disease, hypercalcaemia, severe kidney or liver failure, sensitivity to sulphonamides. *Possible interaction*: NSAIDs, alcohol, antidiabetics, opioids, barbiturates, corticosteroids, cardiac glycosides, lithium, tubocurarine. *Side effects*: gastro-intestinal upset, blood disorders, rash, sensitivity to light, impotence, anorexia, dizziness, pancreatitis, disturbance to metabolism and electrolyte levels. *Manufacturer*: Galen.

XYLOCAINE

Description: a local anaesthetic, lignocaine hydrochloride, available as vials of strength 0.5%, 1% and 2% with or without adrenaline. *Used for*: local anaesthetics. *Dosage*: 200mg maximum (without adrenaline) or 500mg (with). Children: given in proportion to adult dose. See literature. Also, **XYLOCAINE OINTMENT** (5% lignocaine) in tube or accordion syringe. Also, **XYLOCAINE GEL**, 2% lignocaine hydrochloride in tube or accordion syringe, and **XYLOCAINE ANTISEPTIC GEL** containing, in addition, 0.25% chlorhexidine gluconate solution. *Used for*: anaesthesia of urethra or vagina, surface anaesthesia. *Dosage*: women, 3–5ml; men 10ml to start, then 3–5ml. Not for children. Also, **XYLOCAINE 4% TOPICAL** (4% lignocaine hydrochloride). *Used for*: bronchoscopy, dental treatment, reduced sensitivity to pain in oropharyngeal region, surface anaesthesia. *Dosage*: up to 5ml but see literature. Children: up to 3mg/kg. Also, **XYLOCAINE PUMP SPRAY**, 10mg lignocaine per dose. *Used for*: dental treatment, ear, nose and throat surgery, surface anaesthesia in obstetrics. *Dosage*: a maximum of 20 doses. Children: in proportion. *Special care*: epilepsy. *Avoid use*: cardiovascular disease if adrenaline is used, any surgery of the extremities, thyrotoxicosis. *Possible interaction*: phenothiazines, tricyclics, MAOIs (if adrenaline version). *Manufacturer*: Astra.

XYLOCARD

Description: a class I antiarrhythmic, lignocaine hydrochloride, available in preloaded syringes (100mg). *Used for*: arrhythmia of the ventricle associated with myocardial infarction. *Dosage*: 50–100mg over 2 minutes, by intravenous injection. Repeat once or twice after 5 to 10 minutes, if required. Not for children. *Special care*: liver or kidney disease. *Avoid use*: heart block, heart conduction disorders, heart failure. *Possible interaction*: loop diuretics, thiazides, cimetidine, propanolol. *Side effects*: nausea, blurred vision, hypotension, agitation, drowsiness, depression of respiration. *Manufacturer*: Astra.

XYLOPROCT

Description: a combined local anaesthetic and steroid containing 60mg lignocaine, 50mg aluminium acetate, 400mg zinc oxide, and 5mg hydrocortisone acetate in suppository form. *Used for*: haemorrhoids, itching, anal fissure, anal fistula. *Dosage*: 1 at night and after defecation. Also, **XYLOPROCT OINTMENT** containing 5% lignocaine, 18% zinc oxide, 3.5% aluminium acetate and 0.275% hydrocortisone. *Dosage*: use several times per day. *Special care*: pregnancy. Do not use over a long period. *Avoid use*: infections of a viral, fungal or tuberculous nature. *Side effects*: corticosteroid effects. *Manufacturer*: Astra.

Y

YUTOPAR

Description: a ß-agonist for relaxation of uterine smooth muscle, ritodrine hydrochloride, available in yellow tablets (10mg) marked YUTOPAR. *Used for*: premature labour (with no complications), foetal asphyxiation in labour. *Dosage*: 1, half an hour before the end of intravenous therapy. For maintenance, 1 every 2 hours for 24 hours, then 1 or 2 every 4 to 6 hours. Also, **YUTOPAR INJECTION** (10mg/ml in ampoules). *Special care*: diabetes, thyrotoxicosis or cardiovascular disease of the mother, monitor heart rate of mother and foetus. *Avoid use*: if a prolonged pregnancy would be hazardous, toxaemia of pregnancy, cord compression, antepartum haemorrage (bleeding before the birth and after 28th week), threatened abortion. *Possible interactions*: ß-agonists, MAOIs. *Side effects*: anxiety, tachycardia, tremor, higher blood-sugar levels. *Manufacturer*: Solvay.

Z

ZADITEN

Description: an anti-allergic agent and antihistamine, ketotifen, as hydrogen fumarate, available as white, scored tablets (1mg) marked ZADITEN 1. Also **ZADITEN CAPSULES** (1mg white capsules marked CS) and **ZADITEN ELIXIR** (1mg/5ml, sugar-free). *Used for*: prevention of bronchial asthma, allergic rhinitis and conjunctivitis. *Dosage*: 1–2mg twice per day with food. Children over 2 years, 1mg twice per day with food. Not for children under 2 years. *Avoid use*: pregnancy, breast-feeding. *Possible interaction*: antihistamines, oral hypoglycaemics, alcohol, depressants of the CNS. *Side effects*: dry mouth, dizziness, drowsiness, affected reactions. *Manufacturer*: Sandoz.

ZADSTAT

Description: a nitro imidazole and antibacterial/amoeboride/antiprotozoal, metronidazole, available as white tablets (200mg) marked LL and M200. *Used for*: infections caused by anaerobic bacteria, amoebiasis, trichomonal infections, ulcerative gingivitis. *Dosage*: average 600–800mg per day in divided doses, reduced doses for children. See literature for amoebiasis. Partner should also be treated for trichomonal infections when the dose may be up to 2g as a single dose. Also **ZADSTAT SUPPOSITORIES** (500mg and 1g). *Dosage*: see literature. *Special care*: pregnancy, breast-feeding (a high dose treatment is not recommended). *Possible interaction*: oral anticoagulants, alcohol, phenobarbitone. *Side effects*: leucopenia, urticaria, angioneurotic oedema, furred tongue, unpleasant taste, gastro-intestinal upset, dark urine, disturbance to CNS, seizures on prolonged or intensive treatment. *Manufacturer*: Lederle.

ZANTAC

Description: an H_2 blocker, ranitidine hydrochloride, available as white, pentagonal tablets (150mg) and white tablets (300mg) both marked with GLAXO, strength and ZANTAC. Also, **ZANTAC EFFERVESCENT**, 150 and 300mg white effervescent tablets, and **ZANTAC SYRUP**, 150mg/10ml with 7.5% ethanol in a sugar-free syrup. *Used for*: duodenal, benign gastric and post-operative ulcers; ulcers due to NSAIDs. Oesophageal reflux, prevention of ulcers induced by NSAIDs, dyspepsia, oesophagitis. *Dosage*: 150mg 2 times per day or 300mg at bedtime. 150mg 4 times per day for oesophagitis. Also see literature. Not for children under 8 years. Over 8 years, for peptic ulcer, 2–4mg/kg twice per day. Also, **ZANTAC INJECTION**, 50mg/2ml as a solution in ampoules. *Special care*: exclude malignancy first, kidney disease, pregnancy, lactation. *Side ef-*

fects: dizziness, headache, sometimes hepatitis, leucopenia, thrombocytopenia, hypersensitivity, confusion. *Manufacturer*: Glaxo Wellcome.

ZARONTIN

Description: a succinimide and anticonvulsant, ethosuximide, in amber oblong capsules (250mg), marked P-D. Also, **ZARONTIN SYRUP** (250mg/5ml). *Used for*: petit mal. *Dosage*: 500mg per day increasing as required by 250mg at 4 to 7 day intervals to a maximum of 2g per day. Children, 6 to 12 years, adult dose; under 6, 250mg per day adjusted according to response. *Special care*: pregnancy, breast-feeding, liver or kidney disease. Withdrawal should be gradual. *Side effects*: gastric upset, disturbance to CNS, rashes, blood disorders, SLE. *Manufacturer*: Parke-Davis.

ZAVEDOS

Description: a cytotoxic antibiotic, idarubicin hydrochloride, as powder in vials (5 and 10mg). Also, **ZAVEDOS CAPSULES**, 5, 10 and 25mg strengths in capsules coloured orange, red/white and orange/white respectively. Also as powder for reconstitution and injection. *Used for*: acute leukaemia. *Special care*: teratogenic, liver and kidney disease, irritant to skin and tissues (when handling), heart disease, elderly, monitor heart. *Avoid use*: of simultaneous radiotherapy, pregnancy. *Side effects*: nausea, vomiting, hair loss, bone marrow suppression, tissue necrosis upon extravasation, inflammation of mucous membranes. *Manufacturer*: Pharmacia & Upjohn.

ZESTORETIC

Description: an ACE inhibitor and thiazide diuretic containing 20mg lisinopril and 12.5mg hydrochlorothiazide, in white tablets. *Used for*: hypertension. *Dosage*: 1 tablet per day (maximum of 2). Not for children. *Special care*: liver or kidney disease, gout, diabetes, anaesthesia, ischaemic heart or cerebrovascular disease, haemodialysis, imbalance in fluid or electrolyte levels. *Avoid use*: pregnancy, breast-feeding, anuria, angioneurotic oedema in conjunction with previous treatment using ACE inhibitor. *Possible interaction*: lithium, NSAIDs, hypoglycaemics, potassium supplements, potassium-sparing diuretics, tubocurarine. *Side effects*: headache, fatigue, hypotension, cough, dizziness, nausea, impotence, angioneurotic oedema, diarrhoea. *Manufacturer*: Zeneca.

ZESTRIL

Description: an ACE inhibitor, lisinopril, available as tablets, marked with heart shape and strength: 2.5mg (white), 5 and 10mg (pink), and 20mg (red). 2.5, 10 and 20mg have company symbol;10 and 20mg have a trade mark. *Used for*: additional therapy (to digitalis and diuretics) in congestive heart failure, hypertension. *Dosage*: start with 2.5mg per day, increasing gradually to a maintenance dose of 5–20mg once per day. Cease using diuretic 2 to 3 days before treatment for hypertension. Reduce dose of diuretic in treating heart failure and start treatment in hospital. Not for children. *Special care*: renovascular hypertension (increased pressure in hepatic portal vein), kidney disease, haemodialysis, congestive heart failure, anaesthesia, breast-feeding. *Avoid use*: pregnancy, angioneurotic oedema from past treatment with ACE inhibitor, narrowing of aorta, enlargement of right ventricle. *Possible interaction*: potassium supplement, potassium-sparing diuretics, lithium, antihypertensives, indomethacin. *Side effects*: kidney failure, angioneurotic oedema, hypotension, dizziness, headache, diarrhoea, fatigue, cough, nausea, palpitations, rash, weakness. *Manufacturer*: Zeneca.

ZIMOVANE

Description: a cyclopyrrolone and hypnotic, zopiclone, available as white tablets (7.5mg) marked ZM. *Used for*: insomnia. *Dosage*: 1 tablet at bedtime (2 if required). Elderly , ½ tablet. Not for children. *Special care*: liver disorder, check for withdrawal symptoms on completing treatment. *Avoid use*: pregnancy, breastfeeding. *Possible interaction*: trimipramine, alcohol, other depressants of the CNS. *Side effects*: gastro-intestinal upset, metallic aftertaste, allergic reactions, drowsiness, minor behavioural changes, judgement and dexterity may be impaired. *Manufacturer*: R.P.R.

ZINACEF

Description: a cephalosporin and antibacterial, cefuroxime (as sodium salt) available in 250mg, 750mg and 1.5g vials. *Used for*: infections of soft tissue, the respiratory and urinary tracts, meningitis, gonorrhoea, prevention of infection during surgery. *Dosage*: see literature. *Possible interaction*: aminoglycosides, loop diuretics. *Side effects*: gastro-intestinal upset, hypersensitivity reactions. Occasionally leucopenia, neutropenia, candidosis. *Manufacturer*: Glaxo Wellcome.

ZINAMIDE

Description: a derivative of nicotinic acid, pyrazinamide, in white tablets (500mg) marked MSD 504. *Used for*: tuberculosis when used with other anti-tuberculous drugs. *Dosage*: 20–35mg/kg/day in divided doses, to a maximum of 3g. Not for children. *Special care*: past gout or diabetes, check liver function and blood uric acid. *Avoid use*: liver disease. Withdraw if there is liver damage or high blood uric acid with gouty arthritis. *Side effects*: hepatitis. *Manufacturer*: M.S.D.

ZINERYT

Description: an antiobiotic containing erythromycin (4%), zinc acetate (1.2%) in an alcoholic solution. *Used for*: acne. *Dosage*: use twice daily. *Special care*: avoid mucous membranes and eyes. *Side effects*: passing irritation. *Manufacturer*: Yamanouchi.

ZINNAT

Description: a cephalosporin and antibacterial, cefuroxime axetil, in white tables containing 125 or 250mg, marked GLAXO and 125 or 250. Also, **ZINNAT**

SUSPENSION (125mg/5ml). *Used for*: infections of the ear, nose and thorat, respiratory or urinary tracts, skin and soft tissues. *Dosage*: usually 250mg twice per day after food, 500mg for severe infections and a 1g single dose per day for gonorrhoea. Children over 2 years 250mg twice per day; 3 months–2 years, 125mg twice per day. Not for infants under 3 months. *Special care*: pregnancy, breast-feeding, hypersensitivity to penicillin. *Side effects*: colitis, hypersensitivity reactions, headache, gastro-intestinal upset, candidosis, increase in liver enzymes. *Manufacturer*: Glaxo Wellcome.

ZIRTEK

Description: an antihistamine, cetirizine hydrochloride, in white oblong tablets (10mg) marked Y/Y. *Used for*: urticaria, seasonal rhinitis. *Dosage*: 1 tablet per day. Not for children under 6 years; over 6 years, adult dose. Also, **ZIRTEK SOLUTION** (1mg/ml) in banana-flavoured, sugar-free solution. *Dosage*: 10ml per day for adults and children over 6 years. Not for children under 6 years. *Special care*: pregnancy, kidney disease. *Avoid use*: breast-feeding. *Side effects*: agitation, gastro-intestinal upset, dizziness, headache, dry mouth, drowsiness. *Manufacturer*: UCB.

ZITA

Description: an H_2-blocker, cimetidine, in 200, 400 and 800mg tablets. *Used for*: ulcer (stomach, benign gastric and duodenal), reflux oesophagitis, Zollinger-Ellison syndrome. *Dosage*: usually 400mg twice per day or 800mg at night for 4 to 8 weeks, depending upon condition. Children, 20–30mg/kg per day in divided doses. *Special care*: liver or kidney disease, pregnancy, breast-feeding. *Possible interaction*: warfarin, phenytoin, theophylline, pethidine, antiarrhythmics, anticoagulants, rifampicin, antidepressants, antidiabetics, ß-blockers, benzodiazepines, some antipsychotics, chloroquine, carbamazepine. *Side effects*: rash, dizziness, fatigue. Occasionally liver disorder, muscle or joint pain, bradycardia and heart block, gynaecomastia (with high dosages). *Manufacturer*: Eastern.

ZITHROMAX

Description: a macrolide and antibacterial, azithromycin dihydrate, in white capsules (250mg) marked ZTM250 and Pfizer. *Used for*: infections of skin, soft tissue, and respiratory tract, otitis media and certain genital infections. *Dosage*: 2 per day for 3 days taken 1 hour before or 2 hours after food. Also, **ZITHROMAX SUSPENSION**, 200mg/5ml. *Dosage*: children: 12 to 14 years, 10ml; 8 to 11 years, 7.5ml; 3 to 7 years, 5ml; under 3 years, 10mg/kg. *Special care*: pregnancy, breast-feeding, liver or kidney disorder. *Avoid use*: liver disease. *Possible interaction*: antacids, cyclosporin, warfarin, digoxin, ergot derivatives. *Side effects*: allergic reaction, rash, anaphylaxis, gastro-intestinal upset, angioneurotic oedema. *Manufacturer*: Richborough.

ZOCOR

Description: an HMG CoA reductase inhibitor, simvastatin, in oval tablets

(10mg, peach; 20mg, tan) marked with strength and ZOCOR. *Used for*: primary high blood cholesterol levels. *Dosage*: start with 10mg at night, altered to match response, within the range 10–40mg. Not for children. *Special care*: past liver disease, check liver function. *Avoid use*: pregnancy, women should use non-hormonal contraception, breast-feeding, liver disease. *Possible interaction*: cyclosporin, digoxin, coumarin anticoagulants, gemfibrozil, nicotinic acid. *Side effects*: headache, nausea, dyspepsia, diarrhoea, abdominal pain, constipation, flatulence, weakness, myopathy. *Manufacturer*: M.S.D.

ZOFRAN

Description: a 5HT$_3$-antagonist (blocks nausea and vomiting reflexes), ondansetron hydrochloride in yellow, oval tablets (4 and 8mg) marked with GLAXO and strength. Also, **ZOFRAN INJECTION** (2mg/ml). *Used for*: post-operative nausea and vomiting or that due to chemo- and radiotherapy. *Dosage*: see literature. *Special care*: pregnancy. *Avoid use*: breast-feeding. *Side effects*: flushes, headache, constipation. *Manufacturer*: Glaxo Wellcome.

ZOLADEX

Description: a gonadotrophin release hormone analogue, goserelin acetate, as a biodegradable depot (3.6mg). *Used for*: endometriosis, advanced breast cancer, prostate cancer. *Dosage*: 1 depot subcutaneously in abdominal wall every 28 days for up to 6 months. *Special care*: those at risk of osteoporosis, or males at risk of obstruction of the ureter or compression of the spinal cord. *Avoid use*: pregnancy, breast-feeding. Non-hormonal contraception should be used. *Side effects*: headaches, hot flushes, breast swelling or tenderness, rashes, vaginal dryness, hypercalcaemia. *Manufacturer*: Zeneca.

ZOVIRAX

Description: a nucleoside analogue and antiviral, acyclovir, available in shield-shaped tablets; 200mg, blue and marked ZOVIRAX with a triangle; 400mg, pink and marked ZOVIRAX 400 with a triangle. Also 800mg in white, elongated tablet marked ZOVIRAX 800. Also **ZOVIRAX SUSPENSION** (200mg/5ml) and **ZOVIRAX CHICKENPOX TREATMENT** (400mg/5ml). *Used for*: *Herpes simplex* and *Herpes zoster* particularly in immunocompromised patients. *Dosage*: from 800mg–4g per day depending upon condition. Children from 200mg 4 times per day. See literature. Also, **ZOVIRAX INFUSION** (250 and 500mg as powder in vials) and **ZOVIRAX CREAM** (5%). *Dosage*: use 5 times per day at 4-hour intervals, for 5 days. Also ointment, (3%). *Used for*: herpetic keratitis (inflammation of the cornea). *Dosage*: insert 1cm into lower conjuctival sac 5 times per day continuing 3 days after healing. *Special care*: kidney disease, do not use cream in eyes. *Possible interaction*: probenecid. *Side effects*: erythema, flaking skin with topical use, passing irritation, kidney disorder, stinging (with ointment)., *Manufacturer*: Glaxo Wellcome.

ZUMENON

Description: an oestrogen, oestradiol, available as blue tablets (2mg) marked 381 and DUPHAR. *Used for*: symptoms of the menopause. *Dosage*: start with 1 per day, increased to 2 if necessary, reducing to 1 as soon as possible. Commence on fifth day of menstruation (any time if absent). *Special care*: patients at risk of thrombosis or with liver disease. Women with any of the following disorders should be carefully monitored: fibroids in the womb, multiple sclerosis, diabetes, tetany, porphyria, epilepsy, liver disease, hypertension, migraine, otosclerosis, gallstones. Breasts, pelvic organs and blood pressure should be checked at regular intervals during the course of treatment. *Avoid use*: pregnancy, breast-feeding, women with conditions which might lead to thrombosis, thrombophlebitis, serious heart, kidney or liver disease, breast cancer, oestrogen-dependent cancers including those of reproductive system, endometriosis, vaginal bleeding which is undiagnosed. *Possible interaction*: drugs which induce liver enzymes. *Side effects*: tenderness and enlargement of breasts, weight gain, breakthrough bleeding, giddiness, vomiting and nausea, gastro-intestinal upset. Treatment should be halted immediately if severe headaches occur, disturbance of vision, hypertension or any indications of thrombosis, jaundice. Also, in the event of pregnancy and 6 weeks before planned surgery. *Manufacturer*: Solvay.

ZYLORIC

Description: an inhibitor of xanthine oxidase which forms uric acid. Allopurinol is available as white tablets coded U4A (100mg) and ZYLORIC 300 with C9B (300mg). *Used for*: gout, prevention of stones of uric acid and calcium oxalate. *Dosage*: start with 100–300mg per day. Maintenance dose of 200–600mg per day. Not for children. *Special care*: pregnancy, liver or kidney disease, elderly. Anti-inflammatory drug to be given for 1 month at start of treatment. Maintain fluid intake. *Avoid use*: acute gout. *Possible interaction*: anticoagulants, azathioprine, mercaptopurine, chlorpropamide. *Side effects*: nausea, acute gout. Withdraw if there are skin reactions. *Manufacturer*: Glaxo Wellcome.